Place-of-Service Codes for Professional Claims

Listed below are the Place-of-Service codes. The list contains the code, name, and description. These codes should be used on professional claims to specify the entity where service(s) were rendered. Check with your individual payer (eg, Medicare, Medicaid, other private insurance) to determine whether a particular code will be recognized for payment purposes. The codes are maintained by the Centers for Medicare and Medicaid Services (CMS). More information regarding the review and modification process as well as updates to the code set can be found at the CMS Web site http://cms.hhs.gov/states/posdata.pdf. If you would like to comment on a code(s) or description(s), please send your request to posinfo@cms.hhs.gov.

Place of Service Code(s)	Place of Service Name	Place of Service Description
01-02	Unassigned	N/A
03	School	A facility whose primary purpose is education.
04	Homeless Shelter	A facility or location whose primary purpose is to provide temporary housing to homeless individuals (eg, emergency shelters, individual or family shelters).
05	Indian Health Service Free-standing Facility	A facility or location, owned and operated by the Indian Health Service, which provides diagnostic, therapeutic (surgical and non-surgical), and rehabilitation services to American Indians and Alaska Natives who do not require hospitalization.
06	Indian Health Service Provider-based Facility	A facility or location, owned and operated by the Indian Health Service, which provides diagnostic, therapeutic (surgical and non-surgical), and rehabilitation services rendered by, or under the supervision of, physicians to American Indians and Alaska Natives admitted as inpatients or outpatients.
07	Tribal 638 Free-standing Facility	A facility or location owned and operated by a federally recognized American Indian or Alaska Native tribe or tribal organization under a 638 agreement, which provides diagnostic, therapeutic (surgical and non-surgical), and rehabilitation services to tribal members who do not require hospitalization.
08	Tribal 638 Provider-based Facility	A facility or location owned and operated by a federally recognized American Indian or Alaska Native tribe or tribal organization under a 638 agreement, which provides diagnostic, therapeutic (surgical and non-surgical), and rehabilitation services to tribal members admitted as inpatients or outpatients.
09-10	Unassigned	N/A
11	Office	Location, other than a hospital, skilled nursing facility (SNF), military treatment facility, community health center, State or local public health clinic, or intermediate care facility (ICF), where the health professional routinely provides health examinations, diagnosis, and treatment of illness or injury on an ambulatory basis.
12	Home	Location, other than a hospital or other facility, where the patient receives care in a private residence.
13	Assisted Living Facility	Congregate residential facility with self-contained living units providing assessment of each resident's needs and on-site support 24 hours a day, 7 days a week, with the capacity to deliver or arrange for services including some health care and other services.
14	Group Home	A residence, with shared living areas, where clients receive supervision and other services such as social and/or behavioral services, custodial service, and minimal services (eg, medication administration)
15	Mobile Unit	A facility/unit that moves from place-to-place equipped to provide preventive, screening, diagnostic, and/or treatment services.
16-19	Unassigned	N/A
20	Urgent Care Facility	Location, distinct from a hospital emergency room, an office, or a clinic, whose purpose is to diagnose and treat illness or injury for unscheduled, ambulatory patients seeking immediate medical attention.
21	Inpatient Hospital	A facility, other than psychiatric, which primarily provides diagnostic, therapeutic (both surgical and nonsurgical), and rehabilitation services by, or under, the supervision of physicians to patients admitted for a variety of medical conditions.
22	Outpatient Hospital	A portion of a hospital which provides diagnostic, therapeutic (both surgical and nonsurgical), and rehabilitation services to sick or injured persons who do not require hospitalization or institutionalization.
23	Emergency Room — Hospital	A portion of a hospital where emergency diagnosis and treatment of illness or injury is provided.
24	Ambulatory Surgical Center	A freestanding facility, other than a physician's office, where surgical and diagnostic services are provided on an ambulatory basis.
25	Birthing Center	A facility, other than a hospital's maternity facilities or a physician's office, which provides a setting for labor, delivery, and immediate post-partum care as well as immediate care of new-born infants.
26	Military Treatment Facility	A medical facility operated by one or more of the Uniformed Services. Military Treatment Facility (MTF) also refers to certain former U.S. Public Health Service (USPHS) facilities now designated as Uniformed Service Treatment Facilities (USTF).
27-30	Unassigned	N/A
31	Skilled Nursing Facility	A facility that primarily provides inpatient skilled nursing care and related services to patients who require medical, nursing, or rehabilitative services but does not provide the level of care or treatment available in a hospital.

32	Nursing Facility	A facility that primarily provides to residents skilled nursing care and related services for the rehabilitation of injured, disabled, or sick persons, or, on a regular basis, health-related care services above the level of custodial care to other than mentally retarded individuals.
33	Custodial Care Facility	A facility that provides room, board, and other personal assistance services, generally on a long-term basis, and which does not include a medical component.
34	Hospice	A facility, other than a patient's home, in which palliative and supportive care for terminally ill patients and their families are provided.
35-40	Unassigned	N/A
41	Ambulance — Land	A land vehicle specifically designed, equipped, and staffed for lifesaving and transporting the sick or injured.
42	Ambulance — Air or Water	An air or water vehicle specifically designed, equipped, and staffed for lifesaving and transporting the sick or injured.
43-48	Unassigned	N/A
49	Independent Clinic	A location, not part of a hospital and not described by any other Place of Service code, that is organized and operated to provide preventive, diagnostic, therapeutic, rehabilitative, or palliative services to outpatients only.
50	Federally Qualified Health Center	A facility located in a medically underserved area that provides Medicare beneficiaries preventive primary medical care under the general direction of a physician.
51	Inpatient Psychiatric Facility	A facility that provides inpatient psychiatric services for the diagnosis and treatment of mental illness on a 24-hour basis, by or under the supervision of a physician.
52	Psychiatric Facility — Partial Hospitalization	A facility for the diagnosis and treatment of mental illness that provides a planned therapeutic program for patients who do not require full time hospitalization, but who need broader programs than are possible from outpatient visits to a hospital-based or hospital-affiliated facility.
53	Community Mental Health Center	A facility that provides the following services: outpatient services, including specialized outpatient services for children, the elderly, individuals who are chronically ill, and residents of the CMHC's mental health services area who have been discharged from inpatient treatment at a mental health facility; 24 hour a day emergency care services; day treatment, other partial hospitalization services, or psychosocial rehabilitation services; screening for patients being considered for admission to State mental health facilities to determine the appropriateness of such admission; and consultation and education services.
54	Intermediate Care Facility/Mentally Retarded	A facility which primarily provides health-related care and services above the level of custodial care to mentally retarded individuals but does not provide the level of care or treatment available in a hospital or SNF.
55	Residential Substance Abuse Treatment Facility	A facility which provides treatment for substance (alcohol and drug) abuse to live-in residents who do not require acute medical care. Services include individual and group therapy and counseling, family counseling, laboratory tests, drugs and supplies, psychological testing, and room and board.
56	Psychiatric Residential Treatment Center	A facility or distinct part of a facility for psychiatric care which provides a total 24-hour therapeutically planned and professionally staffed group living and learning environment.
57	Non-residential Substance Abuse Treatment Facility	A location which provides treatment for substance (alcohol and drug) abuse on an ambulatory basis. Services include individual and group therapy and counseling, family counseling, laboratory tests, drugs and supplies, and psychological testing.
58-59	Unassigned	N/A
60	Mass Immunization Center	A location where providers administer pneumococcal pneumonia and influenza virus vaccinations and submit these services as electronic media claims, paper claims, or using the roster billing method. This generally takes place in a mass immunization setting, such as a public health center, pharmacy, or mall but may include a physician office setting.
61	Comprehensive Inpatient Rehabilitation Facility	A facility that provides comprehensive rehabilitation services under the supervision of a physician to inpatients with physical disabilities. Services include physical therapy, occupational therapy, speech pathology, social or psychological services, and orthotics and prosthetics services.
62	Comprehensive Outpatient Rehabilitation Facility	A facility that provides comprehensive rehabilitation services under the supervision of a physician to outpatients with physical disabilities. Services include physical therapy, occupational therapy, and speech pathology services.
63-64	Unassigned	N/A
65	End-Stage Renal Disease Treatment Facility	A facility other than a hospital, which provides dialysis treatment, maintenance, and/or training to patients or caregivers on an ambulatory or home-care basis.
66-70	Unassigned	N/A
71	State or Local Public Health Clinic	A facility maintained by either State or local health departments that provides ambulatory primary medical care under the general direction of a physician.
72	Rural Health Clinic	A certified facility which is located in a rural medically underserved area that provides ambulatory primary medical care under the general direction of a physician.
73-80	Unassigned	N/A
81	Independent Laboratory	A laboratory certified to perform diagnostic and/or clinical tests independent of an institution or a physician's office.
82-98	Unassigned	N/A
99	Other Place of Service	Other place of service not identified above.

American Medical Association
Physicians dedicated to the health of America

Current Procedural Terminology

cpt® 2005

Michael Beebe, MS
Joyce A. Dalton
Catherine Duffy, BS, RHIT
Martha Espronceda, AAS
Desiree D. Evans, AAS
Ron Friedmann, BS, RHIA
Rejina L. Glenn

Gloria Green, BA
DeHandro Hayden, BS
Elizabeth Lumakovska, BS, RHIT
Anita Majerowicz, MS, RHIA
Marie L. Mindeman, BA, RHIT
Karen E. O'Hara, BS, CCS-P
Mary R. O'Heron, RHIA, CCS-P

Danielle Pavloski, BS, RHIT, CCS-P
Dan Reyes, BA
Desiree Rozell, MPA
Lianne Stancik, RHIT
Susan Tracy, BA, RHIT
Jennifer Trajkovski, BS, RHIT
Ada Walker, AAS

AMA press

Standard ISBN: 1-57947-578-7
ISSN: 0276-8283

1st Edition printed 1966
2nd Edition printed 1970
3rd Edition printed 1973
4th Edition printed 1977
Revised: 1978, 1979, 1980, 1981, 1982, 1984, 1985,
1986, 1987, 1988, 1989, 1990, 1991, 1992, 1993, 1994,
1995, 1996, 1997, 1998, 1999, 2000, 2001, 2002, 2003, 2004

To purchase additional CPT products, contact the American Medical Association Customer Service
at 800 621-8335.

To request a license for distribution of products containing or reprinting CPT, please see our Web site
at *www.ama-assn.org/go/cpt* or contact the American Medical Association CPT Intellectual Property
Services, 515 N. State Street, Chicago, Illinois 60610, 312 464-5022.

AC25:OP054105:10/04

Foreword

Current Procedural Terminology, Fourth Edition (CPT®) is a listing of descriptive terms and identifying codes for reporting medical services and procedures performed by physicians. The purpose of the terminology is to provide a uniform language that will accurately describe medical, surgical, and diagnostic services, and will thereby provide an effective means for reliable nationwide communication among physicians, patients, and third parties. *CPT 2005* is the most recent revision of a work that first appeared in 1966.

CPT descriptive terms and identifying codes currently serve a wide variety of important functions in the field of medical nomenclature. The *CPT* book is useful for administrative management purposes such as claims processing and for the development of guidelines for medical care review. The uniform language is also applicable to medical education and outcomes, health services and quality research by providing a useful basis for local, regional, and national utilization comparisons. The *CPT* book is the most widely accepted nomenclature for the reporting of physician procedures and services under government and private health insurance programs. In 2000 the CPT Code Set was designated by the Department of Health and Human Services as the national coding standard for physician and other health care professional services and procedures under the Health Insurance Portability and Accountability Act (HIPAA). This means that for all financial and administrative health care transactions sent electronically, the CPT Code Set will need to be used.

The changes that appear in this revision have been prepared by the CPT Editorial Panel with the assistance of physicians representing all specialties of medicine, and with important contributions from many third party payors and governmental agencies.

The American Medical Association trusts that this revision will continue the usefulness of its predecessors in identifying, describing, and coding medical, surgical, and diagnostic services.

Michael D. Maves, MD, MBA
Executive Vice President, CEO

Acknowledgments

Publication of the annual *CPT* book represents many challenges and opportunities. From reconciling the many differences of opinion about the best way to describe a procedure, to the last details on placement of a semicolon, many individuals and organizations devote their energies and expertise to the preparation of this revision.

The editorial staff wishes to express sincere thanks to the many national medical specialty societies, health insurance organizations and agencies, and to the many individual physicians and other health professionals who have made contributions.

Thanks are due to Robert A. Musacchio, PhD, Sr VP, American Medical Association; Claudia Bonnell, Blue Cross and Blue Shield Association; Nelly Leon-Chisen, American Hospital Association; Thomas Musco, America's Health Insurance Plans; and Sue Bowman, RHIA, American Health Information Management Association, for their invaluable assistance in enhancing the CPT Code Set.

And finally, our gratitude to AMA Press of the American Medical Association for their assistance in producing the books, diskettes, and CD-ROMs that contain the CPT Code Set: Anthony J. Frankos, Vice President, Business Products; Mike Desposito, Publisher; Elise Schumacher, Senior Acquisition Editor; J. D. Kinney, Director of Marketing; Jean Roberts, Director, Production and Manufacturing; Erin Kalitowski, Marketing Manager; Pat Lee, Technical Developmental Editor; Rosalyn Carlton, Senior Production Coordinator; Boon Ai Tan, Senior Production Coordinator; Ronnie Summers, Senior Print Coordinator; Angela Boudreau, Technical Project Manager; and Todd Feinstein, Application Developer.

Coding Questions

For questions regarding the use of CPT codes, please contact the American Medical Association CPT Information and Education Services at 800 634-6922.

AMA CPT Editorial Panel

AMA CPT Advisory Committee

American Pediatric Surgical Association
John P. Crow, MD
American Psychiatric Association
Chester W. Schmidt, Jr, MD
American Roentgen Ray Society
Geraldine B. McGinty, MD, MBA
American Society for Aesthetic Plastic Surgery
Paul R. Weiss, MD
American Society for Clinical Pathology
Mark S. Synovec, MD
American Society for Dermatologic Surgery
Pamela K. Phillips, MD
American Society for Gastrointestinal Endoscopy
Klaus Mergener, MD
American Society for Reproductive Medicine
John T. Queenan, Jr, MD
American Society for Surgery of the Hand
Daniel J. Nagle, MD
American Society for Therapeutic Radiology and Oncology
Michael L. Steinberg, MD
American Society of Abdominal Surgeons
Louis F. Alfano, Jr, MD
American Society of Anesthesiologists
H. J. Przybylo, Jr, MD
American Society of Cataract and Refractive Surgery
Stephen S. Lane, MD
American Society of Clinical Oncology
Dean Gesme, MD
William C. Penley, MD*
American Society of Clinical Pathologists
David A. Margolin, MD
American Society of Cytopathology
David C. Hoak, MD
American Society of General Surgeons
Charles Drueck, MD, FACS
American Society of Hematology
Samuel M. Silver, MD, PhD
American Society of Neuroimaging
Mircea A. Morariu, Jr, MD
American Society of Neuroradiology
Robert A. Murray, MD
American Society of Ophthalmic Plastic and Reconstructive Surgery
L. Neal Freeman, MD*
American Society of Plastic Surgeons
Raymond V. Janevicius, MD
American Thoracic Society
Scott Manaker, MD
American Urological Association
Jeffrey A. Dann, MD
Association of University Radiologists
Bob W. Gayler, MD
College of American Pathologists
Stephen N. Bauer, MD
Congress of Neurological Surgeons
R. Patrick Jacob, MD
Contact Lens Association of Ophthalmologists
Charles B. Slonim, MD, FACS
International Spinal Injection Society
Claire Tibiletti, MD*
National Association of Medical Examiners
Paul A. Raslavicus, MD*
North American Spine Society
William Mitchell, MD*
Radiological Society of North America
Richard E. Fulton, MD

Renal Physicians Association
Richard J. Hamburger, MD
Society for Investigative Dermatology
Stephen P. Stone, MD
Society for Vascular Surgery
Anton N. Sidawy, MD
Society of American Gastrointestinal Endoscopic Surgeons
Eric G. Weiss, MD
Paresh C. Shah, MD*
Society of Critical Care Medicine
George A. Sample, MD
Society of Interventional Radiology
Gary S. Dorfman, MD
Society of Nuclear Medicine
Kenneth A. McKusick, MD
Society of Radiologists in Ultrasound
Robert L. Bree, MD
Society of Thoracic Surgeons
Keith S. Naunheim, MD
The Endocrine Society
Richard A. Dickey, MD
The Triological Society
James H. Kelly, MD*
*New Advisors June 2004

AMA Health Care Professionals Advisory Committee (HCPAC)

Tracy R. Gordy, MD, Co-Chair
AMA CPT Editorial Panel
Helene Fearon, PT, Co-Chair
AMA CPT Editorial Panel
American Academy of Physician Assistants
Patrick J. Cafferty, MPAS, PA-C
American Association of Naturopathic Physicians
Wendell B. Milliman, N.D.
American Association for Respiratory Care
Susan Rinaldo-Gallo, Med, RRT
American Chiropractic Association
Craig S. Little, DC
American Dietetic Association
Jane V. White, PhD, RD, FADA
American Massage Therapy Association
Whitney W. Lowe
American Nurses Association
Ann M. Thrailkill, RN
American Occupational Therapy Association
Linda Botten, OTR, CHT, ATP
Leslie F. Davison, Ed.D, OTR/L*
American Optometric Association
Mike Todd, OD
Douglas C. Morrow, OD*
X12 Pharmacy Advisory Panel
Daniel E. Buffington, PharmD, MBA
American Physical Therapy Association
Paul Rockar, PT
American Podiatric Medical Association
Michael J. King, DPM
American Psychological Association
Antonio Puente, PhD
American Speech-Language Hearing Association
R. Wayne Holland, Ed.D
National Association of Social Workers
Nelda Spyres, ACSW, LCSW
National Society of Genetic Counselors
Debra L. Doyle, MS, CGC

Contents

▶ ◀=New or Revised Text

Introduction

Current Procedural Terminology, Fourth Edition (*CPT*®) is a set of codes, descriptions, and guidelines intended to describe procedures and services performed by physicians and other health care providers. Each procedure or service is identified with a five-digit code. The use of CPT codes simplifies the reporting of services.

Inclusion of a descriptor and its associated five-digit code number in the *CPT* book is based on whether the procedure is consistent with contemporary medical practice and is performed by many practitioners in clinical practice in multiple locations. Inclusion in the *CPT* book does not represent endorsement by the American Medical Association of any particular diagnostic or therapeutic procedure. Inclusion or exclusion of a procedure does not imply any health insurance coverage or reimbursement policy.

The CPT code set is published in the late summer or early fall of every year as both electronic data files and books. The release of CPT data files on the internet typically precedes the book by several weeks. In any case, January 1 is the effective date for use of the update of the CPT code set. The interval between the release of the update and the effective date is considered the implementation period and is intended to allow physicians and other providers, payers and vendors to incorporate CPT changes into their systems. The exception to this schedule of release and effective dates are CPT Category II, Category III and vaccine product codes, which are released twice a year on January 1 or July 1 with effective dates for use six months later.

The main body of the material is listed in six sections. Each section is divided into subsections with anatomic, procedural, condition, or descriptor subheadings. The procedures and services with their identifying codes are presented in numeric order with one exception—the entire **Evaluation and Management** section (99201-99499) appears at the beginning of the listed procedures. These items are used by most physicians in reporting a significant portion of their services.

Section Numbers and Their Sequences

Evaluation and Management 99201-99499

Anesthesiology 00100-01999, 99100-99140

Surgery 10021-69990

Radiology (Including Nuclear Medicine and Diagnostic Ultrasound) .70010-79999

Pathology and Laboratory 80048-89356

Medicine
(except Anesthesiology) 90281-99199, 99500-99602

The first and last code numbers and the subsection name of the items appear at the top of most pages (eg, "11055-11313 Surgery/Integumentary System"). The continuous pagination of the *CPT* book is found on the lower, outer margin of each page along with the section name.

Instructions for Use of the *CPT* Book

Select the name of the procedure or service that accurately identifies the service performed. Do not select a CPT code that merely approximates the service provided. If no such procedure or service exists, then report the service using the appropriate unlisted procedure or service code. In surgery, it may be an operation; in medicine, a diagnostic or therapeutic procedure; in radiology, a radiograph. Other additional procedures performed or pertinent special services are also listed. When necessary, any modifying or extenuating circumstances are added. Any service or procedure should be adequately documented in the medical record.

It is important to recognize that the listing of a service or procedure and its code number in a specific section of this book does not restrict its use to a specific specialty group. Any procedure or service in any section of this book may be used to designate the services rendered by any qualified physician or other qualified health care professional.

Format of the Terminology

Current Procedural Terminology (CPT) has been developed as stand-alone descriptions of medical procedures. However, some of the procedures in the *CPT* book are not printed in their entirety, but refer back to a common portion of the procedure listed in a preceding entry. This is evident when an entry is followed by one or more indentations. This is done in an effort to conserve space.

Example

25100   Arthrotomy, wrist joint; with biopsy

25105   with synovectomy

Note that the common part of code 25100 (that part before the semicolon) should be considered part of code 25105. Therefore, the full procedure represented by code 25105 should read:

25105   Arthrotomy, wrist joint; with synovectomy

Requests to Update the CPT Nomenclature

The effectiveness of the *Current Procedural Terminology* (*CPT*®) nomenclature depends on constant updating to reflect changes in medical practice. This can only be accomplished through the interest and timely suggestions of practicing physicians, medical specialty societies, state medical associations, and other organizations and agencies. Accordingly, the American Medical Association welcomes correspondence, inquiries, and suggestions concerning old and new procedures, as well as other matters such as codes and indices.

To submit a suggestion to add, delete, or revise procedures contained in the *CPT* book, please contact:

CPT Editorial Research & Development
American Medical Association
515 North State Street
Chicago, Illinois 60610

Coding change request forms are also available at the AMA/CPT website www.ama-assn.org/ama/pub/article/3866-3846.html.

All proposed changes of the *CPT* book will be considered by the CPT Editorial Panel with consultation of appropriate medical specialty societies.

Guidelines

Specific "Guidelines" are presented at the beginning of each of the six sections. These guidelines define items that are necessary to appropriately interpret and report the procedures and services contained in that section. For example, in the **Medicine** section, specific instructions are provided for handling unlisted services or procedures, special reports, and supplies and materials provided. Guidelines also provide explanations regarding terms that apply only to a particular section. For instance, **Radiology Guidelines** provide a definition of the unique term, "radiological supervision and interpretation." While in **Anesthesia**, a discussion of reporting time is included.

Add-on Codes

Some of the listed procedures are commonly carried out in addition to the primary procedure performed. These additional or supplemental procedures are designated as "add-on" codes with a "**+**" symbol, and are listed in Appendix D of the *CPT* book. Add-on codes in *CPT 2005* can be readily identified by specific descriptor nomenclature which includes phrases such as "each additional" or "(List separately in addition to primary procedure)."

The "add-on" code concept in *CPT 2005* applies only to add-on procedures/services performed by the same physician. Add-on codes describe additional intra-service work associated with the primary procedure (eg, additional digit(s), lesion(s), neurorrhaphy(s), vertebral segment(s), tendon(s), joint(s)).

Add-on codes are always performed in addition to the primary service/procedure, and must never be reported as a stand-alone code. All add-on codes found in the *CPT* book are exempt from the multiple procedure concept (see modifier 51 definition included in **Appendix A**).

Modifiers

A modifier provides the means by which the reporting physician can indicate that a service or procedure that has been performed has been altered by some specific circumstance but not changed in its definition or code. The judicious application of modifiers obviates the necessity for separate procedure listings that may describe the modifying circumstance. Modifiers may be used to indicate to the recipient of a report that:

- A service or procedure has both a professional and technical component.
- A service or procedure was performed by more than one physician and/or in more than one location.
- A service or procedure has been increased or reduced.
- Only part of a service was performed.
- An adjunctive service was performed.
- A bilateral procedure was performed.
- A service or procedure was provided more than once.
- Unusual events occurred.

Example

A physician providing diagnostic or therapeutic radiology services, ultrasound or nuclear medicine services in a hospital would add modifier 26 to report the professional component.

73090-26 = Professional component only for an x-ray of the forearm

Example

Two surgeons may be required to manage a specific surgical problem. When two surgeons work together as primary surgeons performing distinct part(s) of a procedure, each surgeon should report his/her distinct operative work by adding modifier 62 to the procedure code and any associated code(s) for that procedure as long as both surgeons continue to work together as primary surgeons. Each surgeon should report the co-surgery once using the same procedure code. Modifier 62 would be applicable. For instance, a neurological surgeon and an otolaryngologist are working as co-surgeons in performing transsphenoidal excision of a pituitary neoplasm.

61548-62 = Hypophysectomy or excision of pituitary tumor, transnasal or transseptal approach, nonstereotactic + two surgeons modifier

AND the second surgeon would report:

61548-62 = Hypophysectomy or excision of pituitary tumor, transnasal or transseptal approach, nonstereotactic + two surgeons modifier

If additional procedure(s) (including add-on procedure(s)) are performed during the same surgical session, separate code(s) may also be reported with modifier 62 added. **Note:** If a co-surgeon acts as an assistant in the performance of additional procedure(s) during the same surgical session, those services may be reported using separate procedure code(s) with modifier 80 or modifier 82 added, as appropriate. A complete listing of modifiers is found in **Appendix A**.

Unlisted Procedure or Service

It is recognized that there may be services or procedures performed by physicians that are not found in the *CPT* book. Therefore, a number of specific code numbers have been designated for reporting unlisted procedures. When an unlisted procedure number is used, the service or procedure should be described. Each of these unlisted procedural code numbers (with the appropriate accompanying topical entry) relates to a specific section of the book and is presented in the Guidelines of that section.

Special Report

A service that is rarely provided, unusual, variable, or new may require a special report in determining medical appropriateness of the service. Pertinent information should include an adequate definition or description of the nature, extent, and need for the procedure; and the time, effort, and equipment necessary to provide the service. Additional items which may be included are: complexity of symptoms, final diagnosis, pertinent physical findings, diagnostic and therapeutic procedures, concurrent problems, and follow-up care.

Code Changes

A summary listing of additions, deletions, and revisions applicable to the *CPT* book is found in **Appendix B**. New procedure numbers added to the CPT book are identified throughout the text with the symbol "●" placed before the code number. In instances where a code revision has resulted in a substantially altered procedure descriptor, the symbol "▲" is placed before the code number. The symbols "►◄" are used to indicate new and revised text other than the procedure descriptors. CPT add-on codes are annotated by a "✚" symbol and are listed in **Appendix D**. The "⊘" symbol is used to identify codes that are exempt from the use of modifier 51, but have not been designated as CPT add-on procedures/services. A list of codes exempt from modifier 51 usage is included in **Appendix E**. The "⊙" symbol is used to identify the codes which include conscious sedation, listed in **Appendix G**.

Alphabetical Reference Index

An expanded alphabetical index is found in the back of the book. It includes listings by procedure and anatomic site. Procedures and services commonly known by their eponyms or other designations are also included.

CPT in Electronic Formats

CPT 2005 procedure codes and descriptions are also available on CD-ROM as data files and electronic software. Data files are available in ASCII and EBCDIC formats and can be imported into any billing and claims reporting software that accepts a text (TXT) file format. *CPT 2005 Electronic Professional* software is the entire *CPT 2005* Professional Edition on your desktop, in an easy-to-use, fully searchable format. For more information call 800 621-8335 or visit www.amapress.com

CPT Assistant Newsletter and CPT Changes: An Insider's View References

References Contained within *CPT 2005* Professional
The symbol "➋" below many codes throughout the book has been included to indicate that the American Medical Association (AMA) has published reference material on that particular code.

The "➋" symbol refers to two AMA publications — the *CPT Assistant* monthly newsletter and *CPT Changes: An Insider's View*, an annual book with all of the coding changes for the current year.

How to Read the References

Example

✚ **34808**   Endovascular placement of iliac artery occlusion device (List separately in addition to code for primary procedure)
➋ *CPT Assistant* Dec 00:1; *CPT Changes: An Insider's View* 2001

This reference indicates that in the *CPT Assistant* newsletter, December 2000 issue, page 1, and in *CPT Changes: An Insider's View* 2001 edition, material is available that may assist in understanding the application of the code.

How to Obtain the Referenced Publications
CPT Assistant annual subscriptions can be purchased by calling the AMA's Unified Service Center at 800 621-8335. Individual back issues are available for purchase and immediate download at **www.ama-assn.org/go/cpt/online**.

An Archive CD-ROM with every issue of *CPT Assistant* published from the past 14 years is also available. *CPT Assistant Archives 1990-2004* CD-ROM provides a fully searchable electronic library of *CPT Assistant* newsletters right on your desktop. Call 800 621-8335 or visit www.amapress.com for more information.

Current and past editions of *CPT Changes: An Insider's View* can be purchased by calling the AMA's Unified Service Center at 800 621-8335, or online at **www.amapress.com**.

New for 2005! Access all of the content from past and present editions of *CPT Changes: An Insider's View* in a fully searchable electronic software product. More than 2,500 code/guideline changes and explanations from the past six years can now be accessed from your PC with the touch of a button. For more information on *CPT Changes Archives 2000-2005*, call 800 621-8335 or visit www.amapress.com.

Evaluation and Management (E/M) Services Guidelines

In addition to the information presented in the **Introduction,** several other items unique to this section are defined or identified here.

Classification of Evaluation and Management (E/M) Services

The E/M section is divided into broad categories such as office visits, hospital visits, and consultations. Most of the categories are further divided into two or more subcategories of E/M services. For example, there are two subcategories of office visits (new patient and established patient) and there are two subcategories of hospital visits (initial and subsequent). The subcategories of E/M services are further classified into levels of E/M services that are identified by specific codes. This classification is important because the nature of physician work varies by type of service, place of service, and the patient's status.

The basic format of the levels of E/M services is the same for most categories. First, a unique code number is listed. Second, the place and/or type of service is specified, eg, office consultation. Third, the content of the service is defined, eg, comprehensive history and comprehensive examination. (See "Levels of E/M Services," page 2, for details on the content of E/M services.) Fourth, the nature of the presenting problem(s) usually associated with a given level is described. Fifth, the time typically required to provide the service is specified. (A detailed discussion of time is provided on page 3.)

Definitions of Commonly Used Terms

Certain key words and phrases are used throughout the E/M section. The following definitions are intended to reduce the potential for differing interpretations and to increase the consistency of reporting by physicians in differing specialties.

New and Established Patient

Solely for the purposes of distinguishing between new and established patients, **professional services** are those face-to-face services rendered by a physician and reported by a specific CPT code(s). A new patient is one who has not received any professional services from the physician or another physician of the same specialty who belongs to the same group practice, within the past three years.

An established patient is one who has received professional services from the physician or another physician of the same specialty who belongs to the same group practice, within the past three years.

In the instance where a physician is on call for or covering for another physician, the patient's encounter will be classified as it would have been by the physician who is not available.

No distinction is made between new and established patients in the emergency department. E/M services in the emergency department category may be reported for any new or established patient who presents for treatment in the emergency department.

Chief Complaint

A concise statement describing the symptom, problem, condition, diagnosis or other factor that is the reason for the encounter, usually stated in the patient's words.

Concurrent Care

Concurrent care is the provision of similar services, eg, hospital visits, to the same patient by more than one physician on the same day. When concurrent care is provided, no special reporting is required. Modifier 75 has been deleted.

Counseling

Counseling is a discussion with a patient and/or family concerning one or more of the following areas:

- diagnostic results, impressions, and/or recommended diagnostic studies;
- prognosis;
- risks and benefits of management (treatment) options;
- instructions for management (treatment) and/or follow-up;

- importance of compliance with chosen management (treatment) options;
- risk factor reduction; and
- patient and family education.

(For psychotherapy, see 90804-90857)

Family History

A review of medical events in the patient's family that includes significant information about:

- the health status or cause of death of parents, siblings, and children;
- specific diseases related to problems identified in the Chief Complaint or History of the Present Illness, and/or System Review;
- diseases of family members which may be hereditary or place the patient at risk.

History of Present Illness

A chronological description of the development of the patient's present illness from the first sign and/or symptom to the present. This includes a description of location, quality, severity, timing, context, modifying factors and associated signs and symptoms significantly related to the presenting problem(s).

Levels of E/M Services

Within each category or subcategory of E/M service, there are three to five levels of E/M services available for reporting purposes. Levels of E/M services are **not** interchangeable among the different categories or subcategories of service. For example, the first level of E/M services in the subcategory of office visit, new patient, does not have the same definition as the first level of E/M services in the subcategory of office visit, established patient.

The levels of E/M services include examinations, evaluations, treatments, conferences with or concerning patients, preventive pediatric and adult health supervision, and similar medical services, such as the determination of the need and/or location for appropriate care. Medical screening includes the history, examination, and medical decision-making required to determine the need and/or location for appropriate care and treatment of the patient (eg, office and other outpatient setting, emergency department, nursing facility, etc.). The levels of E/M services encompass the wide variations in skill, effort, time, responsibility and medical knowledge required for the prevention or diagnosis and treatment of illness or injury and the promotion of optimal health. Each level of E/M services may be used by all physicians.

The descriptors for the levels of E/M services recognize seven components, six of which are used in defining the levels of E/M services. These components are:

- history;
- examination;

- medical decision making;
- counseling;
- coordination of care;
- nature of presenting problem; and
- time.

The first three of these components (history, examination, and medical decision making) are considered the **key** components in selecting a level of E/M services. (See "Determine the Extent of History Obtained," page 5.)

The next three components (counseling, coordination of care, and the nature of the presenting problem) are considered **contributory** factors in the majority of encounters. Although the first two of these contributory factors are important E/M services, it is not required that these services be provided at every patient encounter.

Coordination of care with other providers or agencies without a patient encounter on that day is reported using the case management codes.

The final component, time, is discussed in detail (see page 3).

Any specifically identifiable procedure (ie, identified with a specific CPT code) performed on or subsequent to the date of initial or subsequent "E/M Services" should be reported separately.

The actual performance and/or interpretation of diagnostic tests/studies ordered during a patient encounter are not included in the levels of E/M services. Physician performance of diagnostic tests/studies for which specific CPT codes are available may be reported separately, in addition to the appropriate E/M code. The physician's interpretation of the results of diagnostic tests/studies (ie, professional component) with preparation of a separate distinctly identifiable signed written report may also be reported separately, using the appropriate CPT code with modifier 26 appended.

The physician may need to indicate that on the day a procedure or service identified by a CPT code was performed, the patient's condition required a significant separately identifiable E/M service above and beyond other services provided or beyond the usual preservice and postservice care associated with the procedure that was performed. The E/M service may be caused or prompted by the symptoms or condition for which the procedure and/or service was provided. This circumstance may be reported by adding modifier 25 to the appropriate level of E/M service. As such, different diagnoses are not required for reporting of the procedure and the E/M services on the same date.

Nature of Presenting Problem

A presenting problem is a disease, condition, illness, injury, symptom, sign, finding, complaint, or other reason for encounter, with or without a diagnosis being established at the time of the encounter. The E/M codes recognize five types of presenting problems that are defined as follows:

Minimal: A problem that may not require the presence of the physician, but service is provided under the physician's supervision.

Self-limited or minor: A problem that runs a definite and prescribed course, is transient in nature, and is not likely to permanently alter health status OR has a good prognosis with management/compliance.

Low severity: A problem where the risk of morbidity without treatment is low; there is little to no risk of mortality without treatment; full recovery without functional impairment is expected.

Moderate severity: A problem where the risk of morbidity without treatment is moderate; there is moderate risk of mortality without treatment; uncertain prognosis OR increased probability of prolonged functional impairment.

High severity: A problem where the risk of morbidity without treatment is high to extreme; there is a moderate to high risk of mortality without treatment OR high probability of severe, prolonged functional impairment.

Past History

A review of the patient's past experiences with illnesses, injuries, and treatments that includes significant information about:

- prior major illnesses and injuries;
- prior operations;
- prior hospitalizations;
- current medications;
- allergies (eg, drug, food);
- age appropriate immunization status;
- age appropriate feeding/dietary status.

Social History

An age appropriate review of past and current activities that includes significant information about:

- marital status and/or living arrangements;
- current employment;
- occupational history;
- use of drugs, alcohol, and tobacco;
- level of education;
- sexual history;
- other relevant social factors.

System Review (Review of Systems)

An inventory of body systems obtained through a series of questions seeking to identify signs and/or symptoms which the patient may be experiencing or has experienced. For the purposes of *CPT* the following elements of a system review have been identified:

- Constitutional symptoms (fever, weight loss, etc.)
- Eyes
- Ears, Nose, Mouth, Throat
- Cardiovascular
- Respiratory
- Gastrointestinal
- Genitourinary
- Musculoskeletal
- Integumentary (skin and/or breast)
- Neurological
- Psychiatric
- Endocrine
- Hematologic/Lymphatic
- Allergic/Immunologic

The review of systems helps define the problem, clarify the differential diagnosis, identify needed testing, or serves as baseline data on other systems that might be affected by any possible management options.

Time

The inclusion of time in the definitions of levels of E/M services has been implicit in prior editions of *CPT.* The inclusion of time as an explicit factor beginning in *CPT 1992* is done to assist physicians in selecting the most appropriate level of E/M services. It should be recognized that the specific times expressed in the visit code descriptors are averages, and therefore represent a range of times which may be higher or lower depending on actual clinical circumstances.

Time is **not** a descriptive component for the emergency department levels of E/M services because emergency department services are typically provided on a variable intensity basis, often involving multiple encounters with several patients over an extended period of time. Therefore, it is often difficult for physicians to provide accurate estimates of the time spent face-to-face with the patient.

Studies to establish levels of E/M services employed surveys of practicing physicians to obtain data on the amount of time and work associated with typical E/M services. Since "work" is not easily quantifiable, the codes must rely on other objective, verifiable measures that correlate with physicians' estimates of their "work". It has been demonstrated that physicians' estimations of **intraservice** time (as explained on the next page), both within and across specialties, is a variable that is predictive of the "work" of E/M services. This same research has shown there is a strong relationship between intra-service time and total time for E/M services. Intra-service time, rather than total time, was chosen for inclusion with the codes because of its relative ease of measurement and because of its direct correlation with measurements of the total amount of time and work associated with typical E/M services.

Intra-service times are defined as **face-to-face** time for office and other outpatient visits and as **unit/floor** time for hospital and other inpatient visits. This distinction is necessary because most of the work of typical office visits takes place during the face-to-face time with the patient, while most of the work of typical hospital visits takes place during the time spent on the patient's floor or unit.

Face-to-face time (office and other outpatient visits and office consultations): For coding purposes, face-to-face time for these services is defined as only that time that the physician spends face-to-face with the patient and/or family. This includes the time in which the physician performs such tasks as obtaining a history, performing an examination, and counseling the patient.

Physicians also spend time doing work before or after the face-to-face time with the patient, performing such tasks as reviewing records and tests, arranging for further services, and communicating further with other professionals and the patient through written reports and telephone contact.

This **non-face-to-face** time for office services—also called pre- and post-encounter time—is not included in the time component described in the E/M codes. However, the pre- and post-face-to-face work associated with an encounter was included in calculating the total work of typical services in physician surveys.

Thus, the face-to-face time associated with the services described by any E/M code is a valid proxy for the total work done before, during, and after the visit.

Unit/floor time (hospital observation services, inpatient hospital care, initial and follow-up hospital consultations, nursing facility): For reporting purposes, intra-service time for these services is defined as unit/floor time, which includes the time that the physician is present on the patient's hospital unit and at the bedside rendering services for that patient. This includes the time in which the physician establishes and/or reviews the patient's chart, examines the patient, writes notes and communicates with other professionals and the patient's family.

In the hospital, pre- and post-time includes time spent off the patient's floor performing such tasks as reviewing pathology and radiology findings in another part of the hospital.

This pre- and post-visit time is not included in the time component described in these codes. However, the pre- and post-work performed during the time spent off the floor or unit was included in calculating the total work of typical services in physician surveys.

Thus, the unit/floor time associated with the services described by any code is a valid proxy for the total work done before, during, and after the visit.

Unlisted Service

An E/M service may be provided that is not listed in this section of *CPT*. When reporting such a service, the appropriate "Unlisted" code may be used to indicate the service, identifying it by "Special Report", as discussed in the following paragraph. The "Unlisted Services" and accompanying codes for the E/M section are as follows:

99429   **Unlisted preventive** medicine service

99499   **Unlisted evaluation and management** service

Special Report

An unlisted service or one that is unusual, variable, or new may require a special report demonstrating the medical appropriateness of the service. Pertinent information should include an adequate definition or description of the nature, extent, and need for the procedure; and the time, effort, and equipment necessary to provide the service. Additional items which may be included are complexity of symptoms, final diagnosis, pertinent physical findings, diagnostic and therapeutic procedures, concurrent problems, and follow-up care.

Clinical Examples

Clinical examples of the codes for E/M services are provided to assist physicians in understanding the meaning of the descriptors and selecting the correct code. The clinical examples are listed in Appendix C. Each example was developed by physicians in the specialties shown.

The same problem, when seen by physicians in different specialties, may involve different amounts of work. Therefore, the appropriate level of encounter should be reported using the descriptors rather than the examples.

The examples have been tested for validity and approved by the CPT Editorial Panel. Physicians were given the examples and asked to assign a code or assess the amount of time and work involved. Only examples that were rated consistently have been included in Appendix C.

Table 1
Categories and Subcategories of Service

Category/Subcategory	Code Numbers	Category/Subcategory	Code Numbers
Office or Other Outpatient Services		Subsequent Nursing Facility Care	99311-99313
New Patient	99201-99205	Nursing Facility Discharge Services	99315-99316
Established Patient	99211-99215	Domiciliary, Rest Home or	
Hospital Observation Discharge Services	99217	Custodial Care Services	
Hospital Observation Services	99218-99220	New Patient	99321-99323
Hospital Observation or Inpatient Care		Established Patient	99331-99333
Services (Including Admission and		Home Services	
Discharge Services)	99234-99236	New Patient	99341-99345
Hospital Inpatient Services		Established Patient	99347-99350
Initial Hospital Care	99221-99223	Prolonged Services	
Subsequent Hospital Care	99231-99233	With Direct Patient Contact	99354-99357
Hospital Discharge Services	99238-99239	Without Direct Patient Contact	99358-99359
Consultations		Standby Services	99360
Office Consultations	99241-99245	Case Management Services	
Initial Inpatient Consultations	99251-99255	Team Conferences	99361-99362
Follow-up Inpatient Consultations	99261-99263	Telephone Calls	99371-99373
Confirmatory Consultations	99271-99275	Care Plan Oversight Services	99374-99380
Emergency Department Services	99281-99288	Preventive Medicine Services	
Pediatric Patient Transport	99289-99290	New Patient	99381-99387
Critical Care Services		Established Patient	99391-99397
Adult (over 24 months of age)	99291-99292	Individual Counseling	99401-99404
Pediatric	99293-99294	Group Counseling	99411-99412
Neonatal	99295-99296	Other	99420-99429
Intensive Care (Low Birth Weight)	99298-99299	Newborn Care	99431-99440
Nursing Facility Services		Special E/M Services	99450-99456
Comprehensive Nursing Facility		Other E/M Services	99499
Assessments	99301-99303		

Instructions for Selecting a Level of E/M Service

Identify the Category and Subcategory of Service

The categories and subcategories of codes available for reporting E/M services are shown in Table 1 above.

Review the Reporting Instructions for the Selected Category or Subcategory

Most of the categories and many of the subcategories of service have special guidelines or instructions unique to that category or subcategory. Where these are indicated, eg, "Inpatient Hospital Care," special instructions will be presented preceding the levels of E/M services.

Review the Level of E/M Service Descriptors and Examples in the Selected Category or Subcategory

The descriptors for the levels of E/M services recognize seven components, six of which are used in defining the levels of E/M services. These components are:

- history;
- examination;
- medical decision making;
- counseling;
- coordination of care;
- nature of presenting problem; and
- time.

The first three of these components (ie, history, examination, and medical decision making) should be considered the **key** components in selecting the level of E/M services. An exception to this rule is in the case of visits which consist predominantly of counseling or coordination of care (See numbered paragraph 3, page 7.)

The nature of the presenting problem and time are provided in some levels to assist the physician in determining the appropriate level of E/M service.

Determine the Extent of History Obtained

The extent of the history is dependent upon clinical judgment and on the nature of the presenting problems(s). The levels of E/M services recognize four types of history that are defined as follows:

Problem focused: chief complaint; brief history of present illness or problem.

Expanded problem focused: chief complaint; brief history of present illness; problem pertinent system review.

Detailed: chief complaint; extended history of present illness; problem pertinent system review extended to include a review of a limited number of additional systems; **pertinent** past, family, and/or social history **directly related to the patient's problems.**

Comprehensive: chief complaint; extended history of present illness; review of systems which is directly related to the problem(s) identified in the history of the present illness plus a review of all additional body systems; **complete** past, family, and social history.

The comprehensive history obtained as part of the preventive medicine evaluation and management service is not problem-oriented and does not involve a chief complaint or present illness. It does, however, include a comprehensive system review and comprehensive or interval past, family, and social history as well as a comprehensive assessment/history of pertinent risk factors.

Determine the Extent of Examination Performed

The extent of the examination performed is dependent on clinical judgment and on the nature of the presenting problem(s). The levels of E/M services recognize four types of examination that are defined as follows:

Problem focused: a limited examination of the affected body area or organ system.

Expanded problem focused: a limited examination of the affected body area or organ system and other symptomatic or related organ system(s).

Detailed: an extended examination of the affected body area(s) and other symptomatic or related organ system(s).

Comprehensive: a general multi-system examination or a complete examination of a single organ system. **Note:** The comprehensive examination performed as part of the preventive medicine evaluation and management service is multisystem, but its extent is based on age and risk factors identified.

For the purposes of these CPT definitions, the following body areas are recognized:

- Head, including the face
- Neck
- Chest, including breasts and axilla
- Abdomen
- Genitalia, groin, buttocks
- Back
- Each extremity

For the purposes of these CPT definitions, the following organ systems are recognized:

- Eyes
- Ears, Nose, Mouth, and Throat
- Cardiovascular
- Respiratory
- Gastrointestinal
- Genitourinary
- Musculoskeletal
- Skin
- Neurologic
- Psychiatric
- Hematologic/Lymphatic/Immunologic

Determine the Complexity of Medical Decision Making

Medical decision making refers to the complexity of establishing a diagnosis and/or selecting a management option as measured by:

- the number of possible diagnoses and/or the number of management options that must be considered;
- the amount and/or complexity of medical records, diagnostic tests, and/or other information that must be obtained, reviewed, and analyzed; and
- the risk of significant complications, morbidity, and/or mortality, as well as comorbidities, associated with the patient's presenting problems(s), the diagnostic procedure(s) and/or the possible management options.

Four types of medical decision making are recognized: straightforward; low complexity; moderate complexity; and high complexity. To qualify for a given type of decision making, two of the three elements in Table 2 on the following page must be met or exceeded.

Comorbidities/underlying diseases, in and of themselves, are not considered in selecting a level of E/M services *unless* their presence significantly increases the complexity of the medical decision making.

Select the Appropriate Level of E/M Services Based on the Following

1. For the following categories/subcategories, **all of the key components,** ie, history, examination, and medical decision making, must meet or exceed the stated requirements to qualify for a particular level of E/M service: office, new patient; hospital observation services; initial hospital care; office consultations; initial inpatient consultations; confirmatory consultations; emergency department services; comprehensive nursing facility assessments; domiciliary care, new patient; and home, new patient.

Table 2
Complexity of Medical Decision Making

Number of Diagnoses or Management Options	Amount and/or Complexity of Data to be Reviewed	Risk of Complications and/or Morbidity or Mortality	Type of Decision Making
minimal	minimal or none	minimal	**straightforward**
limited	limited	low	**low complexity**
multiple	moderate	moderate	**moderate complexity**
extensive	extensive	high	**high complexity**

2. For the following categories/subcategories, **two of the three key components** (ie, history, examination, and medical decision making) must meet or exceed the stated requirements to qualify for a particular level of E/M services: office, established patient; subsequent hospital care; follow-up inpatient consultations; subsequent nursing facility care; domiciliary care, established patient; and home, established patient.

3. When counseling and/or coordination of care dominates (more than 50%) the physician/patient and/or family encounter (face-to-face time in the office or other outpatient setting or floor/unit time in the hospital or nursing facility), then **time** may be considered the key or controlling factor to qualify for a particular level of E/M services. This includes time spent with parties who have assumed responsibility for the care of the patient or decision making whether or not they are family members (eg, foster parents, person acting in locum parentis, legal guardian). The extent of counseling and/or coordination of care must be documented in the medical record.

Notes

⊘=Modifier 51 Exempt   ⊙=Conscious Sedation   ✚=Add-on Code

Evaluation and Management

Office or Other Outpatient Services

The following codes are used to report evaluation and management services provided in the physician's office or in an outpatient or other ambulatory facility. A patient is considered an outpatient until inpatient admission to a health care facility occurs.

To report services provided to a patient who is admitted to a hospital or nursing facility in the course of an encounter in the office or other ambulatory facility, see the notes for initial hospital inpatient care (page 11) or comprehensive nursing facility assessments (page 22).

For services provided by physicians in the emergency department, see 99281-99285.

For observation care, see 99217-99220.

For observation or inpatient care services (including admission and discharge services), see 99234-99236.

New Patient

99201   **Office or other outpatient visit** for the evaluation and management of a new patient, which requires these three key components:

- **a problem focused history;**
- **a problem focused examination; and**
- **straightforward medical decision making.**

Counseling and/or coordination of care with other providers or agencies are provided consistent with the nature of the problem(s) and the patient's and/or family's needs.

Usually, the presenting problems are self limited or minor. Physicians typically spend 10 minutes face-to-face with the patient and/or family.

99202   **Office or other outpatient visit** for the evaluation and management of a new patient, which requires these three key components:

- **an expanded problem focused history;**
- **an expanded problem focused examination; and**
- **straightforward medical decision making.**

Counseling and/or coordination of care with other providers or agencies are provided consistent with the nature of the problem(s) and the patient's and/or family's needs.

Usually, the presenting problem(s) are of low to moderate severity. Physicians typically spend 20 minutes face-to-face with the patient and/or family.

99203   **Office or other outpatient visit** for the evaluation and management of a new patient, which requires these three key components:

- **a detailed history;**
- **a detailed examination; and**
- **medical decision making of low complexity.**

Counseling and/or coordination of care with other providers or agencies are provided consistent with the nature of the problem(s) and the patient's and/or family's needs.

Usually, the presenting problem(s) are of moderate severity. Physicians typically spend 30 minutes face-to-face with the patient and/or family.

99204   **Office or other outpatient visit** for the evaluation and management of a new patient, which requires these three key components:

- **a comprehensive history;**
- **a comprehensive examination; and**
- **medical decision making of moderate complexity.**

Counseling and/or coordination of care with other providers or agencies are provided consistent with the nature of the problem(s) and the patient's and/or family's needs.

Usually, the presenting problem(s) are of moderate to high severity. Physicians typically spend 45 minutes face-to-face with the patient and/or family.

99205   **Office or other outpatient visit** for the evaluation and management of a new patient, which requires these three key components:

- **a comprehensive history;**
- **a comprehensive examination; and**
- **medical decision making of high complexity.**

Counseling and/or coordination of care with other providers or agencies are provided consistent with the nature of the problem(s) and the patient's and/or family's needs.

Usually, the presenting problem(s) are of moderate to high severity. Physicians typically spend 60 minutes face-to-face with the patient and/or family.

Established Patient

99211   **Office or other outpatient visit** for the evaluation and management of an established patient, that may not require the presence of a physician. Usually, the presenting problem(s) are minimal. Typically, 5 minutes are spent performing or supervising these services.

99212 **Office or other outpatient visit** for the evaluation and management of an established patient, which requires at least two of these three key components:

- **a problem focused history;**
- **a problem focused examination;**
- **straightforward medical decision making.**

Counseling and/or coordination of care with other providers or agencies are provided consistent with the nature of the problem(s) and the patient's and/or family's needs.

Usually, the presenting problem(s) are self limited or minor. Physicians typically spend 10 minutes face-to-face with the patient and/or family.

99213 **Office or other outpatient visit** for the evaluation and management of an established patient, which requires at least two of these three key components:

- **an expanded problem focused history;**
- **an expanded problem focused examination;**
- **medical decision making of low complexity.**

Counseling and coordination of care with other providers or agencies are provided consistent with the nature of the problem(s) and the patient's and/or family's needs.

Usually, the presenting problem(s) are of low to moderate severity. Physicians typically spend 15 minutes face-to-face with the patient and/or family.

99214 **Office or other outpatient visit** for the evaluation and management of an established patient, which requires at least two of these three key components:

- **a detailed history;**
- **a detailed examination;**
- **medical decision making of moderate complexity.**

Counseling and/or coordination of care with other providers or agencies are provided consistent with the nature of the problem(s) and the patient's and/or family's needs.

Usually, the presenting problem(s) are of moderate to high severity. Physicians typically spend 25 minutes face-to-face with the patient and/or family.

99215 **Office or other outpatient visit** for the evaluation and management of an established patient, which requires at least two of these three key components:

- **a comprehensive history;**
- **a comprehensive examination;**
- **medical decision making of high complexity.**

Counseling and/or coordination of care with other providers or agencies are provided consistent with the nature of the problem(s) and the patient's and/or family's needs.

Usually, the presenting problem(s) are of moderate to high severity. Physicians typically spend 40 minutes face-to-face with the patient and/or family.

Hospital Observation Services

The following codes are used to report evaluation and management services provided to patients designated/admitted as "observation status" in a hospital. It is not necessary that the patient be located in an observation area designated by the hospital.

If such an area does exist in a hospital (as a separate unit in the hospital, in the emergency department, etc.), these codes are to be utilized if the patient is placed in such an area.

For definitions of key components and commonly used terms, please see **Evaluation and Management Services Guidelines.**

Typical times have not yet been established for this category of services.

Observation Care Discharge Services

Observation care discharge of a patient from "observation status" includes final examination of the patient, discussion of the hospital stay, instructions for continuing care, and preparation of discharge records. For observation or inpatient hospital care including the admission and discharge of the patient on the same date, see codes 99234-99236 as appropriate.

99217 **Observation care discharge** day management (This code is to be utilized by the physician to report all services provided to a patient on discharge from "observation status" if the discharge is on other than the initial date of "observation status." To report services to a patient designated as "observation status" or "inpatient status" and discharged on the same date, use the codes for Observation or Inpatient Care Services [including Admission and Discharge Services, 99234-99236 as appropriate.])

Initial Observation Care

New or Established Patient

The following codes are used to report the encounter(s) by the supervising physician with the patient when designated as "observation status." This refers to the initiation of observation status, supervision of the care plan for observation and performance of periodic reassessments. For observation encounters by other physicians, see Office or Other Outpatient Consultation codes (99241-99245).

To report services provided to a patient who is admitted to the hospital after receiving hospital observation care services on the same date, see the notes for initial hospital inpatient care (page 12). For a patient admitted to the hospital on a date subsequent to the date of observation status, the hospital admission would be reported with the appropriate Initial Hospital Care code (99221-99223).

For a patient admitted and discharged from observation or inpatient status on the same date, the services should be reported with codes 99234-99236 as appropriate. Do not report observation discharge (99217) in conjunction with a hospital admission.

When "observation status" is initiated in the course of an encounter in another site of service (eg, hospital emergency department, physician's office, nursing facility) all evaluation and management services provided by the supervising physician in conjunction with initiating "observation status" are considered part of the initial observation care when performed on the same date. The observation care level of service reported by the supervising physician should include the services related to initiating "observation status" provided in the other sites of service as well as in the observation setting.

Evaluation and management services on the same date provided in sites that are related to initiating "observation status" should NOT be reported separately.

These codes may not be utilized for post-operative recovery if the procedure is considered part of the surgical "package." These codes apply to all evaluation and management services that are provided on the same date of initiating "observation status."

99218 **Initial observation care,** per day, for the evaluation and management of a patient which requires these three key components:

- **a detailed or comprehensive history;**
- **a detailed or comprehensive examination; and**
- **medical decision making that is straightforward or of low complexity.**

Counseling and/or coordination of care with other providers or agencies are provided consistent with the nature of the problem(s) and the patient's and/or family's needs.

Usually, the problem(s) requiring admission to "observation status" are of low severity.

99219 **Initial observation care,** per day, for the evaluation and management of a patient, which requires these three key components:

- **a comprehensive history;**
- **a comprehensive examination; and**
- **medical decision making of moderate complexity.**

Counseling and/or coordination of care with other providers or agencies are provided consistent with the nature of the problem(s) and the patient's and/or family's needs.

Usually, the problem(s) requiring admission to "observation status" are of moderate severity.

99220 **Initial observation care,** per day, for the evaluation and management of a patient, which requires these three key components:

- **a comprehensive history;**
- **a comprehensive examination; and**
- **medical decision making of high complexity.**

Counseling and/or coordination of care with other providers or agencies are provided consistent with the nature of the problem(s) and the patient's and/or family's needs.

Usually, the problem(s) requiring admission to "observation status" are of high severity.

Hospital Inpatient Services

The following codes are used to report evaluation and management services provided to hospital inpatients. Hospital inpatient services include those services provided to patients in a "partial hospital" setting. These codes are to be used to report these partial hospitalization services. See also psychiatry notes in the full text of *CPT.*

For definitions of key components and commonly used terms, please see **Evaluation and Management Services Guidelines.** For Hospital Observation Services, see 99218-99220. For a patient admitted and discharged from observation or inpatient status on the same date, the services should be reported with codes 99234-99236 as appropriate.

Initial Hospital Care

New or Established Patient

The following codes are used to report the first hospital inpatient encounter with the patient by the admitting physician.

For initial inpatient encounters by physicians other than the admitting physician, see initial inpatient consultation codes (99251-99255) or subsequent hospital care codes (99231-99233) as appropriate.

When the patient is admitted to the hospital as an inpatient in the course of an encounter in another site of service (eg, hospital emergency department, observation status in a hospital, physician's office, nursing facility) all evaluation and management services provided by that physician in conjunction with that admission are considered part of the initial hospital care when performed on the same date as the admission. The inpatient care level of service reported by the admitting physician should include the services related to the admission he/she provided in the other sites of service as well as in the inpatient setting.

Evaluation and Management

Evaluation and management services on the same date provided in sites that are related to the admission "observation status" should NOT be reported separately. For a patient admitted and discharged from observation or inpatient status on the same date, the services should be reported with codes 99234-99236 as appropriate.

99221 **Initial hospital care,** per day, for the evaluation and management of a patient which requires these three key components:

- a detailed or comprehensive history;
- a detailed or comprehensive examination; and
- medical decision making that is straightforward or of low complexity.

Counseling and/or coordination of care with other providers or agencies are provided consistent with the nature of the problem(s) and the patient's and/or family's needs.

Usually, the problem(s) requiring admission are of low severity. Physicians typically spend 30 minutes at the bedside and on the patient's hospital floor or unit.

99222 **Initial hospital care,** per day, for the evaluation and management of a patient, which requires these three key components:

- a comprehensive history;
- a comprehensive examination; and
- medical decision making of moderate complexity.

Counseling and/or coordination of care with other providers or agencies are provided consistent with the nature of the problem(s) and the patient's and/or family's needs.

Usually, the problem(s) requiring admission are of moderate severity. Physicians typically spend 50 minutes at the bedside and on the patient's hospital floor or unit.

99223 **Initial hospital care,** per day, for the evaluation and management of a patient, which requires these three key components:

- a comprehensive history;
- a comprehensive examination; and
- medical decision making of high complexity.

Counseling and/or coordination of care with other providers or agencies are provided consistent with the nature of the problem(s) and the patient's and/or family's needs.

Usually, the problem(s) requiring admission are of high severity. Physicians typically spend 70 minutes at the bedside and on the patient's hospital floor or unit.

Subsequent Hospital Care

All levels of subsequent hospital care include reviewing the medical record and reviewing the results of diagnostic studies and changes in the patient's status, (ie, changes in history, physical condition and response to management) since the last assessment by the physician.

99231 **Subsequent hospital care,** per day, for the evaluation and management of a patient, which requires at least two of these three key components:

- a problem focused interval history;
- a problem focused examination;
- medical decision making that is straightforward or of low complexity.

Counseling and/or coordination of care with other providers or agencies are provided consistent with the nature of the problem(s) and the patient's and/or family's needs.

Usually, the patient is stable, recovering or improving. Physicians typically spend 15 minutes at the bedside and on the patient's hospital floor or unit.

99232 **Subsequent hospital care,** per day, for the evaluation and management of a patient, which requires at least two of these three key components:

- an expanded problem focused interval history;
- an expanded problem focused examination;
- medical decision making of moderate complexity.

Counseling and/or coordination of care with other providers or agencies are provided consistent with the nature of the problem(s) and the patient's and/or family's needs.

Usually, the patient is responding inadequately to therapy or has developed a minor complication. Physicians typically spend 25 minutes at the bedside and on the patient's hospital floor or unit.

99233 **Subsequent hospital care,** per day, for the evaluation and management of a patient, which requires at least two of these three key components:

- a detailed interval history;
- a detailed examination;
- medical decision making of high complexity.

Counseling and/or coordination of care with other providers or agencies are provided consistent with the nature of the problem(s) and the patient's and/or family's needs.

Usually, the patient is unstable or has developed a significant complication or a significant new problem. Physicians typically spend 35 minutes at the bedside and on the patient's hospital floor or unit.

Observation or Inpatient Care Services (Including Admission and Discharge Services)

The following codes are used to report observation or inpatient hospital care services provided to patients admitted and discharged on the same date of service. When a patient is admitted to the hospital from observation status on the same date, the physician should report only the initial hospital care code. The initial hospital care code reported by the admitting physician should include the services related to the observation status services he/she provided on the same date of inpatient admission.

When "observation status" is initiated in the course of an encounter in another site of service (eg, hospital emergency department, physician's office, nursing facility) all evaluation and management services provided by the supervising physician in conjunction with initiating "observation status" are considered part of the initial observation care when performed on the same date. The observation care level of service should include the services related to initiating "observation status" provided in the other sites of service as well as in the observation setting when provided by the same physician.

For patients admitted to observation or inpatient care and discharged on a different date, see codes 99218-99220 and 99217, or 99221-99223 and 99238, 99239.

99234 **Observation or inpatient hospital care,** for the evaluation and management of a patient including admission and discharge on the same date which requires these three key components:

- **a detailed or comprehensive history;**
- **a detailed or comprehensive examination; and**
- **medical decision making that is straightforward or of low complexity.**

Counseling and/or coordination of care with other providers or agencies are provided consistent with the nature of the problem(s) and the patient's and/or family's needs.

Usually the presenting problem(s) requiring admission are of low severity.

99235 **Observation or inpatient hospital care,** for the evaluation and management of a patient including admission and discharge on the same date which requires these three key components:

- **a comprehensive history;**
- **a comprehensive examination; and**
- **medical decision making of moderate complexity.**

Counseling and/or coordination of care with other providers or agencies are provided consistent with the nature of the problem(s) and the patient's and/or family's needs.

Usually the presenting problem(s) requiring admission are of moderate severity.

99236 **Observation or inpatient hospital care,** for the evaluation and management of a patient including admission and discharge on the same date which requires these three key components:

- **a comprehensive history;**
- **a comprehensive examination; and**
- **medical decision making of high complexity.**

Counseling and/or coordination of care with other providers or agencies are provided consistent with the nature of the problem(s) and the patient's and/or family's needs.

Usually the presenting problem(s) requiring admission are of high severity.

Hospital Discharge Services

The hospital discharge day management codes are to be used to report the total duration of time spent by a physician for final hospital discharge of a patient. The codes include, as appropriate, final examination of the patient, discussion of the hospital stay, even if the time spent by the physician on that date is not continuous, instructions for continuing care to all relevant caregivers, and preparation of discharge records, prescriptions and referral forms. For a patient admitted and discharged from observation or inpatient status on the same date, the services should be reported with codes 99234-99236 as appropriate.

99238 **Hospital discharge day management;** 30 minutes or less

99239 more than 30 minutes

(These codes are to be utilized by the physician to report all services provided to a patient on the date of discharge, if other than the initial date of inpatient status. To report services to a patient who is admitted as an inpatient, and discharged on the same date, see codes 99234-99236 for observation or inpatient hospital care including the admission and discharge of the patient on the same date. To report concurrent care services provided by a physician(s) other than the attending physician, use subsequent hospital care codes (99231-99233) on the day of discharge.)

(For Observation Care Discharge, use 99217)

(For observation or inpatient hospital care including the admission and discharge of the patient on the same date, see 99234-99236)

(For Nursing Facility Care Discharge, see 99315, 99316)

(For discharge services provided to newborns admitted and discharged on the same date, use 99435)

Consultations

A consultation is a type of service provided by a physician whose opinion or advice regarding evaluation and/or management of a specific problem is requested by another physician or other appropriate source.

A physician consultant may initiate diagnostic and/or therapeutic services at the same or subsequent visit.

The written or verbal request for a consult may be made by a physician or other appropriate source and documented in the patient's medical record. The

Evaluation and Management

consultant's opinion and any services that were ordered or performed must also be documented in the patient's medical record and communicated by written report to the requesting physician or other appropriate source.

A "consultation" initiated by a patient and/or family, and not requested by a physician, is not reported using the initial consultation codes but may be reported using the codes for confirmatory consultation or office visits, as appropriate.

If a confirmatory consultation is required, eg, by a third party payor, modifier 32 should also be reported.

Any specifically identifiable procedure (ie, identified with a specific CPT code) performed on or subsequent to the date of the initial consultation should be reported separately.

If subsequent to the completion of a consultation, the consultant assumes responsibility for management of a portion or all of the patient's condition(s), the follow-up consultation codes should not be used. In the hospital setting, the consulting physician should use the appropriate inpatient hospital consultation code for the initial encounter and then subsequent hospital care codes (not follow-up consultation codes). In the office setting, the appropriate established patient code should be used.

There are four subcategories of consultations: office, initial inpatient, follow-up inpatient, and confirmatory. See each subcategory for specific reporting instructions.

For definitions of key components and commonly used terms, please see **Evaluation and Management Services Guidelines.**

Office or Other Outpatient Consultations

New or Established Patient

The following codes are used to report consultations provided in the physician's office or in an outpatient or other ambulatory facility, including hospital observation services, home services, domiciliary, rest home, custodial care, or emergency department (see consultation definition, above). Follow-up visits in the consultant's office or other outpatient facility that are initiated by the physician consultant are reported using office visit codes for established patients (99211-99215). If an additional request for an opinion or advice regarding the same or a new problem is received from the attending physician and documented in the medical record, the office consultation codes may be used again.

99241 **Office consultation** for a new or established patient, which requires these three key components:

- **a problem focused history;**
- **problem focused examination; and**
- **straightforward medical decision making.**

Counseling and/or coordination of care with other providers or agencies are provided consistent with the nature of the problem(s) and the patient's and/or family's needs.

Usually, the presenting problem(s) are self limited or minor. Physicians typically spend 15 minutes face-to-face with the patient and/or family.

99242 **Office consultation** for a new or established patient, which requires these three key components:

- **an expanded problem focused history;**
- **an expanded problem focused examination; and**
- **straightforward medical decision making.**

Counseling and/or coordination of care with other providers or agencies are provided consistent with the nature of the problem(s) and the patient's and/or family's needs.

Usually, the presenting problem(s) are of low severity. Physicians typically spend 30 minutes face-to-face with the patient and/or family.

99243 **Office consultation** for a new or established patient, which requires these three key components:

- **a detailed history;**
- **a detailed examination; and**
- **medical decision making of low complexity.**

Counseling and/or coordination of care with other providers or agencies are provided consistent with the nature of the problem(s) and the patient's and/or family's needs.

Usually, the presenting problem(s) are of moderate severity. Physicians typically spend 40 minutes face-to-face with the patient and/or family.

99244 **Office consultation** for a new or established patient, which requires these three key components:

- **a comprehensive history;**
- **a comprehensive examination; and**
- **medical decision making of moderate complexity.**

Counseling and/or coordination of care with other providers or agencies are provided consistent with the nature of the problem(s) and the patient's and/or family's needs.

Usually, the presenting problem(s) are of moderate to high severity. Physicians typically spend 60 minutes face-to-face with the patient and/or family.

99245 **Office consultation** for a new or established patient, which requires these three key components:

- **a comprehensive history;**
- **a comprehensive examination; and**
- **medical decision making of high complexity.**

Counseling and/or coordination of care with other providers or agencies are provided consistent with the nature of the problem(s) and the patient's and/or family's needs.

Usually, the presenting problem(s) are of moderate to high severity. Physicians typically spend 80 minutes face-to-face with the patient and/or family.

Initial Inpatient Consultations

New or Established Patient

The following codes are used to report physician consultations provided to hospital inpatients, residents of nursing facilities, or patients in a partial hospital setting. Only one initial consultation should be reported by a consultant per admission.

99251 **Initial inpatient consultation** for a new or established patient, which requires these three key components:

- **a problem focused history;**
- **a problem focused examination; and**
- **straightforward medical decision making.**

Counseling and/or coordination of care with other providers or agencies are provided consistent with the nature of the problem(s) and the patient's and/or family's needs.

Usually, the presenting problem(s) are self limited or minor. Physicians typically spend 20 minutes at the bedside and on the patient's hospital floor or unit.

99252 **Initial inpatient consultation** for a new or established patient, which requires these three key components:

- **an expanded problem focused history;**
- **an expanded problem focused examination; and**
- **straightforward medical decision making.**

Counseling and/or coordination of care with other providers or agencies are provided consistent with the nature of the problem(s) and the patient's and/or family's needs.

Usually, the presenting problem(s) are of low severity. Physicians typically spend 40 minutes at the bedside and on the patient's hospital floor or unit.

99253 **Initial inpatient consultation** for a new or established patient, which requires these three key components:

- **a detailed history;**
- **a detailed examination; and**
- **medical decision making of low complexity.**

Counseling and/or coordination of care with other providers or agencies are provided consistent with the nature of the problem(s) and the patient's and/or family's needs.

Usually, the presenting problem(s) are of moderate severity. Physicians typically spend 55 minutes at the bedside and on the patient's hospital floor or unit.

99254 **Initial inpatient consultation** for a new or established patient, which requires three key components:

- **a comprehensive history;**
- **a comprehensive examination; and**
- **medical decision making of moderate complexity.**

Counseling and/or coordination of care with other providers or agencies are provided consistent with the nature of the problem(s) and the patient's and/or family's needs.

Usually, the presenting problem(s) are of moderate to high severity. Physicians typically spend 80 minutes at the bedside and on the patient's hospital floor or unit.

99255 **Initial inpatient consultation** for a new or established patient, which requires these three key components:

- **a comprehensive history;**
- **a comprehensive examination; and**
- **medical decision making of high complexity.**

Counseling and/or coordination of care with other providers or agencies are provided consistent with the nature of the problem(s) and the patient's and/or family's needs.

Usually, the presenting problem(s) are of moderate to high severity. Physicians typically spend 110 minutes at the bedside and on the patient's hospital floor or unit.

Follow-Up Inpatient Consultations

Established Patient

Follow-up consultations are visits to complete the initial consultation OR subsequent consultative visits requested by the attending physician.

A follow-up consultation includes monitoring progress, recommending management modifications or advising on a new plan of care in response to changes in the patient's status.

If the physician consultant has initiated treatment at the initial consultation, and participates thereafter in the patient's management, the codes for subsequent hospital care should be used (99231-99233).

The following codes are used to report follow-up consultations provided to hospital inpatients or nursing facility residents only. For consultative services provided in other settings, the codes for office or other outpatient consultations should be reported (99241-99245).

99261 **Follow-up inpatient consultation** for an established patient, which requires at least two of these three key components:

- **a problem focused interval history;**
- **a problem focused examination;**
- **medical decision making that is straightforward or of low complexity.**

Evaluation and Management

Counseling and/or coordination of care with other providers or agencies are provided consistent with nature of the problem(s) and the patient's and/or family's needs.

Usually, the patient is stable, recovering or improving. Physicians typically spend 10 minutes at the bedside and on the patient's hospital floor or unit.

99262   **Follow-up inpatient consultation** for an established patient which requires at least two of these three key components:

- **an expanded problem focused interval history;**
- **an expanded problem focused examination;**
- **medical decision making of moderate complexity.**

Counseling and/or coordination of care with other providers or agencies are provided consistent with the nature of the problem(s) and the patient's and/or family's needs.

Usually, the patient is responding inadequately to therapy or has developed a minor complication. Physicians typically spend 20 minutes at the bedside and on the patient's hospital floor or unit.

99263   **Follow-up inpatient consultation** for an established patient which requires at least two of these three key components:

- **a detailed interval history;**
- **a detailed examination;**
- **medical decision making of high complexity.**

Counseling and/or coordination of care with other providers or agencies are provided consistent with the nature of the problem(s) and the patient's and/or family's needs.

Usually, the patient is unstable or has developed a significant complication or a significant new problem. Physicians typically spend 30 minutes at the bedside and on the patient's hospital floor or unit.

Confirmatory Consultations

New or Established Patient

The following codes are used to report the evaluation and management services provided to patients when the consulting physician is aware of the confirmatory nature of the opinion sought (eg, when a second/third opinion is requested or required on the necessity or appropriateness of a previously recommended medical treatment or surgical procedure).

Confirmatory consultations may be provided in any setting.

A physician consultant providing a confirmatory consultation is expected to provide an opinion and/or advice only. Any services subsequent to the opinion are coded at the appropriate level of office visit, established patient, or subsequent hospital care. If a confirmatory

consultation is required, eg, by a third party payor, modifier 32 should also be reported. (See also Consultation notes, page 13.) Typical times have not yet been established for this subcategory of services.

99271   **Confirmatory consultation** for a new or established patient, which requires these three key components:

- **a problem focused history;**
- **a problem focused examination; and**
- **straightforward medical decision making.**

Counseling and/or coordination of care with other providers or agencies are provided consistent with the nature of the problem(s) and the patient's and/or family's needs.

Usually, the presenting problem(s) are self limited or minor.

99272   **Confirmatory consultation** for a new or established patient, which requires these three key components:

- **an expanded problem focused history;**
- **an expanded problem focused examination; and**
- **straightforward medical decision making.**

Counseling and/or coordination of care with other providers or agencies are provided consistent with the nature of the problem(s) and the patient's and/or family's needs.

Usually, the presenting problem(s) are of low severity.

99273   **Confirmatory consultation** for a new or established patient, which requires these three key components:

- **a detailed history;**
- **a detailed examination; and**
- **medical decision making of low complexity.**

Counseling and/or coordination of care with other providers or agencies are provided consistent with the nature of the problem(s) and the patient's and/or family's needs.

Usually, the presenting problem(s) are of moderate severity.

99274   **Confirmatory consultation** for a new or established patient, which requires these three key components:

- **a comprehensive history;**
- **a comprehensive examination; and**
- **medical decision making of moderate complexity.**

Counseling and/or coordination of care with other providers or agencies are provided consistent with the nature of the problem(s) and the patient's and/or family's needs.

Usually, the presenting problem(s) are of moderate to high severity.

99275 **Confirmatory consultation** for a new or established patient, which requires these three key components:

- **a comprehensive history;**
- **a comprehensive examination; and**
- **medical decision making of high complexity.**

Counseling and/or coordination of care with other providers or agencies are provided consistent with the nature of the problem(s) and the patient's and/or family's needs.

Usually, the presenting problem(s) are of moderate to high severity.

Emergency Department Services

New or Established Patient

The following codes are used to report evaluation and management services provided in the emergency department. No distinction is made between new and established patients in the emergency department.

An emergency department is defined as an organized hospital-based facility for the provision of unscheduled episodic services to patients who present for immediate medical attention. The facility must be available 24 hours a day.

For critical care services provided in the emergency department, see Critical Care notes and 99291, 99292.

For evaluation and management services provided to a patient in an observation area of a hospital, see 99217-99220.

For observation or inpatient care services (including admission and discharge services), see 99234-99236.

99281 **Emergency department visit** for the evaluation and management of a patient, which requires these three key components:

- **a problem focused history;**
- **a problem focused examination; and**
- **straightforward medical decision making.**

Counseling and/or coordination of care with other providers or agencies are provided consistent with the nature of the problem(s) and the patient's and/or family's needs.

Usually, the presenting problem(s) are self limited or minor.

99282 **Emergency department visit** for the evaluation and management of a patient, which requires these three key components:

- **an expanded problem focused history;**
- **an expanded problem focused examination; and**
- **medical decision making of low complexity.**

Counseling and/or coordination of care with other providers or agencies are provided consistent with the nature of the problem(s) and the patient's and/or family's needs.

Usually, the presenting problem(s) are of low to moderate severity.

99283 **Emergency department visit** for the evaluation and management of a patient, which requires these three key components:

- **an expanded problem focused history;**
- **an expanded problem focused examination; and**
- **medical decision making of moderate complexity.**

Counseling and/or coordination of care with other providers or agencies are provided consistent with the nature of the problem(s) and the patient's and/or family's needs.

Usually, the presenting problem(s) are of moderate severity.

99284 **Emergency department visit** for the evaluation and management of a patient, which requires these three key components:

- **a detailed history;**
- **a detailed examination; and**
- **medical decision making of moderate complexity.**

Counseling and/or coordination of care with other providers or agencies are provided consistent with the nature of the problem(s) and the patient's and/or family's needs.

Usually, the presenting problem(s) are of high severity, and require urgent evaluation by the physician but do not pose an immediate significant threat to life or physiologic function.

99285 **Emergency department visit** for the evaluation and management of a patient, which requires these three key components within the constraints imposed by the urgency of the patient's clinical condition and/or mental status:

- **a comprehensive history;**
- **a comprehensive examination; and**
- **medical decision making of high complexity.**

Counseling and/or coordination of care with other providers or agencies are provided consistent with the nature of the problem(s) and the patient's and/or family's needs.

Usually, the presenting problem(s) are of high severity and pose an immediate significant threat to life or physiologic function.

Evaluation and Management

Other Emergency Services

In physician directed emergency care, advanced life support, the physician is located in a hospital emergency or critical care department, and is in two-way voice communication with ambulance or rescue personnel outside the hospital. The physician directs the performance of necessary medical procedures, including but not limited to: telemetry of cardiac rhythm; cardiac and/or pulmonary resuscitation; endotracheal or esophageal obturator airway intubation; administration of intravenous fluids and/or administration of intramuscular, intratracheal or subcutaneous drugs; and/or electrical conversion of arrhythmia.

99288 **Physician direction of** emergency medical systems (EMS) emergency care, advanced life support

Pediatric Critical Care Patient Transport

The following codes 99289 and 99290 are used to report the physical attendance and direct face-to-face care by a physician during the interfacility transport of a critically ill or critically injured pediatric patient. For the purpose of reporting codes 99289 and 99290, face-to-face care begins when the physician assumes primary responsibility of the pediatric patient at the referring hospital/facility, and ends when the receiving hospital/facility accepts responsibility for the pediatric patient's care. Only the time the physician spends in direct face-to-face contact with the patient during the transport should be reported. Pediatric patient transport services involving less than 30 minutes of face-to-face physician care should not be reported using codes 99289, 99290. Procedure(s) or service(s) performed by other members of the transporting team may not be reported by the supervising physician.

The following services are included when performed during the pediatric patient transport by the physician providing critical care and may not be reported separately: routine monitoring evaluations (eg, heart rate, respiratory rate, blood pressure, and pulse oximetry), the interpretation of cardiac output measurements (93561, 93562), chest x-rays (71010, 71015, 71020), pulse oximetry (94760, 94761, 94762), blood gases and information data stored in computers (eg, ECGs, blood pressures, hematologic data) (99090), gastric intubation (43752, 91105), temporary transcutaneous pacing (92953), ventilatory management (94656, 94660, 94662) and vascular access procedures (36000, 36400, 36405, 36406, 36410, 36415, 36540, 36600). Any services performed which are not listed above should be reported separately.

Critical care is the direct delivery by a physician(s) of medical care for a critically ill or critically injured patient. A critical illness or injury acutely impairs one or more

vital organ systems such that there is a high probability of imminent or life threatening deterioration in the patient's condition. Critical care involves high complexity decision making to assess, manipulate, and support vital system function(s) to treat single or multiple vital organ system failure and/or to prevent further life threatening deterioration of the patient's condition. Examples of vital organ system failure include, but are not limited to: central nervous system failure, circulatory failure, shock, renal, hepatic, metabolic, and/or respiratory failure.

Providing medical care to a critically ill, injured, or post-operative patient qualifies as a critical care service only if both the illness or injury and the treatment being provided meet the above requirements.

The direction of emergency care to transporting staff by a physician located in a hospital or other facility by two-way communication is not considered direct face-to-face care and should not be reported with codes 99289, 99290. Physician directed emergency care through outside voice communication to transporting staff personnel is reported with code 99288.

The emergency department services codes (99281-99285), initial hospital care codes (99221-99223), hourly critical care codes (99291, 99292), or initial date neonatal intensive care code (99295) are only reported after the patient has been admitted to the emergency department, the inpatient floor or the critical care unit of the receiving facility.

Code 99289 is used to report the first 30-74 minutes of direct face-to-face time with the transport pediatric patient and should be reported only once on a given date. Code 99290 is used to report each additional 30 minutes provided on a given date. Face-to-face services less than 30 minutes should not be reported with these codes.

99289 Critical care services delivered by a physician, face-to-face, during an interfacility transport of critically ill or critically injured pediatric patient, 24 months of age or less; first 30-74 minutes of hands on care during transport

+ 99290 each additional 30 minutes (List separately in addition to code for primary service)

(Use 99290 in conjunction with 99289)

(Critical care of less than 30 minutes total duration should be reported with the appropriate E/M code)

Critical Care Services

Critical care is the direct delivery by a physician(s) of medical care for a critically ill or critically injured patient. A critical illness or injury acutely impairs one or more vital organ systems such that there is a high probability of imminent or life threatening deterioration in the patient's condition. Critical care involves high complexity decision making to assess, manipulate, and support vital system function(s) to treat single or multiple vital organ system failure and/or to prevent further life threatening deterioration of the patient's condition. Examples of vital organ system failure include, but are not limited to: central nervous system failure, circulatory failure, shock, renal, hepatic, metabolic, and/or respiratory failure. Although critical care typically requires interpretation of multiple physiologic parameters and/or application of advanced technology(s), critical care may be provided in life threatening situations when these elements are not present. Critical care may be provided on multiple days, even if no changes are made in the treatment rendered to the patient, provided that the patient's condition continues to require the level of physician attention described above.

Providing medical care to a critically ill, injured, or post-operative patient qualifies as a critical care service only if both the illness or injury and the treatment being provided meet the above requirements. Critical care is usually, but not always, given in a critical care area, such as the coronary care unit, intensive care unit, pediatric intensive care unit, respiratory care unit, or the emergency care facility.

Inpatient critical care services provided to infants ►29◄ days through 24 months of age are reported with pediatric critical care codes 99293 and 99294. The pediatric critical care codes are reported as long as the infant/young child qualifies for critical care services during the hospital stay through 24 months of age. Inpatient critical care services provided to neonates (►28◄ days of age or less) are reported with the neonatal critical care codes 99295 and 99296. The neonatal critical care codes are reported as long as the neonate qualifies for critical care services during the hospital stay through the ►28◄th postnatal day. The reporting of the pediatric and neonatal critical care services is not based on time or the type of unit (eg, pediatric or neonatal critical care unit) and it is not dependent upon the type of provider delivering the care. To report critical care services provided in the outpatient setting (eg, emergency department or office), for neonates and pediatric patients up through 24 months of age, see the hourly Critical Care codes 99291, 99292. If the same physician provides critical care services for a neonatal or pediatric patient in both the outpatient and inpatient settings on the same day, report only the appropriate Neonatal or Pediatric Critical Care code (99293-99296) for all critical care services provided on that day. For additional instructions on reporting these services, see the Neonatal and Pediatric Critical Care section and codes 99293-99296.

Services for a patient who is not critically ill but happens to be in a critical care unit are reported using other appropriate E/M codes.

Critical care and other E/M services may be provided to the same patient on the same date by the same physician.

The following services are included in reporting critical care when performed during the critical period by the physician(s) providing critical care: the interpretation of cardiac output measurements (93561, 93562), chest x-rays (71010, 71015, 71020), pulse oximetry (94760, 94761, 94762), blood gases, and information data stored in computers (eg, ECGs, blood pressures, hematologic data (99090)); gastric intubation (43752, 91105); temporary transcutaneous pacing (92953); ventilatory management (94656, 94657, 94660, 94662); and vascular access procedures (36000, 36410, 36415, 36540, 36600). Any services performed which are not listed above should be reported separately.

Codes 99291, 99292 should be reported for the physician's attendance during the transport of critically ill or critically injured patients over 24 months of age to or from a facility or hospital. For physician transport services of critically ill or critically injured pediatric patients 24 months of age or less see 99289, 99290.

The critical care codes 99291 and 99292 are used to report the total duration of time spent by a physician providing critical care services to a critically ill or critically injured patient, even if the time spent by the physician on that date is not continuous. For any given period of time spent providing critical care services, the physician must devote his or her full attention to the patient and, therefore, cannot provide services to any other patient during the same period of time.

Time spent with the individual patient should be recorded in the patient's record. The time that can be reported as critical care is the time spent engaged in work directly related to the individual patient's care whether that time was spent at the immediate bedside or elsewhere on the floor or unit. For example, time spent on the unit or at the nursing station on the floor reviewing test results or imaging studies, discussing the critically ill patient's care with other medical staff or documenting critical care services in the medical record would be reported as critical care, even though it does not occur at the bedside. Also, when the patient is unable or clinically incompetent to participate in discussions, time spent on the floor or unit with family members or surrogate decision makers obtaining a medical history, reviewing the patient's condition or prognosis, or discussing treatment or limitation(s) of treatment may be reported as critical care, provided that the conversation bears directly on the management of the patient.

Time spent in activities that occur outside of the unit or off the floor (eg, telephone calls, whether taken at home, in the office, or elsewhere in the hospital) may not be reported as critical care since the physician is not immediately available to the patient. Time spent in activities that do not directly contribute to the treatment of the patient may not be reported as critical care, even if they are performed in the critical care unit (eg, participation in administrative meetings or telephone calls to discuss other patients). Time spent performing

Evaluation and Management

Evaluation and Management

separately reportable procedures or services should not be included in the time reported as critical care time.

Code 99291 is used to report the first 30-74 minutes of critical care on a given date. It should be used only once per date even if the time spent by the physician is not continuous on that date. Critical care of less than 30 minutes total duration on a given date should be reported with the appropriate E/M code.

Code 99292 is used to report additional block(s) of time, of up to 30 minutes each beyond the first 74 minutes. (See table below.)

The following examples illustrate the correct reporting of critical care services:

Total Duration of Critical Care	Codes
less than 30 minutes (less than 1/2 hour)	appropriate E/M codes
30-74 minutes (1/2 hr. - 1 hr. 14 min.)	99291 X 1
75-104 minutes (1 hr. 15 min. - 1 hr. 44 min.)	99291 X 1 AND 99292 X 1
105-134 minutes (1 hr. 45 min. - 2 hr. 14 min.)	99291 X 1 AND 99292 X 2
135 - 164 minutes (2 hr. 15 min. - 2 hr. 44 min.)	99291 X 1 AND 99292 X 3
165 - 194 minutes (2 hr. 45 min. - 3 hr. 14 min.)	99291 X 1 AND 99292 X 4
194 minutes or longer (3 hr. 14 min. - etc.)	99291 and 99292 as appropriate (see illustrated reporting examples above)

99291 **Critical care, evaluation and management** of the critically ill or critically injured patient; first 30-74 minutes

+ 99292 each additional 30 minutes (List separately in addition to code for primary service)

(Use 99292 in conjunction with 99291)

Inpatient Neonatal and Pediatric Critical Care Services

The following codes (99293-99296) are used to report services provided by a physician directing the inpatient care of a critically ill neonate/infant. The same definitions for critical care services apply for the adult, child, and neonate.

The initial day neonatal critical care code (99295) can be used in addition to codes 99360, 99436 or 99440 as appropriate, when the physician is present for the delivery (99360 or 99436) and newborn resuscitation (99440) is required. Other procedures performed as a necessary part of the resuscitation (eg, endotracheal intubation (31500)) are also reported separately when performed as part of the pre-admission delivery room care. In order to report these procedures separately, they must be performed as a necessary component of the resuscitation and not simply as a convenience before admission to the neonatal intensive care unit.

Codes 99295, 99296 are used to report services provided by a physician directing the inpatient care of a critically ill neonate through the first ►28◄ days of life. They represent care starting with the date of admission (99295) and subsequent day(s) (99296) and may be reported only once per day, per patient. Once the neonate is no longer considered to be critically ill, the Intensive Low Birth Weight Services codes for those with present body weight of less than 2500 grams (99298, 99299) or the codes for Subsequent Hospital Care (99231-99233) for those with present body weight over 2500 grams should be utilized.

Codes 99293, 99294 are used to report services provided by a physician directing the inpatient care of a critically ill infant or young child from ►29◄ days of postnatal age through 24 months of age. They represent care starting with the date of admission (99293) and subsequent day(s) (99294) and may be reported by a single physician only once per day, per patient in a given setting. The critically ill or critically injured child older than 24 months of age would be reported with hourly critical care service codes (99291, 99292). Once an infant is no longer considered to be critically ill but continues to require intensive care, the Intensive Low Birth Weight Services codes (99298, 99299) should be used to report services for infants with present body weight of less than 2500 grams. When the present body weight of those infants exceeds 2500 grams, the Subsequent Hospital Care (99231-99233) codes should be utilized. To report critical care services provided in the outpatient setting (eg, emergency department or office), for neonates and pediatric patients up through 24 months of age, see the hourly Critical Care codes 99291, 99292. If the same physician provides critical care services for a neonatal or pediatric patient in both the outpatient and inpatient settings on the same day, report only the appropriate Neonatal or Pediatric Critical Care code (99293-99296) for all critical care services provided on that day.

Care rendered under 99293-99296 includes management, monitoring, and treatment of the patient including respiratory, pharmacologic control of the circulatory system, enteral and parenteral nutrition, metabolic and hematologic maintenance, parent/family counseling, case management services, and personal direct supervision of the health care team in the performance of cognitive and procedural activities.

The pediatric and neonatal critical care codes include those procedures listed above for the hourly critical care codes (99291, 99292). In addition, the following procedures are also included in the bundled (global) pediatric and neonatal critical care service codes (99293-99296): umbilical venous (36510) and umbilical arterial (36660) catheters, central (36555) or peripheral vessel catheterization (36000), other arterial catheters (36140, 36620), oral or nasogastric tube placement (43752), endotracheal intubation (31500), lumbar puncture (62270), suprapubic bladder aspiration (51000), bladder catheterization (▶51701, 51702◀), initiation and management of mechanical ventilation (94656, 94657) or continuous positive airway pressure (CPAP) (94660), surfactant administration, intravascular fluid administration (90780, 90781), transfusion of blood components (36430, 36440), vascular punctures (36420, 36600), invasive or non-invasive electronic monitoring of vital signs, bedside pulmonary function testing (94375), and/or monitoring or interpretation of blood gases or oxygen saturation (94760-94762). Any services performed which are not listed above should be reported separately.

For additional instructions, see descriptions listed for 99293-99296

Inpatient Pediatric Critical Care

▲ 99293   **Initial inpatient pediatric critical care,** per day, for the evaluation and management of a critically ill infant or young child, 29 days through 24 months of age

▲ 99294   **Subsequent inpatient pediatric critical care,** per day, for the evaluation and management of a critically ill infant or young child, 29 days through 24 months of age

Inpatient Neonatal Critical Care

▲ 99295   **Initial inpatient neonatal critical care,** per day, for the evaluation and management of a critically ill neonate, 28 days of age or less

This code is reserved for the date of admission for neonates who are critically ill. Critically ill neonates require cardiac and/or respiratory support (including ventilator or nasal CPAP when indicated), continuous or frequent vital sign monitoring, laboratory and blood gas interpretations, follow-up physician reevaluations, and constant observation by the health care team under direct physician supervision. Immediate preoperative evaluation and stabilization of neonates with life threatening surgical or cardiac conditions are included under this code. Neonates with life threatening surgical or cardiac conditions are included under this code.

Care for neonates who require an intensive care setting but who are not critically ill is reported using the initial hospital care codes (99221-99223).

▲ 99296   **Subsequent inpatient neonatal critical care,** per day, for the evaluation and management of a critically ill neonate, 28 days of age or less

A critically ill neonate will require cardiac and/or respiratory support (including ventilator or nasal CPAP when indicated), continuous or frequent vital sign monitoring, laboratory and blood gas interpretations, follow-up physician re-evaluations throughout a 24-hour period, and constant observation by the health care team under direct physician supervision.

(Subsequent care for neonates who require an intensive setting but who are not critically ill is reported using either the intensive low birth weight services codes (99298, 99299) or the subsequent hospital care codes (99231-99233))

(99297 has been deleted. To report, use 99296)

Intensive (Non-Critical) Low Birth Weight Services

Codes 99298, 99299 are used to report services subsequent to the day of admission provided by a physician directing the continuing intensive care of the low birth weight (LBW) or very low birth weight (VLBW) infant who no longer meets the definition of critically ill. They represent subsequent day(s) of care and may be reported only once per day, per patient. Low birth weight services are reported for those neonates less than 2500 grams who do not meet the definition of critical care but continue to require intensive observation and frequent services and interventions only available in an intensive care setting. The level and frequency of services required for the LBW and the VLBW infant exceed those available in less intensive hospital areas or medical floors. Codes 99298, 99299 are global 24-hour codes with the same services bundled as outlined under codes 99293-99296.

For additional instructions, see descriptions listed for 99298, 99299.

99298   **Subsequent intensive care,** per day, for the evaluation and management of the recovering very low birth weight infant (present body weight less than 1500 grams)

Infants with present body weight less than 1500 grams who are no longer critically ill continue to require intensive cardiac and respiratory monitoring, continuous and/or frequent vital sign monitoring, heat maintenance, enteral and/or parenteral nutritional adjustments, laboratory and oxygen monitoring and constant observation by the health care team under direct physician supervision.

99299 **Subsequent intensive care,** per day, for the evaluation and management of the recovering low birth weight infant (present body weight of 1500-2500 grams)

Infants with present body weight of 1500-2500 grams who are no longer critically ill continue to require intensive cardiac and respiratory monitoring, continuous and/or frequent vital sign monitoring, heat maintenance, enteral and/or parenteral nutritional adjustments, laboratory and oxygen monitoring, and constant observation by the health care team under direct physician supervision.

Nursing Facility Services

The following codes are used to report evaluation and management services to patients in Nursing Facilities (formerly called Skilled Nursing Facilities (SNFs), Intermediate Care Facilities (ICFs) or Long Term Care Facilities (LTCFs)).

These codes should also be used to report evaluation and management services provided to a patient in a psychiatric residential treatment center (a facility or a distinct part of a facility for psychiatric care, which provides a 24-hour therapeutically planned and professionally staffed group living and learning environment). If procedures such as medical psychotherapy are provided in addition to evaluation and management services, these should be reported in addition to the evaluation and management services provided.

Nursing facilities that provide convalescent, rehabilitative, or long term care are required to conduct comprehensive, accurate, standardized, and reproducible assessments of each resident's functional capacity using a Resident Assessment Instrument (RAI). All RAIs include the Minimum Data Set (MDS), Resident Assessment Protocols (RAPs) and utilization guidelines. The MDS is the primary screening and assessment tool; the RAPs trigger the identification of potential problems and provide guidelines for follow-up assessments.

Physicians have a central role in assuring that all residents receive thorough assessments and that medical plans of care are instituted or revised to enhance or maintain the residents' physical and psychosocial functioning.

Two subcategories of nursing facility services are recognized: Comprehensive Nursing Facility Assessments and Subsequent Nursing Facility Care. Both subcategories apply to new or established patients. Comprehensive Assessments may be performed at one or more sites in the assessment process: the hospital, observation unit, office, nursing facility, domiciliary/non-nursing facility or patient's home.

For definitions of key components and commonly used terms, please see **Evaluation and Management Services Guidelines.**

Comprehensive Nursing Facility Assessments

New or Established Patient

When the patient is admitted to the nursing facility in the course of an encounter in another site of service (eg, hospital emergency department, physician's office), all evaluation and management services provided by that physician in conjunction with that admission are considered part of the initial nursing facility care when performed on the same date as the admission or readmission. The nursing facility care level of service reported by the admitting physician should include the services related to the admission he/she provided in the other sites of service as well as in the nursing facility setting.

Hospital discharge or observation discharge services performed on the same date of nursing facility admission or readmission may be reported separately. For a patient discharged from inpatient status on the same date of nursing facility admission or readmission, the hospital discharge services should be reported with codes 99238, 99239 as appropriate. For a patient discharged from observation status on the same date of nursing facility admission or readmission, the observation care discharge services should be reported with code 99217. For a patient admitted and discharged from observation or inpatient status on the same date, see codes 99234-99236.

(For nursing facility care discharge, see 99315, 99316)

More than one comprehensive assessment may be necessary during an inpatient confinement.

99301 **Evaluation and management** of a new or established patient involving an annual nursing facility assessment which requires these three key components:

- **a detailed interval history;**
- **a comprehensive examination; and**
- **medical decision making that is straightforward or of low complexity.**

Counseling and/or coordination of care with other providers or agencies are provided consistent with the nature of the problem(s) and the patient's and/or family's needs.

Usually, the patient is stable, recovering or improving. The review and affirmation of the medical plan of care is required. Physicians typically spend 30 minutes at the bedside and on the patient's facility floor or unit.

99302   **Evaluation and management** of a new or established patient involving a nursing facility assessment which requires these three key components:

- **a detailed interval history;**
- **a comprehensive examination; and**
- **medical decision making of moderate to high complexity.**

Counseling and/or coordination of care with other providers or agencies are provided consistent with the nature of the problem(s) and the patient's and/or family's needs.

Usually, the patient has developed a significant complication or a significant new problem and has had a major permanent change in status.

The creation of a new medical plan of care is required. Physicians typically spend 40 minutes at the bedside and on the patient's facility floor or unit.

99303   **Evaluation and management** of a new or established patient involving a nursing facility assessment at the time of initial admission or readmission to the facility, which requires these three key components:

- **a comprehensive history;**
- **a comprehensive examination; and**
- **medical decision making of moderate to high complexity.**

Counseling and/or coordination of care with other providers or agencies are provided consistent with the nature of the problem(s) and the patient's and/or family's needs.

The creation of a medical plan of care is required. Physicians typically spend 50 minutes at the bedside and on the patient's facility floor or unit.

Subsequent Nursing Facility Care

New or Established Patient

The following codes are used to report the services provided to residents of nursing facilities who do not require a comprehensive assessment, and/or who have not had a major, permanent change of status.

All levels include reviewing the medical record, noting changes in the resident's status since the last visit, and reviewing and signing orders.

99311   **Subsequent nursing facility care,** per day, for the evaluation and management of a new or established patient, which requires at least two of these three key components:

- **a problem focused interval history;**
- **a problem focused examination;**
- **medical decision making that is straightforward or of low complexity.**

Counseling and/or coordination of care with other providers or agencies are provided consistent with the nature of the problem(s) and the patient's and/or family's needs.

Usually, the patient is stable, recovering or improving. Physicians typically spend 15 minutes at the bedside and on the patient's facility floor or unit.

99312   **Subsequent nursing facility care,** per day, for the evaluation and management of a new or established patient, which requires at least two of these three key components:

- **an expanded problem focused interval history;**
- **an expanded problem focused examination;**
- **medical decision making of moderate complexity.**

Counseling and/or coordination of care with other providers or agencies are provided consistent with the nature of the problem(s) and the patient's and/or family's needs.

Usually, the patient is responding inadequately to therapy or has developed a minor complication. Physicians typically spend 25 minutes at the bedside and on the patient's facility floor or unit.

99313   **Subsequent nursing facility care,** per day, for the evaluation and management of a new or established patient, which requires at least two of these three key components:

- **a detailed interval history;**
- **a detailed examination;**
- **medical decision making of moderate to high complexity.**

Counseling and/or coordination of care with other providers or agencies are provided consistent with the nature of the problem(s) and the patient's and/or family's needs.

Usually, the patient has developed a significant complication or a significant new problem. Physicians typically spend 35 minutes at the bedside and on the patient's facility floor or unit.

Nursing Facility Discharge Services

The nursing facility discharge day management codes are to be used to report the total duration of time spent by a physician for the final nursing facility discharge of a patient. The codes include, as appropriate, final examination of the patient, discussion of the nursing facility stay, even if the time spent by the physician on that date is not continuous. Instructions are given for continuing care to all relevant caregivers, and preparation of discharge records, prescriptions and referral forms.

99315   Nursing facility discharge day management; 30 minutes or less

99316   more than 30 minutes

Domiciliary, Rest Home (eg, Boarding Home), or Custodial Care Services

The following codes are used to report evaluation and management services in a facility which provides room, board and other personal assistance services, generally on a long-term basis. The facility's services do not include a medical component.

For definitions of key components and commonly used terms, please see **Evaluation and Management Services Guidelines.**

Typical times have not yet been established for this category of services.

New Patient

99321   **Domiciliary or rest home visit** for the evaluation and management of a new patient which requires these three key components:

- **a problem focused history;**
- **a problem focused examination; and**
- **medical decision making that is straightforward or of low complexity.**

Counseling and/or coordination of care with other providers or agencies are provided consistent with the nature of the problem(s) and the patient's and/or family's needs.

Usually, the presenting problem(s) are of low severity.

99322   **Domiciliary or rest home visit** for the evaluation and management of a new patient, which requires these three key components:

- **an expanded problem focused history;**
- **an expanded problem focused examination; and**
- **medical decision making of moderate complexity.**

Counseling and/or coordination of care with other providers or agencies are provided consistent with the nature of the problem(s) and the patient's and/or family's needs.

Usually, the presenting problem(s) are of moderate severity.

99323   **Domiciliary or rest home visit** for the evaluation and management of a new patient, which requires these three key components:

- **a detailed history;**
- **a detailed examination; and**
- **medical decision making of high complexity.**

Counseling and/or coordination of care with other providers or agencies are provided consistent with the nature of the problem(s) and the patient's and/or family's needs.

Usually, the presenting problem(s) are of high complexity.

Established Patient

99331   **Domiciliary or rest home visit** for the evaluation and management of an established patient, which requires at least two of these three key components:

- **a problem focused interval history;**
- **a problem focused examination;**
- **medical decision making that is straightforward or of low complexity.**

Counseling and/or coordination of care with other providers or agencies are provided consistent with the nature of the problem(s) and the patient's and/or family's needs.

Usually, the patient is stable, recovering or improving.

99332   **Domiciliary or rest home visit** for the evaluation and management of an established patient, which requires at least two of these three key components:

- **an expanded problem focused interval history;**
- **an expanded problem focused examination;**
- **medical decision making of moderate complexity.**

Counseling and/or coordination of care with other providers or agencies are provided consistent with the nature of the problem(s) and the patient's and/or family's needs.

Usually, the patient is responding inadequately to therapy or has developed a minor complication.

99333   **Domiciliary or rest home visit** for the evaluation and management of an established patient, which requires at least two of these three key components:

- **a detailed interval history;**
- **a detailed examination;**
- **medical decision making of high complexity.**

Counseling and/or coordination of care with other providers or agencies are provided consistent with the nature of the problem(s) and the patient's and/or family's needs.

Usually, the patient is unstable or has developed a significant complication or a significant new problem.

Home Services

The following codes are used to report evaluation and management services provided in a private residence.

For definitions of key components and commonly used terms, please see **Evaluation and Management Services Guidelines.**

New Patient

99341   **Home visit** for the evaluation and management of a new patient, which requires these three key components:

- **a problem focused history;**
- **a problem focused examination; and**
- **straightforward medical decision making.**

Counseling and/or coordination of care with other providers or agencies are provided consistent with the nature of the problem(s) and the patient's and/or family's needs.

Usually, the presenting problem(s) are of low severity. Physicians typically spend 20 minutes face-to-face with the patient and/or family.

99342   **Home visit** for the evaluation and management of a new patient, which requires these three key components:

- **an expanded problem focused history;**
- **an expanded problem focused examination; and**
- **medical decision making of low complexity.**

Counseling and/or coordination of care with other providers or agencies are provided consistent with the nature of the problem(s) and the patient's and/or family's needs.

Usually, the presenting problem(s) are of moderate severity. Physicians typically spend 30 minutes face-to-face with the patient and/or family.

99343   **Home visit** for the evaluation and management of a new patient, which requires these three key components:

- **a detailed history;**
- **a detailed examination; and**
- **medical decision making of moderate complexity.**

Counseling and/or coordination of care with other providers or agencies are provided consistent with the nature of the problem(s) and the patient's and/or family's needs.

Usually, the presenting problem(s) are of moderate to high severity. Physicians typically spend 45 minutes face-to-face with the patient and/or family.

99344   **Home visit** for the evaluation and management of a new patient, which requires these three components:

- **a comprehensive history;**
- **a comprehensive examination; and**
- **medical decision making of moderate complexity.**

Counseling and/or coordination of care with other providers or agencies are provided consistent with the nature of the problem(s) and the patient's and/or family's needs.

Usually, the presenting problem(s) are of high severity. Physicians typically spend 60 minutes face-to-face with the patient and/or family.

99345   **Home visit** for the evaluation and management of a new patient, which requires these three key components:

- **a comprehensive history;**
- **a comprehensive examination; and**
- **medical decision making of high complexity.**

Counseling and/or coordination of care with other providers or agencies are provided consistent with the nature of the problem(s) and the patient's and/or family's needs.

Usually, the patient is unstable or has developed a significant new problem requiring immediate physician attention. Physicians typically spend 75 minutes face-to-face with the patient and/or family.

Established Patient

99347   **Home visit** for the evaluation and management of an established patient, which requires at least two of these three key components:

- **a problem focused interval history;**
- **a problem focused examination;**
- **straightforward medical decision making.**

Counseling and/or coordination of care with other providers or agencies are provided consistent with the nature of the problem(s) and the patient's and/or family's needs.

Usually, the presenting problem(s) are self limited or minor. Physicians typically spend 15 minutes face-to-face with the patient and/or family.

99348   **Home visit** for the evaluation and management of an established patient, which requires at least two of these three key components:

- **an expanded problem focused interval history;**
- **an expanded problem focused examination;**
- **medical decision making of low complexity.**

Counseling and/or coordination of care with other providers or agencies are provided consistent with the nature of the problem(s) and the patient's and/or family's needs.

Usually, the presenting problem(s) are of low to moderate severity. Physicians typically spend 25 minutes face-to-face with the patient and/or family.

99349   **Home visit** for the evaluation and management of an established patient, which requires at least two of these three key components:

- **a detailed interval history;**
- **a detailed examination;**
- **medical decision making of moderate complexity.**

Counseling and/or coordination of care with other providers or agencies are provided consistent with the nature of the problem(s) and the patient's and/or family's needs.

Evaluation and Management

Usually, the presenting problem(s) are moderate to high severity. Physicians typically spend 40 minutes face-to-face with the patient and/or family.

99350 **Home visit** for the evaluation and management of an established patient, which requires at least two of these three key components:

- **a comprehensive interval history;**
- **a comprehensive examination;**
- **medical decision making of moderate to high complexity.**

Counseling and/or coordination of care with other providers or agencies are provided consistent with the nature of the problem(s) and the patient's and/or family's needs.

Usually, the presenting problem(s) are of moderate to high severity. The patient may be unstable or may have developed a significant new problem requiring immediate physician attention. Physicians typically spend 60 minutes face-to-face with the patient and/or family.

Prolonged Services

Prolonged Physician Service With Direct (Face-To-Face) Patient Contact

Codes 99354-99357 are used when a physician provides prolonged service involving direct (face-to-face) patient contact that is beyond the usual service in either the inpatient or outpatient setting. This service is reported in addition to other physician services, including evaluation and management services at any level. Appropriate codes should be selected for supplies provided or procedures performed in the care of the patient during this period.

Codes 99354-99357 are used to report the total duration of face-to-face time spent by a physician on a given date providing prolonged service, even if the time spent by the physician on that date is not continuous.

Code 99354 or 99356 is used to report the first hour of prolonged service on a given date, depending on the place of service.

Either code also may be used to report a total duration of prolonged service of 30-60 minutes on a given date. Either code should be used only once per date, even if the time spent by the physician is not continuous on that date. Prolonged service of less than 30 minutes total duration on a given date is not separately reported because the work involved is included in the total work of the evaluation and management codes.

Code 99355 or 99357 is used to report each additional 30 minutes beyond the first hour, depending on the place of service. Either code may also be used to report the final 15-30 minutes of prolonged service on a given date.

Prolonged service of less than 15 minutes beyond the first hour or less than 15 minutes beyond the final 30 minutes is not reported separately.

The following examples illustrate the correct reporting of prolonged physician service with direct patient contact in the office setting:

Total Duration of Prolonged Services	Code(s)
less than 30 minutes (less than 1/2 hour)	Not reported separately
30-74 minutes (1/2 hr. - 1 hr. 14 min.)	99354 X 1
75-104 minutes (1 hr. 15 min. - 1 hr. 44 min.)	99354 X 1 AND 99355 X 1
105-134 minutes (1 hr. 45 min. - 2 hr. 14 min.)	99354 X 1 AND 99355 X 2
135-164 minutes (2 hr. 15 min. - 2 hr. 44 min.)	99354 X 1 AND 99355 X 3
165-194 minutes (2 hr. 45 min. - 3 hr. 14 min.)	99354 X 1 AND 99355 X 4

+ 99354 Prolonged physician service in the office or other outpatient setting requiring direct (face-to-face) patient contact beyond the usual service (eg, prolonged care and treatment of an acute asthmatic patient in an outpatient setting); first hour (List separately in addition to code for office or other outpatient Evaluation and Management service)

(Use 99354 in conjunction with 99201-99215, 99241-99245, 99301-99350)

+ 99355 each additional 30 minutes (List separately in addition to code for prolonged physician service)

(Use 99355 in conjunction with 99354)

+ 99356 Prolonged physician service in the inpatient setting, requiring direct (face-to-face) patient contact beyond the usual service (eg, maternal fetal monitoring for high risk delivery or other physiological monitoring, prolonged care of an acutely ill inpatient); first hour (List separately in addition to code for inpatient Evaluation and Management service)

(Use 99356 in conjunction with 99221-99233, 99251-99255, 99261-99263)

+ 99357 each additional 30 minutes (List separately in addition to code for prolonged physician service)

(Use 99357 in conjunction with 99356)

Prolonged Physician Service Without Direct (Face-To-Face) Patient Contact

Codes 99358 and 99359 are used when a physician provides prolonged service not involving direct (face-to-face) care that is beyond the usual service in either the inpatient or outpatient setting.

This service is to be reported in addition to other physician service, including evaluation and management services at any level.

Codes 99358 and 99359 are used to report the total duration of non-face-to-face time spent by a physician on a given date providing prolonged service, even if the time spent by the physician on that date is not continuous. Code 99358 is used to report the first hour of prolonged service on a given date regardless of the place of service.

It may also be used to report a total duration of prolonged service of 30-60 minutes on a given date. It should be used only once per date even if the time spent by the physician is not continuous on that date.

Prolonged service of less than 30 minutes total duration on a given date is not separately reported.

Code 99359 is used to report each additional 30 minutes beyond the first hour regardless of the place of service. It may also be used to report the final 15-30 minutes of prolonged service on a given date.

Prolonged service of less than 15 minutes beyond the first hour or less than 15 minutes beyond the final 30 minutes is not reported separately.

+ **99358** **Prolonged evaluation and management service** before and/or after direct (face-to-face) patient care (eg, review of extensive records and tests, communication with other professionals and/or the patient/family); first hour (List separately in addition to code(s) for other physician service(s) and/or inpatient or outpatient Evaluation and Management service)

+ **99359** each additional 30 minutes (List separately in addition to code for prolonged physician service)

(Use 99359 in conjunction with 99358)

(To report telephone calls, see 99371-99373)

Physician Standby Services

Code 99360 is used to report physician standby service that is requested by another physician and that involves prolonged physician attendance without direct (face-to-face) patient contact. The physician may not be providing care or services to other patients during this period. This code is not used to report time spent proctoring another physician. It is also not used if the period of standby ends with the performance of a procedure subject to a "surgical" package by the physician who was on standby.

Code 99360 is used to report the total duration of time spent by a physician on a given date on standby. Standby service of less than 30 minutes total duration on a given date is not reported separately.

Second and subsequent periods of standby beyond the first 30 minutes may be reported only if a full 30 minutes of standby was provided for each unit of service reported.

99360 **Physician standby service,** requiring prolonged physician attendance, each 30 minutes (eg, operative standby, standby for frozen section, for cesarean/high risk delivery, for monitoring EEG)

(For hospital mandated on call services, see 99026, 99027)

(99360 may be reported in addition to 99431, 99440 as appropriate)

(Do not report 99360 in conjunction with 99436)

Case Management Services

Physician case management is a process in which a physician is responsible for direct care of a patient, and for coordinating and controlling access to or initiating and/or supervising other health care services needed by the patient.

Team Conferences

99361 **Medical conference** by a physician with interdisciplinary team of health professionals or representatives of community agencies to coordinate activities of patient care (patient not present); approximately 30 minutes

99362   approximately 60 minutes

Telephone Calls

99371 **Telephone call** by a physician to patient or for consultation or medical management or for coordinating medical management with other health care professionals (eg, nurses, therapists, social workers, nutritionists, physicians, pharmacists); simple or brief (eg, to report on tests and/or laboratory results, to clarify or alter previous instructions, to integrate new information from other health professionals into the medical treatment plan, or to adjust therapy)

99372   intermediate (eg, to provide advice to an established patient on a new problem, to initiate therapy that can be handled by telephone, to discuss test results in detail, to coordinate medical management of a new problem in an established patient, to discuss and evaluate new information and details, or to initiate new plan of care)

Evaluation and Management

99373   complex or lengthy (eg, lengthy counseling session with anxious or distraught patient, detailed or prolonged discussion with family members regarding seriously ill patient, lengthy communication necessary to coordinate complex services of several different health professionals working on different aspects of the total patient care plan)

Care Plan Oversight Services

Care Plan Oversight Services are reported separately from codes for office/outpatient, hospital, home, nursing facility or domiciliary services. The complexity and approximate physician time of the care plan oversight services provided within a 30-day period determine code selection. Only one physician may report services for a given period of time, to reflect that physician's sole or predominant supervisory role with a particular patient. These codes should not be reported for supervision of patients in nursing facilities or under the care of home health agencies unless they require recurrent supervision of therapy.

The work involved in providing very low intensity or infrequent supervision services is included in the pre- and post-encounter work for home, office/outpatient and nursing facility or domiciliary visit codes.

99374   **Physician supervision** of a patient under care of home health agency (patient not present) in home, domiciliary or equivalent environment (eg, Alzheimer's facility) requiring complex and multidisciplinary care modalities involving regular physician development and/or revision of care plans, review of subsequent reports of patient status, review of related laboratory and other studies, communication (including telephone calls) for purposes of assessment or care decisions with health care professional(s), family member(s), surrogate decision maker(s) (eg, legal guardian) and/or key caregiver(s) involved in patient's care, integration of new information into the medical treatment plan and/or adjustment of medical therapy, within a calendar month; 15-29 minutes

99375   30 minutes or more

99377   **Physician supervision** of a hospice patient (patient not present) requiring complex and multidisciplinary care modalities involving regular physician development and/or revision of care plans, review of subsequent reports of patient status, review of related laboratory and other studies, communication (including telephone calls) for purposes of assessment or care decisions with health care professional(s), family member(s), surrogate decision maker(s) (eg, legal guardian) and/or key caregiver(s) involved in patient's care, integration of new information into the medical treatment plan and/or adjustment of medical therapy, within a calendar month; 15-29 minutes

99378   30 minutes or more

99379   **Physician supervision** of a nursing facility patient (patient not present) requiring complex and multidisciplinary care modalities involving regular physician development and/or revision of care plans, review of subsequent reports of patient status, review of related laboratory and other studies, communication (including telephone calls) for purposes of assessment or care decisions with health care professional(s), family member(s), surrogate decision maker(s) (eg, legal guardian) and/or key caregiver(s) involved in patient's care, integration of new information into the medical treatment plan and/or adjustment of medical therapy, within a calendar month; 15-29 minutes

99380   30 minutes or more

Preventive Medicine Services

The following codes are used to report the preventive medicine evaluation and management of infants, children, adolescents and adults.

The extent and focus of the services will largely depend on the age of the patient.

If an abnormality/ies is encountered or a preexisting problem is addressed in the process of performing this preventive medicine evaluation and management service, and if the problem/abnormality is significant enough to require additional work to perform the key components of a problem-oriented E/M service, then the appropriate Office/Outpatient code 99201-99215 should also be reported. Modifier 25 should be added to the Office/Outpatient code to indicate that a significant, separately identifiable Evaluation and Management service was provided by the same physician on the same day as the preventive medicine service. The appropriate preventive medicine service is additionally reported.

An insignificant or trivial problem/abnormality that is encountered in the process of performing the preventive medicine evaluation and management service and which does not require additional work and the performance of the key components of a problem-oriented E/M service should not be reported.

The "comprehensive" nature of the Preventive Medicine Services codes 99381-99397 reflects an age and gender appropriate history/exam and is NOT synonymous with the "comprehensive" examination required in Evaluation and Management codes 99201-99350.

Codes 99381-99397 include counseling/anticipatory guidance/risk factor reduction interventions which are provided at the time of the initial or periodic comprehensive preventive medicine examination. (Refer to codes 99401-99412 for reporting those counseling/anticipatory guidance/risk factor reduction interventions that are provided at an encounter separate from the preventive medicine examination.)

Immunizations and ancillary studies involving laboratory, radiology, other procedures, or screening tests identified with a specific CPT code are reported separately. For immunizations, see ▶90465◀-90474 and 90476-90749.

New Patient

99381   **Initial comprehensive preventive medicine** evaluation and management of an individual including an age and gender appropriate history, examination, counseling/anticipatory guidance/risk factor reduction interventions, and the ordering of appropriate immunization(s), laboratory/diagnostic procedures, new patient; infant (age under 1 year)

99382   early childhood (age 1 through 4 years)

99383   late childhood (age 5 through 11 years)

99384   adolescent (age 12 through 17 years)

99385   18-39 years

99386   40-64 years

99387   65 years and over

Established Patient

99391   **Periodic comprehensive preventive medicine** reevaluation and management of an individual including an age and gender appropriate history, examination, counseling/anticipatory guidance/risk factor reduction interventions, and the ordering of appropriate immunization(s), laboratory/diagnostic procedures, established patient; infant (age under 1 year)

99392   early childhood (age 1 through 4 years)

99393   late childhood (age 5 through 11 years)

99394   adolescent (age 12 through 17 years)

99395   18-39 years

99396   40-64 years

99397   65 years and over

Counseling and/or Risk Factor Reduction Intervention

New or Established Patient

These codes are used to report services provided to individuals at a separate encounter for the purpose of promoting health and preventing illness or injury.

Preventive medicine counseling and risk factor reduction interventions provided as a separate encounter will vary with age and should address such issues as family problems, diet and exercise, substance abuse, sexual practices, injury prevention, dental health, and diagnostic and laboratory test results available at the time of the encounter.

These codes are not to be used to report counseling and risk factor reduction interventions provided to patients with symptoms or established illness. For counseling

individual patients with symptoms or established illness, use the appropriate office, hospital or consultation or other evaluation and management codes. For counseling groups of patients with symptoms or established illness, use 99078.

Preventive Medicine, Individual Counseling

99401   **Preventive medicine counseling** and/or risk factor reduction intervention(s) provided to an individual (separate procedure); approximately 15 minutes

99402   approximately 30 minutes

99403   approximately 45 minutes

99404   approximately 60 minutes

Preventive Medicine, Group Counseling

99411   **Preventive medicine counseling** and/or risk factor reduction intervention(s) provided to individuals in a group setting (separate procedure); approximately 30 minutes

99412   approximately 60 minutes

Other Preventive Medicine Services

99420   **Administration and interpretation** of health risk assessment instrument (eg, health hazard appraisal)

99429   **Unlisted preventive** medicine service

Newborn Care

The following codes are used to report the services provided to newborns in several different settings.

For newborn hospital discharge services provided on a date subsequent to the admission date of the newborn, use 99238.

For discharge services provided to newborns admitted and discharged on the same date, use 99435.

99431   **History and examination** of the normal newborn infant, initiation of diagnostic and treatment programs and preparation of hospital records. (This code should also be used for birthing room deliveries.)

99432   **Normal newborn care** in other than hospital or birthing room setting, including physical examination of baby and conference(s) with parent(s)

99433   **Subsequent hospital care,** for the evaluation and management of a normal newborn, per day

99435   **History and examination** of the normal newborn infant, including the preparation of medical records. (This code should only be used for newborns assessed and discharged from the hospital or birthing room on the same date.)

Evaluation and Management

Evaluation and Management

99436   **Attendance** at delivery (when requested by delivering physician) and initial stabilization of newborn

(99436 may be reported in addition to 99431)

(Do not report 99436 in conjunction with 99440)

99440   **Newborn resuscitation**: provision of positive pressure ventilation and/or chest compressions in the presence of acute inadequate ventilation and/or cardiac output

Special Evaluation and Management Services

The following codes are used to report evaluations performed to establish baseline information prior to life or disability insurance certificates being issued. This service is performed in the office or other setting, and applies to both new and established patients. When using these codes, no active management of the problem(s) is undertaken during the encounter.

If other evaluation and management services and/or procedures are performed on the same date, the appropriate E/M or procedure code(s) should be reported in addition to these codes.

Basic Life and/or Disability Evaluation Services

99450   **Basic life** and/or disability examination that includes:

- **measurement of height, weight and blood pressure;**
- **completion of a medical history following a life insurance pro forma;**
- **collection of blood sample and/or urinalysis complying with "chain of custody" protocols; and**
- **completion of necessary documentation/certificates.**

Work Related or Medical Disability Evaluation Services

99455   **Work related** or medical disability examination by the treating physician that includes:

- **completion of a medical history commensurate with the patient's condition;**
- **performance of an examination commensurate with the patient's condition;**
- **formulation of a diagnosis, assessment of capabilities and stability, and calculation of impairment;**
- **development of future medical treatment plan; and**
- **completion of necessary documentation/certificates and report.**

99456   **Work related** or medical disability examination by other than the treating physician that includes:

- **completion of a medical history commensurate with the patient's condition;**
- **performance of an examination commensurate with the patient's condition;**
- **formulation of a diagnosis, assessment of capabilities and stability, and calculation of impairment;**
- **development of future medical treatment plan; and**
- **completion of necessary documentation/certificates and report.**

(Do not report 99455, 99456 in conjunction with 99080 for the completion of Workman's Compensation forms)

Other Evaluation and Management Services

99499   **Unlisted evaluation and management** service

Anesthesia Guidelines

Services involving administration of anesthesia are reported by the use of the anesthesia five digit procedure code (00100-01999) plus modifier codes (defined under "Anesthesia Modifiers" later in these Guidelines).

The reporting of anesthesia services is appropriate by or under the responsible supervision of a physician. These services may include but are not limited to general, regional, supplementation of local anesthesia, or other supportive services in order to afford the patient the anesthesia care deemed optimal by the anesthesiologist during any procedure. These services include the usual preoperative and postoperative visits, the anesthesia care during the procedure, the administration of fluids and/or blood and the usual monitoring services (eg, ECG, temperature, blood pressure, oximetry, capnography, and mass spectrometry). Unusual forms of monitoring (eg, intra-arterial, central venous, and Swan-Ganz) are not included.

Items used by all physicians in reporting their services are presented in the **Introduction.** Some of the commonalities are repeated here for the convenience of those physicians referring to this section on **Anesthesia.** Other definitions and items unique to anesthesia are also listed.

To report sedation with or without analgesia (conscious sedation) provided by a physician also performing the service for which conscious sedation is being provided, see codes 99141, 99142. ▶When any physician, other than the physician performing the procedure, provides anesthesia services as specified in *CPT* guidelines (conscious sedation or otherwise), the Anesthesia codes should be reported.◀

To report regional or general anesthesia provided by a physician also performing the services for which the anesthesia is being provided, see modifier 47 in Appendix A.

Time Reporting

Time for anesthesia procedures may be reported as is customary in the local area. Anesthesia time begins when the anesthesiologist begins to prepare the patient for the induction of anesthesia in the operating room or in an equivalent area and ends when the anesthesiologist is no longer in personal attendance, that is, when the patient may be safely placed under postoperative supervision.

Physician's Services

Physician's services rendered in the office, home, or hospital, consultation, and other medical services are listed in the section entitled **Evaluation and Management Services** (99200 series) found in the front of the book, beginning on page 1. "Special Services and Reporting" (99000 series) are presented in the **Medicine** section.

Materials Supplied by Physician

Supplies and materials provided by the physician (eg, sterile trays, drugs) over and above those usually included with the office visit or other services rendered may be listed separately. List drugs, tray supplies, and materials provided. Identify as 99070.

Separate or Multiple Procedures

When multiple surgical procedures are performed during a single anesthetic administration, the anesthesia code representing the most complex procedure is reported. The time reported is the combined total for all procedures.

Special Report

A service that is rarely provided, unusual, variable, or new may require a special report in determining medical appropriateness of the service. Pertinent information should include an adequate definition or description of the nature, extent, and need for the procedure; and the time, effort, and equipment necessary to provide the service. Additional items which may be included are:

- complexity of symptoms;
- final diagnosis;
- pertinent physical findings;
- diagnostic and therapeutic procedures;
- concurrent problems;
- follow-up care.

Anesthesia Modifiers

All anesthesia services are reported by use of the anesthesia five digit procedure code (00100-01999) plus the addition of a physical status modifier. The use of other optional modifiers may be appropriate.

Physical Status Modifiers

Physical Status modifiers are represented by the initial letter 'P' followed by a single digit from 1 to 6 defined below.

P1-A normal healthy patient.

P2-A patient with mild systemic disease.

P3-A patient with severe systemic disease.

P4-A patient with severe systemic disease that is a constant threat to life.

P5-A moribund patient who is not expected to survive without the operation.

P6-A declared brain-dead patient whose organs are being removed for donor purposes.

The above six levels are consistent with the American Society of Anesthesiologists (ASA) ranking of patient physical status. Physical status is included in *CPT* to distinguish among various levels of complexity of the anesthesia service provided.

Example: 00100-P1

Qualifying Circumstances

More than one may be selected.

Many anesthesia services are provided under particularly difficult circumstances, depending on factors such as extraordinary condition of patient, notable operative conditions, and/or unusual risk factors. This section includes a list of important qualifying circumstances that significantly impact on the character of the anesthesia service provided. These procedures would not be reported alone but would be reported as additional procedure numbers qualifying an anesthesia procedure or service.

+ 99100   Anesthesia for patient of extreme age, under 1 year and over 70 (List separately in addition to code for primary anesthesia procedure)

(For procedure performed on infants less than 1 year of age at time of surgery, see 00326, 00834, 00836)

+ 99116   Anesthesia complicated by utilization of total body hypothermia (List separately in addition to code for primary anesthesia procedure)

+ 99135   Anesthesia complicated by utilization of controlled hypotension (List separately in addition to code for primary anesthesia procedure)

+ 99140   Anesthesia complicated by emergency conditions (specify) (List separately in addition to code for primary anesthesia procedure)

(An emergency is defined as existing when delay in treatment of the patient would lead to a significant increase in the threat to life or body part.)

Anesthesia

Head

00100   Anesthesia for procedures on salivary glands, including biopsy

00102   Anesthesia for procedures involving plastic repair of cleft lip

00103   Anesthesia for reconstructive procedures of eyelid (eg, blepharoplasty, ptosis surgery)

00104   Anesthesia for electroconvulsive therapy

00120   Anesthesia for procedures on external, middle, and inner ear including biopsy; not otherwise specified

00124   otoscopy

00126   tympanotomy

00140   Anesthesia for procedures on eye; not otherwise specified

00142   lens surgery

00144   corneal transplant

00145   vitreoretinal surgery

00147   iridectomy

00148   ophthalmoscopy

00160   Anesthesia for procedures on nose and accessory sinuses; not otherwise specified

00162   radical surgery

00164   biopsy, soft tissue

00170   Anesthesia for intraoral procedures, including biopsy; not otherwise specified

00172   repair of cleft palate

00174   excision of retropharyngeal tumor

00176   radical surgery

00190   Anesthesia for procedures on facial bones or skull; not otherwise specified

00192   radical surgery (including prognathism)

00210   Anesthesia for intracranial procedures; not otherwise specified

00212   subdural taps

00214   burr holes, including ventriculography

00215   cranioplasty or elevation of depressed skull fracture, extradural (simple or compound)

00216   vascular procedures

00218   procedures in sitting position

00220   cerebrospinal fluid shunting procedures

00222   electrocoagulation of intracranial nerve

Neck

00300   Anesthesia for all procedures on the integumentary system, muscles and nerves of head, neck, and posterior trunk, not otherwise specified

00320   Anesthesia for all procedures on esophagus, thyroid, larynx, trachea and lymphatic system of neck; not otherwise specified, age 1 year or older

00322   needle biopsy of thyroid

(For procedures on cervical spine and cord, see 00600, 00604, 00670)

00326   Anesthesia for all procedures on the larynx and trachea in children less than 1 year of age

(Do not report 00326 in conjunction with 99100)

00350   Anesthesia for procedures on major vessels of neck; not otherwise specified

00352   simple ligation

(For arteriography, use 01916)

Thorax (Chest Wall and Shoulder Girdle)

00400   Anesthesia for procedures on the integumentary system on the extremities, anterior trunk and perineum; not otherwise specified

00402   reconstructive procedures on breast (eg, reduction or augmentation mammoplasty, muscle flaps)

00404   radical or modified radical procedures on breast

00406   radical or modified radical procedures on breast with internal mammary node dissection

00410   electrical conversion of arrhythmias

00450   Anesthesia for procedures on clavicle and scapula; not otherwise specified

00452   radical surgery

00454   biopsy of clavicle

Anesthesia

00470 Anesthesia for partial rib resection; not otherwise specified

00472 thoracoplasty (any type)

00474 radical procedures (eg, pectus excavatum)

Intrathoracic

00500 Anesthesia for all procedures on esophagus

00520 Anesthesia for closed chest procedures; (including bronchoscopy) not otherwise specified

00522 needle biopsy of pleura

00524 pneumocentesis

00528 mediastinoscopy and diagnostic thoracoscopy not utilizing one lung ventilation

(For tracheobronchial reconstruction, use 00539)

00529 mediastinoscopy and diagnostic thoracoscopy utilizing one lung ventilation

00530 Anesthesia for permanent transvenous pacemaker insertion

00532 Anesthesia for access to central venous circulation

00534 Anesthesia for transvenous insertion or replacement of pacing cardioverter-defibrillator

(For transthoracic approach, use 00560)

00537 Anesthesia for cardiac electrophysiologic procedures including radiofrequency ablation

00539 Anesthesia for tracheobronchial reconstruction

00540 Anesthesia for thoracotomy procedures involving lungs, pleura, diaphragm, and mediastinum (including surgical thoracoscopy); not otherwise specified

00541 utilizing one lung ventilation

00542 decortication

(00544 has been deleted. To report, use 00542)

00546 pulmonary resection with thoracoplasty

00548 intrathoracic procedures on the trachea and bronchi

00550 Anesthesia for sternal debridement

00560 Anesthesia for procedures on heart, pericardial sac, and great vessels of chest; without pump oxygenator

● 00561 with pump oxygenator, under one year of age

▶(Do not report 00561 in conjunction with 99100, 99116, and 99135)◀

00562 with pump oxygenator

00563 with pump oxygenator with hypothermic circulatory arrest

00566 Anesthesia for direct coronary artery bypass grafting without pump oxygenator

00580 Anesthesia for heart transplant or heart/lung transplant

Spine and Spinal Cord

00600 Anesthesia for procedures on cervical spine and cord; not otherwise specified

(For myelography and diskography, see radiological procedures 01905)

00604 procedures with patient in the sitting position

00620 Anesthesia for procedures on thoracic spine and cord; not otherwise specified

00622 thoracolumbar sympathectomy

00630 Anesthesia for procedures in lumbar region; not otherwise specified

00632 lumbar sympathectomy

00634 chemonucleolysis

00635 diagnostic or therapeutic lumbar puncture

00640 Anesthesia for manipulation of the spine or for closed procedures on the cervical, thoracic or lumbar spine

00670 Anesthesia for extensive spine and spinal cord procedures (eg, spinal instrumentation or vascular procedures)

Upper Abdomen

00700 Anesthesia for procedures on upper anterior abdominal wall; not otherwise specified

00702 percutaneous liver biopsy

00730 Anesthesia for procedures on upper posterior abdominal wall

00740 Anesthesia for upper gastrointestinal endoscopic procedures, endoscope introduced proximal to duodenum

00750 Anesthesia for hernia repairs in upper abdomen; not otherwise specified

00752 lumbar and ventral (incisional) hernias and/or wound dehiscence

00754 omphalocele

00756 transabdominal repair of diaphragmatic hernia

00770 Anesthesia for all procedures on major abdominal blood vessels

00790 Anesthesia for intraperitoneal procedures in upper abdomen including laparoscopy; not otherwise specified

00792 partial hepatectomy or management of liver hemorrhage (excluding liver biopsy)

00794 pancreatectomy, partial or total (eg, Whipple procedure)

00796 liver transplant (recipient)

(For harvesting of liver, use 01990)

00797 gastric restrictive procedure for morbid obesity

Lower Abdomen

00800 Anesthesia for procedures on lower anterior abdominal wall; not otherwise specified

00802   panniculectomy

00810 Anesthesia for lower intestinal endoscopic procedures, endoscope introduced distal to duodenum

00820 Anesthesia for procedures on lower posterior abdominal wall

00830 Anesthesia for hernia repairs in lower abdomen; not otherwise specified

00832   ventral and incisional hernias

(For hernia repairs in the infant 1 year of age or younger, see 00834, 00836)

00834 Anesthesia for hernia repairs in the lower abdomen not otherwise specified, under 1 year of age

(Do not report 00834 in conjunction with 99100)

00836 Anesthesia for hernia repairs in the lower abdomen not otherwise specified, infants less than 37 weeks gestational age at birth and less than 50 weeks gestational age at time of surgery

(Do not report 00836 in conjunction with 99100)

00840 Anesthesia for intraperitoneal procedures in lower abdomen including laparoscopy; not otherwise specified

00842   amniocentesis

00844   abdominoperineal resection

00846   radical hysterectomy

00848   pelvic exenteration

00851   tubal ligation/transection

00860 Anesthesia for extraperitoneal procedures in lower abdomen, including urinary tract; not otherwise specified

00862   renal procedures, including upper 1/3 of ureter, or donor nephrectomy

00864   total cystectomy

00865   radical prostatectomy (suprapubic, retropubic)

00866   adrenalectomy

00868   renal transplant (recipient)

(For donor nephrectomy, use 00862)

(For harvesting kidney from brain-dead patient, use 01990)

(00869 has been deleted. To report, use 00921)

00870   cystolithotomy

00872 Anesthesia for lithotripsy, extracorporeal shock wave; with water bath

00873   without water bath

00880 Anesthesia for procedures on major lower abdominal vessels; not otherwise specified

00882   inferior vena cava ligation

Perineum

(For perineal procedures on integumentary system, muscles and nerves, see 00300, 00400)

00902 Anesthesia for; anorectal procedure

00904   radical perineal procedure

00906   vulvectomy

00908   perineal prostatectomy

00910 Anesthesia for transurethral procedures (including urethrocystoscopy); not otherwise specified

00912   transurethral resection of bladder tumor(s)

00914   transurethral resection of prostate

00916   post-transurethral resection bleeding

00918   with fragmentation, manipulation and/or removal of ureteral calculus

00920 Anesthesia for procedures on male genitalia (including open urethral procedures); not otherwise specified

00921   vasectomy, unilateral or bilateral

00922   seminal vesicles

00924   undescended testis, unilateral or bilateral

00926   radical orchiectomy, inguinal

00928   radical orchiectomy, abdominal

00930   orchiopexy, unilateral or bilateral

00932   complete amputation of penis

00934   radical amputation of penis with bilateral inguinal lymphadenectomy

00936   radical amputation of penis with bilateral inguinal and iliac lymphadenectomy

00938   insertion of penile prosthesis (perineal approach)

00940 Anesthesia for vaginal procedures (including biopsy of labia, vagina, cervix or endometrium); not otherwise specified

00942   colpotomy, vaginectomy, colporrhaphy, and open urethral procedures

00944   vaginal hysterectomy

00948   cervical cerclage

00950   culdoscopy

00952   hysteroscopy and/or hysterosalpingography

Anesthesia

Pelvis (Except Hip)

01112	Anesthesia for bone marrow aspiration and/or biopsy, anterior or posterior iliac crest
01120	Anesthesia for procedures on bony pelvis
01130	Anesthesia for body cast application or revision
01140	Anesthesia for interpelviabdominal (hindquarter) amputation
01150	Anesthesia for radical procedures for tumor of pelvis, except hindquarter amputation
01160	Anesthesia for closed procedures involving symphysis pubis or sacroiliac joint
01170	Anesthesia for open procedures involving symphysis pubis or sacroiliac joint
01173	Anesthesia for open repair of fracture disruption of pelvis or column fracture involving acetabulum
01180	Anesthesia for obturator neurectomy; extrapelvic
01190	intrapelvic

Upper Leg (Except Knee)

01200	Anesthesia for all closed procedures involving hip joint
01202	Anesthesia for arthroscopic procedures of hip joint
01210	Anesthesia for open procedures involving hip joint; not otherwise specified
01212	hip disarticulation
01214	total hip arthroplasty
01215	revision of total hip arthroplasty
01220	Anesthesia for all closed procedures involving upper 2/3 of femur
01230	Anesthesia for open procedures involving upper 2/3 of femur; not otherwise specified
01232	amputation
01234	radical resection
01250	Anesthesia for all procedures on nerves, muscles, tendons, fascia, and bursae of upper leg
01260	Anesthesia for all procedures involving veins of upper leg, including exploration
01270	Anesthesia for procedures involving arteries of upper leg, including bypass graft; not otherwise specified
01272	femoral artery ligation
01274	femoral artery embolectomy

Knee and Popliteal Area

Surgical endoscopy/arthroscopy always includes a diagnostic endoscopy/arthroscopy.

01320	Anesthesia for all procedures on nerves, muscles, tendons, fascia, and bursae of knee and/or popliteal area
01340	Anesthesia for all closed procedures on lower 1/3 of femur
01360	Anesthesia for all open procedures on lower 1/3 of femur
01380	Anesthesia for all closed procedures on knee joint
01382	Anesthesia for diagnostic arthroscopic procedures of knee joint
01390	Anesthesia for all closed procedures on upper ends of tibia, fibula, and/or patella
01392	Anesthesia for all open procedures on upper ends of tibia, fibula, and/or patella
01400	Anesthesia for open or surgical arthroscopic procedures on knee joint; not otherwise specified
01402	total knee arthroplasty
01404	disarticulation at knee
01420	Anesthesia for all cast applications, removal, or repair involving knee joint
01430	Anesthesia for procedures on veins of knee and popliteal area; not otherwise specified
01432	arteriovenous fistula
01440	Anesthesia for procedures on arteries of knee and popliteal area; not otherwise specified
01442	popliteal thromboendarterectomy, with or without patch graft
01444	popliteal excision and graft or repair for occlusion or aneurysm

Lower Leg (Below Knee, Includes Ankle and Foot)

Surgical endoscopy/arthroscopy always includes a diagnostic endoscopy/arthroscopy.

01462	Anesthesia for all closed procedures on lower leg, ankle, and foot
01464	Anesthesia for arthroscopic procedures of ankle and/or foot
01470	Anesthesia for procedures on nerves, muscles, tendons, and fascia of lower leg, ankle, and foot; not otherwise specified
01472	repair of ruptured Achilles tendon, with or without graft
01474	gastrocnemius recession (eg, Strayer procedure)

01480 Anesthesia for open procedures on bones of lower leg, ankle, and foot; not otherwise specified

01482 radical resection (including below knee amputation)

01484 osteotomy or osteoplasty of tibia and/or fibula

01486 total ankle replacement

01490 Anesthesia for lower leg cast application, removal, or repair

01500 Anesthesia for procedures on arteries of lower leg, including bypass graft; not otherwise specified

01502 embolectomy, direct or with catheter

01520 Anesthesia for procedures on veins of lower leg; not otherwise specified

01522 venous thrombectomy, direct or with catheter

Shoulder and Axilla

Surgical endoscopy/arthroscopy always includes a diagnostic endoscopy/arthroscopy.

Includes humeral head and neck, sternoclavicular joint, acromioclavicular joint, and shoulder joint.

01610 Anesthesia for all procedures on nerves, muscles, tendons, fascia, and bursae of shoulder and axilla

01620 Anesthesia for all closed procedures on humeral head and neck, sternoclavicular joint, acromioclavicular joint, and shoulder joint

01622 Anesthesia for diagnostic arthroscopic procedures of shoulder joint

01630 Anesthesia for open or surgical arthroscopic procedures on humeral head and neck, sternoclavicular joint, acromioclavicular joint, and shoulder joint; not otherwise specified

01632 radical resection

01634 shoulder disarticulation

01636 interthoracoscapular (forequarter) amputation

01638 total shoulder replacement

01650 Anesthesia for procedures on arteries of shoulder and axilla; not otherwise specified

01652 axillary-brachial aneurysm

01654 bypass graft

01656 axillary-femoral bypass graft

01670 Anesthesia for all procedures on veins of shoulder and axilla

01680 Anesthesia for shoulder cast application, removal or repair; not otherwise specified

01682 shoulder spica

Upper Arm and Elbow

Surgical endoscopy/arthroscopy always includes a diagnostic endoscopy/arthroscopy.

01710 Anesthesia for procedures on nerves, muscles, tendons, fascia, and bursae of upper arm and elbow; not otherwise specified

01712 tenotomy, elbow to shoulder, open

01714 tenoplasty, elbow to shoulder

01716 tenodesis, rupture of long tendon of biceps

01730 Anesthesia for all closed procedures on humerus and elbow

01732 Anesthesia for diagnostic arthroscopic procedures of elbow joint

01740 Anesthesia for open or surgical arthroscopic procedures of the elbow; not otherwise specified

01742 osteotomy of humerus

01744 repair of nonunion or malunion of humerus

01756 radical procedures

01758 excision of cyst or tumor of humerus

01760 total elbow replacement

01770 Anesthesia for procedures on arteries of upper arm and elbow; not otherwise specified

01772 embolectomy

01780 Anesthesia for procedures on veins of upper arm and elbow; not otherwise specified

01782 phleborrhaphy

Forearm, Wrist, and Hand

01810 Anesthesia for all procedures on nerves, muscles, tendons, fascia, and bursae of forearm, wrist, and hand

01820 Anesthesia for all closed procedures on radius, ulna, wrist, or hand bones

01829 Anesthesia for diagnostic arthroscopic procedures on the wrist

01830 Anesthesia for open or surgical arthroscopic/endoscopic procedures on distal radius, distal ulna, wrist, or hand joints; not otherwise specified

01832 total wrist replacement

01840 Anesthesia for procedures on arteries of forearm, wrist, and hand; not otherwise specified

01842 embolectomy

01844 Anesthesia for vascular shunt, or shunt revision, any type (eg, dialysis)

Anesthesia

01850   Anesthesia for procedures on veins of forearm, wrist, and hand; not otherwise specified

01852   phleborrhaphy

01860   Anesthesia for forearm, wrist, or hand cast application, removal, or repair

Radiological Procedures

01905   Anesthesia for myelography, diskography, vertebroplasty

01916   Anesthesia for diagnostic arteriography/venography

(Do not report 01916 in conjunction with therapeutic codes 01924-01926, 01930-01933)

01920   Anesthesia for cardiac catheterization including coronary angiography and ventriculography (not to include Swan-Ganz catheter)

01922   Anesthesia for non-invasive imaging or radiation therapy

01924   Anesthesia for therapeutic interventional radiologic procedures involving the arterial system; not otherwise specified

01925   carotid or coronary

01926   intracranial, intracardiac, or aortic

01930   Anesthesia for therapeutic interventional radiologic procedures involving the venous/lymphatic system (not to include access to the central circulation); not otherwise specified

01931   intrahepatic or portal circulation (eg, transcutaneous porto-caval shunt (TIPS))

01932   intrathoracic or jugular

01933   intracranial

Burn Excisions or Debridement

01951   Anesthesia for second and third degree burn excision or debridement with or without skin grafting, any site, for total body surface area (TBSA) treated during anesthesia and surgery; less than four percent total body surface area

01952   between four and nine percent of total body surface area

+ 01953   each additional nine percent total body surface area or part thereof (List separately in addition to code for primary procedure)

(Use 01953 in conjunction with 01952)

Obstetric

01958   Anesthesia for external cephalic version procedure

01960   Anesthesia for vaginal delivery only

01961   Anesthesia for cesarean delivery only

01962   Anesthesia for urgent hysterectomy following delivery

01963   Anesthesia for cesarean hysterectomy without any labor analgesia/anesthesia care

01964   Anesthesia for abortion procedures

01967   Neuraxial labor analgesia/anesthesia for planned vaginal delivery (this includes any repeat subarachnoid needle placement and drug injection and/or any necessary replacement of an epidural catheter during labor)

+ 01968   Anesthesia for cesarean delivery following neuraxial labor analgesia/anesthesia (List separately in addition to code for primary procedure performed)

(Use 01968 in conjunction with 01967)

+ 01969   Anesthesia for cesarean hysterectomy following neuraxial labor analgesia/anesthesia (List separately in addition to code for primary procedure performed)

(Use 01969 in conjunction with 01967)

Other Procedures

01990   Physiological support for harvesting of organ(s) from brain-dead patient

01991   Anesthesia for diagnostic or therapeutic nerve blocks and injections (when block or injection is performed by a different provider); other than the prone position

01992   prone position

(Do not report 01991or 01992 in conjunction with 99141)

01995   Regional intravenous administration of local anesthetic agent or other medication (upper or lower extremity)

(For intra-arterial or intravenous therapy for pain management, see 90783, 90784)

01996   Daily hospital management of epidural or subarachnoid continuous drug administration

(Report code 01996 for daily hospital management of continuous epidural or subarachnoid drug administration performed after insertion of an epidural or subarachnoid catheter)

01999   Unlisted anesthesia procedure(s)

Surgery Guidelines

Items used by all physicians in reporting their services are presented in the **Introduction.** Some of the commonalities are repeated here for the convenience of those physicians referring to this section on **Surgery.** Other definitions and items unique to Surgery are also listed.

Physicians' Services

Physicians' services rendered in the office, home, or hospital, consultations, and other medical services are listed in the section entitled **Evaluation and Management Services** (▶99201-99499◀) found in the front of the book, beginning on page 9. "Special Services and Reports" (99000 series) is presented in the **Medicine** section.

CPT Surgical Package Definition

The services provided by the physician to any patient by their very nature are variable. The CPT codes that represent a readily identifiable surgical procedure thereby include, on a procedure-by-procedure basis, a variety of services. In defining the specific services "included" in a given CPT surgical code, the following services are always included in addition to the operation per se:

- local infiltration, metacarpal/metatarsal/digital block or topical anesthesia;
- subsequent to the decision for surgery, one related E/M encounter on the date immediately prior to or on the date of procedure (including history and physical);
- immediate postoperative care, including dictating operative notes, talking with the family and other physicians;
- writing orders;
- evaluating the patient in the postanesthesia recovery area;
- typical postoperative follow-up care.

Follow-Up Care for Diagnostic Procedures

Follow-up care for diagnostic procedures (eg, endoscopy, arthroscopy, injection procedures for radiography) includes only that care related to recovery from the diagnostic procedure itself. Care of the condition for which the diagnostic procedure was performed or of other concomitant conditions is not included and may be listed separately.

Follow-Up Care for Therapeutic Surgical Procedures

Follow-up care for therapeutic surgical procedures includes only that care which is usually a part of the surgical service. Complications, exacerbations, recurrence, or the presence of other diseases or injuries requiring additional services should be separately reported.

Materials Supplied by Physician

Supplies and materials provided by the physician (eg, sterile trays/drugs), over and above those usually included with the procedure(s) rendered are reported separately. List drugs, trays, supplies, and materials provided. Identify as 99070 or specific supply code.

Reporting More Than One Procedure/Service

When a physician performs more than one procedure/service on the same date, same session or during a post-operative period (subject to the "surgical package" concept), several CPT modifiers may apply. (See Appendix A for definition.)

27 Multiple Outpatient Hospital E/M Encounters on the Same Date

For hospital outpatient reporting purposes, utilization of hospital resources related to separate and distinct E/M encounters performed in multiple outpatient hospital settings on the same date may be reported by adding modifier 27 to each appropriate level outpatient and/or emergency department E/M code(s). This modifier provides a means of reporting circumstances involving evaluation and management services provided by physician(s) in more than one (multiple) outpatient hospital setting(s) (eg, hospital emergency department, clinic). **Note:** This modifier is not to be used for physician reporting of multiple E/M services performed by the same physician on the same date. For physician reporting of all outpatient evaluation and management services provided by the same physician on the same date and performed in multiple outpatient setting(s) (eg, hospital emergency department, clinic), see **Evaluation and Management, Emergency Department,** or **Preventive Medicine Services** codes.

51 Multiple Procedures

When multiple procedures/services (other than evaluation and management) are performed at the same session, report the most significant procedure first, with all other procedures listed with modifier 51 appended. For a list of procedures exempt from the use of modifier 51, see Appendices D and E.

58 Staged or Related Procedure or Service by the Same Physician During the Postoperative Period

When a procedure(s) is prospectively planned as a staged procedure, or when the secondary and subsequent procedure(s) is more extensive, or to indicate therapy following a diagnostic surgical procedure, use modifier 58 with the staged procedure(s).

59 Distinct Procedural Service

For procedure(s)/service(s) not ordinarily performed or encountered on the same day by the same physician, but appropriate under certain circumstances (eg, different site or organ system, separate excision or lesion), use modifier 59.

76 Repeat Procedure by Same Physician

When a procedure or service is repeated by the same physician subsequent to the original service, use modifier 76.

77 Repeat Procedure by Another Physician

When a procedure is repeated by another physician subsequent to the original service, use modifier 77.

78 Return to the Operating Room for a Related Procedure During the Postoperative Period

When a procedure, related to the initial procedure, requires a return to the operating room during the postoperative period of that initial procedure, use modifier 78.

79 Unrelated Procedure or Service by the Same Physician During the Postoperative Period

When a procedure, unrelated to the initial procedure, is performed by the same physician during the postoperative period of the initial procedure, use modifier 79.

91 Repeat Clinical Diagnostic Laboratory Test

In the course of treatment of the patient, it may be necessary to repeat the same laboratory test on the same day to obtain subsequent (multiple) test results. Under these circumstances, the laboratory test performed can be identified by its usual procedure number and the addition of modifier 91. **Note:** This modifier may not be used when tests are rerun to confirm initial results; due to testing problems with specimens or equipment; or for any other reason when a normal, one-time, reportable result is all that is required. This modifier may not be used when other code(s) describe a series of test results (eg, glucose tolerance tests, evocative/suppression testing). This modifier may only be used for laboratory test(s) performed more than once on the same day on the same patient.

Separate Procedure

Some of the procedures or services listed in *CPT* that are commonly carried out as an integral component of a total service or procedure have been identified by the inclusion of the term "separate procedure." The codes designated as "separate procedure" should not be reported in addition to the code for the total procedure or service of which it is considered an integral component.

However, when a procedure or service that is designated as a "separate procedure" is carried out independently or considered to be unrelated or distinct from other procedures/services provided at that time, it may be reported by itself, or in addition to other procedures/services by appending modifier 59 to the specific "separate procedure" code to indicate that the procedure is not considered to be a component of another procedure, but is a distinct, independent procedure. This may represent a different session or patient encounter, different procedure or surgery, different site or organ system, separate incision/excision, separate lesion, or separate injury (or area of injury in extensive injuries).

Subsection Information

Several of the subheadings or subsections have special needs or instructions unique to that section. Where these are indicated (eg, "Maternity Care and Delivery"), special **"Notes"** will be presented preceding those procedural terminology listings, referring to that subsection specifically. If there is an "Unlisted Procedure" code number (see below) for the individual subsection, it will also be shown. Those subsections within the **Surgery** section that have **"Notes"** are as follows:

►◄=New or Revised Text

Surgery Guidelines

Excision 67800-67820

Reconstruction 67930-67999

Operating Microscope 69990

Unlisted Service or Procedure

A service or procedure may be provided that is not listed in this edition of *CPT*. When reporting such a service, the appropriate "Unlisted Procedure" code may be used to indicate the service, identifying it by "Special Report" as discussed in the section below. The "Unlisted Procedures" and accompanying codes for **Surgery** are as follows:

15999 Unlisted procedure, excision pressure ulcer

17999 Unlisted procedure, skin, mucous membrane and subcutaneous tissue

19499 Unlisted procedure, breast

20999 Unlisted procedure, musculoskeletal system, general

21089 Unlisted maxillofacial prosthetic procedure

21299 Unlisted craniofacial and maxillofacial procedure

21499 Unlisted musculoskeletal procedure, head

21899 Unlisted procedure, neck or thorax

22899 Unlisted procedure, spine

22999 Unlisted procedure, abdomen, musculoskeletal system

23929 Unlisted procedure, shoulder

24999 Unlisted procedure, humerus or elbow

25999 Unlisted procedure, forearm or wrist

26989 Unlisted procedure, hands or fingers

27299 Unlisted procedure, pelvis or hip joint

27599 Unlisted procedure, femur or knee

27899 Unlisted procedure, leg or ankle

28899 Unlisted procedure, foot or toes

29799 Unlisted procedure, casting or strapping

29999 Unlisted procedure, arthroscopy

30999 Unlisted procedure, nose

31299 Unlisted procedure, accessory sinuses

31599 Unlisted procedure, larynx

31899 Unlisted procedure, trachea, bronchi

32999 Unlisted procedure, lungs and pleura

33999 Unlisted procedure, cardiac surgery

36299 Unlisted procedure, vascular injection

37501 Unlisted vascular endoscopy procedure

37799 Unlisted procedure, vascular surgery

38129 Unlisted laparoscopy procedure, spleen

38589 Unlisted laparoscopy procedure, lymphatic system

38999 Unlisted procedure, hemic or lymphatic system

39499 Unlisted procedure, mediastinum

39599 Unlisted procedure, diaphragm

40799 Unlisted procedure, lips

40899 Unlisted procedure, vestibule of mouth

41599 Unlisted procedure, tongue, floor of mouth

41899 Unlisted procedure, dentoalveolar structures

42299 Unlisted procedure, palate, uvula

42699 Unlisted procedure, salivary glands or ducts

42999 Unlisted procedure, pharynx, adenoids, or tonsils

43289 Unlisted laparoscopy procedure, esophagus

43499 Unlisted procedure, esophagus

43659 Unlisted laparoscopy procedure, stomach

43999 Unlisted procedure, stomach

44238 Unlisted laparoscopy procedure, intestine (except rectum)

44239 Unlisted laparoscopy procedure, rectum

44799 Unlisted procedure, intestine

44899 Unlisted procedure, Meckel's diverticulum and the mesentery

44979 Unlisted laparoscopy procedure, appendix

45999 Unlisted procedure, rectum

46999 Unlisted procedure, anus

47379 Unlisted laparoscopic procedure, liver

47399 Unlisted procedure, liver

47579 Unlisted laparoscopy procedure, biliary tract

47999 Unlisted procedure, biliary tract

48999 Unlisted procedure, pancreas

49329 Unlisted laparoscopy procedure, abdomen, peritoneum and omentum

49659 Unlisted laparoscopy procedure, hernioplasty, herniorrhaphy, herniotomy

49999 Unlisted procedure, abdomen, peritoneum and omentum

50549 Unlisted laparoscopy procedure, renal

50949 Unlisted laparoscopy procedure, ureter

53899 Unlisted procedure, urinary system

54699 Unlisted laparoscopy procedure, testis

55559 Unlisted laparoscopy procedure, spermatic cord

55899 Unlisted procedure, male genital system

58578 Unlisted laparoscopy procedure, uterus

58579 Unlisted hysteroscopy procedure, uterus

58679 Unlisted laparoscopy procedure, oviduct, ovary

58999 Unlisted procedure, female genital system (nonobstetrical)

59897 Unlisted fetal invasive procedure, including ultrasound guidance

59898 Unlisted laparoscopy procedure, maternity care and delivery

59899 Unlisted procedure, maternity care and delivery

60659 Unlisted laparoscopy procedure, endocrine system

60699 Unlisted procedure, endocrine system

64999 Unlisted procedure, nervous system

66999 Unlisted procedure, anterior segment of eye

67299 Unlisted procedure, posterior segment

67399 Unlisted procedure, ocular muscle

67599 Unlisted procedure, orbit

67999 Unlisted procedure, eyelids

68399 Unlisted procedure, conjunctiva

68899 Unlisted procedure, lacrimal system

69399	Unlisted procedure, external ear
69799	Unlisted procedure, middle ear
69949	Unlisted procedure, inner ear
69979	Unlisted procedure, temporal bone, middle fossa approach

Special Report

A service that is rarely provided, unusual, variable, or new may require a special report in determining medical appropriateness of the service. Pertinent information should include an adequate definition or description of the nature, extent, and need for the procedure, and the time, effort, and equipment necessary to provide the service. Additional items which may be included are:

- complexity of symptoms;
- final diagnosis;
- pertinent physical findings (such as size, locations, and number of lesion(s), if appropriate);
- diagnostic and therapeutic procedures (including major and supplementary surgical procedures, if appropriate);
- concurrent problems;
- follow-up care.

Surgical Destruction

Surgical destruction is a part of a surgical procedure and different methods of destruction are not ordinarily listed separately unless the technique substantially alters the standard management of a problem or condition. Exceptions under special circumstances are provided for by separate code numbers.

Notes

Surgery

General

10021   Fine needle aspiration; without imaging guidance

10022   with imaging guidance

(For radiological supervision and interpretation, see 76003, 76360, 76393, 76942)

(For percutaneous needle biopsy other than fine needle aspiration, see 20206 for muscle, 32400 for pleura, 32405 for lung or mediastinum, 42400 for salivary gland, 47000, 47001 for liver, 48102 for pancreas, 49180 for abdominal or retroperitoneal mass, 60100 for thyroid, 62269 for spinal cord)

(For evaluation of fine needle aspirate, see 88172, 88173)

Integumentary System

Skin, Subcutaneous and Accessory Structures

Incision and Drainage

(For excision, see 11400, et seq)

10040   Acne surgery (eg, marsupialization, opening or removal of multiple milia, comedones, cysts, pustules)

10060   Incision and drainage of abscess (eg, carbuncle, suppurative hidradenitis, cutaneous or subcutaneous abscess, cyst, furuncle, or paronychia); simple or single

10061   complicated or multiple

10080   Incision and drainage of pilonidal cyst; simple

10081   complicated

(For excision of pilonidal cyst, see 11770-11772)

10120   Incision and removal of foreign body, subcutaneous tissues; simple

10121   complicated

(To report wound exploration due to penetrating trauma without laparotomy or thoracotomy, see 20100-20103, as appropriate)

(To report debridement associated with open fracture(s) and/or dislocation(s), use 11010-11012, as appropriate)

10140   Incision and drainage of hematoma, seroma or fluid collection

(If imaging guidance is performed, see 76360, 76393, 76942)

10160   Puncture aspiration of abscess, hematoma, bulla, or cyst

(If imaging guidance is performed, see 76360, 76393, 76942)

10180   Incision and drainage, complex, postoperative wound infection

(For secondary closure of surgical wound, see 12020, 12021, 13160)

Excision—Debridement

(For dermabrasions, see 15780-15783)

(For nail debridement, see 11720-11721)

(For burn(s), see 16000-16035)

11000   Debridement of extensive eczematous or infected skin; up to 10% of body surface

►(For abdominal wall or genitalia debridement for necrotizing soft tissue infection, see 11004-11006)◄

+ 11001   each additional 10% of the body surface (List separately in addition to code for primary procedure)

(Use 11001 in conjunction with 11000)

● 11004   Debridement of skin, subcutaneous tissue, muscle and fascia for necrotizing soft tissue infection; external genitalia and perineum

● 11005   abdominal wall, with or without fascial closure

● 11006   external genitalia, perineum and abdominal wall, with or without fascial closure

+● 11008   Removal of prosthetic material or mesh, abdominal wall for necrotizing soft tissue infection (List separately in addition to code for primary procedure)

►(Use 11008 in conjunction with 11004-11006)◄

►(Do not report 11008 in conjunction with 11000-11001, 11010-11044)◄

►(Report skin grafts or flaps separately when performed for closure at the same session as 11004-11008)◄

►(If orchiectomy is performed, use 54520)◄

►(If testicular transplantation is performed, use 54680)◄

11010   Debridement including removal of foreign material associated with open fracture(s) and/or dislocation(s); skin and subcutaneous tissues

11011   skin, subcutaneous tissue, muscle fascia, and muscle

11012   skin, subcutaneous tissue, muscle fascia, muscle, and bone

Surgery: Integumentary System

11040	Debridement; skin, partial thickness
11041	skin, full thickness
11042	skin, and subcutaneous tissue
11043	skin, subcutaneous tissue, and muscle
11044	skin, subcutaneous tissue, muscle, and bone

(Do not report 11040-11044 in conjunction with ▶97597-◀97602)

Paring or Cutting

(To report destruction, see 17000-17004)

11055	Paring or cutting of benign hyperkeratotic lesion (eg, corn or callus); single lesion
11056	two to four lesions
11057	more than four lesions

Biopsy

During certain surgical procedures in the integumentary system, such as excision, destruction, or shave removals, the removed tissue is often submitted for pathologic examination. The obtaining of tissue for pathology during the course of these procedures is a routine component of such procedures. This obtaining of tissue is not considered a separate biopsy procedure and is not separately reported. The use of a biopsy procedure code (eg, 11100, 11101) indicates that the procedure to obtain tissue for pathologic examination was performed independently, or was unrelated or distinct from other procedures/services provided at that time. Such biopsies are not considered components of other procedures when performed on different lesions or different sites on the same date, and are to be reported separately.

(For biopsy of conjunctiva, use 68100; eyelid, use 67810)

| 11100 | Biopsy of skin, subcutaneous tissue and/or mucous membrane (including simple closure), unless otherwise listed; single lesion |
| + 11101 | each separate/additional lesion (List separately in addition to code for primary procedure) |

(Use 11101 in conjunction with 11100)

Removal of Skin Tags

Removal by scissoring or any sharp method, ligature strangulation, electrosurgical destruction or combination of treatment modalities including chemical or electrocauterization of wound, with or without local anesthesia.

| 11200 | Removal of skin tags, multiple fibrocutaneous tags, any area; up to and including 15 lesions |
| + 11201 | each additional ten lesions (List separately in addition to code for primary procedure) |

(Use 11201 in conjunction with 11200)

Shaving of Epidermal or Dermal Lesions

Shaving is the sharp removal by transverse incision or horizontal slicing to remove epidermal and dermal lesions without a full-thickness dermal excision. This includes local anesthesia, chemical or electrocauterization of the wound. The wound does not require suture closure.

11300	Shaving of epidermal or dermal lesion, single lesion, trunk, arms or legs; lesion diameter 0.5 cm or less
11301	lesion diameter 0.6 to 1.0 cm
11302	lesion diameter 1.1 to 2.0 cm
11303	lesion diameter over 2.0 cm
11305	Shaving of epidermal or dermal lesion, single lesion, scalp, neck, hands, feet, genitalia; lesion diameter 0.5 cm or less
11306	lesion diameter 0.6 to 1.0 cm
11307	lesion diameter 1.1 to 2.0 cm
11308	lesion diameter over 2.0 cm
11310	Shaving of epidermal or dermal lesion, single lesion, face, ears, eyelids, nose, lips, mucous membrane; lesion diameter 0.5 cm or less
11311	lesion diameter 0.6 to 1.0 cm
11312	lesion diameter 1.1 to 2.0 cm
11313	lesion diameter over 2.0 cm

Excision—Benign Lesions

Excision (including simple closure) of benign lesions of skin (eg, neoplasm, cicatricial, fibrous, inflammatory, congenital, cystic lesions), includes local anesthesia. See appropriate size and area below. For shave removal, see 11300 et seq., and for electrosurgical and other methods see 17000 et seq.

Excision is defined as full-thickness (through the dermis) removal of a lesion, including margins, and includes simple (non-layered) closure when performed. Report separately each benign lesion excised. Code selection is determined by measuring the greatest clinical diameter of the apparent lesion plus that margin required for complete excision (lesion diameter plus the most narrow margins required equals the excised diameter). The margins refer to the most narrow margin required to adequately excise the lesion, based on the physician's judgment. The measurement of lesion plus margin is made prior to excision. The excised diameter is the same whether the surgical defect is repaired in a linear fashion, or reconstructed (eg, with a skin graft).

The closure of defects created by incision, excision, or trauma may require intermediate or complex closure. Repair by intermediate or complex closure should be reported separately. For excision of benign lesions requiring more than simple closure, ie, requiring intermediate or complex closure, report 11400-11446 in addition to appropriate intermediate (12031-12057) or complex closure (13100-13153) codes. For reconstructive closure, see 14000-14300, 15000-15261, 15570-15770. See page 49 for definition of intermediate or complex closure.

11400 Excision, benign lesion including margins, except skin tag (unless listed elsewhere), trunk, arms or legs; excised diameter 0.5 cm or less

11401   excised diameter 0.6 to 1.0 cm

11402   excised diameter 1.1 to 2.0 cm

11403   excised diameter 2.1 to 3.0 cm

11404   excised diameter 3.1 to 4.0 cm

11406   excised diameter over 4.0 cm

           (For unusual or complicated excision, add modifier 22)

11420 Excision, benign lesion including margins, except skin tag (unless listed elsewhere), scalp, neck, hands, feet, genitalia; excised diameter 0.5 cm or less

11421   excised diameter 0.6 to 1.0 cm

11422   excised diameter 1.1 to 2.0 cm

11423   excised diameter 2.1 to 3.0 cm

11424   excised diameter 3.1 to 4.0 cm

11426   excised diameter over 4.0 cm

           (For unusual or complicated excision, add modifier 22)

11440 Excision, other benign lesion including margins (unless listed elsewhere), face, ears, eyelids, nose, lips, mucous membrane; excised diameter 0.5 cm or less

11441   excised diameter 0.6 to 1.0 cm

11442   excised diameter 1.1 to 2.0 cm

11443   excised diameter 2.1 to 3.0 cm

11444   excised diameter 3.1 to 4.0 cm

11446   excised diameter over 4.0 cm

           (For unusual or complicated excision, add modifier 22)

           (For eyelids involving more than skin, see also 67800 et seq)

11450 Excision of skin and subcutaneous tissue for hidradenitis, axillary; with simple or intermediate repair

11451   with complex repair

11462 Excision of skin and subcutaneous tissue for hidradenitis, inguinal; with simple or intermediate repair

11463   with complex repair

11470 Excision of skin and subcutaneous tissue for hidradenitis, perianal, perineal, or umbilical; with simple or intermediate repair

11471   with complex repair

           (When skin graft or flap is used for closure, use appropriate procedure code in addition)

           (For bilateral procedure, add modifier 50)

Excision—Malignant Lesions

Excision (including simple closure) of malignant lesions of skin (eg, basal cell carcinoma, squamous cell carcinoma, melanoma) includes local anesthesia. (See appropriate size and body area below.) For destruction of malignant lesions of skin, see destruction codes 17260-17286.

Excision is defined as full-thickness (through the dermis) removal of a lesion including margins, and includes simple (non-layered) closure when performed. Report separately each malignant lesion excised. Code selection is determined by measuring the greatest clinical diameter of the apparent lesion plus that margin required for complete excision (lesion diameter plus the most narrow margins required equals the excised diameter). The margins refer to the most narrow margin required to adequately excise the lesion, based on the physician's judgment. The measurement of lesion plus margin is made prior to excision. The excised diameter is the same whether the surgical defect is repaired in a linear fashion, or reconstructed (eg, with a skin graft).

The closure of defects created by incision, excision, or trauma may require intermediate or complex closure. Repair by intermediate or complex closure should be reported separately. For excision of malignant lesions requiring more than simple closure, ie, requiring intermediate or complex closure, report 11600-11646 in addition to appropriate intermediate (12031-12057) or complex closure (13100-13153) codes. For reconstructive closure, see 14000-14300, 15000-15261, 15570-15770. See page 49 for definition of intermediate or complex closure.

When frozen section pathology shows the margins of excision were not adequate, an additional excision may be necessary for complete tumor removal. Use only one code to report the additional excision and re-excision(s) based on the final widest excised diameter required for complete tumor removal at the same operative session. To report a re-excision procedure performed to widen margins at a subsequent operative session, see codes 11600-11646, as appropriate. Append modifier 58 if the re-excision procedure is performed during the postoperative period of the primary excision procedure.

11600 Excision, malignant lesion including margins, trunk, arms, or legs; excised diameter 0.5 cm or less

11601   excised diameter 0.6 to 1.0 cm

11602   excised diameter 1.1 to 2.0 cm

11603   excised diameter 2.1 to 3.0 cm

11604   excised diameter 3.1 to 4.0 cm

11606   excised diameter over 4.0 cm

Surgery: Integumentary System

Surgery: Integumentary System

11620 Excision, malignant lesion including margins, scalp, neck, hands, feet, genitalia; excised diameter 0.5 cm or less

11621 excised diameter 0.6 to 1.0 cm

11622 excised diameter 1.1 to 2.0 cm

11623 excised diameter 2.1 to 3.0 cm

11624 excised diameter 3.1 to 4.0 cm

11626 excised diameter over 4.0 cm

11640 Excision, malignant lesion including margins, face, ears, eyelids, nose, lips; excised diameter 0.5 cm or less

11641 excised diameter 0.6 to 1.0 cm

11642 excised diameter 1.1 to 2.0 cm

11643 excised diameter 2.1 to 3.0 cm

11644 excised diameter 3.1 to 4.0 cm

11646 excised diameter over 4.0 cm

(For eyelids involving more than skin, see also 67800 et seq)

Nails

(For drainage of paronychia or onychia, see 10060, 10061)

11719 Trimming of nondystrophic nails, any number

11720 Debridement of nail(s) by any method(s); one to five

11721 six or more

11730 Avulsion of nail plate, partial or complete, simple; single

+ 11732 each additional nail plate (List separately in addition to code for primary procedure)

(Use 11732 in conjunction with 11730)

11740 Evacuation of subungual hematoma

11750 Excision of nail and nail matrix, partial or complete, (eg, ingrown or deformed nail) for permanent removal;

11752 with amputation of tuft of distal phalanx

(For skin graft, if used, use 15050)

11755 Biopsy of nail unit (eg, plate, bed, matrix, hyponychium, proximal and lateral nail folds) (separate procedure)

11760 Repair of nail bed

11762 Reconstruction of nail bed with graft

11765 Wedge excision of skin of nail fold (eg, for ingrown toenail)

Pilonidal Cyst

11770 Excision of pilonidal cyst or sinus; simple

11771 extensive

11772 complicated

(For incision of pilonidal cyst, see 10080, 10081)

Introduction

11900 Injection, intralesional; up to and including seven lesions

11901 more than seven lesions

(11900, 11901 are not to be used for preoperative local anesthetic injection)

(For veins, see 36470, 36471)

(For intralesional chemotherapy administration, see 96405, 96406)

11920 Tattooing, intradermal introduction of insoluble opaque pigments to correct color defects of skin, including micropigmentation; 6.0 sq cm or less

11921 6.1 to 20.0 sq cm

+ 11922 each additional 20.0 sq cm (List separately in addition to code for primary procedure)

(Use 11922 in conjunction with 11921)

11950 Subcutaneous injection of filling material (eg, collagen); 1 cc or less

11951 1.1 to 5.0 cc

11952 5.1 to 10.0 cc

11954 over 10.0 cc

11960 Insertion of tissue expander(s) for other than breast, including subsequent expansion

(For breast reconstruction with tissue expander(s), use 19357)

11970 Replacement of tissue expander with permanent prosthesis

11971 Removal of tissue expander(s) without insertion of prosthesis

11975 Insertion, implantable contraceptive capsules

11976 Removal, implantable contraceptive capsules

11977 Removal with reinsertion, implantable contraceptive capsules

11980 Subcutaneous hormone pellet implantation (implantation of estradiol and/or testosterone pellets beneath the skin)

11981 Insertion, non-biodegradable drug delivery implant

11982 Removal, non-biodegradable drug delivery implant

11983 Removal with reinsertion, non-biodegradable drug delivery implant

Repair (Closure)

Use the codes in this section to designate wound closure utilizing sutures, staples, or tissue adhesives (eg, 2-cyanoacrylate), either singly or in combination with each other, or in combination with adhesive strips. Wound closure utilizing adhesive strips as the sole repair material should be coded using the appropriate E/M code.

Definitions

The repair of wounds may be classified as Simple, Intermediate, or Complex.

Simple repair is used when the wound is superficial; eg, involving primarily epidermis or dermis, or subcutaneous tissues without significant involvement of deeper structures, and requires simple one layer closure. This includes local anesthesia and chemical or electrocauterization of wounds not closed.

Intermediate repair includes the repair of wounds that, in addition to the above, require layered closure of one or more of the deeper layers of subcutaneous tissue and superficial (non-muscle) fascia, in addition to the skin (epidermal and dermal) closure. Single-layer closure of heavily contaminated wounds that have required extensive cleaning or removal of particulate matter also constitutes intermediate repair.

Complex repair includes the repair of wounds requiring more than layered closure, viz., scar revision, debridement, (eg, traumatic lacerations or avulsions), extensive undermining, stents or retention sutures. Necessary preparation includes creation of a defect for repairs (eg, excision of a scar requiring a complex repair) or the debridement of complicated lacerations or avulsions. Complex repair does not include excision of benign (11400-11446) or malignant (11600-11646) lesions.

Instructions for listing services at time of wound repair:

1. The repaired wound(s) should be measured and recorded in centimeters, whether curved, angular, or stellate.

2. When multiple wounds are repaired, add together the lengths of those in the same classification (see above) and from all anatomic sites that are grouped together into the same code descriptor. For example, add together the lengths of intermediate repairs to the trunk and extremities. Do not add lengths of repairs from different groupings of anatomic sites (eg, face and extremities). Also, do not add together lengths of different classifications (eg, intermediate and complex repairs).

When more than one classification of wounds is repaired, list the more complicated as the primary procedure and the less complicated as the secondary procedure, using modifier 51.

3. Decontamination and/or debridement: Debridement is considered a separate procedure only when gross contamination requires prolonged cleansing, when appreciable amounts of devitalized or contaminated tissue are removed, or when debridement is carried out separately without immediate primary closure. (For extensive debridement of soft tissue and/or bone, see 11040-11044.)

(For extensive debridement of soft tissue and/or bone, not associated with open fracture(s) and/or dislocation(s) resulting from penetrating and/or blunt trauma, see 11040-11044.)

(For extensive debridement of subcutaneous tissue, muscle fascia, muscle, and/or bone associated with open fracture(s) and/or dislocation(s), see 11010-11012.)

4. Involvement of nerves, blood vessels and tendons: Report under appropriate system (Nervous, Cardiovascular, Musculoskeletal) for repair of these structures. The repair of these associated wounds is included in the primary procedure unless it qualifies as a complex wound, in which case modifier 51 applies.

Simple ligation of vessels in an open wound is considered as part of any wound closure.

Simple "exploration" of nerves, blood vessels or tendons exposed in an open wound is also considered part of the essential treatment of the wound and is not a separate procedure unless appreciable dissection is required. If the wound requires enlargement, extension of dissection (to determine penetration), debridement, removal of foreign body(s), ligation or coagulation of minor subcutaneous and/or muscular blood vessel(s) of the subcutaneous tissue, muscle fascia, and/or muscle, not requiring thoracotomy or laparotomy, use codes 20100-20103, as appropriate.

Repair—Simple

Sum of lengths of repairs for each group of anatomic sites.

12001	Simple repair of superficial wounds of scalp, neck, axillae, external genitalia, trunk and/or extremities (including hands and feet); 2.5 cm or less
12002	2.6 cm to 7.5 cm
12004	7.6 cm to 12.5 cm
12005	12.6 cm to 20.0 cm
12006	20.1 cm to 30.0 cm
12007	over 30.0 cm
12011	Simple repair of superficial wounds of face, ears, eyelids, nose, lips and/or mucous membranes; 2.5 cm or less
12013	2.6 cm to 5.0 cm
12014	5.1 cm to 7.5 cm
12015	7.6 cm to 12.5 cm
12016	12.6 cm to 20.0 cm
12017	20.1 cm to 30.0 cm
12018	over 30.0 cm
12020	Treatment of superficial wound dehiscence; simple closure
12021	with packing

(For extensive or complicated secondary wound closure, use 13160)

Surgery: Integumentary System

Repair—Intermediate

Sum of lengths of repairs for each group of anatomic sites.

12031   Layer closure of wounds of scalp, axillae, trunk and/or extremities (excluding hands and feet); 2.5 cm or less

12032   2.6 cm to 7.5 cm

12034   7.6 cm to 12.5 cm

12035   12.6 cm to 20.0 cm

12036   20.1 cm to 30.0 cm

12037   over 30.0 cm

12041   Layer closure of wounds of neck, hands, feet and/or external genitalia; 2.5 cm or less

12042   2.6 cm to 7.5 cm

12044   7.6 cm to 12.5 cm

12045   12.6 cm to 20.0 cm

12046   20.1 cm to 30.0 cm

12047   over 30.0 cm

12051   Layer closure of wounds of face, ears, eyelids, nose, lips and/or mucous membranes; 2.5 cm or less

12052   2.6 cm to 5.0 cm

12053   5.1 cm to 7.5 cm

12054   7.6 cm to 12.5 cm

12055   12.6 cm to 20.0 cm

12056   20.1 cm to 30.0 cm

12057   over 30.0 cm

Repair—Complex

Reconstructive procedures, complicated wound closure.

Sum of lengths of repairs for each group of anatomic sites.

(For full thickness repair of lip or eyelid, see respective anatomical subsections)

13100   Repair, complex, trunk; 1.1 cm to 2.5 cm

(For 1.0 cm or less, see simple or intermediate repairs)

13101   2.6 cm to 7.5 cm

+ 13102   each additional 5 cm or less (List separately in addition to code for primary procedure)

(Use 13102 in conjunction with 13101)

13120   Repair, complex, scalp, arms, and/or legs; 1.1 cm to 2.5 cm

(For 1.0 cm or less, see simple or intermediate repairs)

13121   2.6 cm to 7.5 cm

+ 13122   each additional 5 cm or less (List separately in addition to code for primary procedure)

(Use 13122 in conjunction with 13121)

13131   Repair, complex, forehead, cheeks, chin, mouth, neck, axillae, genitalia, hands and/or feet; 1.1 cm to 2.5 cm

(For 1.0 cm or less, see simple or intermediate repairs)

13132   2.6 cm to 7.5 cm

+ 13133   each additional 5 cm or less (List separately in addition to code for primary procedure)

(Use 13133 in conjunction with 13132)

13150   Repair, complex, eyelids, nose, ears and/or lips; 1.0 cm or less

(See also 40650-40654, 67961-67975)

13151   1.1 cm to 2.5 cm

13152   2.6 cm to 7.5 cm

+ 13153   each additional 5 cm or less (List separately in addition to code for primary procedure)

(Use 13153 in conjunction with 13152)

13160   Secondary closure of surgical wound or dehiscence, extensive or complicated

(For packing or simple secondary wound closure, see 12020, 12021)

Adjacent Tissue Transfer or Rearrangement

For full thickness repair of lip or eyelid, see respective anatomical subsections.

Excision (including lesion) and/or repair by adjacent tissue transfer or rearrangement (eg, Z-plasty, W-plasty, V-Y plasty, rotation flap, advancement flap, double pedicle flap). When applied in repairing lacerations, the procedures listed must be developed by the surgeon to accomplish the repair. They do not apply when direct closure or rearrangement of traumatic wounds incidentally result in these configurations.

Skin graft necessary to close secondary defect is considered an additional procedure. For purposes of code selection, the term "defect" includes the primary and secondary defects. The primary defect resulting from the excision and the secondary defect resulting from flap design to perform the reconstruction are measured together to determine the code.

14000   Adjacent tissue transfer or rearrangement, trunk; defect 10 sq cm or less

14001   defect 10.1 sq cm to 30.0 sq cm

14020   Adjacent tissue transfer or rearrangement, scalp, arms and/or legs; defect 10 sq cm or less

14021   defect 10.1 sq cm to 30.0 sq cm

14040   Adjacent tissue transfer or rearrangement, forehead, cheeks, chin, mouth, neck, axillae, genitalia, hands and/or feet; defect 10 sq cm or less

14041   defect 10.1 sq cm to 30.0 sq cm

14060   Adjacent tissue transfer or rearrangement, eyelids, nose, ears and/or lips; defect 10 sq cm or less

14061   defect 10.1 sq cm to 30.0 sq cm

       (For eyelid, full thickness, see 67961 et seq)

14300   Adjacent tissue transfer or rearrangement, more than 30 sq cm, unusual or complicated, any area

14350   Filleted finger or toe flap, including preparation of recipient site

Free Skin Grafts

Identify by size and location of the defect (recipient area) and the type of graft; includes simple debridement of granulations or recent avulsion.

When a primary procedure such as orbitectomy, radical mastectomy, or deep tumor removal requires skin graft for definitive closure, see appropriate anatomical subsection for primary procedure and this section for skin graft.

Use 15000 for initial wound preparation.

Use 15100-15261 for autogenous skin grafts. For autogenous tissue-cultured skin grafts, use 15100-15121. These codes include harvesting of keratinocytes and their subsequent application. Procedures are coded by recipient site. Use codes 15342 and 15343 for application of skin substitute/neodermis. Use modifier 58 for staged application procedure(s).

Repair of donor site requiring skin graft or local flaps is to be added as an additional procedure.

Codes 15000, 15001, 15350, 15351, 15400, 15401 describe burn and wound preparation and management procedures. The following definition should be applied to codes 15000, 15001, 15100, 15101, 15120, 15121 when determining the involvement of body size. The measurement of 100 sq cm is applicable to adults and children age 10 and over, percentages apply to infants and children under the age of 10.

       (For microvascular flaps, see 15756-15758)

15000   Surgical preparation or creation of recipient site by excision of open wounds, burn eschar, or scar (including subcutaneous tissues); first 100 sq cm or one percent of body area of infants and children

       (For appropriate skin grafts, see 15050-15261; list the free graft separately by its procedure number when the graft, immediate or delayed, is applied)

+ 15001   each additional 100 sq cm or each additional one percent of body area of infants and children (List separately in addition to code for primary procedure)

       (Use 15001 in conjunction with 15000)

       (For excision of benign lesions, see 11400-11471)

       (For excision of malignant lesions, see 11600-11646)

       (For excision with alloplastic dressing, use 15000 only)

       (For excision with immediate skin grafting use 15050-15261 in addition to 15000)

       (For excision with immediate allograft placement use 15350 in addition to 15000)

       (For excision with immediate xenograft placement use 15400 in addition to 15000)

15050   Pinch graft, single or multiple, to cover small ulcer, tip of digit, or other minimal open area (except on face), up to defect size 2 cm diameter

15100   Split graft, trunk, arms, legs; first 100 sq cm or less, or one percent of body area of infants and children (except 15050)

+ 15101   each additional 100 sq cm, or each additional one percent of body area of infants and children, or part thereof (List separately in addition to code for primary procedure)

       (Use 15101 in conjunction with 15100)

15120   Split graft, face, scalp, eyelids, mouth, neck, ears, orbits, genitalia, hands, feet and/or multiple digits; first 100 sq cm or less, or one percent of body area of infants and children (except 15050)

+ 15121   each additional 100 sq cm, or each additional one percent of body area of infants and children, or part thereof (List separately in addition to code for primary procedure)

       (Use 15121 in conjunction with 15120)

       (For eyelids, see also 67961 et seq)

15200   Full thickness graft, free, including direct closure of donor site, trunk; 20 sq cm or less

+ 15201   each additional 20 sq cm (List separately in addition to code for primary procedure)

       (Use 15201 in conjunction with 15200)

15220   Full thickness graft, free, including direct closure of donor site, scalp, arms, and/or legs; 20 sq cm or less

+ 15221   each additional 20 sq cm (List separately in addition to code for primary procedure)

       (Use 15221 in conjunction with 15220)

15240   Full thickness graft, free, including direct closure of donor site, forehead, cheeks, chin, mouth, neck, axillae, genitalia, hands, and/or feet; 20 sq cm or less

       (For finger tip graft, use 15050)

       (For repair of syndactyly, fingers, see 26560-26562)

+ 15241   each additional 20 sq cm (List separately in addition to code for primary procedure)

       (Use 15241 in conjunction with 15240)

Surgery: Integumentary System

Surgery: Integumentary System

15260   Full thickness graft, free, including direct closure of donor site, nose, ears, eyelids, and/or lips; 20 sq cm or less

+ 15261   each additional 20 sq cm (List separately in addition to code for primary procedure)

        (Use 15261 in conjunction with 15260)

        (For eyelids, see also 67961 et seq)

        (Repair of donor site requiring skin graft or local flaps, to be added as additional separate procedure)

15342   Application of bilaminate skin substitute/neodermis; 25 sq cm

+ 15343   each additional 25 sq cm (List separately in addition to code for primary procedure)

        (Use 15343 in conjunction with 15342)

15350   Application of allograft, skin; 100 sq cm or less

        (For staged tissue graft implantation, use modifier 58)

+ 15351   each additional 100 sq cm (List separately in addition to code for primary procedure)

        (Use 15351 in conjunction with 15350)

15400   Application of xenograft, skin; 100 sq cm or less

+ 15401   each additional 100 sq cm (List separately in addition to code for primary procedure)

        (Use 15401 in conjunction with 15400)

Flaps (Skin and/or Deep Tissues)

Regions listed refer to recipient area (not donor site) when flap is being attached in transfer or to final site.

Regions listed refer to donor site when tube is formed for later or when "delay" of flap is prior to transfer.

Procedures 15570-15738 do not include extensive immobilization (eg, large plaster casts and other immobilizing devices are considered additional separate procedures).

Repair of donor site requiring skin graft or local flaps is considered an additional separate procedure.

        (For microvascular flaps, see 15756-15758)

15570   Formation of direct or tubed pedicle, with or without transfer; trunk

15572   scalp, arms, or legs

15574   forehead, cheeks, chin, mouth, neck, axillae, genitalia, hands or feet

15576   eyelids, nose, ears, lips, or intraoral

15600   Delay of flap or sectioning of flap (division and inset); at trunk

15610   at scalp, arms, or legs

15620   at forehead, cheeks, chin, neck, axillae, genitalia, hands, or feet

15630   at eyelids, nose, ears, or lips

15650   Transfer, intermediate, of any pedicle flap (eg, abdomen to wrist, Walking tube), any location

        (For eyelids, nose, ears, or lips, see also anatomical area)

        (For revision, defatting or rearranging of transferred pedicle flap or skin graft, see 13100-14300)

        (Procedures 15732-15738 are described by donor site of the muscle, myocutaneous, or fasciocutaneous flap)

15732   Muscle, myocutaneous, or fasciocutaneous flap; head and neck (eg, temporalis, masseter muscle, sternocleidomastoid, levator scapulae)

15734   trunk

15736   upper extremity

15738   lower extremity

Other Flaps and Grafts

Repair of donor site requiring skin graft or local flaps should be reported as an additional procedure.

15740   Flap; island pedicle

15750   neurovascular pedicle

15756   Free muscle or myocutaneous flap with microvascular anastomosis

        (Do not report code 69990 in addition to code 15756)

15757   Free skin flap with microvascular anastomosis

        (Do not report code 69990 in addition to code 15757)

15758   Free fascial flap with microvascular anastomosis

        (Do not report code 69990 in addition to code 15758)

15760   Graft; composite (eg, full thickness of external ear or nasal ala), including primary closure, donor area

15770   derma-fat-fascia

15775   Punch graft for hair transplant; 1 to 15 punch grafts

15776   more than 15 punch grafts

        (For strip transplant, use 15220)

Other Procedures

15780   Dermabrasion; total face (eg, for acne scarring, fine wrinkling, rhytids, general keratosis)

15781   segmental, face

15782   regional, other than face

15783   superficial, any site, (eg, tattoo removal)

15786   Abrasion; single lesion (eg, keratosis, scar)

+ 15787   each additional four lesions or less (List separately in addition to code for primary procedure)

        (Use 15787 in conjunction with 15786)

15788   Chemical peel, facial; epidermal

15789   dermal

15792   Chemical peel, nonfacial; epidermal

15793   dermal

15810   Salabrasion; 20 sq cm or less

15811   over 20 sq cm

15819   Cervicoplasty

15820   Blepharoplasty, lower eyelid;

15821   with extensive herniated fat pad

15822   Blepharoplasty, upper eyelid;

15823   with excessive skin weighting down lid

      (For bilateral blepharoplasty, add modifier 50)

15824   Rhytidectomy; forehead

      (For repair of brow ptosis, use 67900)

15825   neck with platysmal tightening (platysmal flap, P-flap)

15826   glabellar frown lines

15828   cheek, chin, and neck

15829   superficial musculoaponeurotic system (SMAS) flap

      (For bilateral rhytidectomy, add modifier 50)

15831   Excision, excessive skin and subcutaneous tissue (including lipectomy); abdomen (abdominoplasty)

15832   thigh

15833   leg

15834   hip

15835   buttock

15836   arm

15837   forearm or hand

15838   submental fat pad

15839   other area

      (For bilateral procedure, add modifier 50)

15840   Graft for facial nerve paralysis; free fascia graft (including obtaining fascia)

      (For bilateral procedure, add modifier 50)

15841   free muscle graft (including obtaining graft)

15842   free muscle flap by microsurgical technique

      (Do not report code 69990 in addition to code 15842)

15845   regional muscle transfer

      (For intravenous fluorescein examination of blood flow in graft or flap, use 15860)

      (For nerve transfers, decompression, or repair, see 64831-64876, 64905, 64907, 69720, 69725, 69740, 69745, 69955)

15850   Removal of sutures under anesthesia (other than local), same surgeon

15851   Removal of sutures under anesthesia (other than local), other surgeon

15852   Dressing change (for other than burns) under anesthesia (other than local)

15860   Intravenous injection of agent (eg, fluorescein) to test vascular flow in flap or graft

15876   Suction assisted lipectomy; head and neck

15877   trunk

15878   upper extremity

15879   lower extremity

Pressure Ulcers (Decubitus Ulcers)

15920   Excision, coccygeal pressure ulcer, with coccygectomy; with primary suture

15922   with flap closure

15931   Excision, sacral pressure ulcer, with primary suture;

15933   with ostectomy

15934   Excision, sacral pressure ulcer, with skin flap closure;

15935   with ostectomy

15936   Excision, sacral pressure ulcer, in preparation for muscle or myocutaneous flap or skin graft closure;

15937   with ostectomy

      (For repair of defect using muscle or myocutaneous flap, use code(s) 15734 and/or 15738 in addition to 15936, 15937. For repair of defect using split skin graft, use codes 15100 and/or 15101 in addition to 15936, 15937)

15940   Excision, ischial pressure ulcer, with primary suture;

15941   with ostectomy (ischiectomy)

15944   Excision, ischial pressure ulcer, with skin flap closure;

15945   with ostectomy

15946   Excision, ischial pressure ulcer, with ostectomy, in preparation for muscle or myocutaneous flap or skin graft closure

      (For repair of defect using muscle or myocutaneous flap, use code(s) 15734 and/or 15738 in addition to 15946. For repair of defect using split skin graft, use codes 15100 and/or 15101 in addition to 15946)

15950   Excision, trochanteric pressure ulcer, with primary suture;

15951   with ostectomy

15952   Excision, trochanteric pressure ulcer, with skin flap closure;

15953   with ostectomy

Surgery: Integumentary System

Surgery: Integumentary System

15956   Excision, trochanteric pressure ulcer, in preparation for muscle or myocutaneous flap or skin graft closure;

15958   with ostectomy

(For repair of defect using muscle or myocutaneous flap, use code(s) 15734 and/or 15738 in addition to 15956, 15958. For repair of defect using split skin graft, use codes 15100 and/or 15101 in addition to 15956, 15958)

15999   Unlisted procedure, excision pressure ulcer

(For free skin graft to close ulcer or donor site, see 15000 et seq)

Burns, Local Treatment

Procedures 16000-16036 refer to local treatment of burned surface only.

List percentage of body surface involved and depth of burn.

For necessary related medical services (eg, hospital visits, detention) in management of burned patients, see appropriate services in **Evaluation and Management** and **Medicine** sections.

(For skin graft, see 15100-15650)

16000   Initial treatment, first degree burn, when no more than local treatment is required

16010   Dressings and/or debridement, initial or subsequent; under anesthesia, small

16015   under anesthesia, medium or large, or with major debridement

16020   without anesthesia, office or hospital, small

16025   without anesthesia, medium (eg, whole face or whole extremity)

16030   without anesthesia, large (eg, more than one extremity)

16035   Escharotomy; initial incision

+ 16036   each additional incision (List separately in addition to code for primary procedure)

(Use 16036 in conjunction with 16035)

(For debridement, curettement of burn wound, see 16010-16030)

Destruction

Destruction means the ablation of benign, premalignant or malignant tissues by any method, with or without curettement, including local anesthesia, and not usually requiring closure.

Any method includes electrosurgery, cryosurgery, laser and chemical treatment. Lesions include condylomata, papillomata, molluscum contagiosum, herpetic lesions, warts (ie, common, plantar, flat), milia, or other benign, premalignant (eg, actinic keratoses), or malignant lesions.

(For destruction of lesion(s) in specific anatomic sites, see 40820, 46900-46917, 46924, 54050-54057, 54065, 56501, 56515, 57061, 57065, 67850, 68135)

(For paring or cutting of benign hyperkeratotic lesions (eg, corns or calluses), see 11055-11057)

(For sharp removal or electrosurgical destruction of skin tags and fibrocutaneous tags, see 11200, 11201)

(For cryotherapy of acne, use 17340)

(For initiation or follow-up care of topical chemotherapy (eg, 5-FU or similar agents), see appropriate office visits)

(For shaving of epidermal or dermal lesions, see 11300-11313)

Destruction, Benign or Premalignant Lesions

17000   Destruction (eg, laser surgery, electrosurgery, cryosurgery, chemosurgery, surgical curettement), all benign or premalignant lesions (eg, actinic keratoses) other than skin tags or cutaneous vascular proliferative lesions; first lesion

+ 17003   second through 14 lesions, each (List separately in addition to code for first lesion)

(Use 17003 in conjunction with 17000)

⊘ **17004**   Destruction (eg, laser surgery, electrosurgery, cryosurgery, chemosurgery, surgical curettement), all benign or premalignant lesions (eg, actinic keratoses) other than skin tags or cutaneous vascular proliferative lesions, 15 or more lesions

(Do not report 17004 in conjunction with 17000-17003)

17106   Destruction of cutaneous vascular proliferative lesions (eg, laser technique); less than 10 sq cm

17107   10.0 to 50.0 sq cm

17108   over 50.0 sq cm

17110   Destruction (eg, laser surgery, electrosurgery, cryosurgery, chemosurgery, surgical curettement), of flat warts, molluscum contagiosum, or milia; up to 14 lesions

17111   15 or more lesions

(For destruction of common or plantar warts, see 17000, 17003, 17004)

17250   Chemical cauterization of granulation tissue (proud flesh, sinus or fistula)

(17250 is not to be used with removal or excision codes for the same lesion)

Destruction, Malignant Lesions, Any Method

17260   Destruction, malignant lesion (eg, laser surgery, electrosurgery, cryosurgery, chemosurgery, surgical curettement), trunk, arms or legs; lesion diameter 0.5 cm or less

17261   lesion diameter 0.6 to 1.0 cm

17262   lesion diameter 1.1 to 2.0 cm

17263   lesion diameter 2.1 to 3.0 cm

17264   lesion diameter 3.1 to 4.0 cm

17266   lesion diameter over 4.0 cm

17270   Destruction, malignant lesion (eg, laser surgery, electrosurgery, cryosurgery, chemosurgery, surgical curettement), scalp, neck, hands, feet, genitalia; lesion diameter 0.5 cm or less

17271   lesion diameter 0.6 to 1.0 cm

17272   lesion diameter 1.1 to 2.0 cm

17273   lesion diameter 2.1 to 3.0 cm

17274   lesion diameter 3.1 to 4.0 cm

17276   lesion diameter over 4.0 cm

17280   Destruction, malignant lesion (eg, laser surgery, electrosurgery, cryosurgery, chemosurgery, surgical curettement), face, ears, eyelids, nose, lips, mucous membrane; lesion diameter 0.5 cm or less

17281   lesion diameter 0.6 to 1.0 cm

17282   lesion diameter 1.1 to 2.0 cm

17283   lesion diameter 2.1 to 3.0 cm

17284   lesion diameter 3.1 to 4.0 cm

17286   lesion diameter over 4.0 cm

Mohs Micrographic Surgery

Mohs micrographic surgery, for the removal of complex or ill-defined skin cancer, requires a single physician to act in two integrated, but separate and distinct capacities: surgeon and pathologist. If either of these responsibilities are delegated to another physician who reports his services separately, these codes are not appropriate. If repair is performed, use separate repair, flap, or graft codes. If a biopsy of a suspected skin cancer is performed on the same day as Mohs surgery because there was no prior pathology confirmation of a diagnosis, then report diagnostic skin biopsy (11100, 11101) and frozen section pathology (88331) with modifier 59 to distinguish from the subsequent definitive surgical procedure of Mohs surgery.

⊘ **17304**   Chemosurgery (Mohs micrographic technique), including removal of all gross tumor, surgical excision of tissue specimens, mapping, color coding of specimens, microscopic examination of specimens by the surgeon, and complete histopathologic preparation including the first routine stain (eg, hematoxylin and eosin, toluidine blue); first stage, fresh tissue technique, up to 5 specimens

(If additional special pathology procedures, stains or immunostains are required, use 88311-88314, 88342)

⊘ **17305**   second stage, fixed or fresh tissue, up to 5 specimens

⊘ **17306**   third stage, fixed or fresh tissue, up to 5 specimens

⊘ **17307**   additional stage(s), up to 5 specimens, each stage

+ **17310**   each additional specimen, after the first 5 specimens, fixed or fresh tissue, any stage (List separately in addition to code for primary procedure)

(Use 17310 in conjunction with 17304-17307)

Other Procedures

17340   Cryotherapy (CO_2 slush, liquid N_2) for acne

17360   Chemical exfoliation for acne (eg, acne paste, acid)

17380   Electrolysis epilation, each 1/2 hour

(For actinotherapy, use 96900)

17999   Unlisted procedure, skin, mucous membrane and subcutaneous tissue

Breast

Incision

19000   Puncture aspiration of cyst of breast;

+ **19001**   each additional cyst (List separately in addition to code for primary procedure)

(Use 19001 in conjunction with 19000)

(If imaging guidance is performed, see 76095, 76096, 76393, 76942)

19020   Mastotomy with exploration or drainage of abscess, deep

19030   Injection procedure only for mammary ductogram or galactogram

(For radiological supervision and interpretation, see 76086, 76088)

(For catheter lavage of mammary ducts for collection of cytology specimens, use Category III codes 0046T, 0047T)

Surgery: Integumentary System

Excision

(To report bilateral procedures, report modifier 50 with the procedure code)

►Excisional breast surgery includes certain biopsy procedures, the removal of cysts or other benign or malignant tumors or lesions, and the surgical treatment of breast and chest wall malignancies. Biopsy procedures may be percutaneous or open, and they involve the removal of differing amounts of tissue for diagnosis.◄

►Breast biopsies are reported using codes 19100-19103. The open excision of breast lesions (eg, lesions of the breast ducts, cysts, benign or malignant tumors), without specific attention to adequate surgical margins, with or without the preoperative placement of radiological markers, is reported using codes 19110-19126. Partial mastectomy procedures (eg, lumpectomy, tylectomy, quadrantectomy, or segmentectomy) describe open excisions of breast tissue with specific attention to adequate surgical margins.◄

►Partial mastectomy procedures are reported using codes 19160 or 19162 as appropriate. Documentation for partial mastectomy procedures includes attention to the removal of adequate surgical margins surrounding the breast mass or lesion.◄

►Total mastectomy procedures include simple mastectomy, complete mastectomy, subcutaneous mastectomy, modified radical mastectomy, radical mastectomy, and more extended procedures (eg, Urban type operation). Total mastectomy procedures are reported using codes 19180, 19182, 19200, 19220, or 19240 as appropriate.◄

►Excisions or resections of chest wall tumors including ribs, with or without reconstruction, with or without mediastinal lymphadenectomy, are reported using codes 19260, 19271, or 19272. Codes 19260-19272 are not restricted to breast tumors and are used to report resections of chest wall tumors originating from any chest wall component. (For excision of lung or pleura, see 32310 et seq.)◄

19100   Biopsy of breast; percutaneous, needle core, not using imaging guidance (separate procedure)

(For fine needle aspiration, use 10021)

(For image guided breast biopsy, see 19102, 19103, 10022)

19101   open, incisional

19102   percutaneous, needle core, using imaging guidance

(For placement of percutaneous localization clip, use 19295)

19103   percutaneous, automated vacuum assisted or rotating biopsy device, using imaging guidance

(For imaging guidance performed in conjunction with 19102, 19103, see 76095, 76096, 76360, 76393, 76942)

(For placement of percutaneous localization clip, use 19295)

19110   Nipple exploration, with or without excision of a solitary lactiferous duct or a papilloma lactiferous duct

19112   Excision of lactiferous duct fistula

19120   Excision of cyst, fibroadenoma, or other benign or malignant tumor, aberrant breast tissue, duct lesion, nipple or areolar lesion (except 19140), open, male or female, one or more lesions

19125   Excision of breast lesion identified by preoperative placement of radiological marker, open; single lesion

+ 19126   each additional lesion separately identified by a preoperative radiological marker (List separately in addition to code for primary procedure)

(Use 19126 in conjunction with 19125)

19140   Mastectomy for gynecomastia

▲ **19160**   Mastectomy, partial (eg, lumpectomy, tylectomy, quadrantectomy, segmentectomy);

19162   with axillary lymphadenectomy

►(For placement of radiotherapy afterloading balloon/brachytherapy catheters, see 19296-19298)◄

19180   Mastectomy, simple, complete

(For immediate or delayed insertion of implant, use 19340 or 19342)

(For gynecomastia, use 19140)

19182   Mastectomy, subcutaneous

(For immediate or delayed insertion of implant, use 19340 or 19342)

19200   Mastectomy, radical, including pectoral muscles, axillary lymph nodes

(For immediate or delayed insertion of implant, use 19340 or 19342)

19220   Mastectomy, radical, including pectoral muscles, axillary and internal mammary lymph nodes (Urban type operation)

(For immediate or delayed insertion of implant, use 19340 or 19342)

19240   Mastectomy, modified radical, including axillary lymph nodes, with or without pectoralis minor muscle, but excluding pectoralis major muscle

(For immediate or delayed insertion of implant, use 19340 or 19342)

19260 Excision of chest wall tumor including ribs

19271 Excision of chest wall tumor involving ribs, with plastic reconstruction; without mediastinal lymphadenectomy

19272   with mediastinal lymphadenectomy

Introduction

19290 Preoperative placement of needle localization wire, breast;

+ **19291**   each additional lesion (List separately in addition to code for primary procedure)

(Use 19291 in conjunction with 19290)

(For radiological supervision and interpretation, see 76095, 76096, 76942)

+ **19295** Image guided placement, metallic localization clip, percutaneous, during breast biopsy (List separately in addition to code for primary procedure)

(Use 19295 in conjunction with 19102, 19103)

● **19296** Placement of radiotherapy afterloading balloon catheter into the breast for interstitial radioelement application following partial mastectomy, includes imaging guidance; on date separate from partial mastectomy

+● **19297**   concurrent with partial mastectomy (List separately in addition to code for primary procedure)

►(Use 19297 in conjunction with 19160 or 19162)◄

⊙● **19298** Placement of radiotherapy afterloading brachytherapy catheters (multiple tube and button type) into the breast for interstitial radioelement application following (at the time of or subsequent to) partial mastectomy, includes imaging guidance

Repair and/or Reconstruction

(To report bilateral procedures, report modifier 50 with the procedure code)

19316 Mastopexy

19318 Reduction mammaplasty

19324 Mammaplasty, augmentation; without prosthetic implant

19325   with prosthetic implant

(For flap or graft, use also appropriate number)

19328 Removal of intact mammary implant

19330 Removal of mammary implant material

19340 Immediate insertion of breast prosthesis following mastopexy, mastectomy or in reconstruction

19342 Delayed insertion of breast prosthesis following mastopexy, mastectomy or in reconstruction

(For supply of implant, use 99070)

(For preparation of custom breast implant, use 19396)

19350 Nipple/areola reconstruction

19355 Correction of inverted nipples

19357 Breast reconstruction, immediate or delayed, with tissue expander, including subsequent expansion

19361 Breast reconstruction with latissimus dorsi flap, with or without prosthetic implant

19364 Breast reconstruction with free flap

(Do not report code 69990 in addition to code 19364)

(19364 includes harvesting of the flap, microvascular transfer, closure of the donor site, and inset shaping the flap into a breast)

19366 Breast reconstruction with other technique

(For operating microscope, use 69990)

(For insertion of prosthesis, use also 19340 or 19342)

19367 Breast reconstruction with transverse rectus abdominis myocutaneous flap (TRAM), single pedicle, including closure of donor site;

19368   with microvascular anastomosis (supercharging)

(Do not report code 69990 in addition to code 19368)

19369 Breast reconstruction with transverse rectus abdominis myocutaneous flap (TRAM), double pedicle, including closure of donor site

19370 Open periprosthetic capsulotomy, breast

19371 Periprosthetic capsulectomy, breast

19380 Revision of reconstructed breast

19396 Preparation of moulage for custom breast implant

Other Procedures

(For microwave thermotherapy of the breast, use Category III code 0061T)

19499 Unlisted procedure, breast

Surgery: Integumentary System

Notes

Musculoskeletal System

Cast and strapping procedures appear at the end of this section.

The services listed below include the application and removal of the first cast or traction device only. Subsequent replacement of cast and/or traction device may require an additional listing.

Definitions

The terms "closed treatment," "open treatment," and "percutaneous skeletal fixation" have been carefully chosen to accurately reflect current orthopaedic procedural treatments.

Closed treatment specifically means that the fracture site is not surgically opened (exposed to the external environment and directly visualized). This terminology is used to describe procedures that treat fractures by three methods: 1) without manipulation 2) with manipulation 3) with or without traction.

Open treatment is used when the fractured bone is either (1) surgically opened (exposed to the external environment) and the fracture (bone ends) visualized and internal fixation may be used or (2) the fractured bone is opened remote from the fracture site in order to insert an intramedullary nail across the fracture site (the fracture site is not opened and visualized).

Percutaneous skeletal fixation describes fracture treatment which is neither open nor closed. In this procedure, the fracture fragments are not visualized, but fixation (eg, pins) is placed across the fracture site, usually under x-ray imaging.

The type of fracture (eg, open, compound, closed) does not have any coding correlation with the type of treatment (eg, closed, open, or percutaneous) provided.

The codes for treatment of fractures and joint injuries (dislocations) are categorized by the type of manipulation (reduction) and stabilization (fixation or immobilization). These codes can apply to either open (compound) or closed fractures or joint injuries.

Skeletal traction is the application of a force (distracting or traction force) to a limb segment through a wire, pin, screw, or clamp that is attached (eg, penetrates) to bone.

Skin traction is the application of a force (longitudinal) to a limb using felt or strapping applied directly to skin only.

External fixation is the usage of skeletal pins plus an attaching mechanism/device used for temporary or definitive treatment of acute or chronic bony deformity.

Codes for obtaining autogenous bone grafts, cartilage, tendon, fascia lata grafts or other tissues through separate incisions are to be used only when the graft is not already listed as part of the basic procedure.

Re-reduction of a fracture and/or dislocation performed by the primary physician may be identified by the addition of the modifier 76 to the usual procedure number to indicate "Repeat Procedure by Same Physician." (See guidelines.)

Codes for external fixation are to be used only when external fixation is not already listed as part of the basic procedure.

All codes for suction irrigation have been deleted. To report, list only the primary surgical procedure performed (eg, sequestrectomy, deep incision).

Manipulation is used throughout the musculoskeletal fracture and dislocation subsections to specifically mean the attempted reduction or restoration of a fracture or joint dislocation to its normal anatomic alignment by the application of manually applied forces.

(For computer assisted musculoskeletal surgical navigational orthopedic procedures, report 0054T-0056T)

General

Incision

20000   Incision of soft tissue abscess (eg, secondary to osteomyelitis); superficial

20005   deep or complicated

Wound Exploration—Trauma (eg, Penetrating Gunshot, Stab Wound)

20100-20103 relate to wound(s) resulting from penetrating trauma. These codes describe surgical exploration and enlargement of the wound, extension of dissection (to determine penetration), debridement, removal of foreign body(s), ligation or coagulation of minor subcutaneous and/or muscular blood vessel(s), of the subcutaneous tissue, muscle fascia, and/or muscle, not requiring thoracotomy or laparotomy. If a repair is done to major structure(s) or major blood vessel(s) requiring thoracotomy or laparotomy, then those specific code(s) would supersede the use of codes 20100-20103. To report Simple, Intermediate, or Complex repair of wound(s) that do not require enlargement of the wound, extension of dissection, etc., as stated above, use specific Repair code(s) in the Integumentary System section.

20100   Exploration of penetrating wound (separate procedure); neck

20101   chest

20102   abdomen/flank/back

20103   extremity

Surgery: Musculoskeletal System

Excision

20150 Excision of epiphyseal bar, with or without autogenous soft tissue graft obtained through same fascial incision

(For aspiration of bone marrow, use 38220)

20200 Biopsy, muscle; superficial

20205   deep

20206 Biopsy, muscle, percutaneous needle

(If imaging guidance is performed, see 76360, 76393, 76942)

(For fine needle aspiration, use 10021 or 10022)

(For evaluation of fine needle aspirate, see 88172-88173)

(For excision of muscle tumor, deep, see specific anatomic section)

20220 Biopsy, bone, trocar, or needle; superficial (eg, ilium, sternum, spinous process, ribs)

20225   deep (eg, vertebral body, femur)

(For bone marrow biopsy, use 38221)

(For radiologic supervision and interpretation, see 76003, 76360, 76393)

20240 Biopsy, bone, open; superficial (eg, ilium, sternum, spinous process, ribs, trochanter of femur)

20245   deep (eg, humerus, ischium, femur)

20250 Biopsy, vertebral body, open; thoracic

20251   lumbar or cervical

(For sequestrectomy, osteomyelitis or drainage of bone abscess, see anatomical area)

Introduction or Removal

(For injection procedure for arthrography, see anatomical area)

20500 Injection of sinus tract; therapeutic (separate procedure)

20501   diagnostic (sinogram)

(For radiological supervision and interpretation, use 76080)

20520 Removal of foreign body in muscle or tendon sheath; simple

20525   deep or complicated

20526 Injection, therapeutic (eg, local anesthetic, corticosteroid), carpal tunnel

20550 Injection(s); single tendon sheath, or ligament, aponeurosis (eg, plantar "fascia")

20551   single tendon origin/insertion

20552 Injection(s); single or multiple trigger point(s), one or two muscle(s)

20553   single or multiple trigger point(s), three or more muscle(s)

(If imaging guidance is performed, see 76003, 76393, 76942)

20600 Arthrocentesis, aspiration and/or injection; small joint or bursa (eg, fingers, toes)

20605   intermediate joint or bursa (eg, temporomandibular, acromioclavicular, wrist, elbow or ankle, olecranon bursa)

20610   major joint or bursa (eg, shoulder, hip, knee joint, subacromial bursa)

(If imaging guidance is performed, see 76003, 76360, 76393, 76942)

20612 Aspiration and/or injection of ganglion cyst(s) any location

(To report multiple ganglion cyst aspirations/injections, use 20612 and append modifier 59)

20615 Aspiration and injection for treatment of bone cyst

20650 Insertion of wire or pin with application of skeletal traction, including removal (separate procedure)

⊘ **20660** Application of cranial tongs, caliper, or stereotactic frame, including removal (separate procedure)

20661 Application of halo, including removal; cranial

20662   pelvic

20663   femoral

20664 Application of halo, including removal, cranial, 6 or more pins placed, for thin skull osteology (eg, pediatric patients, hydrocephalus, osteogenesis imperfecta), requiring general anesthesia

20665 Removal of tongs or halo applied by another physician

20670 Removal of implant; superficial, (eg, buried wire, pin or rod) (separate procedure)

20680   deep (eg, buried wire, pin, screw, metal band, nail, rod or plate)

⊘ **20690** Application of a uniplane (pins or wires in one plane), unilateral, external fixation system

⊘ **20692** Application of a multiplane (pins or wires in more than one plane), unilateral, external fixation system (eg, Ilizarov, Monticelli type)

20693 Adjustment or revision of external fixation system requiring anesthesia (eg, new pin(s) or wire(s) and/or new ring(s) or bar(s))

20694 Removal, under anesthesia, of external fixation system

Replantation

20802   Replantation, arm (includes surgical neck of humerus through elbow joint), complete amputation

(To report replantation of incomplete arm amputation, see specific code(s) for repair of bone(s), ligament(s), tendon(s), nerve(s), or blood vessel(s) with modifier 52)

20805   Replantation, forearm (includes radius and ulna to radial carpal joint), complete amputation

(To report replantation of incomplete forearm amputation, see specific code(s) for repair of bone(s), ligament(s), tendon(s), nerve(s), or blood vessel(s) with modifier 52)

20808   Replantation, hand (includes hand through metacarpophalangeal joints), complete amputation

(To report replantation of incomplete hand amputation, see specific code(s) for repair of bone(s), ligament(s), tendon(s), nerve(s), or blood vessel(s) with modifier 52)

20816   Replantation, digit, excluding thumb (includes metacarpophalangeal joint to insertion of flexor sublimis tendon), complete amputation

(To report replantation of incomplete digit amputation, excluding thumb, see specific code(s) for repair of bone(s), ligament(s), tendon(s), nerve(s), or blood vessel(s) with modifier 52)

20822   Replantation, digit, excluding thumb (includes distal tip to sublimis tendon insertion), complete amputation

(To report replantation of incomplete digit amputation, excluding thumb, see specific code(s) for repair of bone(s), ligament(s), tendon(s), nerve(s), or blood vessel(s) with modifier 52)

20824   Replantation, thumb (includes carpometacarpal joint to MP joint), complete amputation

(To report replantation of incomplete thumb amputation, see specific code(s) for repair of bone(s), ligament(s), tendon(s), nerve(s), or blood vessel(s) with modifier 52)

20827   Replantation, thumb (includes distal tip to MP joint), complete amputation

(To report replantation of incomplete thumb amputation, see specific code(s) for repair of bone(s), ligament(s), tendon(s), nerve(s), or blood vessel(s) with modifier 52)

(To report replantation of complete leg amputation, see specific code(s) for repair of bone(s), ligament(s), tendon(s), nerve(s), or blood vessel(s) with modifier 52)

(To report replantation of incomplete leg amputation, see specific code(s) for repair of bone(s), ligament(s), tendon(s), nerve(s), or blood vessel(s) with modifier 52)

20838   Replantation, foot, complete amputation

(To report replantation of incomplete foot amputation, see specific code(s) for repair of bone(s), ligament(s), tendon(s), nerve(s), or blood vessel(s) with modifier 52)

Grafts (or Implants)

Codes for obtaining autogenous bone, cartilage, tendon, fascia lata grafts, or other tissues through separate skin/fascial incisions should be reported separately unless the code descriptor references the harvesting of the graft or implant (eg, includes obtaining graft).

Do not append modifier 62 to bone graft codes 20900-20938.

(For spinal surgery bone graft(s) see codes 20930-20938)

⊘ **20900**   Bone graft, any donor area; minor or small (eg, dowel or button)

⊘ **20902**   major or large

⊘ **20910**   Cartilage graft; costochondral

⊘ **20912**   nasal septum

(For ear cartilage, use 21235)

⊘ **20920**   Fascia lata graft; by stripper

⊘ **20922**   by incision and area exposure, complex or sheet

⊘ **20924**   Tendon graft, from a distance (eg, palmaris, toe extensor, plantaris)

⊘ **20926**   Tissue grafts, other (eg, paratenon, fat, dermis)

(Codes 20930-20938 are reported in addition to codes for the definitive procedure(s) without modifier 51)

⊘ **20930**   Allograft for spine surgery only; morselized

⊘ **20931**   structural

⊘ **20936**   Autograft for spine surgery only (includes harvesting the graft); local (eg, ribs, spinous process, or laminar fragments) obtained from same incision

⊘ **20937**   morselized (through separate skin or fascial incision)

⊘ **20938**   structural, bicortical or tricortical (through separate skin or fascial incision)

(For needle aspiration of bone marrow for the purpose of bone grafting, use 38220)

Other Procedures

20950   Monitoring of interstitial fluid pressure (includes insertion of device, eg, wick catheter technique, needle manometer technique) in detection of muscle compartment syndrome

20955   Bone graft with microvascular anastomosis; fibula

20956   iliac crest

20957   metatarsal

20962   other than fibula, iliac crest, or metatarsal

(Do not report code 69990 in addition to codes 20955-20962)

Surgery: Musculoskeletal System

20969 Free osteocutaneous flap with microvascular anastomosis; other than iliac crest, metatarsal, or great toe

20970 iliac crest

20972 metatarsal

20973 great toe with web space

(Do not report code 69990 in addition to codes 20969-20973)

(For great toe, wrap-around procedure, use 26551)

⊘ **20974** Electrical stimulation to aid bone healing; noninvasive (nonoperative)

⊘ **20975** invasive (operative)

20979 Low intensity ultrasound stimulation to aid bone healing, noninvasive (nonoperative)

⊙ **20982** Ablation, bone tumor(s) (eg, osteoid osteoma, metastasis) radiofrequency, percutaneous, including computed tomographic guidance

20999 Unlisted procedure, musculoskeletal system, general

Head

Skull, facial bones and temporomandibular joint.

Incision

(For drainage of superficial abscess and hematoma, use 20000)

(For removal of embedded foreign body from dentoalveolar structure, see 41805, 41806)

21010 Arthrotomy, temporomandibular joint

(To report bilateral procedures, report 21010 with modifier 50)

Excision

21015 Radical resection of tumor (eg, malignant neoplasm), soft tissue of face or scalp

(To report excision of skull tumor for osteomyelitis, use 61501)

21025 Excision of bone (eg, for osteomyelitis or bone abscess); mandible

21026 facial bone(s)

21029 Removal by contouring of benign tumor of facial bone (eg, fibrous dysplasia)

21030 Excision of benign tumor or cyst of maxilla or zygoma by enucleation and curettage

21031 Excision of torus mandibularis

21032 Excision of maxillary torus palatinus

21034 Excision of malignant tumor of maxilla or zygoma

21040 Excision of benign tumor or cyst of mandible, by enucleation and/or curettage

(21041 has been deleted)

(For enucleation and/or curettage of benign cysts or tumors of mandible not requiring osteotomy, use 21040)

(For excision of benign tumor or cyst of mandible requiring osteotomy, see 21046-21047)

21044 Excision of malignant tumor of mandible;

21045 radical resection

(For bone graft, use 21215)

21046 Excision of benign tumor or cyst of mandible; requiring intra-oral osteotomy (eg, locally aggressive or destructive lesion(s))

21047 requiring extra-oral osteotomy and partial mandibulectomy (eg, locally aggressive or destructive lesion(s))

21048 Excision of benign tumor or cyst of maxilla; requiring intra-oral osteotomy (eg, locally aggressive or destructive lesion(s))

21049 requiring extra-oral osteotomy and partial maxillectomy (eg, locally aggressive or destructive lesion(s))

21050 Condylectomy, temporomandibular joint (separate procedure)

(For bilateral procedures, report 21050 with modifier 50)

21060 Meniscectomy, partial or complete, temporomandibular joint (separate procedure)

(For bilateral procedures, report 21060 with modifier 50)

21070 Coronoidectomy (separate procedure)

(For bilateral procedures, report 21070 with modifier 50)

Introduction or Removal

(For application or removal of caliper or tongs, see 20660, 20665.) Codes 21076-21089 describe professional services for the rehabilitation of patients with oral, facial or other anatomical deficiencies by means of prostheses such as an artificial eye, ear, or nose or intraoral obturator to close a cleft. Codes 21076-21089 should only be used when the physician actually designs and prepares the prosthesis (ie, not prepared by an outside laboratory).

21076 Impression and custom preparation; surgical obturator prosthesis

21077 orbital prosthesis

21079 interim obturator prosthesis

21080 definitive obturator prosthesis

21081 mandibular resection prosthesis

21082 palatal augmentation prosthesis

21083	palatal lift prosthesis	

21083   palatal lift prosthesis

21084   speech aid prosthesis

21085   oral surgical splint

21086   auricular prosthesis

21087   nasal prosthesis

21088   facial prosthesis

21089   Unlisted maxillofacial prosthetic procedure

21100   Application of halo type appliance for maxillofacial fixation, includes removal (separate procedure)

21110   Application of interdental fixation device for conditions other than fracture or dislocation, includes removal

      (For removal of interdental fixation by another physician, see 20670-20680)

21116   Injection procedure for temporomandibular joint arthrography

      (For radiological supervision and interpretation, use 70332. Do not report 76003 in addition to 70332)

Repair, Revision, and/or Reconstruction

      (For cranioplasty, see 21179, 21180 and 62116, 62120, 62140-62147)

21120   Genioplasty; augmentation (autograft, allograft, prosthetic material)

21121   sliding osteotomy, single piece

21122   sliding osteotomies, two or more osteotomies (eg, wedge excision or bone wedge reversal for asymmetrical chin)

21123   sliding, augmentation with interpositional bone grafts (includes obtaining autografts)

21125   Augmentation, mandibular body or angle; prosthetic material

21127   with bone graft, onlay or interpositional (includes obtaining autograft)

21137   Reduction forehead; contouring only

21138   contouring and application of prosthetic material or bone graft (includes obtaining autograft)

21139   contouring and setback of anterior frontal sinus wall

21141   Reconstruction midface, LeFort I; single piece, segment movement in any direction (eg, for Long Face Syndrome), without bone graft

21142   two pieces, segment movement in any direction, without bone graft

21143   three or more pieces, segment movement in any direction, without bone graft

21145   single piece, segment movement in any direction, requiring bone grafts (includes obtaining autografts)

21146   two pieces, segment movement in any direction, requiring bone grafts (includes obtaining autografts) (eg, ungrafted unilateral alveolar cleft)

21147   three or more pieces, segment movement in any direction, requiring bone grafts (includes obtaining autografts) (eg, ungrafted bilateral alveolar cleft or multiple osteotomies)

21150   Reconstruction midface, LeFort II; anterior intrusion (eg, Treacher-Collins Syndrome)

21151   any direction, requiring bone grafts (includes obtaining autografts)

21154   Reconstruction midface, LeFort III (extracranial), any type, requiring bone grafts (includes obtaining autografts); without LeFort I

21155   with LeFort I

21159   Reconstruction midface, LeFort III (extra and intracranial) with forehead advancement (eg, mono bloc), requiring bone grafts (includes obtaining autografts); without LeFort I

21160   with LeFort I

21172   Reconstruction superior-lateral orbital rim and lower forehead, advancement or alteration, with or without grafts (includes obtaining autografts)

      (For frontal or parietal craniotomy performed for craniosynostosis, use 61556)

21175   Reconstruction, bifrontal, superior-lateral orbital rims and lower forehead, advancement or alteration (eg, plagiocephaly, trigonocephaly, brachycephaly), with or without grafts (includes obtaining autografts)

      (For bifrontal craniotomy performed for craniosynostosis, use 61557)

21179   Reconstruction, entire or majority of forehead and/or supraorbital rims; with grafts (allograft or prosthetic material)

21180   with autograft (includes obtaining grafts)

      (For extensive craniectomy for multiple suture craniosynostosis, use only 61558 or 61559)

21181   Reconstruction by contouring of benign tumor of cranial bones (eg, fibrous dysplasia), extracranial

21182   Reconstruction of orbital walls, rims, forehead, nasoethmoid complex following intra- and extracranial excision of benign tumor of cranial bone (eg, fibrous dysplasia), with multiple autografts (includes obtaining grafts); total area of bone grafting less than 40 sq cm

21183   total area of bone grafting greater than 40 sq cm but less than 80 sq cm

21184   total area of bone grafting greater than 80 sq cm

      (For excision of benign tumor of cranial bones, see 61563, 61564)

Surgery: Musculoskeletal System

21188   Reconstruction midface, osteotomies (other than LeFort type) and bone grafts (includes obtaining autografts)

21193   Reconstruction of mandibular rami, horizontal, vertical, C, or L osteotomy; without bone graft

21194   with bone graft (includes obtaining graft)

21195   Reconstruction of mandibular rami and/or body, sagittal split; without internal rigid fixation

21196   with internal rigid fixation

21198   Osteotomy, mandible, segmental;

21199   with genioglossus advancement

(To report total osteotomy of the maxilla, see 21141-21160)

21206   Osteotomy, maxilla, segmental (eg, Wassmund or Schuchard)

21208   Osteoplasty, facial bones; augmentation (autograft, allograft, or prosthetic implant)

21209   reduction

21210   Graft, bone; nasal, maxillary or malar areas (includes obtaining graft)

(For cleft palate repair, see 42200-42225)

21215   mandible (includes obtaining graft)

21230   Graft; rib cartilage, autogenous, to face, chin, nose or ear (includes obtaining graft)

21235   ear cartilage, autogenous, to nose or ear (includes obtaining graft)

(To report graft augmentation of facial bones, use 21208)

21240   Arthroplasty, temporomandibular joint, with or without autograft (includes obtaining graft)

21242   Arthroplasty, temporomandibular joint, with allograft

21243   Arthroplasty, temporomandibular joint, with prosthetic joint replacement

21244   Reconstruction of mandible, extraoral, with transosteal bone plate (eg, mandibular staple bone plate)

21245   Reconstruction of mandible or maxilla, subperiosteal implant; partial

21246   complete

21247   Reconstruction of mandibular condyle with bone and cartilage autografts (includes obtaining grafts) (eg, for hemifacial microsomia)

21248   Reconstruction of mandible or maxilla, endosteal implant (eg, blade, cylinder); partial

21249   complete

(To report midface reconstruction, see 21141-21160)

21255   Reconstruction of zygomatic arch and glenoid fossa with bone and cartilage (includes obtaining autografts)

21256   Reconstruction of orbit with osteotomies (extracranial) and with bone grafts (includes obtaining autografts) (eg, micro-ophthalmia)

21260   Periorbital osteotomies for orbital hypertelorism, with bone grafts; extracranial approach

21261   combined intra- and extracranial approach

21263   with forehead advancement

21267   Orbital repositioning, periorbital osteotomies, unilateral, with bone grafts; extracranial approach

21268   combined intra- and extracranial approach

21270   Malar augmentation, prosthetic material

(For malar augmentation with bone graft, use 21210)

21275   Secondary revision of orbitocraniofacial reconstruction

21280   Medial canthopexy (separate procedure)

(For medial canthoplasty, use 67950)

21282   Lateral canthopexy

21295   Reduction of masseter muscle and bone (eg, for treatment of benign masseteric hypertrophy); extraoral approach

21296   intraoral approach

Other Procedures

21299   Unlisted craniofacial and maxillofacial procedure

Fracture and/or Dislocation

21300   Closed treatment of skull fracture without operation

(For operative repair, see 62000-62010)

21310   Closed treatment of nasal bone fracture without manipulation

21315   Closed treatment of nasal bone fracture; without stabilization

21320   with stabilization

21325   Open treatment of nasal fracture; uncomplicated

21330   complicated, with internal and/or external skeletal fixation

21335   with concomitant open treatment of fractured septum

21336   Open treatment of nasal septal fracture, with or without stabilization

21337   Closed treatment of nasal septal fracture, with or without stabilization

21338   Open treatment of nasoethmoid fracture; without external fixation

21339   with external fixation

21340   Percutaneous treatment of nasoethmoid complex fracture, with splint, wire or headcap fixation, including repair of canthal ligaments and/or the nasolacrimal apparatus

21343   Open treatment of depressed frontal sinus fracture

21344   Open treatment of complicated (eg, comminuted or involving posterior wall) frontal sinus fracture, via coronal or multiple approaches

21345   Closed treatment of nasomaxillary complex fracture (LeFort II type), with interdental wire fixation or fixation of denture or splint

21346   Open treatment of nasomaxillary complex fracture (LeFort II type); with wiring and/or local fixation

21347   requiring multiple open approaches

21348   with bone grafting (includes obtaining graft)

21355   Percutaneous treatment of fracture of malar area, including zygomatic arch and malar tripod, with manipulation

21356   Open treatment of depressed zygomatic arch fracture (eg, Gillies approach)

21360   Open treatment of depressed malar fracture, including zygomatic arch and malar tripod

21365   Open treatment of complicated (eg, comminuted or involving cranial nerve foramina) fracture(s) of malar area, including zygomatic arch and malar tripod; with internal fixation and multiple surgical approaches

21366   with bone grafting (includes obtaining graft)

21385   Open treatment of orbital floor blowout fracture; transantral approach (Caldwell-Luc type operation)

21386   periorbital approach

21387   combined approach

21390   periorbital approach, with alloplastic or other implant

21395   periorbital approach with bone graft (includes obtaining graft)

21400   Closed treatment of fracture of orbit, except blowout; without manipulation

21401   with manipulation

21406   Open treatment of fracture of orbit, except blowout; without implant

21407   with implant

21408   with bone grafting (includes obtaining graft)

21421   Closed treatment of palatal or maxillary fracture (LeFort I type), with interdental wire fixation or fixation of denture or splint

21422   Open treatment of palatal or maxillary fracture (LeFort I type);

21423   complicated (comminuted or involving cranial nerve foramina), multiple approaches

21431   Closed treatment of craniofacial separation (LeFort III type) using interdental wire fixation of denture or splint

21432   Open treatment of craniofacial separation (LeFort III type); with wiring and/or internal fixation

21433   complicated (eg, comminuted or involving cranial nerve foramina), multiple surgical approaches

21435   complicated, utilizing internal and/or external fixation techniques (eg, head cap, halo device, and/or intermaxillary fixation)

(For removal of internal or external fixation device, use 20670)

21436   complicated, multiple surgical approaches, internal fixation, with bone grafting (includes obtaining graft)

21440   Closed treatment of mandibular or maxillary alveolar ridge fracture (separate procedure)

21445   Open treatment of mandibular or maxillary alveolar ridge fracture (separate procedure)

21450   Closed treatment of mandibular fracture; without manipulation

21451   with manipulation

21452   Percutaneous treatment of mandibular fracture, with external fixation

21453   Closed treatment of mandibular fracture with interdental fixation

21454   Open treatment of mandibular fracture with external fixation

21461   Open treatment of mandibular fracture; without interdental fixation

21462   with interdental fixation

21465   Open treatment of mandibular condylar fracture

21470   Open treatment of complicated mandibular fracture by multiple surgical approaches including internal fixation, interdental fixation, and/or wiring of dentures or splints

21480   Closed treatment of temporomandibular dislocation; initial or subsequent

21485   complicated (eg, recurrent requiring intermaxillary fixation or splinting), initial or subsequent

21490   Open treatment of temporomandibular dislocation

(For interdental wire fixation, use 21497)

21493   Closed treatment of hyoid fracture; without manipulation

21494   with manipulation

21495   Open treatment of hyoid fracture

(For treatment of fracture of larynx, see 31584-31586)

21497   Interdental wiring, for condition other than fracture

Other Procedures

21499   Unlisted musculoskeletal procedure, head

(For unlisted craniofacial or maxillofacial procedure, use 21299)

Surgery: Musculoskeletal System

Neck (Soft Tissues) and Thorax

(For cervical spine and back, see 21920 et seq)

(For injection of fracture site or trigger point, use 20550)

Incision

(For incision and drainage of abscess or hematoma, superficial, see 10060, 10140)

21501   Incision and drainage, deep abscess or hematoma, soft tissues of neck or thorax;

21502   with partial rib ostectomy

21510   Incision, deep, with opening of bone cortex (eg, for osteomyelitis or bone abscess), thorax

Excision

(For bone biopsy, see 20220-20251)

21550   Biopsy, soft tissue of neck or thorax

(For needle biopsy of soft tissue, use 20206)

21555   Excision tumor, soft tissue of neck or thorax; subcutaneous

21556   deep, subfascial, intramuscular

21557   Radical resection of tumor (eg, malignant neoplasm), soft tissue of neck or thorax

21600   Excision of rib, partial

(For radical resection of chest wall and rib cage for tumor, use 19260)

(For radical debridement of chest wall and rib cage for injury, see 11040-11044)

21610   Costotransversectomy (separate procedure)

21615   Excision first and/or cervical rib;

21616   with sympathectomy

21620   Ostectomy of sternum, partial

21627   Sternal debridement

(For debridement and closure, use 21750)

21630   Radical resection of sternum;

21632   with mediastinal lymphadenectomy

Repair, Revision, and/or Reconstruction

(For superficial wound, see **Integumentary System** section under Repair—Simple)

21685   Hyoid myotomy and suspension

21700   Division of scalenus anticus; without resection of cervical rib

21705   with resection of cervical rib

21720   Division of sternocleidomastoid for torticollis, open operation; without cast application

(For transection of spinal accessory and cervical nerves, see 63191, 64722)

21725   with cast application

21740   Reconstructive repair of pectus excavatum or carinatum; open

21742   minimally invasive approach (Nuss procedure), without thoracoscopy

21743   minimally invasive approach (Nuss procedure), with thoracoscopy

21750   Closure of median sternotomy separation with or without debridement (separate procedure)

Fracture and/or Dislocation

21800   Closed treatment of rib fracture, uncomplicated, each

21805   Open treatment of rib fracture without fixation, each

21810   Treatment of rib fracture requiring external fixation (flail chest)

21820   Closed treatment of sternum fracture

21825   Open treatment of sternum fracture with or without skeletal fixation

(For sternoclavicular dislocation, see 23520-23532)

Other Procedures

21899   Unlisted procedure, neck or thorax

Back and Flank

Excision

21920   Biopsy, soft tissue of back or flank; superficial

21925   deep

(For needle biopsy of soft tissue, use 20206)

21930   Excision, tumor, soft tissue of back or flank

21935   Radical resection of tumor (eg, malignant neoplasm), soft tissue of back or flank

Spine (Vertebral Column)

Cervical, thoracic, and lumbar spine.

Within the SPINE section, bone grafting procedures are reported separately and in addition to arthrodesis. For bone grafts in other Musculoskeletal sections, see specific code(s) descriptor(s) and/or accompanying guidelines.

To report bone grafts performed after arthrodesis, see codes 20930-20938. Bone graft codes are reported without modifier 51 (multiple procedure). Do not append modifier 62 to bone graft codes 20900-20938.

Example:

Posterior arthrodesis of L5-S1 for degenerative disc disease utilizing morselized autogenous iliac bone graft harvested through a separate fascial incision.

Report as 22612 and 20937.

Within the SPINE section, instrumentation is reported separately and in addition to arthrodesis. To report instrumentation procedures performed with definitive vertebral procedure(s), see codes 22840-22855. Instrumentation procedure codes 22840-22848 and 22851 are reported in addition to the definitive procedure(s) without modifier 51. Modifier 62 may not be appended to the definitive or add-on spinal instrumentation procedure code(s) 22840-22848 and 22850-22852.

Example:

Posterior arthrodesis of L4-S1, utilizing morselized autogenous iliac bone graft harvested through separate fascial incision, and pedicle screw fixation.

Report as 22612, 22614, 22842, and 20937.

Vertebral procedures are sometimes followed by arthrodesis and in addition may include bone grafts and instrumentation.

When arthrodesis is performed in addition to another procedure, the arthrodesis should be reported in addition to the original procedure with modifier 51 (multiple procedures). Examples are after osteotomy, fracture care, vertebral corpectomy and laminectomy. Since bone grafts and instrumentation are never performed without arthrodesis, modifier 51 (multiple procedures) is not used.

Arthrodesis, however, may be performed in the absence of other procedures and therefore when it is combined with another definitive procedure, modifier 51 (multiple procedure) is appropriate.

Example:

Treatment of a burst fracture of L2 by corpec tomy followed by arthrodesis of L1-L3, utilizing anterior instrumentation L1-L3 and structural allograft.

Report as 63090, 22558-51, 22585, 22845, and 20931.

When two surgeons work together as primary surgeons performing distinct part(s) of a single reportable procedure, each surgeon should report his/her distinct operative work by appending modifier 62 to the single definitive procedure code. If additional procedure(s) (including add-on procedure(s)) are performed during the same surgical session, separate code(s) may be reported by each co-surgeon, with modifier 62 appended (see Appendix A).

Example:

A 42-year-old male with a history of posttraumatic degenerative disc disease at L3-4 and L4-5 (internal disc disruption) underwent surgical repair. Surgeon A performed an anterior exposure of the spine with mobilization of the great vessels. Surgeon B performed anterior (minimal) diskectomy and fusion at L3-4 and L4-5 using anterior interbody technique.

Report surgeon A: 22558 append modifier 62, 22585 append modifier 62
Report surgeon B: 22558 append modifier 62, 22585 append modifier 62, 20931

> (Do not append modifier 62 to bone graft code 20931)
>
> (For injection procedure for myelography, use 62284)
>
> (For injection procedure for diskography, see 62290, 62291)
>
> (For injection procedure, chemonucleolysis, single or multiple levels, use 62292)
>
> (For injection procedure for facet joints, see 64470-64476, 64622-64627)
>
> (For needle or trocar biopsy, see 20220-20225)

Excision

For the following codes, when two surgeons work together as primary surgeons performing distinct part(s) of partial vertebral body excision, each surgeon should report his/her distinct operative work by appending modifier 62 to the procedure code. In this situation, modifier 62 may be appended to the procedure code(s) 22100-22102, 22110-22114 and, as appropriate, to the associated additional vertebral segment add-on code(s) 22103, 22116 as long as both surgeons continue to work together as primary surgeons.

> (For bone biopsy, see 20220-20251)
>
> (To report soft tissue biopsy of back or flank, see 21920-21925)
>
> (For needle biopsy of soft tissue, use 20206)
>
> (To report excision of soft tissue tumor of back or flank, use 21930)

22100	Partial excision of posterior vertebral component (eg, spinous process, lamina or facet) for intrinsic bony lesion, single vertebral segment; cervical
22101	thoracic
22102	lumbar
+ 22103	each additional segment (List separately in addition to code for primary procedure)

> (Use 22103 in conjunction with 22100, 22101, 22102)

Surgery: Musculoskeletal System

22110   Partial excision of vertebral body, for intrinsic bony lesion, without decompression of spinal cord or nerve root(s), single vertebral segment; cervical

22112   thoracic

22114   lumbar

+ 22116   each additional vertebral segment (List separately in addition to code for primary procedure)

(Use 22116 in conjunction with 22110, 22112, 22114)

(For complete or near complete resection of vertebral body, see vertebral corpectomy, 63081-63091)

(For spinal reconstruction with bone graft (autograft, allograft) and/or methylmethacrylate of cervical vertebral body, use 63081 and 22554 and 20931 or 20938)

(For spinal reconstruction with bone graft (autograft, allograft) and/or methylmethacrylate of thoracic vertebral body, use 63085 or 63087 and 22556 and 20931 or 20938)

(For spinal reconstruction with bone graft (autograft, allograft) and/or methylmethacrylate of lumbar vertebral body, use 63087 or 63090 and 22558 and 20931 or 20938)

(For spinal reconstruction following vertebral body resection, use 63082 or 63086 or 63088 or 63091, and 22585)

(For harvest of bone autograft for vertebral reconstruction, see 20931 or 20938)

(For cervical spinal reconstruction with prosthetic replacement of resected vertebral bodies, see codes 63081 and 22554 and 20931 or 20938 and 22851)

(For thoracic spinal reconstruction with prosthetic replacement of resected vertebral bodies, see codes 63085 or 63087 and 22556 and 20931 or 20938 and 22851)

(For lumbar spinal reconstruction with prosthetic replacement of resected vertebral bodies, see codes 63087 or 63090 and 22558, and 20931 or 20938 and 22851)

(For osteotomy of spine, see 22210-22226)

Osteotomy

To report arthrodesis, see codes 22590-22632. (Report in addition to code(s) for the definitive procedure with modifier 51.)

To report instrumentation procedures, see codes 22840-22855. (Report in addition to code(s) for the definitive procedure(s) without modifier 51.) Do not append modifier 62 to spinal instrumentation codes 22840-22848 and 22850-22852.

To report bone graft procedures, see codes 20930-20938. (Report in addition to code(s) for the definitive procedure(s) without modifier 51.) Do not append modifier 62 to bone graft codes 20900-20938.

For the following codes, when two surgeons work together as primary surgeons performing distinct part(s) of an anterior spine osteotomy, each surgeon should report his/her distinct operative work by appending modifier 62 to the procedure code. In this situation, modifier 62 may be appended to the procedure code(s) 22210-22214, 22220-22224 and, as appropriate, to associated additional segment add-on code(s) 22216, 22226 as long as both surgeons continue to work together as primary surgeons.

22210   Osteotomy of spine, posterior or posterolateral approach, one vertebral segment; cervical

22212   thoracic

22214   lumbar

+ 22216   each additional vertebral segment (List separately in addition to primary procedure)

(Use 22216 in conjunction with 22210, 22212, 22214)

22220   Osteotomy of spine, including diskectomy, anterior approach, single vertebral segment; cervical

22222   thoracic

22224   lumbar

+ 22226   each additional vertebral segment (List separately in addition to code for primary procedure)

(Use 22226 in conjunction with 22220, 22222, 22224)

(For vertebral corpectomy, see 63081-63091)

Fracture and/or Dislocation

To report arthrodesis, see codes 22590-22632. (Report in addition to code(s) for the definitive procedure with modifier 51.)

To report instrumentation procedures, see codes 22840-22855. (Report in addition to code(s) for the definitive procedure(s) without modifier 51.) Do not append modifier 62 to spinal instrumentation codes 22840-22848 and 22850-22852.

To report bone graft procedures, see codes 20930-20938. (Report in addition to code(s) for the definitive procedure(s) without modifier 51.) Do not append modifier 62 to bone graft codes 20900-20938.

For the following codes, when two surgeons work together as primary surgeons performing distinct part(s) of open fracture and/or dislocation procedure(s), each surgeon should report his/her distinct operative work by appending modifier 62 to the procedure code. In this situation, modifier 62 may be appended to the procedure code(s) 22318-22327 and, as appropriate, the associated additional fracture vertebrae or dislocated segment add-on code 22328 as long as both surgeons continue to work together as primary surgeons.

22305	Closed treatment of vertebral process fracture(s)
22310	Closed treatment of vertebral body fracture(s), without manipulation, requiring and including casting or bracing
22315	Closed treatment of vertebral fracture(s) and/or dislocation(s) requiring casting or bracing, with and including casting and/or bracing, with or without anesthesia, by manipulation or traction

(For spinal subluxation, use 97140)

22318	Open treatment and/or reduction of odontoid fracture(s) and or dislocation(s) (including os odontoideum), anterior approach, including placement of internal fixation; without grafting
22319	with grafting
22325	Open treatment and/or reduction of vertebral fracture(s) and/or dislocation(s), posterior approach, one fractured vertebrae or dislocated segment; lumbar
22326	cervical
22327	thoracic
+ 22328	each additional fractured vertebrae or dislocated segment (List separately in addition to code for primary procedure)

(Use 22328 in conjunction with 22325, 22326, 22327)

(For treatment of vertebral fracture by the anterior approach, see corpectomy 63081-63091, and appropriate arthrodesis, bone graft and instrument codes)

(For decompression of spine following fracture, see 63001-63091; for arthrodesis of spine following fracture, see 22548-22632)

Manipulation

(For spinal manipulation without anesthesia, use 97140)

22505	Manipulation of spine requiring anesthesia, any region

Vertebral Body, Embolization or Injection

22520	Percutaneous vertebroplasty, one vertebral body, unilateral or bilateral injection; thoracic
22521	lumbar
+ 22522	each additional thoracic or lumbar vertebral body (List separately in addition to code for primary procedure)

(Use 22522 in conjunction with 22520, 22521 as appropriate)

(For radiological supervision and interpretation, see 76012, 76013)

Lateral Extracavitary Approach Technique

22532	Arthrodesis, lateral extracavitary technique, including minimal diskectomy to prepare interspace (other than for decompression); thoracic
22533	lumbar
+ 22534	thoracic or lumbar, each additional vertebral segment (List separately in addition to code for primary procedure)

(Use 22534 in conjunction with 22532 and 22533)

Arthrodesis

Arthrodesis may be performed in the absence of other procedures and therefore when it is combined with another definitive procedure (eg, osteotomy, fracture care, vertebral corpectomy or laminectomy), modifier 51 is appropriate. However, arthrodesis codes 22585, 22614, and 22632 are considered add-on procedure codes and should not be used with modifier 51.

▶To report instrumentation procedures, see 22840-22855. (Codes 22840-22848, 22851 are reported in conjunction with code(s) for the definitive procedure(s) without modifier 51. When instrumentation reinsertion or removal is reported in conjunction with other definitive procedures including arthrodesis, decompression, and exploration of fusion, append modifier 51 to 22849, 22850, 22852, and 22855.) To report exploration of fusion, use 22830. (When exploration is reported in conjunction with other definitive procedures, including arthrodesis and decompression, append modifier 51 to 22830.) Do not append modifier 62 to spinal instrumentation codes 22840-22848 and 22850-22852.◀

To report bone graft procedures, see codes 20930-20938. (Report in addition to code(s) for the definitive procedure(s) without modifier 51.) Do not append modifier 62 to bone graft codes 20900-20938.

Anterior or Anterolateral Approach Technique

Procedure codes 22554-22558 are for SINGLE interspace; for additional interspaces, use 22585. A vertebral interspace is the non-bony compartment between two adjacent vertebral bodies, which contains the intervertebral disk, and includes the nucleus pulposus, annulus fibrosus, and two cartilagenous endplates.

For the following codes, when two surgeons work together as primary surgeons performing distinct part(s) of an anterior interbody arthrodesis, each surgeon should report his/her distinct operative work by appending

Surgery: Musculoskeletal System

Surgery: Musculoskeletal System

modifier 62 to the procedure code. In this situation, modifier 62 may be appended to the procedure code(s) 22548-22558 and, as appropriate, to the associated additional interspace add-on code 22585 as long as both surgeons continue to work together as primary surgeons.

22548 Arthrodesis, anterior transoral or extraoral technique, clivus-C1-C2 (atlas-axis), with or without excision of odontoid process

(For intervertebral disk excision by laminotomy or laminectomy, see 63020-63042)

22554 Arthrodesis, anterior interbody technique, including minimal diskectomy to prepare interspace (other than for decompression); cervical below C2

22556 thoracic

22558 lumbar

+ 22585 each additional interspace (List separately in addition to code for primary procedure)

(Use 22585 in conjunction with 22554, 22556, 22558)

Posterior, Posterolateral or Lateral Transverse Process Technique

To report instrumentation procedures, see codes 22840-22855. (Report in addition to code(s) for the definitive procedure(s) without modifier 51.) Do not append modifier 62 to spinal instrumentation codes 22840-22848 and 22850-22852.

To report bone graft procedures, see codes 20930-20938. (Report in addition to code(s) for the definitive procedure(s) without modifier 51.) Do not append modifier 62 to bone graft codes 20900-20938.

A vertebral segment describes the basic constituent part into which the spine may be divided. It represents a single complete vertebral bone with its associated articular processes and laminae. A vertebral interspace is the non-bony compartment between two adjacent vertebral bodies which contains the intervertebral disk, and includes the nucleus pulposus, annulus fibrosus, and two cartilagenous endplates.

22590 Arthrodesis, posterior technique, craniocervical (occiput-C2)

22595 Arthrodesis, posterior technique, atlas-axis (C1-C2)

22600 Arthrodesis, posterior or posterolateral technique, single level; cervical below C2 segment

22610 thoracic (with or without lateral transverse technique)

22612 lumbar (with or without lateral transverse technique)

+ 22614 each additional vertebral segment (List separately in addition to code for primary procedure)

(Use 22614 in conjunction with 22600, 22610, 22612)

22630 Arthrodesis, posterior interbody technique, including laminectomy and/or diskectomy to prepare interspace (other than for decompression), single interspace; lumbar

+ 22632 each additional interspace (List separately in addition to code for primary procedure)

(Use 22632 in conjunction with 22630)

Spine Deformity (eg, Scoliosis, Kyphosis)

To report instrumentation procedures, see codes 22840-22855. (Report in addition to code(s) for the definitive procedure(s) without modifier 51.) Do not append modifier 62 to spinal instrumentation codes 22840-22848 and 22850-22852.

To report bone graft procedures, see codes 20930-20938. (Report in addition to code(s) for the definitive procedure(s) without modifier 51.) Do not append modifier 62 to bone graft codes 20900-20938.

A vertebral segment describes the basic constituent part into which the spine may be divided. It represents a single complete vertebral bone with its associated articular processes and laminae.

For the following codes, when two surgeons work together as primary surgeons performing distinct part(s) of an arthrodesis for spinal deformity, each surgeon should report his/her distinct operative work by appending modifier 62 to the procedure code. In this situation, modifier 62 may be appended to procedure code(s) 22800-22819 as long as both surgeons continue to work together as primary surgeons.

22800 Arthrodesis, posterior, for spinal deformity, with or without cast; up to 6 vertebral segments

22802 7 to 12 vertebral segments

22804 13 or more vertebral segments

22808 Arthrodesis, anterior, for spinal deformity, with or without cast; 2 to 3 vertebral segments

22810 4 to 7 vertebral segments

22812 8 or more vertebral segments

22818 Kyphectomy, circumferential exposure of spine and resection of vertebral segment(s) (including body and posterior elements); single or 2 segments

22819 3 or more segments

(To report arthrodesis, see 22800-22804 and add modifier 51)

Exploration

▶To report instrumentation procedures, see 22840-22855. (Codes 22840-22848, 22851 are reported in conjunction with code(s) for the definitive procedure(s) without modifier 51. When instrumentation reinsertion or removal is reported in conjunction with other definitive procedures including arthrodesis, decompression, and exploration of fusion, append modifier 51 to 22849, 22850, 22852 and 22855.) To report exploration of fusion, see 22830. (When exploration is reported in conjunction with other definitive procedures, including arthrodesis and decompression, append modifier 51 to 22830.)◄

(To report bone graft procedures, see 20930-20938)

22830   Exploration of spinal fusion

Spinal Instrumentation

Segmental instrumentation is defined as fixation at each end of the construct and at least one additional interposed bony attachment.

Non-segmental instrumentation is defined as fixation at each end of the construct and may span several vertebral segments without attachment to the intervening segments.

Insertion of spinal instrumentation is reported separately and in addition to arthrodesis. Instrumentation procedure codes 22840-22848, 22851 are reported in addition to the definitive procedure(s) without modifier 51. Do not append modifier 62 to spinal instrumentation codes 22840-22848 and 22850-22852.

To report bone graft procedures, see codes 20930-20938. (Report in addition to code(s) for definitive procedure(s) without modifier 51.) Do not append modifier 62 to bone graft codes 20900-20938.

A vertebral segment describes the basic constituent part into which the spine may be divided. It represents a single complete vertebral bone with its associated articular processes and laminae. A vertebral interspace is the non-bony compartment between two adjacent vertebral bodies, which contains the intervertebral disk, and includes the nucleus pulposus, annulus fibrosus, and two cartilagenous endplates.

►List 22840-22855 separately, in conjunction with code(s) for fracture, dislocation, arthrodesis or exploration of fusion of the spine 22325-22328, 22548-22812, and 22830. Codes 22840-22848, 22851 are reported in conjunction with code(s) for the definitive procedure(s) without modifier 51. Codes 22849, 22850, 22852, and 22855 are subject to modifier 51 if reported with other definitive procedure(s), including arthrodesis, decompression, and exploration of fusion. Code 22849 should not be reported with 22850, 22852, and 22855 at the same spinal levels.◄

⊘ **22840**   Posterior non-segmental instrumentation (eg, Harrington rod technique, pedicle fixation across one interspace, atlantoaxial transarticular screw fixation, sublaminar wiring at C1, facet screw fixation)

⊘ **22841**   Internal spinal fixation by wiring of spinous processes

⊘ **22842**   Posterior segmental instrumentation (eg, pedicle fixation, dual rods with multiple hooks and sublaminar wires); 3 to 6 vertebral segments

⊘ **22843**   7 to 12 vertebral segments

⊘ **22844**   13 or more vertebral segments

⊘ **22845**   Anterior instrumentation; 2 to 3 vertebral segments

⊘ **22846**   4 to 7 vertebral segments

⊘ **22847**   8 or more vertebral segments

⊘ **22848**   Pelvic fixation (attachment of caudal end of instrumentation to pelvic bony structures) other than sacrum

22849   Reinsertion of spinal fixation device

22850   Removal of posterior nonsegmental instrumentation (eg, Harrington rod)

⊘ **22851**   Application of intervertebral biomechanical device(s) (eg, synthetic cage(s), threaded bone dowel(s), methylmethacrylate) to vertebral defect or interspace

22852   Removal of posterior segmental instrumentation

22855   Removal of anterior instrumentation

Other Procedures

22899   Unlisted procedure, spine

Abdomen

Excision

22900   Excision, abdominal wall tumor, subfascial (eg, desmoid)

Other Procedures

22999   Unlisted procedure, abdomen, musculoskeletal system

Shoulder

Clavicle, scapula, humerus head and neck, sterno-clavicular joint, acromioclavicular joint and shoulder joint.

Incision

23000   Removal of subdeltoid calcareous deposits, open

(For arthroscopic removal of bursal deposits, use 29999)

23020   Capsular contracture release (eg, Sever type procedure)

(For incision and drainage procedures, superficial, see 10040-10160)

23030   Incision and drainage, shoulder area; deep abscess or hematoma

23031   infected bursa

Surgery: Musculoskeletal System

23035 Incision, bone cortex (eg, osteomyelitis or bone abscess), shoulder area

23040 Arthrotomy, glenohumeral joint, including exploration, drainage, or removal of foreign body

23044 Arthrotomy, acromioclavicular, sternoclavicular joint, including exploration, drainage, or removal of foreign body

Excision

23065 Biopsy, soft tissue of shoulder area; superficial

23066 deep

(For needle biopsy of soft tissue, use 20206)

23075 Excision, soft tissue tumor, shoulder area; subcutaneous

23076 deep, subfascial, or intramuscular

23077 Radical resection of tumor (eg, malignant neoplasm), soft tissue of shoulder area

23100 Arthrotomy, glenohumeral joint, including biopsy

23101 Arthrotomy, acromioclavicular joint or sternoclavicular joint, including biopsy and/or excision of torn cartilage

23105 Arthrotomy; glenohumeral joint, with synovectomy, with or without biopsy

23106 sternoclavicular joint, with synovectomy, with or without biopsy

23107 Arthrotomy, glenohumeral joint, with joint exploration, with or without removal of loose or foreign body

23120 Claviculectomy; partial

(For arthroscopic procedure, use 29824)

23125 total

23130 Acromioplasty or acromionectomy, partial, with or without coracoacromial ligament release

23140 Excision or curettage of bone cyst or benign tumor of clavicle or scapula;

23145 with autograft (includes obtaining graft)

23146 with allograft

23150 Excision or curettage of bone cyst or benign tumor of proximal humerus;

23155 with autograft (includes obtaining graft)

23156 with allograft

23170 Sequestrectomy (eg, for osteomyelitis or bone abscess), clavicle

23172 Sequestrectomy (eg, for osteomyelitis or bone abscess), scapula

23174 Sequestrectomy (eg, for osteomyelitis or bone abscess), humeral head to surgical neck

23180 Partial excision (craterization, saucerization, or diaphysectomy) bone (eg, osteomyelitis), clavicle

23182 Partial excision (craterization, saucerization, or diaphysectomy) bone (eg, osteomyelitis), scapula

23184 Partial excision (craterization, saucerization, or diaphysectomy) bone (eg, osteomyelitis), proximal humerus

23190 Ostectomy of scapula, partial (eg, superior medial angle)

23195 Resection, humeral head

(For replacement with implant, use 23470)

23200 Radical resection for tumor; clavicle

23210 scapula

23220 Radical resection of bone tumor, proximal humerus;

23221 with autograft (includes obtaining graft)

23222 with prosthetic replacement

Introduction or Removal

(For arthrocentesis or needling of bursa, use 20610)

(For K-wire or pin insertion or removal, see 20650, 20670, 20680)

23330 Removal of foreign body, shoulder; subcutaneous

23331 deep (eg, Neer hemiarthroplasty removal)

23332 complicated (eg, total shoulder)

23350 Injection procedure for shoulder arthrography or enhanced CT/MRI shoulder arthrography

(For radiographic arthrography, radiological supervision and interpretation, use 73040. Fluoroscopy (76003) is inclusive of radiographic arthrography)

(When fluoroscopic guided injection is performed for enhanced CT arthrography, use 23350, 76003, and 73201 or 73202)

(When fluoroscopic guided injection is performed for enhanced MR arthrography, use 23350, 76003, and 73222 or 73223)

(For enhanced CT or enhanced MRI arthrography, use 76003 and either 73201, 73202, 73222 or 73223)

(To report biopsy of the shoulder and joint, see 29805-29826)

Repair, Revision, and/or Reconstruction

23395 Muscle transfer, any type, shoulder or upper arm; single

23397 multiple

23400 Scapulopexy (eg, Sprengels deformity or for paralysis)

23405 Tenotomy, shoulder area; single tendon

23406 multiple tendons through same incision

23410   Repair of ruptured musculotendinous cuff (eg, rotator cuff) open; acute

23412   chronic

           (For arthroscopic procedure, use 29827)

23415   Coracoacromial ligament release, with or without acromioplasty

           (For arthroscopic procedure, use 29826)

23420   Reconstruction of complete shoulder (rotator) cuff avulsion, chronic (includes acromioplasty)

23430   Tenodesis of long tendon of biceps

23440   Resection or transplantation of long tendon of biceps

23450   Capsulorrhaphy, anterior; Putti-Platt procedure or Magnuson type operation

           (To report arthroscopic thermal capsulorrhaphy, use 29999)

23455   with labral repair (eg, Bankart procedure)

           (For arthroscopic procedure, use 29806)

23460   Capsulorrhaphy, anterior, any type; with bone block

23462   with coracoid process transfer

           (To report open thermal capsulorrhaphy, use 23929)

23465   Capsulorrhaphy, glenohumeral joint, posterior, with or without bone block

           (For sternoclavicular and acromioclavicular reconstruction, see 23530, 23550)

23466   Capsulorrhaphy, glenohumeral joint, any type multi-directional instability

23470   Arthroplasty, glenohumeral joint; hemiarthroplasty

23472   total shoulder (glenoid and proximal humeral replacement (eg, total shoulder))

           (For removal of total shoulder implants, see 23331, 23332)

           (For osteotomy, proximal humerus, use 24400)

23480   Osteotomy, clavicle, with or without internal fixation;

23485   with bone graft for nonunion or malunion (includes obtaining graft and/or necessary fixation)

23490   Prophylactic treatment (nailing, pinning, plating or wiring) with or without methylmethacrylate; clavicle

23491   proximal humerus

Fracture and/or Dislocation

23500   Closed treatment of clavicular fracture; without manipulation

23505   with manipulation

23515   Open treatment of clavicular fracture, with or without internal or external fixation

23520   Closed treatment of sternoclavicular dislocation; without manipulation

23525   with manipulation

23530   Open treatment of sternoclavicular dislocation, acute or chronic;

23532   with fascial graft (includes obtaining graft)

23540   Closed treatment of acromioclavicular dislocation; without manipulation

23545   with manipulation

23550   Open treatment of acromioclavicular dislocation, acute or chronic;

23552   with fascial graft (includes obtaining graft)

23570   Closed treatment of scapular fracture; without manipulation

23575   with manipulation, with or without skeletal traction (with or without shoulder joint involvement)

23585   Open treatment of scapular fracture (body, glenoid or acromion) with or without internal fixation

23600   Closed treatment of proximal humeral (surgical or anatomical neck) fracture; without manipulation

23605   with manipulation, with or without skeletal traction

23615   Open treatment of proximal humeral (surgical or anatomical neck) fracture, with or without internal or external fixation, with or without repair of tuberosity(s);

23616   with proximal humeral prosthetic replacement

23620   Closed treatment of greater humeral tuberosity fracture; without manipulation

23625   with manipulation

23630   Open treatment of greater humeral tuberosity fracture, with or without internal or external fixation

23650   Closed treatment of shoulder dislocation, with manipulation; without anesthesia

23655   requiring anesthesia

23660   Open treatment of acute shoulder dislocation

           (Repairs for recurrent dislocations, see 23450-23466)

23665   Closed treatment of shoulder dislocation, with fracture of greater humeral tuberosity, with manipulation

23670   Open treatment of shoulder dislocation, with fracture of greater humeral tuberosity, with or without internal or external fixation

23675   Closed treatment of shoulder dislocation, with surgical or anatomical neck fracture, with manipulation

23680   Open treatment of shoulder dislocation, with surgical or anatomical neck fracture, with or without internal or external fixation

Surgery: Musculoskeletal System

Manipulation

23700 Manipulation under anesthesia, shoulder joint, including application of fixation apparatus (dislocation excluded)

Arthrodesis

23800 Arthrodesis, glenohumeral joint;

23802 with autogenous graft (includes obtaining graft)

Amputation

23900 Interthoracoscapular amputation (forequarter)

23920 Disarticulation of shoulder;

23921 secondary closure or scar revision

Other Procedures

23929 Unlisted procedure, shoulder

Humerus (Upper Arm) and Elbow

Elbow area includes head and neck of radius and olecranon process.

Incision

(For incision and drainage procedures, superficial, see 10040-10160)

23930 Incision and drainage, upper arm or elbow area; deep abscess or hematoma

23931 bursa

23935 Incision, deep, with opening of bone cortex (eg, for osteomyelitis or bone abscess), humerus or elbow

24000 Arthrotomy, elbow, including exploration, drainage, or removal of foreign body

24006 Arthrotomy of the elbow, with capsular excision for capsular release (separate procedure)

Excision

24065 Biopsy, soft tissue of upper arm or elbow area; superficial

24066 deep (subfascial or intramuscular)

(For needle biopsy of soft tissue, use 20206)

24075 Excision, tumor, soft tissue of upper arm or elbow area; subcutaneous

24076 deep (subfascial or intramuscular)

24077 Radical resection of tumor (eg, malignant neoplasm), soft tissue of upper arm or elbow area

24100 Arthrotomy, elbow; with synovial biopsy only

24101 with joint exploration, with or without biopsy, with or without removal of loose or foreign body

24102 with synovectomy

24105 Excision, olecranon bursa

24110 Excision or curettage of bone cyst or benign tumor, humerus;

24115 with autograft (includes obtaining graft)

24116 with allograft

24120 Excision or curettage of bone cyst or benign tumor of head or neck of radius or olecranon process;

24125 with autograft (includes obtaining graft)

24126 with allograft

24130 Excision, radial head

(For replacement with implant, use 24366)

24134 Sequestrectomy (eg, for osteomyelitis or bone abscess), shaft or distal humerus

24136 Sequestrectomy (eg, for osteomyelitis or bone abscess), radial head or neck

24138 Sequestrectomy (eg, for osteomyelitis or bone abscess), olecranon process

24140 Partial excision (craterization, saucerization, or diaphysectomy) bone (eg, osteomyelitis), humerus

24145 Partial excision (craterization, saucerization, or diaphysectomy) bone (eg, osteomyelitis), radial head or neck

24147 Partial excision (craterization, saucerization, or diaphysectomy) bone (eg, osteomyelitis), olecranon process

24149 Radical resection of capsule, soft tissue, and heterotopic bone, elbow, with contracture release (separate procedure)

(For capsular and soft tissue release only, use 24006)

24150 Radical resection for tumor, shaft or distal humerus;

24151 with autograft (includes obtaining graft)

24152 Radical resection for tumor, radial head or neck;

24153 with autograft (includes obtaining graft)

24155 Resection of elbow joint (arthrectomy)

Introduction or Removal

(For K-wire or pin insertion or removal, see 20650, 20670, 20680)

(For arthrocentesis or needling of bursa or joint, use 20605)

24160 Implant removal; elbow joint

24164 radial head

24200 Removal of foreign body, upper arm or elbow area; subcutaneous

24201 deep (subfascial or intramuscular)

24220   Injection procedure for elbow arthrography

(For radiological supervision and interpretation, use 73085. Do not report 76003 in addition to 73085)

(For injection for tennis elbow, use 20550)

Repair, Revision, and/or Reconstruction

24300   Manipulation, elbow, under anesthesia

(For application of external fixation, see 20690 or 20692)

24301   Muscle or tendon transfer, any type, upper arm or elbow, single (excluding 24320-24331)

24305   Tendon lengthening, upper arm or elbow, each tendon

24310   Tenotomy, open, elbow to shoulder, each tendon

24320   Tenoplasty, with muscle transfer, with or without free graft, elbow to shoulder, single (Seddon-Brookes type procedure)

24330   Flexor-plasty, elbow (eg, Steindler type advancement);

24331   with extensor advancement

24332   Tenolysis, triceps

24340   Tenodesis of biceps tendon at elbow (separate procedure)

24341   Repair, tendon or muscle, upper arm or elbow, each tendon or muscle, primary or secondary (excludes rotator cuff)

24342   Reinsertion of ruptured biceps or triceps tendon, distal, with or without tendon graft

24343   Repair lateral collateral ligament, elbow, with local tissue

24344   Reconstruction lateral collateral ligament, elbow, with tendon graft (includes harvesting of graft)

24345   Repair medial collateral ligament, elbow, with local tissue

24346   Reconstruction medial collateral ligament, elbow, with tendon graft (includes harvesting of graft)

24350   Fasciotomy, lateral or medial (eg, tennis elbow or epicondylitis);

24351   with extensor origin detachment

24352   with annular ligament resection

24354   with stripping

24356   with partial ostectomy

24360   Arthroplasty, elbow; with membrane (eg, fascial)

24361   with distal humeral prosthetic replacement

24362   with implant and fascia lata ligament reconstruction

24363   with distal humerus and proximal ulnar prosthetic replacement (eg, total elbow)

24365   Arthroplasty, radial head;

24366   with implant

24400   Osteotomy, humerus, with or without internal fixation

24410   Multiple osteotomies with realignment on intramedullary rod, humeral shaft (Sofield type procedure)

24420   Osteoplasty, humerus (eg, shortening or lengthening) (excluding 64876)

24430   Repair of nonunion or malunion, humerus; without graft (eg, compression technique)

24435   with iliac or other autograft (includes obtaining graft)

(For proximal radius and/or ulna, see 25400-25420)

24470   Hemiepiphyseal arrest (eg, cubitus varus or valgus, distal humerus)

24495   Decompression fasciotomy, forearm, with brachial artery exploration

24498   Prophylactic treatment (nailing, pinning, plating or wiring), with or without methylmethacrylate, humeral shaft

Fracture and/or Dislocation

24500   Closed treatment of humeral shaft fracture; without manipulation

24505   with manipulation, with or without skeletal traction

24515   Open treatment of humeral shaft fracture with plate/screws, with or without cerclage

24516   Treatment of humeral shaft fracture, with insertion of intramedullary implant, with or without cerclage and/or locking screws

24530   Closed treatment of supracondylar or transcondylar humeral fracture, with or without intercondylar extension; without manipulation

24535   with manipulation, with or without skin or skeletal traction

24538   Percutaneous skeletal fixation of supracondylar or transcondylar humeral fracture, with or without intercondylar extension

24545   Open treatment of humeral supracondylar or transcondylar fracture, with or without internal or external fixation; without intercondylar extension

24546   with intercondylar extension

24560   Closed treatment of humeral epicondylar fracture, medial or lateral; without manipulation

24565   with manipulation

24566   Percutaneous skeletal fixation of humeral epicondylar fracture, medial or lateral, with manipulation

24575   Open treatment of humeral epicondylar fracture, medial or lateral, with or without internal or external fixation

24576   Closed treatment of humeral condylar fracture, medial or lateral; without manipulation

24577   with manipulation

24579   Open treatment of humeral condylar fracture, medial or lateral, with or without internal or external fixation

(To report closed treatment of fractures without manipulation, see 24530, 24560, 24576, 24650, 24670)

(To report closed treatment of fractures with manipulation, see 24535, 24565, 24577, 24675)

24582   Percutaneous skeletal fixation of humeral condylar fracture, medial or lateral, with manipulation

24586   Open treatment of periarticular fracture and/or dislocation of the elbow (fracture distal humerus and proximal ulna and/or proximal radius);

24587   with implant arthroplasty

(See also 24361)

24600   Treatment of closed elbow dislocation; without anesthesia

24605   requiring anesthesia

24615   Open treatment of acute or chronic elbow dislocation

24620   Closed treatment of Monteggia type of fracture dislocation at elbow (fracture proximal end of ulna with dislocation of radial head), with manipulation

24635   Open treatment of Monteggia type of fracture dislocation at elbow (fracture proximal end of ulna with dislocation of radial head), with or without internal or external fixation

24640   Closed treatment of radial head subluxation in child, nursemaid elbow, with manipulation

24650   Closed treatment of radial head or neck fracture; without manipulation

24655   with manipulation

24665   Open treatment of radial head or neck fracture, with or without internal fixation or radial head excision;

24666   with radial head prosthetic replacement

24670   Closed treatment of ulnar fracture, proximal end (olecranon process); without manipulation

24675   with manipulation

24685   Open treatment of ulnar fracture proximal end (olecranon process), with or without internal or external fixation

Arthrodesis

24800   Arthrodesis, elbow joint; local

24802   with autogenous graft (includes obtaining graft)

Amputation

24900   Amputation, arm through humerus; with primary closure

24920   open, circular (guillotine)

24925   secondary closure or scar revision

24930   re-amputation

24931   with implant

24935   Stump elongation, upper extremity

24940   Cineplasty, upper extremity, complete procedure

Other Procedures

24999   Unlisted procedure, humerus or elbow

Forearm and Wrist

Radius, ulna, carpal bones and joints.

Incision

25000   Incision, extensor tendon sheath, wrist (eg, deQuervains disease)

(For decompression median nerve or for carpal tunnel syndrome, use 64721)

25001   Incision, flexor tendon sheath, wrist (eg, flexor carpi radialis)

25020   Decompression fasciotomy, forearm and/or wrist, flexor OR extensor compartment; without debridement of nonviable muscle and/or nerve

25023   with debridement of nonviable muscle and/or nerve

(For decompression fasciotomy with brachial artery exploration, use 24495)

(For incision and drainage procedures, superficial, see 10060-10160)

(For debridement, see also 11000-11044)

25024   Decompression fasciotomy, forearm and/or wrist, flexor AND extensor compartment; without debridement of nonviable muscle and/or nerve

25025   with debridement of nonviable muscle and/or nerve

25028   Incision and drainage, forearm and/or wrist; deep abscess or hematoma

25031   bursa

25035   Incision, deep, bone cortex, forearm and/or wrist (eg, osteomyelitis or bone abscess)

25040   Arthrotomy, radiocarpal or midcarpal joint, with exploration, drainage, or removal of foreign body

Excision

25065   Biopsy, soft tissue of forearm and/or wrist; superficial

25066   deep (subfascial or intramuscular)

(For needle biopsy of soft tissue, use 20206)

25075   Excision, tumor, soft tissue of forearm and/or wrist area; subcutaneous

25076   deep (subfascial or intramuscular)

25077   Radical resection of tumor (eg, malignant neoplasm), soft tissue of forearm and/or wrist area

25085   Capsulotomy, wrist (eg, contracture)

25100   Arthrotomy, wrist joint; with biopsy

25101   with joint exploration, with or without biopsy, with or without removal of loose or foreign body

25105   with synovectomy

25107   Arthrotomy, distal radioulnar joint including repair of triangular cartilage, complex

25110   Excision, lesion of tendon sheath, forearm and/or wrist

25111   Excision of ganglion, wrist (dorsal or volar); primary

25112   recurrent

(For hand or finger, use 26160)

25115   Radical excision of bursa, synovia of wrist, or forearm tendon sheaths (eg, tenosynovitis, fungus, Tbc, or other granulomas, rheumatoid arthritis); flexors

25116   extensors, with or without transposition of dorsal retinaculum

(For finger synovectomies, use 26145)

25118   Synovectomy, extensor tendon sheath, wrist, single compartment;

25119   with resection of distal ulna

25120   Excision or curettage of bone cyst or benign tumor of radius or ulna (excluding head or neck of radius and olecranon process);

(For head or neck of radius or olecranon process, see 24120-24126)

25125   with autograft (includes obtaining graft)

25126   with allograft

25130   Excision or curettage of bone cyst or benign tumor of carpal bones;

25135   with autograft (includes obtaining graft)

25136   with allograft

25145   Sequestrectomy (eg, for osteomyelitis or bone abscess), forearm and/or wrist

25150   Partial excision (craterization, saucerization, or diaphysectomy) of bone (eg, for osteomyelitis); ulna

25151   radius

(For head or neck of radius or olecranon process, see 24145, 24147)

25170   Radical resection for tumor, radius or ulna

25210   Carpectomy; one bone

(For carpectomy with implant, see 25441-25445)

25215   all bones of proximal row

25230   Radial styloidectomy (separate procedure)

25240   Excision distal ulna partial or complete (eg, Darrach type or matched resection)

(For implant replacement, distal ulna, use 25442)

(For obtaining fascia for interposition, see 20920, 20922)

Introduction or Removal

(For K-wire, pin or rod insertion or removal, see 20650, 20670, 20680)

25246   Injection procedure for wrist arthrography

(For radiological supervision and interpretation, use 73115. Do not report 76003 in addition to 73115)

(For foreign body removal, superficial use 20520)

25248   Exploration with removal of deep foreign body, forearm or wrist

25250   Removal of wrist prosthesis; (separate procedure)

25251   complicated, including total wrist

25259   Manipulation, wrist, under anesthesia

(For application of external fixation, see 20690 or 20692)

Repair, Revision, and/or Reconstruction

25260   Repair, tendon or muscle, flexor, forearm and/or wrist; primary, single, each tendon or muscle

25263   secondary, single, each tendon or muscle

25265   secondary, with free graft (includes obtaining graft), each tendon or muscle

25270   Repair, tendon or muscle, extensor, forearm and/or wrist; primary, single, each tendon or muscle

25272   secondary, single, each tendon or muscle

25274   secondary, with free graft (includes obtaining graft), each tendon or muscle

25275   Repair, tendon sheath, extensor, forearm and/or wrist, with free graft (includes obtaining graft) (eg, for extensor carpi ulnaris subluxation)

25280   Lengthening or shortening of flexor or extensor tendon, forearm and/or wrist, single, each tendon

25290   Tenotomy, open, flexor or extensor tendon, forearm and/or wrist, single, each tendon

25295   Tenolysis, flexor or extensor tendon, forearm and/or wrist, single, each tendon

25300   Tenodesis at wrist; flexors of fingers

25301   extensors of fingers

25310   Tendon transplantation or transfer, flexor or extensor, forearm and/or wrist, single; each tendon

25312   with tendon graft(s) (includes obtaining graft), each tendon

25315   Flexor origin slide (eg, for cerebral palsy, Volkmann contracture), forearm and/or wrist;

25316   with tendon(s) transfer

25320   Capsulorrhaphy or reconstruction, wrist, open (eg, capsulodesis, ligament repair, tendon transfer or graft) (includes synovectomy, capsulotomy and open reduction) for carpal instability

25332   Arthroplasty, wrist, with or without interposition, with or without external or internal fixation

(For obtaining fascia for interposition, see 20920, 20922)

(For prosthetic replacement arthroplasty, see 25441-25446)

25335   Centralization of wrist on ulna (eg, radial club hand)

25337   Reconstruction for stabilization of unstable distal ulna or distal radioulnar joint, secondary by soft tissue stabilization (eg, tendon transfer, tendon graft or weave, or tenodesis) with or without open reduction of distal radioulnar joint

(For harvesting of fascia lata graft, see 20920, 20922)

25350   Osteotomy, radius; distal third

25355   middle or proximal third

25360   Osteotomy; ulna

25365   radius AND ulna

25370   Multiple osteotomies, with realignment on intramedullary rod (Sofield type procedure); radius OR ulna

25375   radius AND ulna

25390   Osteoplasty, radius OR ulna; shortening

25391   lengthening with autograft

25392   Osteoplasty, radius AND ulna; shortening (excluding 64876)

25393   lengthening with autograft

25394   Osteoplasty, carpal bone, shortening

25400   Repair of nonunion or malunion, radius OR ulna; without graft (eg, compression technique)

25405   with autograft (includes obtaining graft)

25415   Repair of nonunion or malunion, radius AND ulna; without graft (eg, compression technique)

25420   with autograft (includes obtaining graft)

25425   Repair of defect with autograft; radius OR ulna

25426   radius AND ulna

25430   Insertion of vascular pedicle into carpal bone (eg, Hori procedure)

25431   Repair of nonunion of carpal bone (excluding carpal scaphoid (navicular)) (includes obtaining graft and necessary fixation), each bone

25440   Repair of nonunion, scaphoid carpal (navicular) bone, with or without radial styloidectomy (includes obtaining graft and necessary fixation)

25441   Arthroplasty with prosthetic replacement; distal radius

25442   distal ulna

25443   scaphoid carpal (navicular)

25444   lunate

25445   trapezium

25446   distal radius and partial or entire carpus (total wrist)

25447   Arthroplasty, interposition, intercarpal or carpometacarpal joints

(For wrist arthroplasty, use 25332)

25449   Revision of arthroplasty, including removal of implant, wrist joint

25450   Epiphyseal arrest by epiphysiodesis or stapling; distal radius OR ulna

25455   distal radius AND ulna

25490   Prophylactic treatment (nailing, pinning, plating or wiring) with or without methylmethacrylate; radius

25491   ulna

25492   radius AND ulna

Fracture and/or Dislocation

25500   Closed treatment of radial shaft fracture; without manipulation

25505   with manipulation

25515   Open treatment of radial shaft fracture, with or without internal or external fixation

25520   Closed treatment of radial shaft fracture and closed treatment of dislocation of distal radioulnar joint (Galeazzi fracture/dislocation)

25525   Open treatment of radial shaft fracture, with internal and/ or external fixation and closed treatment of dislocation of distal radioulnar joint (Galeazzi fracture/dislocation), with or without percutaneous skeletal fixation

25526   Open treatment of radial shaft fracture, with internal and/or external fixation and open treatment, with or without internal or external fixation of distal radioulnar joint (Galeazzi fracture/dislocation), includes repair of triangular fibrocartilage complex

25530   Closed treatment of ulnar shaft fracture; without manipulation

25535   with manipulation

25545   Open treatment of ulnar shaft fracture, with or without internal or external fixation

25560   Closed treatment of radial and ulnar shaft fractures; without manipulation

25565   with manipulation

25574   Open treatment of radial AND ulnar shaft fractures, with internal or external fixation; of radius OR ulna

25575   of radius AND ulna

25600   Closed treatment of distal radial fracture (eg, Colles or Smith type) or epiphyseal separation, with or without fracture of ulnar styloid; without manipulation

25605   with manipulation

25611   Percutaneous skeletal fixation of distal radial fracture (eg, Colles or Smith type) or epiphyseal separation, with or without fracture of ulnar styloid, requiring manipulation, with or without external fixation

25620   Open treatment of distal radial fracture (eg, Colles or Smith type) or epiphyseal separation, with or without fracture of ulnar styloid, with or without internal or external fixation

25622   Closed treatment of carpal scaphoid (navicular) fracture; without manipulation

25624   with manipulation

25628   Open treatment of carpal scaphoid (navicular) fracture, with or without internal or external fixation

25630   Closed treatment of carpal bone fracture (excluding carpal scaphoid (navicular)); without manipulation, each bone

25635   with manipulation, each bone

25645   Open treatment of carpal bone fracture (other than carpal scaphoid (navicular)), each bone

25650   Closed treatment of ulnar styloid fracture

25651   Percutaneous skeletal fixation of ulnar styloid fracture

25652   Open treatment of ulnar styloid fracture

25660   Closed treatment of radiocarpal or intercarpal dislocation, one or more bones, with manipulation

25670   Open treatment of radiocarpal or intercarpal dislocation, one or more bones

25671   Percutaneous skeletal fixation of distal radioulnar dislocation

25675   Closed treatment of distal radioulnar dislocation with manipulation

25676   Open treatment of distal radioulnar dislocation, acute or chronic

25680   Closed treatment of trans-scaphoperilunar type of fracture dislocation, with manipulation

25685   Open treatment of trans-scaphoperilunar type of fracture dislocation

25690   Closed treatment of lunate dislocation, with manipulation

25695   Open treatment of lunate dislocation

Arthrodesis

25800   Arthrodesis, wrist; complete, without bone graft (includes radiocarpal and/or intercarpal and/or carpometacarpal joints)

25805   with sliding graft

25810   with iliac or other autograft (includes obtaining graft)

25820   Arthrodesis, wrist; limited, without bone graft (eg, intercarpal or radiocarpal)

25825   with autograft (includes obtaining graft)

25830   Arthrodesis, distal radioulnar joint with segmental resection of ulna, with or without bone graft (eg, Sauve-Kapandji procedure)

Amputation

25900   Amputation, forearm, through radius and ulna;

25905   open, circular (guillotine)

25907   secondary closure or scar revision

25909   re-amputation

25915   Krukenberg procedure

25920   Disarticulation through wrist;

25922   secondary closure or scar revision

25924   re-amputation

25927   Transmetacarpal amputation;

25929   secondary closure or scar revision

25931   re-amputation

Other Procedures

25999   Unlisted procedure, forearm or wrist

Hand and Fingers

Incision

26010	Drainage of finger abscess; simple
26011	complicated (eg, felon)
26020	Drainage of tendon sheath, digit and/or palm, each
26025	Drainage of palmar bursa; single, bursa
26030	multiple bursa
26034	Incision, bone cortex, hand or finger (eg, osteomyelitis or bone abscess)
26035	Decompression fingers and/or hand, injection injury (eg, grease gun)
26037	Decompressive fasciotomy, hand (excludes 26035)
	(For injection injury, use 26035)
26040	Fasciotomy, palmar (eg, Dupuytren's contracture); percutaneous
26045	open, partial
	(For fasciectomy, see 26121-26125)
26055	Tendon sheath incision (eg, for trigger finger)
26060	Tenotomy, percutaneous, single, each digit
26070	Arthrotomy, with exploration, drainage, or removal of loose or foreign body; carpometacarpal joint
26075	metacarpophalangeal joint, each
26080	interphalangeal joint, each

Excision

26100	Arthrotomy with biopsy; carpometacarpal joint, each
26105	metacarpophalangeal joint, each
26110	interphalangeal joint, each
26115	Excision, tumor or vascular malformation, soft tissue of hand or finger; subcutaneous
26116	deep (subfascial or intramuscular)
26117	Radical resection of tumor (eg, malignant neoplasm), soft tissue of hand or finger
26121	Fasciectomy, palm only, with or without Z-plasty, other local tissue rearrangement, or skin grafting (includes obtaining graft)
26123	Fasciectomy, partial palmar with release of single digit including proximal interphalangeal joint, with or without Z-plasty, other local tissue rearrangement, or skin grafting (includes obtaining graft);
+ 26125	each additional digit (List separately in addition to code for primary procedure)
	(Use 26125 in conjunction with 26123)
	(For fasciotomy, see 26040, 26045)

26130	Synovectomy, carpometacarpal joint
26135	Synovectomy, metacarpophalangeal joint including intrinsic release and extensor hood reconstruction, each digit
26140	Synovectomy, proximal interphalangeal joint, including extensor reconstruction, each interphalangeal joint
26145	Synovectomy, tendon sheath, radical (tenosynovectomy), flexor tendon, palm and/or finger, each tendon
	(For tendon sheath synovectomies at wrist, see 25115, 25116)
26160	Excision of lesion of tendon sheath or joint capsule (eg, cyst, mucous cyst, or ganglion), hand or finger
	(For wrist ganglion, see 25111, 25112)
	(For trigger digit, use 26055)
26170	Excision of tendon, palm, flexor, single (separate procedure), each
26180	Excision of tendon, finger, flexor (separate procedure), each tendon
26185	Sesamoidectomy, thumb or finger (separate procedure)
26200	Excision or curettage of bone cyst or benign tumor of metacarpal;
26205	with autograft (includes obtaining graft)
26210	Excision or curettage of bone cyst or benign tumor of proximal, middle, or distal phalanx of finger;
26215	with autograft (includes obtaining graft)
26230	Partial excision (craterization, saucerization, or diaphysectomy) bone (eg, osteomyelitis); metacarpal
26235	proximal or middle phalanx of finger
26236	distal phalanx of finger
26250	Radical resection, metacarpal (eg, tumor);
26255	with autograft (includes obtaining graft)
26260	Radical resection, proximal or middle phalanx of finger (eg, tumor);
26261	with autograft (includes obtaining graft)
26262	Radical resection, distal phalanx of finger (eg, tumor)

Introduction or Removal

26320	Removal of implant from finger or hand
	(For removal of foreign body in hand or finger, see 20520, 20525)

Repair, Revision, and/or Reconstruction

26340   Manipulation, finger joint, under anesthesia, each joint

(For application of external fixation, see 20690 or 20692)

26350   Repair or advancement, flexor tendon, not in zone 2 digital flexor tendon sheath (eg, no man's land); primary or secondary without free graft, each tendon

26352   secondary with free graft (includes obtaining graft), each tendon

26356   Repair or advancement, flexor tendon, in zone 2 digital flexor tendon sheath (eg, no man's land); primary, without free graft, each tendon

26357   secondary, without free graft, each tendon

26358   secondary, with free graft (includes obtaining graft), each tendon

26370   Repair or advancement of profundus tendon, with intact superficialis tendon; primary, each tendon

26372   secondary with free graft (includes obtaining graft), each tendon

26373   secondary without free graft, each tendon

26390   Excision flexor tendon, with implantation of synthetic rod for delayed tendon graft, hand or finger, each rod

26392   Removal of synthetic rod and insertion of flexor tendon graft, hand or finger (includes obtaining graft), each rod

26410   Repair, extensor tendon, hand, primary or secondary; without free graft, each tendon

26412   with free graft (includes obtaining graft), each tendon

26415   Excision of extensor tendon, with implantation of synthetic rod for delayed tendon graft, hand or finger, each rod

26416   Removal of synthetic rod and insertion of extensor tendon graft (includes obtaining graft), hand or finger, each rod

26418   Repair, extensor tendon, finger, primary or secondary; without free graft, each tendon

26420   with free graft (includes obtaining graft) each tendon

26426   Repair of extensor tendon, central slip, secondary (eg, boutonniere deformity); using local tissue(s), including lateral band(s), each finger

26428   with free graft (includes obtaining graft), each finger

26432   Closed treatment of distal extensor tendon insertion, with or without percutaneous pinning (eg, mallet finger)

26433   Repair of extensor tendon, distal insertion, primary or secondary; without graft (eg, mallet finger)

26434   with free graft (includes obtaining graft)

(For tenovaginotomy for trigger finger, use 26055)

26437   Realignment of extensor tendon, hand, each tendon

26440   Tenolysis, flexor tendon; palm OR finger, each tendon

26442   palm AND finger, each tendon

26445   Tenolysis, extensor tendon, hand OR finger, each tendon

26449   Tenolysis, complex, extensor tendon, finger, including forearm, each tendon

26450   Tenotomy, flexor, palm, open, each tendon

26455   Tenotomy, flexor, finger, open, each tendon

26460   Tenotomy, extensor, hand or finger, open, each tendon

26471   Tenodesis; of proximal interphalangeal joint, each joint

26474   of distal joint, each joint

26476   Lengthening of tendon, extensor, hand or finger, each tendon

26477   Shortening of tendon, extensor, hand or finger, each tendon

26478   Lengthening of tendon, flexor, hand or finger, each tendon

26479   Shortening of tendon, flexor, hand or finger, each tendon

26480   Transfer or transplant of tendon, carpometacarpal area or dorsum of hand; without free graft, each tendon

26483   with free tendon graft (includes obtaining graft), each tendon

26485   Transfer or transplant of tendon, palmar; without free tendon graft, each tendon

26489   with free tendon graft (includes obtaining graft), each tendon

26490   Opponensplasty; superficialis tendon transfer type, each tendon

26492   tendon transfer with graft (includes obtaining graft), each tendon

26494   hypothenar muscle transfer

26496   other methods

(For thumb fusion in opposition, use 26820)

26497   Transfer of tendon to restore intrinsic function; ring and small finger

26498   all four fingers

26499   Correction claw finger, other methods

26500   Reconstruction of tendon pulley, each tendon; with local tissues (separate procedure)

26502   with tendon or fascial graft (includes obtaining graft) (separate procedure)

26504   with tendon prosthesis (separate procedure)

26508   Release of thenar muscle(s) (eg, thumb contracture)

26510   Cross intrinsic transfer, each tendon

Surgery: Musculoskeletal System

Surgery: Musculoskeletal System

26516	Capsulodesis, metacarpophalangeal joint; single digit
26517	two digits
26518	three or four digits
26520	Capsulectomy or capsulotomy; metacarpophalangeal joint, each joint
26525	interphalangeal joint, each joint

(To report carpometacarpal joint arthroplasty, use 25447)

26530	Arthroplasty, metacarpophalangeal joint; each joint
26531	with prosthetic implant, each joint
26535	Arthroplasty, interphalangeal joint; each joint
26536	with prosthetic implant, each joint
26540	Repair of collateral ligament, metacarpophalangeal or interphalangeal joint
26541	Reconstruction, collateral ligament, metacarpophalangeal joint, single; with tendon or fascial graft (includes obtaining graft)
26542	with local tissue (eg, adductor advancement)
26545	Reconstruction, collateral ligament, interphalangeal joint, single, including graft, each joint
26546	Repair non-union, metacarpal or phalanx, (includes obtaining bone graft with or without external or internal fixation)
26548	Repair and reconstruction, finger, volar plate, interphalangeal joint
26550	Pollicization of a digit
26551	Transfer, toe-to-hand with microvascular anastomosis; great toe wrap-around with bone graft

(For great toe with web space, use 20973)

26553	other than great toe, single
26554	other than great toe, double

(Do not report code 69990 in addition to codes 26551-26554)

26555	Transfer, finger to another position without microvascular anastomosis
26556	Transfer, free toe joint, with microvascular anastomosis

(Do not report code 69990 in addition to code 26556)

(To report great toe-to-hand transfer, use 20973)

26560	Repair of syndactyly (web finger) each web space; with skin flaps
26561	with skin flaps and grafts
26562	complex (eg, involving bone, nails)
26565	Osteotomy; metacarpal, each
26567	phalanx of finger, each
26568	Osteoplasty, lengthening, metacarpal or phalanx
26580	Repair cleft hand

26587	Reconstruction of polydactylous digit, soft tissue and bone

(For excision of polydactylous digit, soft tissue only, use 11200)

26590	Repair macrodactylia, each digit
26591	Repair, intrinsic muscles of hand, each muscle
26593	Release, intrinsic muscles of hand, each muscle
26596	Excision of constricting ring of finger, with multiple Z-plasties

(To report release of scar contracture or graft repairs see 11041-11042, 14040-14041, or 15120, 15240)

Fracture and/or Dislocation

26600	Closed treatment of metacarpal fracture, single; without manipulation, each bone
26605	with manipulation, each bone
26607	Closed treatment of metacarpal fracture, with manipulation, with external fixation, each bone
26608	Percutaneous skeletal fixation of metacarpal fracture, each bone
26615	Open treatment of metacarpal fracture, single, with or without internal or external fixation, each bone
26641	Closed treatment of carpometacarpal dislocation, thumb, with manipulation
26645	Closed treatment of carpometacarpal fracture dislocation, thumb (Bennett fracture), with manipulation
26650	Percutaneous skeletal fixation of carpometacarpal fracture dislocation, thumb (Bennett fracture), with manipulation, with or without external fixation
26665	Open treatment of carpometacarpal fracture dislocation, thumb (Bennett fracture), with or without internal or external fixation
26670	Closed treatment of carpometacarpal dislocation, other than thumb, with manipulation, each joint; without anesthesia
26675	requiring anesthesia
26676	Percutaneous skeletal fixation of carpometacarpal dislocation, other than thumb, with manipulation, each joint
26685	Open treatment of carpometacarpal dislocation, other than thumb; with or without internal or external fixation, each joint
26686	complex, multiple or delayed reduction
26700	Closed treatment of metacarpophalangeal dislocation, single, with manipulation; without anesthesia
26705	requiring anesthesia
26706	Percutaneous skeletal fixation of metacarpophalangeal dislocation, single, with manipulation

26715   Open treatment of metacarpophalangeal dislocation, single, with or without internal or external fixation

26720   Closed treatment of phalangeal shaft fracture, proximal or middle phalanx, finger or thumb; without manipulation, each

26725   with manipulation, with or without skin or skeletal traction, each

26727   Percutaneous skeletal fixation of unstable phalangeal shaft fracture, proximal or middle phalanx, finger or thumb, with manipulation, each

26735   Open treatment of phalangeal shaft fracture, proximal or middle phalanx, finger or thumb, with or without internal or external fixation, each

26740   Closed treatment of articular fracture, involving metacarpophalangeal or interphalangeal joint; without manipulation, each

26742   with manipulation, each

26746   Open treatment of articular fracture, involving metacarpophalangeal or interphalangeal joint, with or without internal or external fixation, each

26750   Closed treatment of distal phalangeal fracture, finger or thumb; without manipulation, each

26755   with manipulation, each

26756   Percutaneous skeletal fixation of distal phalangeal fracture, finger or thumb, each

26765   Open treatment of distal phalangeal fracture, finger or thumb, with or without internal or external fixation, each

26770   Closed treatment of interphalangeal joint dislocation, single, with manipulation; without anesthesia

26775   requiring anesthesia

26776   Percutaneous skeletal fixation of interphalangeal joint dislocation, single, with manipulation

26785   Open treatment of interphalangeal joint dislocation, with or without internal or external fixation, single

Arthrodesis

26820   Fusion in opposition, thumb, with autogenous graft (includes obtaining graft)

26841   Arthrodesis, carpometacarpal joint, thumb, with or without internal fixation;

26842   with autograft (includes obtaining graft)

26843   Arthrodesis, carpometacarpal joint, digit, other than thumb, each;

26844   with autograft (includes obtaining graft)

26850   Arthrodesis, metacarpophalangeal joint, with or without internal fixation;

26852   with autograft (includes obtaining graft)

26860   Arthrodesis, interphalangeal joint, with or without internal fixation;

+ 26861   each additional interphalangeal joint (List separately in addition to code for primary procedure)

(Use 26861 in conjunction with 26860)

26862   with autograft (includes obtaining graft)

+ 26863   with autograft (includes obtaining graft), each additional joint (List separately in addition to code for primary procedure)

(Use 26863 in conjunction with 26862)

Amputation

(For hand through metacarpal bones, use 25927)

26910   Amputation, metacarpal, with finger or thumb (ray amputation), single, with or without interosseous transfer

(For repositioning, see 26550, 26555)

26951   Amputation, finger or thumb, primary or secondary, any joint or phalanx, single, including neurectomies; with direct closure

26952   with local advancement flaps (V-Y, hood)

(For repair of soft tissue defect requiring split or full thickness graft or other pedicle flaps, see 15050-15758)

Other Procedures

26989   Unlisted procedure, hands or fingers

Pelvis and Hip Joint

Including head and neck of femur.

Incision

(For incision and drainage procedures, superficial, see 10040-10160)

26990   Incision and drainage, pelvis or hip joint area; deep abscess or hematoma

26991   infected bursa

26992   Incision, bone cortex, pelvis and/or hip joint (eg, osteomyelitis or bone abscess)

27000   Tenotomy, adductor of hip, percutaneous (separate procedure)

27001   Tenotomy, adductor of hip, open

(To report bilateral procedures, report 27001 with modifier 50)

27003   Tenotomy, adductor, subcutaneous, open, with obturator neurectomy

(To report bilateral procedures, report 27003 with modifier 50)

Surgery: Musculoskeletal System

Surgery: Musculoskeletal System

27005 Tenotomy, hip flexor(s), open (separate procedure)

27006 Tenotomy, abductors and/or extensor(s) of hip, open (separate procedure)

27025 Fasciotomy, hip or thigh, any type

(To report bilateral procedures, report 27025 with modifier 50)

27030 Arthrotomy, hip, with drainage (eg, infection)

27033 Arthrotomy, hip, including exploration or removal of loose or foreign body

27035 Denervation, hip joint, intrapelvic or extrapelvic intra-articular branches of sciatic, femoral, or obturator nerves

(For obturator neurectomy, see 64763, 64766)

27036 Capsulectomy or capsulotomy, hip, with or without excision of heterotopic bone, with release of hip flexor muscles (ie, gluteus medius, gluteus minimus, tensor fascia latae, rectus femoris, sartorius, iliopsoas)

Excision

27040 Biopsy, soft tissue of pelvis and hip area; superficial

27041 deep, subfascial or intramuscular

(For needle biopsy of soft tissue, use 20206)

27047 Excision, tumor, pelvis and hip area; subcutaneous tissue

27048 deep, subfascial, intramuscular

27049 Radical resection of tumor, soft tissue of pelvis and hip area (eg, malignant neoplasm)

27050 Arthrotomy, with biopsy; sacroiliac joint

27052 hip joint

27054 Arthrotomy with synovectomy, hip joint

27060 Excision; ischial bursa

27062 trochanteric bursa or calcification

(For arthrocentesis or needling of bursa, use 20610)

27065 Excision of bone cyst or benign tumor; superficial (wing of ilium, symphysis pubis, or greater trochanter of femur) with or without autograft

27066 deep, with or without autograft

27067 with autograft requiring separate incision

27070 Partial excision (craterization, saucerization) (eg, osteomyelitis or bone abscess); superficial (eg, wing of ilium, symphysis pubis, or greater trochanter of femur)

27071 deep (subfascial or intramuscular)

27075 Radical resection of tumor or infection; wing of ilium, one pubic or ischial ramus or symphysis pubis

27076 ilium, including acetabulum, both pubic rami, or ischium and acetabulum

27077 innominate bone, total

27078 ischial tuberosity and greater trochanter of femur

27079 ischial tuberosity and greater trochanter of femur, with skin flaps

27080 Coccygectomy, primary

(For pressure (decubitus) ulcer, see 15920, 15922 and 15931-15958)

Introduction or Removal

27086 Removal of foreign body, pelvis or hip; subcutaneous tissue

27087 deep (subfascial or intramuscular)

27090 Removal of hip prosthesis; (separate procedure)

27091 complicated, including total hip prosthesis, methylmethacrylate with or without insertion of spacer

27093 Injection procedure for hip arthrography; without anesthesia

(For radiological supervision and interpretation, use 73525. Do not report 76003 in addition to 73525)

27095 with anesthesia

(For radiological supervision and interpretation, use 73525. Do not report 76003 in addition to 73525)

27096 Injection procedure for sacroiliac joint, arthrography and/or anesthetic/steroid

(27096 is to be used only with imaging confirmation of intra-articular needle positioning)

(For radiological supervision and interpretation of sacroiliac joint arthrography, use 73542)

(For fluoroscopic guidance without formal arthrography, use 76005)

(Code 27096 is a unilateral procedure. For bilateral procedure, use modifier 50)

Repair, Revision, and/or Reconstruction

27097 Release or recession, hamstring, proximal

27098 Transfer, adductor to ischium

27100 Transfer external oblique muscle to greater trochanter including fascial or tendon extension (graft)

27105 Transfer paraspinal muscle to hip (includes fascial or tendon extension graft)

27110 Transfer iliopsoas; to greater trochanter of femur

27111 to femoral neck

27120 Acetabuloplasty; (eg, Whitman, Colonna, Haygroves, or cup type)

27122 resection, femoral head (eg, Girdlestone procedure)

27125 Hemiarthroplasty, hip, partial (eg, femoral stem prosthesis, bipolar arthroplasty)

(For prosthetic replacement following fracture of the hip, use 27236)

27130 Arthroplasty, acetabular and proximal femoral prosthetic replacement (total hip arthroplasty), with or without autograft or allograft

27132 Conversion of previous hip surgery to total hip arthroplasty, with or without autograft or allograft

27134 Revision of total hip arthroplasty; both components, with or without autograft or allograft

27137   acetabular component only, with or without autograft or allograft

27138   femoral component only, with or without allograft

27140 Osteotomy and transfer of greater trochanter of femur (separate procedure)

27146 Osteotomy, iliac, acetabular or innominate bone;

27147   with open reduction of hip

27151   with femoral osteotomy

27156   with femoral osteotomy and with open reduction of hip

27158 Osteotomy, pelvis, bilateral (eg, congenital malformation)

27161 Osteotomy, femoral neck (separate procedure)

27165 Osteotomy, intertrochanteric or subtrochanteric including internal or external fixation and/or cast

27170 Bone graft, femoral head, neck, intertrochanteric or subtrochanteric area (includes obtaining bone graft)

27175 Treatment of slipped femoral epiphysis; by traction, without reduction

27176   by single or multiple pinning, in situ

27177 Open treatment of slipped femoral epiphysis; single or multiple pinning or bone graft (includes obtaining graft)

27178   closed manipulation with single or multiple pinning

27179   osteoplasty of femoral neck (Heyman type procedure)

27181   osteotomy and internal fixation

27185 Epiphyseal arrest by epiphysiodesis or stapling, greater trochanter of femur

27187 Prophylactic treatment (nailing, pinning, plating or wiring) with or without methylmethacrylate, femoral neck and proximal femur

Fracture and/or Dislocation

27193 Closed treatment of pelvic ring fracture, dislocation, diastasis or subluxation; without manipulation

27194   with manipulation, requiring more than local anesthesia

27200 Closed treatment of coccygeal fracture

27202 Open treatment of coccygeal fracture

27215 Open treatment of iliac spine(s), tuberosity avulsion, or iliac wing fracture(s) (eg, pelvic fracture(s) which do not disrupt the pelvic ring), with internal fixation

27216 Percutaneous skeletal fixation of posterior pelvic ring fracture and/or dislocation (includes ilium, sacroiliac joint and/or sacrum)

27217 Open treatment of anterior ring fracture and/or dislocation with internal fixation (includes pubic symphysis and/or rami)

27218 Open treatment of posterior ring fracture and/or dislocation with internal fixation (includes ilium, sacroiliac joint and/or sacrum)

27220 Closed treatment of acetabulum (hip socket) fracture(s); without manipulation

27222   with manipulation, with or without skeletal traction

27226 Open treatment of posterior or anterior acetabular wall fracture, with internal fixation

27227 Open treatment of acetabular fracture(s) involving anterior or posterior (one) column, or a fracture running transversely across the acetabulum, with internal fixation

27228 Open treatment of acetabular fracture(s) involving anterior and posterior (two) columns, includes T-fracture and both column fracture with complete articular detachment, or single column or transverse fracture with associated acetabular wall fracture, with internal fixation

27230 Closed treatment of femoral fracture, proximal end, neck; without manipulation

27232   with manipulation, with or without skeletal traction

27235 Percutaneous skeletal fixation of femoral fracture, proximal end, neck

27236 Open treatment of femoral fracture, proximal end, neck, internal fixation or prosthetic replacement

27238 Closed treatment of intertrochanteric, pertrochanteric, or subtrochanteric femoral fracture; without manipulation

27240   with manipulation, with or without skin or skeletal traction

27244 Treatment of intertrochanteric, pertrochanteric, or subtrochanteric femoral fracture; with plate/screw type implant, with or without cerclage

27245   with intramedullary implant, with or without interlocking screws and/or cerclage

27246 Closed treatment of greater trochanteric fracture, without manipulation

27248 Open treatment of greater trochanteric fracture, with or without internal or external fixation

Surgery: Musculoskeletal System

27250 Closed treatment of hip dislocation, traumatic; without anesthesia

27252   requiring anesthesia

27253 Open treatment of hip dislocation, traumatic, without internal fixation

27254 Open treatment of hip dislocation, traumatic, with acetabular wall and femoral head fracture, with or without internal or external fixation

(For treatment of acetabular fracture with fixation, see 27226, 27227)

27256 Treatment of spontaneous hip dislocation (developmental, including congenital or pathological), by abduction, splint or traction; without anesthesia, without manipulation

27257   with manipulation, requiring anesthesia

27258 Open treatment of spontaneous hip dislocation (developmental, including congenital or pathological), replacement of femoral head in acetabulum (including tenotomy, etc);

27259   with femoral shaft shortening

27265 Closed treatment of post hip arthroplasty dislocation; without anesthesia

27266   requiring regional or general anesthesia

Manipulation

27275 Manipulation, hip joint, requiring general anesthesia

Arthrodesis

27280 Arthrodesis, sacroiliac joint (including obtaining graft)

(To report bilateral procedures, report 27280 with modifier 50)

27282 Arthrodesis, symphysis pubis (including obtaining graft)

27284 Arthrodesis, hip joint (including obtaining graft);

27286   with subtrochanteric osteotomy

Amputation

27290 Interpelviabdominal amputation (hindquarter amputation)

27295 Disarticulation of hip

Other Procedures

27299 Unlisted procedure, pelvis or hip joint

Femur (Thigh Region) and Knee Joint

Including tibial plateaus.

Incision

(For incision and drainage of abscess or hematoma, superficial, see 10040-10160)

27301 Incision and drainage, deep abscess, bursa, or hematoma, thigh or knee region

27303 Incision, deep, with opening of bone cortex, femur or knee (eg, osteomyelitis or bone abscess)

27305 Fasciotomy, iliotibial (tenotomy), open

(For combined Ober-Yount fasciotomy, use 27025)

27306 Tenotomy, percutaneous, adductor or hamstring; single tendon (separate procedure)

27307   multiple tendons

27310 Arthrotomy, knee, with exploration, drainage, or removal of foreign body (eg, infection)

27315 Neurectomy, hamstring muscle

27320 Neurectomy, popliteal (gastrocnemius)

Excision

27323 Biopsy, soft tissue of thigh or knee area; superficial

27324   deep (subfascial or intramuscular)

(For needle biopsy of soft tissue, use 20206)

27327 Excision, tumor, thigh or knee area; subcutaneous

27328   deep, subfascial, or intramuscular

27329 Radical resection of tumor (eg, malignant neoplasm), soft tissue of thigh or knee area

27330 Arthrotomy, knee; with synovial biopsy only

27331   including joint exploration, biopsy, or removal of loose or foreign bodies

27332 Arthrotomy, with excision of semilunar cartilage (meniscectomy) knee; medial OR lateral

27333   medial AND lateral

27334 Arthrotomy, with synovectomy, knee; anterior OR posterior

27335   anterior AND posterior including popliteal area

27340 Excision, prepatellar bursa

27345 Excision of synovial cyst of popliteal space (eg, Baker's cyst)

27347 Excision of lesion of meniscus or capsule (eg, cyst, ganglion), knee

27350 Patellectomy or hemipatellectomy

27355 Excision or curettage of bone cyst or benign tumor of femur;

27356   with allograft

27357   with autograft (includes obtaining graft)

+ 27358   with internal fixation (List in addition to code for primary procedure)

(Use 27358 in conjunction with 27355, 27356, or 27357)

27360 Partial excision (craterization, saucerization, or diaphysectomy) bone, femur, proximal tibia and/or fibula (eg, osteomyelitis or bone abscess)

27365 Radical resection of tumor, bone, femur or knee

(For radical resection of tumor, soft tissue, use 27329)

Introduction or Removal

27370 Injection procedure for knee arthrography

(For radiological supervision and interpretation, use 73580. Do not report 76003 in addition to 73580)

27372 Removal of foreign body, deep, thigh region or knee area

(For removal of knee prosthesis including "total knee," use 27488)

(For surgical arthroscopic knee procedures, see 29870-29887)

Repair, Revision, and/or Reconstruction

27380 Suture of infrapatellar tendon; primary

27381   secondary reconstruction, including fascial or tendon graft

27385 Suture of quadriceps or hamstring muscle rupture; primary

27386   secondary reconstruction, including fascial or tendon graft

27390 Tenotomy, open, hamstring, knee to hip; single tendon

27391   multiple tendons, one leg

27392   multiple tendons, bilateral

27393 Lengthening of hamstring tendon; single tendon

27394   multiple tendons, one leg

27395   multiple tendons, bilateral

27396 Transplant, hamstring tendon to patella; single tendon

27397   multiple tendons

27400 Transfer, tendon or muscle, hamstrings to femur (eg, Egger's type procedure)

27403 Arthrotomy with meniscus repair, knee

(For arthroscopic repair, use 29882)

27405 Repair, primary, torn ligament and/or capsule, knee; collateral

27407   cruciate

(For cruciate ligament reconstruction, use 27427)

27409   collateral and cruciate ligaments

(For ligament reconstruction, see 27427-27429)

● 27412 Autologous chondrocyte implantation, knee

►(Do not report 27412 in conjunction with 20926, 27331, 27570)◄

►(For harvesting of chondrocytes, use 29870)◄

● 27415 Osteochondral allograft, knee, open

►(For arthroscopic implant of osteochondral allograft, use 29867)◄

27418 Anterior tibial tubercleplasty (eg, Maquet type procedure)

27420 Reconstruction of dislocating patella; (eg, Hauser type procedure)

27422   with extensor realignment and/or muscle advancement or release (eg, Campbell, Goldwaite type procedure)

27424   with patellectomy

27425 Lateral retinacular release, open

(For arthroscopic lateral release, use 29873)

27427 Ligamentous reconstruction (augmentation), knee; extra-articular

27428   intra-articular (open)

27429   intra-articular (open) and extra-articular

(For primary repair of ligament(s) performed in conjunction with reconstruction, report 27405, 27407 or 27409 in conjunction with 27427, 27428 or 27429)

27430 Quadricepsplasty (eg, Bennett or Thompson type)

27435 Capsulotomy, posterior capsular release, knee

27437 Arthroplasty, patella; without prosthesis

27438   with prosthesis

27440 Arthroplasty, knee, tibial plateau;

27441   with debridement and partial synovectomy

27442 Arthroplasty, femoral condyles or tibial plateau(s), knee;

27443   with debridement and partial synovectomy

27445 Arthroplasty, knee, hinge prosthesis (eg, Walldius type)

27446 Arthroplasty, knee, condyle and plateau; medial OR lateral compartment

27447   medial AND lateral compartments with or without patella resurfacing (total knee arthroplasty)

(For revision of total knee arthroplasty, use 27487)

(For removal of total knee prosthesis, use 27488)

27448 Osteotomy, femur, shaft or supracondylar; without fixation

(To report bilateral procedures, report 27448 with modifier 50)

27450 with fixation

(To report bilateral procedures, report 27450 with modifier 50)

27454 Osteotomy, multiple, with realignment on intramedullary rod, femoral shaft (eg, Sofield type procedure)

27455 Osteotomy, proximal tibia, including fibular excision or osteotomy (includes correction of genu varus (bowleg) or genu valgus (knock-knee)); before epiphyseal closure

(To report bilateral procedures, report 27455 with modifier 50)

27457 after epiphyseal closure

(To report bilateral procedures, report 27457 with modifier 50)

27465 Osteoplasty, femur; shortening (excluding 64876)

27466 lengthening

27468 combined, lengthening and shortening with femoral segment transfer

27470 Repair, nonunion or malunion, femur, distal to head and neck; without graft (eg, compression technique)

27472 with iliac or other autogenous bone graft (includes obtaining graft)

27475 Arrest, epiphyseal, any method (eg, epiphysiodesis); distal femur

27477 tibia and fibula, proximal

27479 combined distal femur, proximal tibia and fibula

27485 Arrest, hemiepiphyseal, distal femur or proximal tibia or fibula (eg, genu varus or valgus)

27486 Revision of total knee arthroplasty, with or without allograft; one component

27487 femoral and entire tibial component

27488 Removal of prosthesis, including total knee prosthesis, methylmethacrylate with or without insertion of spacer, knee

27495 Prophylactic treatment (nailing, pinning, plating or wiring) with or without methylmethacrylate, femur

27496 Decompression fasciotomy, thigh and/or knee, one compartment (flexor or extensor or adductor);

27497 with debridement of nonviable muscle and/or nerve

27498 Decompression fasciotomy, thigh and/or knee, multiple compartments;

27499 with debridement of nonviable muscle and/or nerve

Fracture and/or Dislocation

(For arthroscopic treatment of intercondylar spine(s) and tuberosity fracture(s) of the knee, see 29850, 29851)

(For arthroscopic treatment of tibial fracture, see 29855, 29856)

27500 Closed treatment of femoral shaft fracture, without manipulation

27501 Closed treatment of supracondylar or transcondylar femoral fracture with or without intercondylar extension, without manipulation

27502 Closed treatment of femoral shaft fracture, with manipulation, with or without skin or skeletal traction

27503 Closed treatment of supracondylar or transcondylar femoral fracture with or without intercondylar extension, with manipulation, with or without skin or skeletal traction

27506 Open treatment of femoral shaft fracture, with or without external fixation, with insertion of intramedullary implant, with or without cerclage and/or locking screws

27507 Open treatment of femoral shaft fracture with plate/screws, with or without cerclage

27508 Closed treatment of femoral fracture, distal end, medial or lateral condyle, without manipulation

27509 Percutaneous skeletal fixation of femoral fracture, distal end, medial or lateral condyle, or supracondylar or transcondylar, with or without intercondylar extension, or distal femoral epiphyseal separation

27510 Closed treatment of femoral fracture, distal end, medial or lateral condyle, with manipulation

27511 Open treatment of femoral supracondylar or transcondylar fracture without intercondylar extension, with or without internal or external fixation

27513 Open treatment of femoral supracondylar or transcondylar fracture with intercondylar extension, with or without internal or external fixation

27514 Open treatment of femoral fracture, distal end, medial or lateral condyle, with or without internal or external fixation

27516 Closed treatment of distal femoral epiphyseal separation; without manipulation

27517 with manipulation, with or without skin or skeletal traction

27519 Open treatment of distal femoral epiphyseal separation, with or without internal or external fixation

27520 Closed treatment of patellar fracture, without manipulation

27524 Open treatment of patellar fracture, with internal fixation and/or partial or complete patellectomy and soft tissue repair

27530   Closed treatment of tibial fracture, proximal (plateau); without manipulation

27532   with or without manipulation, with skeletal traction

(For arthroscopic treatment, see 29855, 29856)

27535   Open treatment of tibial fracture, proximal (plateau); unicondylar, with or without internal or external fixation

27536   bicondylar, with or without internal fixation

(For arthroscopic treatment, see 29855, 29856)

27538   Closed treatment of intercondylar spine(s) and/or tuberosity fracture(s) of knee, with or without manipulation

(For arthroscopic treatment, see 29850, 29851)

27540   Open treatment of intercondylar spine(s) and/or tuberosity fracture(s) of the knee, with or without internal or external fixation

27550   Closed treatment of knee dislocation; without anesthesia

27552   requiring anesthesia

27556   Open treatment of knee dislocation, with or without internal or external fixation; without primary ligamentous repair or augmentation/reconstruction

27557   with primary ligamentous repair

27558   with primary ligamentous repair, with augmentation/reconstruction

27560   Closed treatment of patellar dislocation; without anesthesia

(For recurrent dislocation, see 27420-27424)

27562   requiring anesthesia

27566   Open treatment of patellar dislocation, with or without partial or total patellectomy

Manipulation

27570   Manipulation of knee joint under general anesthesia (includes application of traction or other fixation devices)

Arthrodesis

27580   Arthrodesis, knee, any technique

Amputation

27590   Amputation, thigh, through femur, any level;

27591   immediate fitting technique including first cast

27592   open, circular (guillotine)

27594   secondary closure or scar revision

27596   re-amputation

27598   Disarticulation at knee

Other Procedures

27599   Unlisted procedure, femur or knee

Leg (Tibia and Fibula) and Ankle Joint

Incision

27600   Decompression fasciotomy, leg; anterior and/or lateral compartments only

27601   posterior compartment(s) only

27602   anterior and/or lateral, and posterior compartment(s)

(For incision and drainage procedures, superficial, see 10040-10160)

(For decompression fasciotomy with debridement, see 27892-27894)

27603   Incision and drainage, leg or ankle; deep abscess or hematoma

27604   infected bursa

27605   Tenotomy, percutaneous, Achilles tendon (separate procedure); local anesthesia

27606   general anesthesia

27607   Incision (eg, osteomyelitis or bone abscess), leg or ankle

27610   Arthrotomy, ankle, including exploration, drainage, or removal of foreign body

27612   Arthrotomy, posterior capsular release, ankle, with or without Achilles tendon lengthening

(See also 27685)

Excision

27613   Biopsy, soft tissue of leg or ankle area; superficial

27614   deep (subfascial or intramuscular)

(For needle biopsy of soft tissue, use 20206)

27615   Radical resection of tumor (eg, malignant neoplasm), soft tissue of leg or ankle area

27618   Excision, tumor, leg or ankle area; subcutaneous tissue

27619   deep (subfascial or intramuscular)

27620   Arthrotomy, ankle, with joint exploration, with or without biopsy, with or without removal of loose or foreign body

27625   Arthrotomy, with synovectomy, ankle;

27626   including tenosynovectomy

Surgery: Musculoskeletal System

27630 Excision of lesion of tendon sheath or capsule (eg, cyst or ganglion), leg and/or ankle

27635 Excision or curettage of bone cyst or benign tumor, tibia or fibula;

27637 with autograft (includes obtaining graft)

27638 with allograft

27640 Partial excision (craterization, saucerization, or diaphysectomy) bone (eg, osteomyelitis or exostosis); tibia

27641 fibula

27645 Radical resection of tumor, bone; tibia

27646 fibula

27647 talus or calcaneus

Introduction or Removal

27648 Injection procedure for ankle arthrography

(For radiological supervision and interpretation, use 73615. Do not report 76003 in addition to 73615)

(For ankle arthroscopy, see 29894-29898)

Repair, Revision, and/or Reconstruction

27650 Repair, primary, open or percutaneous, ruptured Achilles tendon;

27652 with graft (includes obtaining graft)

27654 Repair, secondary, Achilles tendon, with or without graft

27656 Repair, fascial defect of leg

27658 Repair, flexor tendon, leg; primary, without graft, each tendon

27659 secondary, with or without graft, each tendon

27664 Repair, extensor tendon, leg; primary, without graft, each tendon

27665 secondary, with or without graft, each tendon

27675 Repair, dislocating peroneal tendons; without fibular osteotomy

27676 with fibular osteotomy

27680 Tenolysis, flexor or extensor tendon, leg and/or ankle; single, each tendon

27681 multiple tendons (through separate incision(s))

27685 Lengthening or shortening of tendon, leg or ankle; single tendon (separate procedure)

27686 multiple tendons (through same incision), each

27687 Gastrocnemius recession (eg, Strayer procedure)

(Toe extensors are considered as a group to be a single tendon when transplanted into midfoot)

27690 Transfer or transplant of single tendon (with muscle redirection or rerouting); superficial (eg, anterior tibial extensors into midfoot)

27691 deep (eg, anterior tibial or posterior tibial through interosseous space, flexor digitorum longus, flexor hallucis longus, or peroneal tendon to midfoot or hindfoot)

+ 27692 each additional tendon (List separately in addition to code for primary procedure)

(Use 27692 in conjunction with 27690, 27691)

27695 Repair, primary, disrupted ligament, ankle; collateral

27696 both collateral ligaments

27698 Repair, secondary, disrupted ligament, ankle, collateral (eg, Watson-Jones procedure)

27700 Arthroplasty, ankle;

27702 with implant (total ankle)

27703 revision, total ankle

27704 Removal of ankle implant

27705 Osteotomy; tibia

27707 fibula

27709 tibia and fibula

27712 multiple, with realignment on intramedullary rod (eg, Sofield type procedure)

(For osteotomy to correct genu varus (bowleg) or genu valgus (knock-knee), see 27455-27457)

27715 Osteoplasty, tibia and fibula, lengthening or shortening

27720 Repair of nonunion or malunion, tibia; without graft, (eg, compression technique)

27722 with sliding graft

27724 with iliac or other autograft (includes obtaining graft)

27725 by synostosis, with fibula, any method

27727 Repair of congenital pseudarthrosis, tibia

27730 Arrest, epiphyseal (epiphysiodesis), open; distal tibia

27732 distal fibula

27734 distal tibia and fibula

27740 Arrest, epiphyseal (epiphysiodesis), any method, combined, proximal and distal tibia and fibula;

27742 and distal femur

(For epiphyseal arrest of proximal tibia and fibula, use 27477)

27745 Prophylactic treatment (nailing, pinning, plating or wiring) with or without methylmethacrylate, tibia

Fracture and/or Dislocation

27750   Closed treatment of tibial shaft fracture (with or without fibular fracture); without manipulation

27752   with manipulation, with or without skeletal traction

27756   Percutaneous skeletal fixation of tibial shaft fracture (with or without fibular fracture) (eg, pins or screws)

27758   Open treatment of tibial shaft fracture, (with or without fibular fracture) with plate/screws, with or without cerclage

27759   Treatment of tibial shaft fracture (with or without fibular fracture) by intramedullary implant, with or without interlocking screws and/or cerclage

27760   Closed treatment of medial malleolus fracture; without manipulation

27762   with manipulation, with or without skin or skeletal traction

27766   Open treatment of medial malleolus fracture, with or without internal or external fixation

27780   Closed treatment of proximal fibula or shaft fracture; without manipulation

27781   with manipulation

27784   Open treatment of proximal fibula or shaft fracture, with or without internal or external fixation

27786   Closed treatment of distal fibular fracture (lateral malleolus); without manipulation

27788   with manipulation

27792   Open treatment of distal fibular fracture (lateral malleolus), with or without internal or external fixation

(For treatment of tibia and fibula shaft fractures, see 27750-27759)

27808   Closed treatment of bimalleolar ankle fracture, (including Potts); without manipulation

27810   with manipulation

27814   Open treatment of bimalleolar ankle fracture, with or without internal or external fixation

27816   Closed treatment of trimalleolar ankle fracture; without manipulation

27818   with manipulation

27822   Open treatment of trimalleolar ankle fracture, with or without internal or external fixation, medial and/or lateral malleolus; without fixation of posterior lip

27823   with fixation of posterior lip

27824   Closed treatment of fracture of weight bearing articular portion of distal tibia (eg, pilon or tibial plafond), with or without anesthesia; without manipulation

27825   with skeletal traction and/or requiring manipulation

27826   Open treatment of fracture of weight bearing articular surface/portion of distal tibia (eg, pilon or tibial plafond), with internal or external fixation; of fibula only

27827   of tibia only

27828   of both tibia and fibula

27829   Open treatment of distal tibiofibular joint (syndesmosis) disruption, with or without internal or external fixation

27830   Closed treatment of proximal tibiofibular joint dislocation; without anesthesia

27831   requiring anesthesia

27832   Open treatment of proximal tibiofibular joint dislocation, with or without internal or external fixation, or with excision of proximal fibula

27840   Closed treatment of ankle dislocation; without anesthesia

27842   requiring anesthesia, with or without percutaneous skeletal fixation

27846   Open treatment of ankle dislocation, with or without percutaneous skeletal fixation; without repair or internal fixation

27848   with repair or internal or external fixation

(For surgical or diagnostic arthroscopic procedures, see 29894-29898)

Manipulation

27860   Manipulation of ankle under general anesthesia (includes application of traction or other fixation apparatus)

Arthrodesis

27870   Arthrodesis, ankle, open

(For arthroscopic ankle arthrodesis, use 29899)

27871   Arthrodesis, tibiofibular joint, proximal or distal

Amputation

27880   Amputation, leg, through tibia and fibula;

27881   with immediate fitting technique including application of first cast

27882   open, circular (guillotine)

27884   secondary closure or scar revision

27886   re-amputation

27888   Amputation, ankle, through malleoli of tibia and fibula (eg, Syme, Pirogoff type procedures), with plastic closure and resection of nerves

27889   Ankle disarticulation

Other Procedures

27892 Decompression fasciotomy, leg; anterior and/or lateral compartments only, with debridement of nonviable muscle and/or nerve

(For decompression fasciotomy of the leg without debridement, use 27600)

27893 posterior compartment(s) only, with debridement of nonviable muscle and/or nerve

(For decompression fasciotomy of the leg without debridement, use 27601)

27894 anterior and/or lateral, and posterior compartment(s), with debridement of nonviable muscle and/or nerve

(For decompression fasciotomy of the leg without debridement, use 27602)

27899 Unlisted procedure, leg or ankle

Foot and Toes

Incision

(For incision and drainage procedures, superficial, see 10040-10160)

28001 Incision and drainage, bursa, foot

28002 Incision and drainage below fascia, with or without tendon sheath involvement, foot; single bursal space

28003 multiple areas

28005 Incision, bone cortex (eg, osteomyelitis or bone abscess), foot

28008 Fasciotomy, foot and/or toe

(See also 28060, 28062, 28250)

28010 Tenotomy, percutaneous, toe; single tendon

28011 multiple tendons

(For open tenotomy, see 28230-28234)

28020 Arthrotomy, including exploration, drainage, or removal of loose or foreign body; intertarsal or tarsometatarsal joint

28022 metatarsophalangeal joint

28024 interphalangeal joint

28030 Neurectomy, intrinsic musculature of foot

28035 Release, tarsal tunnel (posterior tibial nerve decompression)

(For other nerve entrapments, see 64704, 64722)

Excision

28043 Excision, tumor, foot; subcutaneous tissue

28045 deep, subfascial, intramuscular

28046 Radical resection of tumor (eg, malignant neoplasm), soft tissue of foot

28050 Arthrotomy with biopsy; intertarsal or tarsometatarsal joint

28052 metatarsophalangeal joint

28054 interphalangeal joint

28060 Fasciectomy, plantar fascia; partial (separate procedure)

28062 radical (separate procedure)

(For plantar fasciotomy, see 28008, 28250)

28070 Synovectomy; intertarsal or tarsometatarsal joint, each

28072 metatarsophalangeal joint, each

28080 Excision, interdigital (Morton) neuroma, single, each

28086 Synovectomy, tendon sheath, foot; flexor

28088 extensor

28090 Excision of lesion, tendon, tendon sheath, or capsule (including synovectomy) (eg, cyst or ganglion); foot

28092 toe(s), each

28100 Excision or curettage of bone cyst or benign tumor, talus or calcaneus;

28102 with iliac or other autograft (includes obtaining graft)

28103 with allograft

28104 Excision or curettage of bone cyst or benign tumor, tarsal or metatarsal, except talus or calcaneus;

28106 with iliac or other autograft (includes obtaining graft)

28107 with allograft

28108 Excision or curettage of bone cyst or benign tumor, phalanges of foot

(For ostectomy, partial (eg, hallux valgus, Silver type procedure), use 28290)

28110 Ostectomy, partial excision, fifth metatarsal head (bunionette) (separate procedure)

28111 Ostectomy, complete excision; first metatarsal head

28112 other metatarsal head (second, third or fourth)

28113 fifth metatarsal head

28114 all metatarsal heads, with partial proximal phalangectomy, excluding first metatarsal (eg, Clayton type procedure)

28116 Ostectomy, excision of tarsal coalition

28118 Ostectomy, calcaneus;

28119 for spur, with or without plantar fascial release

28120 Partial excision (craterization, saucerization, sequestrectomy, or diaphysectomy) bone (eg, osteomyelitis or bossing); talus or calcaneus

28122 tarsal or metatarsal bone, except talus or calcaneus

(For partial excision of talus or calcaneus, use 28120)

(For cheilectomy for hallux rigidus, use 28289)

28124 phalanx of toe

28126   Resection, partial or complete, phalangeal base, each toe

28130   Talectomy (astragalectomy)

         (For calcanectomy, use 28118)

28140   Metatarsectomy

28150   Phalangectomy, toe, each toe

28153   Resection, condyle(s), distal end of phalanx, each toe

28160   Hemiphalangectomy or interphalangeal joint excision, toe, proximal end of phalanx, each

28171   Radical resection of tumor, bone; tarsal (except talus or calcaneus)

28173   metatarsal

28175   phalanx of toe

         (For talus or calcaneus, use 27647)

Introduction or Removal

28190   Removal of foreign body, foot; subcutaneous

28192   deep

28193   complicated

Repair, Revision, and/or Reconstruction

28200   Repair, tendon, flexor, foot; primary or secondary, without free graft, each tendon

28202   secondary with free graft, each tendon (includes obtaining graft)

28208   Repair, tendon, extensor, foot; primary or secondary, each tendon

28210   secondary with free graft, each tendon (includes obtaining graft)

28220   Tenolysis, flexor, foot; single tendon

28222   multiple tendons

28225   Tenolysis, extensor, foot; single tendon

28226   multiple tendons

28230   Tenotomy, open, tendon flexor; foot, single or multiple tendon(s) (separate procedure)

28232   toe, single tendon (separate procedure)

28234   Tenotomy, open, extensor, foot or toe, each tendon

         (For tendon transfer to midfoot or hindfoot, see 27690, 27691)

28238   Reconstruction (advancement), posterior tibial tendon with excision of accessory tarsal navicular bone (eg, Kidner type procedure)

         (For subcutaneous tenotomy, see 28010, 28011)

         (For transfer or transplant of tendon with muscle redirection or rerouting, see 27690-27692)

         (For extensor hallucis longus transfer with great toe IP fusion (Jones procedure), use 28760)

28240   Tenotomy, lengthening, or release, abductor hallucis muscle

28250   Division of plantar fascia and muscle (eg, Steindler stripping) (separate procedure)

28260   Capsulotomy, midfoot; medial release only (separate procedure)

28261   with tendon lengthening

28262   extensive, including posterior talotibial capsulotomy and tendon(s) lengthening (eg, resistant clubfoot deformity)

28264   Capsulotomy, midtarsal (eg, Heyman type procedure)

28270   Capsulotomy; metatarsophalangeal joint, with or without tenorrhaphy, each joint (separate procedure)

28272   interphalangeal joint, each joint (separate procedure)

28280   Syndactylization, toes (eg, webbing or Kelikian type procedure)

28285   Correction, hammertoe (eg, interphalangeal fusion, partial or total phalangectomy)

28286   Correction, cock-up fifth toe, with plastic skin closure (eg, Ruiz-Mora type procedure)

28288   Ostectomy, partial, exostectomy or condylectomy, metatarsal head, each metatarsal head

28289   Hallux rigidus correction with cheilectomy, debridement and capsular release of the first metatarsophalangeal joint

28290   Correction, hallux valgus (bunion), with or without sesamoidectomy; simple exostectomy (eg, Silver type procedure)

28292   Keller, McBride, or Mayo type procedure

28293   resection of joint with implant

28294   with tendon transplants (eg, Joplin type procedure)

28296   with metatarsal osteotomy (eg, Mitchell, Chevron, or concentric type procedures)

28297   Lapidus type procedure

28298   by phalanx osteotomy

28299   by double osteotomy

28300   Osteotomy; calcaneus (eg, Dwyer or Chambers type procedure), with or without internal fixation

28302   talus

28304   Osteotomy, tarsal bones, other than calcaneus or talus;

28305   with autograft (includes obtaining graft) (eg, Fowler type)

28306   Osteotomy, with or without lengthening, shortening or angular correction, metatarsal; first metatarsal

28307   first metatarsal with autograft (other than first toe)

28308   other than first metatarsal, each

28309   multiple (eg, Swanson type cavus foot procedure)

Surgery: Musculoskeletal System

Surgery: Musculoskeletal System

28310   Osteotomy, shortening, angular or rotational correction; proximal phalanx, first toe (separate procedure)

28312   other phalanges, any toe

28313   Reconstruction, angular deformity of toe, soft tissue procedures only (eg, overlapping second toe, fifth toe, curly toes)

28315   Sesamoidectomy, first toe (separate procedure)

28320   Repair, nonunion or malunion; tarsal bones

28322   metatarsal, with or without bone graft (includes obtaining graft)

28340   Reconstruction, toe, macrodactyly; soft tissue resection

28341   requiring bone resection

28344   Reconstruction, toe(s); polydactyly

28345   syndactyly, with or without skin graft(s), each web

28360   Reconstruction, cleft foot

Fracture and/or Dislocation

28400   Closed treatment of calcaneal fracture; without manipulation

28405   with manipulation

28406   Percutaneous skeletal fixation of calcaneal fracture, with manipulation

28415   Open treatment of calcaneal fracture, with or without internal or external fixation;

28420   with primary iliac or other autogenous bone graft (includes obtaining graft)

28430   Closed treatment of talus fracture; without manipulation

28435   with manipulation

28436   Percutaneous skeletal fixation of talus fracture, with manipulation

28445   Open treatment of talus fracture, with or without internal or external fixation

28450   Treatment of tarsal bone fracture (except talus and calcaneus); without manipulation, each

28455   with manipulation, each

28456   Percutaneous skeletal fixation of tarsal bone fracture (except talus and calcaneus), with manipulation, each

28465   Open treatment of tarsal bone fracture (except talus and calcaneus), with or without internal or external fixation, each

28470   Closed treatment of metatarsal fracture; without manipulation, each

28475   with manipulation, each

28476   Percutaneous skeletal fixation of metatarsal fracture, with manipulation, each

28485   Open treatment of metatarsal fracture, with or without internal or external fixation, each

28490   Closed treatment of fracture great toe, phalanx or phalanges; without manipulation

28495   with manipulation

28496   Percutaneous skeletal fixation of fracture great toe, phalanx or phalanges, with manipulation

28505   Open treatment of fracture great toe, phalanx or phalanges, with or without internal or external fixation

28510   Closed treatment of fracture, phalanx or phalanges, other than great toe; without manipulation, each

28515   with manipulation, each

28525   Open treatment of fracture, phalanx or phalanges, other than great toe, with or without internal or external fixation, each

28530   Closed treatment of sesamoid fracture

28531   Open treatment of sesamoid fracture, with or without internal fixation

28540   Closed treatment of tarsal bone dislocation, other than talotarsal; without anesthesia

28545   requiring anesthesia

28546   Percutaneous skeletal fixation of tarsal bone dislocation, other than talotarsal, with manipulation

28555   Open treatment of tarsal bone dislocation, with or without internal or external fixation

28570   Closed treatment of talotarsal joint dislocation; without anesthesia

28575   requiring anesthesia

28576   Percutaneous skeletal fixation of talotarsal joint dislocation, with manipulation

28585   Open treatment of talotarsal joint dislocation, with or without internal or external fixation

28600   Closed treatment of tarsometatarsal joint dislocation; without anesthesia

28605   requiring anesthesia

28606   Percutaneous skeletal fixation of tarsometatarsal joint dislocation, with manipulation

28615   Open treatment of tarsometatarsal joint dislocation, with or without internal or external fixation

28630   Closed treatment of metatarsophalangeal joint dislocation; without anesthesia

28635   requiring anesthesia

28636   Percutaneous skeletal fixation of metatarsophalangeal joint dislocation, with manipulation

28645   Open treatment of metatarsophalangeal joint dislocation, with or without internal or external fixation

28660   Closed treatment of interphalangeal joint dislocation; without anesthesia

28665   requiring anesthesia

28666   Percutaneous skeletal fixation of interphalangeal joint dislocation, with manipulation

28675   Open treatment of interphalangeal joint dislocation, with or without internal or external fixation

Arthrodesis

28705   Arthrodesis; pantalar

28715   triple

28725   subtalar

28730   Arthrodesis, midtarsal or tarsometatarsal, multiple or transverse;

28735   with osteotomy (eg, flatfoot correction)

28737   Arthrodesis, with tendon lengthening and advancement, midtarsal, tarsal navicular-cuneiform (eg, Miller type procedure)

28740   Arthrodesis, midtarsal or tarsometatarsal, single joint

28750   Arthrodesis, great toe; metatarsophalangeal joint

28755   interphalangeal joint

28760   Arthrodesis, with extensor hallucis longus transfer to first metatarsal neck, great toe, interphalangeal joint (eg, Jones type procedure)

          (For hammertoe operation or interphalangeal fusion, use 28285)

Amputation

28800   Amputation, foot; midtarsal (eg, Chopart type procedure)

28805   transmetatarsal

28810   Amputation, metatarsal, with toe, single

28820   Amputation, toe; metatarsophalangeal joint

28825   interphalangeal joint

          (For amputation of tuft of distal phalanx, use 11752)

Other Procedures

          (For extracorporeal shock wave therapy involving musculoskeletal system, or plantar fascia, see Category III codes 0019T, 0020T)

28899   Unlisted procedure, foot or toes

Application of Casts and Strapping

The listed procedures apply when the cast application or strapping is a replacement procedure used during or after the period of follow-up care, or when the cast application or strapping is an initial service performed without a restorative treatment or procedure(s) to stabilize or protect a fracture, injury, or dislocation and/or to afford comfort to a patient. Restorative treatment or procedure(s) rendered by another physician following the application of the initial cast/splint/strap may be reported with a treatment of fracture and/or dislocation code.

A physician who applies the initial cast, strap or splint and also assumes all of the subsequent fracture, dislocation, or injury care cannot use the application of casts and strapping codes as an initial service, since the first cast/splint or strap application is included in the treatment of fracture and/or dislocation codes. (See notes under Musculoskeletal System, page 59. A temporary cast/splint/strap is not considered to be part of the preoperative care, and the use of the modifier 56 is not applicable. Additional evaluation and management services are reportable only if signifi cant identifiable further services are provided at the time of the cast application or strapping.

If cast application or strapping is provided as an initial service (eg, casting of a sprained ankle or knee) in which no other procedure or treatment (eg, surgical repair, reduction of a fracture or joint dislocation) is performed or is expected to be performed by a physician rendering the initial care only, use the casting, strapping and/or supply code (99070) in addition to an evaluation and management code as appropriate.

Listed procedures include removal of cast or strapping.

          (For orthotics fitting and training, use 97504)

Body and Upper Extremity

Casts

29000   Application of halo type body cast (see 20661-20663 for insertion)

29010   Application of Risser jacket, localizer, body; only

29015   including head

29020   Application of turnbuckle jacket, body; only

29025   including head

29035   Application of body cast, shoulder to hips;

29040   including head, Minerva type

29044   including one thigh

29046   including both thighs

29049   Application, cast; figure-of-eight

29055   shoulder spica

29058   plaster Velpeau

29065   shoulder to hand (long arm)

29075   elbow to finger (short arm)

Surgery: Musculoskeletal System

29085	hand and lower forearm (gauntlet)
29086	finger (eg, contracture)

Splints

29105	Application of long arm splint (shoulder to hand)
29125	Application of short arm splint (forearm to hand); static
29126	dynamic
29130	Application of finger splint; static
29131	dynamic

Strapping—Any Age

29200	Strapping; thorax
29220	low back
29240	shoulder (eg, Velpeau)
29260	elbow or wrist
29280	hand or finger

Lower Extremity

Casts

29305	Application of hip spica cast; one leg
29325	one and one-half spica or both legs

(For hip spica (body) cast, including thighs only, use 29046)

29345	Application of long leg cast (thigh to toes);
29355	walker or ambulatory type
29358	Application of long leg cast brace
29365	Application of cylinder cast (thigh to ankle)
29405	Application of short leg cast (below knee to toes);
29425	walking or ambulatory type
29435	Application of patellar tendon bearing (PTB) cast
29440	Adding walker to previously applied cast
29445	Application of rigid total contact leg cast
29450	Application of clubfoot cast with molding or manipulation, long or short leg

(To report bilateral procedure, use 29450 with modifier 50)

Splints

29505	Application of long leg splint (thigh to ankle or toes)
29515	Application of short leg splint (calf to foot)

Strapping—Any Age

29520	Strapping; hip
29530	knee
29540	ankle and/or foot
29550	toes
29580	Unna boot
29590	Denis-Browne splint strapping

Removal or Repair

Codes for cast removals should be employed only for casts applied by another physician.

29700	Removal or bivalving; gauntlet, boot or body cast
29705	full arm or full leg cast
29710	shoulder or hip spica, Minerva, or Risser jacket, etc.
29715	turnbuckle jacket
29720	Repair of spica, body cast or jacket
29730	Windowing of cast
29740	Wedging of cast (except clubfoot casts)
29750	Wedging of clubfoot cast

(To report bilateral procedure, use 29750 with modifier 50)

Other Procedures

29799	Unlisted procedure, casting or strapping

Endoscopy/Arthroscopy

Surgical endoscopy/arthroscopy always includes a diagnostic endoscopy/arthroscopy.

When arthroscopy is performed in conjunction with arthrotomy, add modifier 51.

29800	Arthroscopy, temporomandibular joint, diagnostic, with or without synovial biopsy (separate procedure)
29804	Arthroscopy, temporomandibular joint, surgical

(For open procedure, use 21010)

29805	Arthroscopy, shoulder, diagnostic, with or without synovial biopsy (separate procedure)

(For open procedure, see 23065-23066, 23100-23101)

29806	Arthroscopy, shoulder, surgical; capsulorrhaphy

(For open procedure, see 23450-23466)

(To report thermal capsulorrhaphy, use 29999)

29807	repair of SLAP lesion
29819	with removal of loose body or foreign body

(For open procedure, see 23040-23044, 23107)

29820   synovectomy, partial

(For open procedure, see 23105)

29821   synovectomy, complete

(For open procedure, see 23105)

29822   debridement, limited

(For open procedure, see specific open shoulder procedure performed)

29823   debridement, extensive

(For open procedure, see specific open shoulder procedure performed)

29824   distal claviculectomy including distal articular surface (Mumford procedure)

(For open procedure, use 23120)

29825   with lysis and resection of adhesions, with or without manipulation

(For open procedure, see specific open shoulder procedure performed)

29826   decompression of subacromial space with partial acromioplasty, with or without coracoacromial release

(For open procedure, use 23130 or 23415)

29827   with rotator cuff repair

(For open or mini-open rotator cuff repair, use 23412)

(When arthroscopic subacromial decompression is performed at the same setting, use 29826 and append modifier 51)

(When arthroscopic distal clavicle resection is performed at the same setting, use 29824 and append modifier 51)

29830   Arthroscopy, elbow, diagnostic, with or without synovial biopsy (separate procedure)

29834   Arthroscopy, elbow, surgical; with removal of loose body or foreign body

29835   synovectomy, partial

29836   synovectomy, complete

29837   debridement, limited

29838   debridement, extensive

29840   Arthroscopy, wrist, diagnostic, with or without synovial biopsy (separate procedure)

29843   Arthroscopy, wrist, surgical; for infection, lavage and drainage

29844   synovectomy, partial

29845   synovectomy, complete

29846   excision and/or repair of triangular fibrocartilage and/or joint debridement

29847   internal fixation for fracture or instability

29848   Endoscopy, wrist, surgical, with release of transverse carpal ligament

(For open procedure, use 64721)

29850   Arthroscopically aided treatment of intercondylar spine(s) and/or tuberosity fracture(s) of the knee, with or without manipulation; without internal or external fixation (includes arthroscopy)

29851   with internal or external fixation (includes arthroscopy)

(For bone graft, use 20900, 20902)

29855   Arthroscopically aided treatment of tibial fracture, proximal (plateau); unicondylar, with or without internal or external fixation (includes arthroscopy)

29856   bicondylar, with or without internal or external fixation (includes arthroscopy)

(For bone graft, use 20900, 20902)

29860   Arthroscopy, hip, diagnostic with or without synovial biopsy (separate procedure)

29861   Arthroscopy, hip, surgical; with removal of loose body or foreign body

29862   with debridement/shaving of articular cartilage (chondroplasty), abrasion arthroplasty, and/or resection of labrum

29863   with synovectomy

● **29866**   Arthroscopy, knee, surgical; osteochondral autograft(s) (eg, mosaicplasty) (includes harvesting of the autograft)

▶(Do not report 29866 in conjunction with 29870, 29871, 29874, 29875, 29877, 29884 when performed at the same session and/or 29879, 29885-29887 when performed in the same compartment)◀

● **29867**   osteochondral allograft (eg, mosaicplasty)

▶(Do not report 29867 in conjunction with 27570, 29870, 29871, 29874, 29875, 29877, 29884 when performed at the same session and/or 29879, 29885-29887 when performed in the same compartment)◀

▶(Do not report 29867 in conjunction with 27415)◀

● **29868**   meniscal transplantation (includes arthrotomy for meniscal insertion), medial or lateral

▶(Do not report 29868 in conjunction with 29870, 29871, 29874, 29875, 29880, 29883, 29884 when performed at the same session or 29881, 29882 when performed in the same compartment)◀

29870   Arthroscopy, knee, diagnostic, with or without synovial biopsy (separate procedure)

▶(For open autologous chondrocyte implantation of the knee, use 27412)◀

Surgery: Musculoskeletal System

Surgery: Musculoskeletal System

29871   Arthroscopy, knee, surgical; for infection, lavage and drainage

▶(For implantation of osteochondral graft for treatment of articular surface defect, see 27412, 27415, 29866, 29867)◀

29873   with lateral release

(For open lateral release, use 27425)

29874   for removal of loose body or foreign body (eg, osteochondritis dissecans fragmentation, chondral fragmentation)

29875   synovectomy, limited (eg, plica or shelf resection) (separate procedure)

29876   synovectomy, major, two or more compartments (eg, medial or lateral)

29877   debridement/shaving of articular cartilage (chondroplasty)

29879   abrasion arthroplasty (includes chondroplasty where necessary) or multiple drilling or microfracture

29880   with meniscectomy (medial AND lateral, including any meniscal shaving)

29881   with meniscectomy (medial OR lateral, including any meniscal shaving)

29882   with meniscus repair (medial OR lateral)

29883   with meniscus repair (medial AND lateral)

▶(For meniscal transplantation, medial or lateral, knee, use 29868)◀

29884   with lysis of adhesions, with or without manipulation (separate procedure)

29885   drilling for osteochondritis dissecans with bone grafting, with or without internal fixation (including debridement of base of lesion)

29886   drilling for intact osteochondritis dissecans lesion

29887   drilling for intact osteochondritis dissecans lesion with internal fixation

29888   Arthroscopically aided anterior cruciate ligament repair/augmentation or reconstruction

29889   Arthroscopically aided posterior cruciate ligament repair/augmentation or reconstruction

(Procedures 29888 and 29889 should not be used with reconstruction procedures 27427-27429)

29891   Arthroscopy, ankle, surgical, excision of osteochondral defect of talus and/or tibia, including drilling of the defect

29892   Arthroscopically aided repair of large osteochondritis dissecans lesion, talar dome fracture, or tibial plafond fracture, with or without internal fixation (includes arthroscopy)

29893   Endoscopic plantar fasciotomy

29894   Arthroscopy, ankle (tibiotalar and fibulotalar joints), surgical; with removal of loose body or foreign body

29895   synovectomy, partial

29897   debridement, limited

29898   debridement, extensive

29899   with ankle arthrodesis

(For open ankle arthrodesis, use 27870)

29900   Arthroscopy, metacarpophalangeal joint, diagnostic, includes synovial biopsy

(Do not report 29900 with 29901, 29902)

29901   Arthroscopy, metacarpophalangeal joint, surgical; with debridement

29902   with reduction of displaced ulnar collateral ligament (eg, Stenar lesion)

29999   Unlisted procedure, arthroscopy

Respiratory System

Nose

Incision

30000   Drainage abscess or hematoma, nasal, internal approach

   (For external approach, see 10060, 10140)

30020   Drainage abscess or hematoma, nasal septum

   (For lateral rhinotomy, see specific application (eg, 30118, 30320))

Excision

30100   Biopsy, intranasal

   (For biopsy skin of nose, see 11100, 11101)

30110   Excision, nasal polyp(s), simple

   (30110 would normally be completed in an office setting)

   (To report bilateral procedure, use 30110 with modifier 50)

30115   Excision, nasal polyp(s), extensive

   (30115 would normally require the facilities available in a hospital setting)

   (To report bilateral procedure, use 30115 with modifier 50)

30117   Excision or destruction (eg, laser), intranasal lesion; internal approach

30118   external approach (lateral rhinotomy)

30120   Excision or surgical planing of skin of nose for rhinophyma

30124   Excision dermoid cyst, nose; simple, skin, subcutaneous

30125   complex, under bone or cartilage

30130   Excision turbinate, partial or complete, any method

30140   Submucous resection turbinate, partial or complete, any method

   (For submucous resection of nasal septum, use 30520)

   (For reduction of turbinates, use 30140 with modifier 52)

30150   Rhinectomy; partial

30160   total

   (For closure and/or reconstruction, primary or delayed, see **Integumentary System,** 13150-13160, 14060-14300, 15120, 15121, 15260, 15261, 15760, 20900-20912)

Introduction

30200   Injection into turbinate(s), therapeutic

30210   Displacement therapy (Proetz type)

30220   Insertion, nasal septal prosthesis (button)

Removal of Foreign Body

30300   Removal foreign body, intranasal; office type procedure

30310   requiring general anesthesia

30320   by lateral rhinotomy

Repair

   (For obtaining tissues for graft, see 20900-20926, 21210)

30400   Rhinoplasty, primary; lateral and alar cartilages and/or elevation of nasal tip

   (For columellar reconstruction, see 13150 et seq)

30410   complete, external parts including bony pyramid, lateral and alar cartilages, and/or elevation of nasal tip

30420   including major septal repair

30430   Rhinoplasty, secondary; minor revision (small amount of nasal tip work)

30435   intermediate revision (bony work with osteotomies)

30450   major revision (nasal tip work and osteotomies)

30460   Rhinoplasty for nasal deformity secondary to congenital cleft lip and/or palate, including columellar lengthening; tip only

30462   tip, septum, osteotomies

30465   Repair of nasal vestibular stenosis (eg, spreader grafting, lateral nasal wall reconstruction)

   (30465 excludes obtaining graft. For graft procedure, see 20900-20926, 21210)

   (30465 is used to report a bilateral procedure. For unilateral procedure, use modifier 52)

30520   Septoplasty or submucous resection, with or without cartilage scoring, contouring or replacement with graft

   (For submucous resection of turbinates, use 30140)

30540   Repair choanal atresia; intranasal

30545   transpalatine

   (Do not report modifier 63 in conjunction with 30540, 30545)

30560   Lysis intranasal synechia

30580   Repair fistula; oromaxillary (combine with 31030 if antrotomy is included)

30600   oronasal

Surgery: Respiratory System

Surgery: Respiratory System

30620 Septal or other intranasal dermatoplasty (does not include obtaining graft)

30630 Repair nasal septal perforations

Destruction

30801 Cautery and/or ablation, mucosa of turbinates, unilateral or bilateral, any method, (separate procedure); superficial

30802   intramural

Other Procedures

30901 Control nasal hemorrhage, anterior, simple (limited cautery and/or packing) any method

(To report bilateral procedure, use 30901 with modifier 50)

30903 Control nasal hemorrhage, anterior, complex (extensive cautery and/or packing) any method

(To report bilateral procedure, use 30903 with modifier 50)

30905 Control nasal hemorrhage, posterior, with posterior nasal packs and/or cautery, any method; initial

30906   subsequent

30915 Ligation arteries; ethmoidal

30920   internal maxillary artery, transantral

(For ligation external carotid artery, use 37600)

30930 Fracture nasal turbinate(s), therapeutic

30999 Unlisted procedure, nose

Accessory Sinuses

Incision

31000 Lavage by cannulation; maxillary sinus (antrum puncture or natural ostium)

(To report bilateral procedure, use 31000 with modifier 50)

31002   sphenoid sinus

31020 Sinusotomy, maxillary (antrotomy); intranasal

(To report bilateral procedure, use 31020 with modifier 50)

31030   radical (Caldwell-Luc) without removal of antrochoanal polyps

(To report bilateral procedure, use 31030 with modifier 50)

31032   radical (Caldwell-Luc) with removal of antrochoanal polyps

(To report bilateral procedure, use 31032 with modifier 50)

31040 Pterygomaxillary fossa surgery, any approach

(For transantral ligation of internal maxillary artery, use 30920)

31050 Sinusotomy, sphenoid, with or without biopsy;

31051   with mucosal stripping or removal of polyp(s)

31070 Sinusotomy frontal; external, simple (trephine operation)

(For frontal intranasal sinusotomy, use 31276)

31075   transorbital, unilateral (for mucocele or osteoma, Lynch type)

31080   obliterative without osteoplastic flap, brow incision (includes ablation)

31081   obliterative, without osteoplastic flap, coronal incision (includes ablation)

31084   obliterative, with osteoplastic flap, brow incision

31085   obliterative, with osteoplastic flap, coronal incision

31086   nonobliterative, with osteoplastic flap, brow incision

31087   nonobliterative, with osteoplastic flap, coronal incision

31090 Sinusotomy, unilateral, three or more paranasal sinuses (frontal, maxillary, ethmoid, sphenoid)

Excision

31200 Ethmoidectomy; intranasal, anterior

31201   intranasal, total

31205   extranasal, total

31225 Maxillectomy; without orbital exenteration

31230   with orbital exenteration (en bloc)

(For orbital exenteration only, see 65110 et seq)

(For skin grafts, see 15120 et seq)

Endoscopy

A surgical sinus endoscopy includes a sinusotomy (when appropriate) and diagnostic endoscopy.

Codes 31231-31294 are used to report unilateral procedures unless otherwise specified.

The codes 31231-31235 for diagnostic evaluation refer to employing a nasal/sinus endoscope to inspect the interior of the nasal cavity and the middle and superior meatus, the turbinates, and the spheno-ethmoid recess. Any time a diagnostic evaluation is performed all these areas would be inspected and a separate code is not reported for each area.

31231 Nasal endoscopy, diagnostic, unilateral or bilateral (separate procedure)

31233 Nasal/sinus endoscopy, diagnostic with maxillary sinusoscopy (via inferior meatus or canine fossa puncture)

31235   Nasal/sinus endoscopy, diagnostic with sphenoid sinusoscopy (via puncture of sphenoidal face or cannulation of ostium)

31237   Nasal/sinus endoscopy, surgical; with biopsy, polypectomy or debridement (separate procedure)

31238   with control of nasal hemorrhage

31239   with dacryocystorhinostomy

31240   with concha bullosa resection

(For endoscopic osteomeatal complex (OMC) resection with antrostomy and/or anterior ethmoidectomy, with or without removal of polyp(s), use 31254 and 31256)

(For endoscopic osteomeatal complex (OMC) resection with antrostomy, removal of antral mucosal disease, and/or anterior ethmoidectomy, with or without removal of polyp(s), use 31254 and 31267)

(For endoscopic frontal sinus exploration, osteomeatal complex (OMC) resection and/or anterior ethmoidectomy, with or without removal of polyp(s), use 31254 and 31276)

(For endoscopic frontal sinus exploration, osteomeatal complex (OMC) resection, antrostomy, and/or anterior ethmoidectomy, with or without removal of polyp(s), use 31254, 31256, and 31276)

(For endoscopic nasal diagnostic endoscopy, see 31231-31235)

(For endoscopic osteomeatal complex (OMC) resection, frontal sinus exploration, antrostomy, removal of antral mucosal disease, and/or anterior ethmoidectomy, with or without removal of polyp(s), use 31254, 31267, and 31276)

31254   Nasal/sinus endoscopy, surgical; with ethmoidectomy, partial (anterior)

31255   with ethmoidectomy, total (anterior and posterior)

31256   Nasal/sinus endoscopy, surgical, with maxillary antrostomy;

(For endoscopic anterior and posterior ethmoidectomy (APE) and antrostomy, with or without removal of polyp(s), use 31255 and 31256)

(For endoscopic anterior and posterior ethmoidectomy (APE), antrostomy and removal of antral mucosal disease, with or without removal of polyp(s), use 31255 and 31267)

(For endoscopic anterior and posterior ethmoidectomy (APE), and frontal sinus exploration, with or without removal of polyp(s), use 31255 and 31276)

31267   with removal of tissue from maxillary sinus

(For endoscopic anterior and posterior ethmoidectomy (APE), and frontal sinus exploration and antrostomy, with or without removal of polyp(s), use 31255, 31256, and 31276)

(For endoscopic anterior and posterior ethmoidectomy (APE), frontal sinus exploration, antrostomy, and removal of antral mucosal disease, with or without removal of polyp(s), use 31255, 31267, and 31276)

31276   Nasal/sinus endoscopy, surgical with frontal sinus exploration, with or without removal of tissue from frontal sinus

(For endoscopic anterior and posterior ethmoidectomy and sphenoidotomy (APS), with or without removal of polyp(s), use 31255, 31287 or 31288)

(For endoscopic anterior and posterior ethmoidectomy and sphenoidotomy (APS), and antrostomy, with or without removal of polyp(s), use 31255, 31256, and 31287 or 31288)

(For endoscopic anterior and posterior ethmoidectomy and sphenoidotomy (APS), antrostomy and removal of antral mucosal disease, with or without removal of polyp(s), use 31255, 31267, and 31287 or 31288)

(For endoscopic anterior and posterior ethmoidectomy and sphenoidotomy (APS), and frontal sinus exploration with or without removal of polyp(s), use 31255, 31287 or 31288, and 31276)

(For endoscopic anterior and posterior ethmoidectomy and sphenoidotomy (APS), with or without removal of polyp(s), with frontal sinus exploration and antrostomy, use 31255, 31256, 31287 or 31288, and 31276)

(For unilateral endoscopy of two or more sinuses, see 31231-31235)

(For endoscopic anterior and posterior ethmoidectomy and sphenoidotomy (APS), frontal sinus exploration, antrostomy and removal of antral mucosal disease, with or without removal of polyp(s), see 31255, 31267, 31287 or 31288 and 31276)

31287   Nasal/sinus endoscopy, surgical, with sphenoidotomy;

31288   with removal of tissue from the sphenoid sinus

31290   Nasal/sinus endoscopy, surgical, with repair of cerebrospinal fluid leak; ethmoid region

31291   sphenoid region

31292   Nasal/sinus endoscopy, surgical; with medial or inferior orbital wall decompression

31293   with medial orbital wall and inferior orbital wall decompression

31294   with optic nerve decompression

Other Procedures

(For hypophysectomy, transantral or transeptal approach, use 61548)

(For transcranial hypophysectomy, use 61546)

31299   Unlisted procedure, accessory sinuses

Surgery: Respiratory System

Larynx

Excision

31300 Laryngotomy (thyrotomy, laryngofissure); with removal of tumor or laryngocele, cordectomy

31320   diagnostic

31360 Laryngectomy; total, without radical neck dissection

31365   total, with radical neck dissection

31367   subtotal supraglottic, without radical neck dissection

31368   subtotal supraglottic, with radical neck dissection

31370 Partial laryngectomy (hemilaryngectomy); horizontal

31375   laterovertical

31380   anterovertical

31382   antero-latero-vertical

31390 Pharyngolaryngectomy, with radical neck dissection; without reconstruction

31395   with reconstruction

31400 Arytenoidectomy or arytenoidopexy, external approach

(For endoscopic arytenoidectomy, use 31560)

31420 Epiglottidectomy

Introduction

⊘ **31500** Intubation, endotracheal, emergency procedure

(For injection procedure for bronchography, see 31656, 31708, 31710)

31502 Tracheotomy tube change prior to establishment of fistula tract

Endoscopy

For endoscopic procedures, code appropriate endoscopy of each anatomic site examined.

31505 Laryngoscopy, indirect; diagnostic (separate procedure)

31510   with biopsy

31511   with removal of foreign body

31512   with removal of lesion

31513   with vocal cord injection

31515 Laryngoscopy direct, with or without tracheoscopy; for aspiration

31520   diagnostic, newborn

(Do not report modifier 63 in conjunction with 31520)

31525   diagnostic, except newborn

31526   diagnostic, with operating microscope

(Do not report code 69990 in addition to code 31526)

31527   with insertion of obturator

31528   with dilation, initial

31529   with dilation, subsequent

31530 Laryngoscopy, direct, operative, with foreign body removal;

31531   with operating microscope

(Do not report code 69990 in addition to code 31531)

31535 Laryngoscopy, direct, operative, with biopsy;

31536   with operating microscope

(Do not report code 69990 in addition to code 31536)

31540 Laryngoscopy, direct, operative, with excision of tumor and/or stripping of vocal cords or epiglottis;

31541   with operating microscope

(Do not report code 69990 in addition to code 31541)

● **31545** Laryngoscopy, direct, operative, with operating microscope or telescope, with submucosal removal of non-neoplastic lesion(s) of vocal cord; reconstruction with local tissue flap(s)

● **31546**   reconstruction with graft(s) (includes obtaining autograft)

▶(Do not report 31546 in addition to 20926 for graft harvest)◀

▶(For reconstruction of vocal cord with allograft, use 31599)◀

▶(Do not report 31545 or 31546 in conjunction with 31540, 31541, 69990)◀

31560 Laryngoscopy, direct, operative, with arytenoidectomy;

31561   with operating microscope

(Do not report code 69990 in addition to code 31561)

31570 Laryngoscopy, direct, with injection into vocal cord(s), therapeutic;

31571   with operating microscope

(Do not report code 69990 in addition to code 31571)

31575 Laryngoscopy, flexible fiberoptic; diagnostic

31576   with biopsy

31577   with removal of foreign body

31578   with removal of lesion

(To report flexible fiberoptic endoscopic evaluation of swallowing, see 92612-92613)

(To report flexible fiberoptic endoscopic evaluation with sensory testing, see 92614-92615)

(To report flexible fiberoptic endoscopic evaluation of swallowing with sensory testing, see 92616-92617)

(For flexible fiberoptic laryngoscopy as part of flexible fiberoptic endoscopic evaluation of swallowing and/or laryngeal sensory testing by cine or video recording, see 92612-92617)

31579   Laryngoscopy, flexible or rigid fiberoptic, with stroboscopy

Repair

31580   Laryngoplasty; for laryngeal web, two stage, with keel insertion and removal

31582   for laryngeal stenosis, with graft or core mold, including tracheotomy

31584   with open reduction of fracture

31585   Treatment of closed laryngeal fracture; without manipulation

31586   with closed manipulative reduction

31587   Laryngoplasty, cricoid split

31588   Laryngoplasty, not otherwise specified (eg, for burns, reconstruction after partial laryngectomy)

31590   Laryngeal reinnervation by neuromuscular pedicle

Destruction

31595   Section recurrent laryngeal nerve, therapeutic (separate procedure), unilateral

Other Procedures

31599   Unlisted procedure, larynx

Trachea and Bronchi

Incision

31600   Tracheostomy, planned (separate procedure);

31601   under two years

31603   Tracheostomy, emergency procedure; transtracheal

31605   cricothyroid membrane

31610   Tracheostomy, fenestration procedure with skin flaps

(For endotracheal intubation, use 31500)

(For tracheal aspiration under direct vision, use 31515)

31611   Construction of tracheoesophageal fistula and subsequent insertion of an alaryngeal speech prosthesis (eg, voice button, Blom-Singer prosthesis)

31612   Tracheal puncture, percutaneous with transtracheal aspiration and/or injection

31613   Tracheostoma revision; simple, without flap rotation

31614   complex, with flap rotation

Endoscopy

For endoscopy procedures, code appropriate endoscopy of each anatomic site examined. Surgical bronchoscopy always includes diagnostic bronchoscopy when performed by the same physician. Codes 31622-31646 include fluoroscopic guidance, when performed.

(For tracheoscopy, see laryngoscopy codes 31515-31578)

⊙ **31615**   Tracheobronchoscopy through established tracheostomy incision

⊙+● **31620**   Endobronchial ultrasound (EBUS) during bronchoscopic diagnostic or therapeutic intervention(s) (List separately in addition to code for primary procedure(s))

▶(Use 31620 in conjunction with 31622-31638)◀

⊙ **31622**   Bronchoscopy, rigid or flexible, with or without fluoroscopic guidance; diagnostic, with or without cell washing (separate procedure)

⊙ **31623**   with brushing or protected brushings

⊙ **31624**   with bronchial alveolar lavage

⊙ **31625**   with bronchial or endobronchial biopsy(s), single or multiple sites

⊙ **31628**   with transbronchial lung biopsy(s), single lobe

(31628 should be reported only once regardless of how many transbronchial lung biopsies are performed in a lobe)

(To report transbronchial lung biopsies performed on additional lobe, use 31632)

⊙ **31629**   with transbronchial needle aspiration biopsy(s), trachea, main stem and/or lobar bronchus(i)

(31629 should be reported only once for upper airway biopsies regardless of how many transbronchial needle aspiration biopsies are performed in the upper airway or in a lobe)

(To report transbronchial needle aspiration biopsies performed on additional lobe(s), use 31633)

▲ **31630**   with tracheal/bronchial dilation or closed reduction of fracture

▲ **31631**   with placement of tracheal stent(s) (includes tracheal/bronchial dilation as required)

▶(For placement of bronchial stent, see 31636, 31637)◀

▶(For revision of tracheal/bronchial stent, use 31638)◀

+ **31632**   with transbronchial lung biopsy(s), each additional lobe (List separately in addition to code for primary procedure)

(Use 31632 in conjunction with 31628)

(31632 should be reported only once regardless of how many transbronchial lung biopsies are performed in a lobe)

+ **31633**   with transbronchial needle aspiration biopsy(s), each additional lobe (List separately in addition to code for primary procedure)

Surgery: Respiratory System

Surgery: Respiratory System

(Use 31633 in conjunction with 31629)

(31633 should be reported only once regardless of how many transbronchial needle aspiration biopsies are performed in the trachea or the additional lobe)

⊙ **31635**   with removal of foreign body

● **31636**   with placement of bronchial stent(s) (includes tracheal/bronchial dilation as required), initial bronchus

+● **31637**   each additional major bronchus stented (List separately in addition to code for primary procedure)

►(Use 31637 in conjunction with 31636)◄

● **31638**   with revision of tracheal or bronchial stent inserted at previous session (includes tracheal/bronchial dilation as required)

31640   with excision of tumor

31641   Bronchoscopy, (rigid or flexible); with destruction of tumor or relief of stenosis by any method other than excision (eg, laser therapy, cryotherapy)

(For bronchoscopic photodynamic therapy, report 31641 in addition to 96570, 96571 as appropriate)

31643   with placement of catheter(s) for intracavitary radioelement application

(For intracavitary radioelement application, see 77761-77763, 77781-77784)

⊙ **31645**   with therapeutic aspiration of tracheobronchial tree, initial (eg, drainage of lung abscess)

⊙ **31646**   with therapeutic aspiration of tracheobronchial tree, subsequent

(For catheter aspiration of tracheobronchial tree at bedside, use 31725)

⊙ **31656**   with injection of contrast material for segmental bronchography (fiberscope only)

(For radiological supervision and interpretation, see 71040, 71060)

Introduction

(For endotracheal intubation, use 31500)

(For tracheal aspiration under direct vision, see 31515)

31700   Catheterization, transglottic (separate procedure)

31708   Instillation of contrast material for laryngography or bronchography, without catheterization

(For radiological supervision and interpretation, see 70373, 71040, 71060)

31710   Catheterization for bronchography, with or without instillation of contrast material

(For bronchoscopic catheterization for bronchography, fiberscope only, use 31656)

(For radiological supervision and interpretation, see 71040, 71060)

31715   Transtracheal injection for bronchography

(For radiological supervision and interpretation, see 71040, 71060)

(For prolonged services, see 99354-99360)

31717   Catheterization with bronchial brush biopsy

31720   Catheter aspiration (separate procedure); nasotracheal

⊙ **31725**   tracheobronchial with fiberscope, bedside

31730   Transtracheal (percutaneous) introduction of needle wire dilator/stent or indwelling tube for oxygen therapy

Repair

31750   Tracheoplasty; cervical

31755   tracheopharyngeal fistulization, each stage

31760   intrathoracic

31766   Carinal reconstruction

31770   Bronchoplasty; graft repair

31775   excision stenosis and anastomosis

(For lobectomy and bronchoplasty, use 32501)

31780   Excision tracheal stenosis and anastomosis; cervical

31781   cervicothoracic

31785   Excision of tracheal tumor or carcinoma; cervical

31786   thoracic

31800   Suture of tracheal wound or injury; cervical

31805   intrathoracic

31820   Surgical closure tracheostomy or fistula; without plastic repair

31825   with plastic repair

(For repair tracheoesophageal fistula, see 43305, 43312)

31830   Revision of tracheostomy scar

Other Procedures

31899   Unlisted procedure, trachea, bronchi

Lungs and Pleura

Incision

⊘ **32000**   Thoracentesis, puncture of pleural cavity for aspiration, initial or subsequent

(If imaging guidance is performed, see 76003, 76360, 76942)

(For total lung lavage, use 32997)

⊘ **32002**   Thoracentesis with insertion of tube with or without water seal (eg, for pneumothorax) (separate procedure)

(If imaging guidance is performed, see 76003, 76360, 76942)

32005 Chemical pleurodesis (eg, for recurrent or persistent pneumothorax)

⊙● **32019** Insertion of indwelling tunneled pleural catheter with cuff

▶(Do not report 32019 in conjunction with 32000-32005, 32020, 36000, 36410, 62318, 62319, 64450, 64470, 64475)◀

▶(If imaging guidance is performed, use 75989)◀

⊙⊘ **32020** Tube thoracostomy with or without water seal (eg, for abscess, hemothorax, empyema) (separate procedure)

(If imaging guidance is performed, use 75989)

32035 Thoracostomy; with rib resection for empyema

32036 with open flap drainage for empyema

32095 Thoracotomy, limited, for biopsy of lung or pleura

(To report wound exploration due to penetrating trauma without thoractomy, use 20102)

32100 Thoracotomy, major; with exploration and biopsy

32110 with control of traumatic hemorrhage and/or repair of lung tear

32120 for postoperative complications

32124 with open intrapleural pneumonolysis

32140 with cyst(s) removal, with or without a pleural procedure

32141 with excision-plication of bullae, with or without any pleural procedure

(For lung volume reduction, use 32491)

32150 with removal of intrapleural foreign body or fibrin deposit

32151 with removal of intrapulmonary foreign body

32160 with cardiac massage

(For segmental or other resections of lung, see 32480-32525)

32200 Pneumonostomy; with open drainage of abscess or cyst

⊙ **32201** with percutaneous drainage of abscess or cyst

(For radiological supervision and interpretation, use 75989)

32215 Pleural scarification for repeat pneumothorax

32220 Decortication, pulmonary (separate procedure); total

32225 partial

Excision

32310 Pleurectomy, parietal (separate procedure)

32320 Decortication and parietal pleurectomy

32400 Biopsy, pleura; percutaneous needle

(If imaging guidance is performed, see 76003, 76360, 76393, 76942)

(For fine needle aspiration, use 10021 or 10022)

(For evaluation of fine needle aspirate, see 88172, 88173)

32402 open

32405 Biopsy, lung or mediastinum, percutaneous needle

(For radiological supervision and interpretation, see 76003, 76360, 76393, 76942)

(For fine needle aspiration, use 10022)

(For evaluation of fine needle aspirate, see 88172, 88173)

32420 Pneumocentesis, puncture of lung for aspiration

32440 Removal of lung, total pneumonectomy;

32442 with resection of segment of trachea followed by broncho-tracheal anastomosis (sleeve pneumonectomy)

32445 extrapleural

(For extrapleural pneumonectomy, with empyemectomy, use 32445 and 32540)

32480 Removal of lung, other than total pneumonectomy; single lobe (lobectomy)

32482 two lobes (bilobectomy)

32484 single segment (segmentectomy)

(For removal of lung with bronchoplasty, use 32501)

32486 with circumferential resection of segment of bronchus followed by broncho-bronchial anastomosis (sleeve lobectomy)

32488 all remaining lung following previous removal of a portion of lung (completion pneumonectomy)

(For total or segmental lobectomy, with concomitant decortication, use 32320 and the appropriate removal of lung code)

32491 excision-plication of emphysematous lung(s) (bullous or non-bullous) for lung volume reduction, sternal split or transthoracic approach, with or without any pleural procedure

32500 wedge resection, single or multiple

+ **32501** Resection and repair of portion of bronchus (bronchoplasty) when performed at time of lobectomy or segmentectomy (List separately in addition to code for primary procedure)

(Use 32501 in conjunction with 32480, 32482, 32484)

(32501 is to be used when a portion of the bronchus to preserved lung is removed and requires plastic closure to preserve function of that preserved lung. It is not to be used for closure for the proximal end of a resected bronchus)

Surgery: Respiratory System

Surgery: Respiratory System

32520	Resection of lung; with resection of chest wall
32522	with reconstruction of chest wall, without prosthesis
32525	with major reconstruction of chest wall, with prosthesis
32540	Extrapleural enucleation of empyema (empyemectomy)

(For extrapleural enucleation of empyema (empyemectomy) with lobectomy, use 32540 and the appropriate removal of lung code)

Endoscopy

Surgical thoracoscopy always includes diagnostic thoracoscopy.

For endoscopic procedures, code appropriate endoscopy of each anatomic site examined.

32601	Thoracoscopy, diagnostic (separate procedure); lungs and pleural space, without biopsy
32602	lungs and pleural space, with biopsy
32603	pericardial sac, without biopsy
32604	pericardial sac, with biopsy
32605	mediastinal space, without biopsy
32606	mediastinal space, with biopsy

(Surgical thoracoscopy always includes diagnostic thoracoscopy)

32650	Thoracoscopy, surgical; with pleurodesis (eg, mechanical or chemical)
32651	with partial pulmonary decortication
32652	with total pulmonary decortication, including intrapleural pneumonolysis
32653	with removal of intrapleural foreign body or fibrin deposit
32654	with control of traumatic hemorrhage
32655	with excision-plication of bullae, including any pleural procedure
32656	with parietal pleurectomy
32657	with wedge resection of lung, single or multiple
32658	with removal of clot or foreign body from pericardial sac
32659	with creation of pericardial window or partial resection of pericardial sac for drainage
32660	with total pericardiectomy
32661	with excision of pericardial cyst, tumor, or mass
32662	with excision of mediastinal cyst, tumor, or mass
32663	with lobectomy, total or segmental
32664	with thoracic sympathectomy
32665	with esophagomyotomy (Heller type)

(For exploratory thoracoscopy, and exploratory thoracoscopy with biopsy, see 32601-32606)

Repair

32800	Repair lung hernia through chest wall
32810	Closure of chest wall following open flap drainage for empyema (Clagett type procedure)
32815	Open closure of major bronchial fistula
32820	Major reconstruction, chest wall (posttraumatic)

Lung Transplantation

►Lung allotransplantation involves three distinct components of physician work:◄

►1) *Cadaver donor pneumonectomy(s)*, which include(s) harvesting the allograft and cold preservation of the allograft (perfusing with cold preservation solution and cold maintenance) (use 32850).◄

►2) *Backbench work*:◄

►Preparation of a cadaver donor single lung allograft prior to transplantation, including dissection of the allograft from surrounding soft tissues to prepare the pulmonary venous/atrial cuff, pulmonary artery, and bronchus unilaterally (use 32855).◄

►Preparation of a cadaver donor double lung allograft prior to transplantation, including dissection of the allograft from surrounding soft tissues to prepare the pulmonary venous/atrial cuff, pulmonary artery, and bronchus bilaterally (use 32856).◄

►3) *Recipient lung allotransplantation*, which includes transplantation of a single or double lung allograft and care of the recipient (see 32851-32854).◄

▲ 32850	Donor pneumonectomy (including cold preservation), from cadaver donor
32851	Lung transplant, single; without cardiopulmonary bypass
32852	with cardiopulmonary bypass
32853	Lung transplant, double (bilateral sequential or en bloc); without cardiopulmonary bypass
32854	with cardiopulmonary bypass
● 32855	Backbench standard preparation of cadaver donor lung allograft prior to transplantation, including dissection of allograft from surrounding soft tissues to prepare pulmonary venous/atrial cuff, pulmonary artery, and bronchus; unilateral
● 32856	bilateral

►(For repair or resection procedures on the donor lung, see 32491, 32500, 35216, or 35276)◄

Surgical Collapse Therapy; Thoracoplasty

(See also 32520-32525)

32900   Resection of ribs, extrapleural, all stages

32905   Thoracoplasty, Schede type or extrapleural (all stages);

32906   with closure of bronchopleural fistula

(For open closure of major bronchial fistula, use 32815)

(For resection of first rib for thoracic outlet compression, see 21615, 21616)

32940   Pneumonolysis, extraperiosteal, including filling or packing procedures

32960   Pneumothorax, therapeutic, intrapleural injection of air

Other Procedures

32997   Total lung lavage (unilateral)

(For bronchoscopic bronchial alveolar lavage, use 31624)

32999   Unlisted procedure, lungs and pleura

Surgery: Respiratory System

Notes

⊘=Modifier 51 Exempt   ⊙=Conscious Sedation   ✚=Add-on Code

Cardiovascular System

Selective vascular catheterizations should be coded to include introduction and all lesser order selective catheterizations used in the approach (eg, the description for a selective right middle cerebral artery catheterization includes the introduction and placement catheterization of the right common and internal carotid arteries).

Additional second and/or third order arterial catheterizations within the same family of arteries supplied by a single first order artery should be expressed by 36218 or 36248. Additional first order or higher catheterizations in vascular families supplied by a first order vessel different from a previously selected and coded family should be separately coded using the conventions described above.

(For monitoring, operation of pump and other nonsurgical services, see 99190-99192, 99291, 99292, 99354-99360)

(For other medical or laboratory related services, see appropriate section)

(For radiological supervision and interpretation, see 75600-75978)

Heart and Pericardium

Pericardium

⊙ **33010** Pericardiocentesis; initial

(For radiological supervision and interpretation, use 76930)

⊙ **33011** subsequent

(For radiological supervision and interpretation, use 76930)

33015 Tube pericardiostomy

33020 Pericardiotomy for removal of clot or foreign body (primary procedure)

33025 Creation of pericardial window or partial resection for drainage

33030 Pericardiectomy, subtotal or complete; without cardiopulmonary bypass

33031 with cardiopulmonary bypass

33050 Excision of pericardial cyst or tumor

Cardiac Tumor

33120 Excision of intracardiac tumor, resection with cardiopulmonary bypass

33130 Resection of external cardiac tumor

Transmyocardial Revascularization

33140 Transmyocardial laser revascularization, by thoracotomy; (separate procedure)

+ **33141** performed at the time of other open cardiac procedure(s) (List separately in addition to code for primary procedure)

(Use 33141 in conjunction with 33400-33496, 33510-33536, 33542)

Pacemaker or Pacing Cardioverter-Defibrillator

A pacemaker system includes a pulse generator containing electronics and a battery, and one or more electrodes (leads). Pulse generators are placed in a subcutaneous "pocket" created in either a subclavicular site or underneath the abdominal muscles just below the ribcage. Electrodes may be inserted through a vein (transvenous) or they may be placed on the surface of the heart (epicardial). The epicardial location of electrodes requires a thoracotomy for electrode insertion.

A single chamber pacemaker system includes a pulse generator and one electrode inserted in either the atrium or ventricle. A dual chamber pacemaker system includes a pulse generator and one electrode inserted in the right atrium and one electrode inserted in the right ventricle. In certain circumstances, an additional electrode may be required to achieve pacing of the left ventricle (bi-ventricular pacing). In this event, transvenous (cardiac vein) placement of the electrode should be separately reported using code 33224 or 33225.

Like a pacemaker system, a pacing cardioverter-defibrillator system includes a pulse generator and electrodes, although pacing cardioverter-defibrillators may require multiple leads, even when only a single chamber is being paced. A pacing cardioverter-defibrillator system may be inserted in a single chamber (pacing in the ventricle) or in dual chambers (pacing in atrium and ventricle). These devices use a combination of antitachycardia pacing, low energy cardioversion or defibrillating shocks to treat ventricular tachycardia or ventricular fibrillation.

Pacing cardioverter-defibrillator pulse generators may be implanted in a subcutaneous infraclavicular pocket or in an abdominal pocket. Removal of a pacing cardioverter-defibrillator pulse generator requires opening of the existing subcutaneous pocket and disconnection of the pulse generator from its electrode(s). A thoracotomy (or laparotomy in the case of abdominally placed pulse generators) is not required to remove the pulse generator.

The electrodes (leads) of a pacing cardioverter-defibrillator system are positioned in the heart via the venous system (transvenously), in most circumstances. In certain circumstances, an additional electrode may be required to achieve pacing of the left ventricle (biventricular pacing). In this event, transvenous (cardiac vein) placement of the electrode should be separately reported using code 33224 or 33225.

Electrode positioning on the epicardial surface of the heart requires a thoracotomy (codes 33245-33246). Removal of electrode(s) may first be attempted by transvenous extraction (code 33244). However, if transvenous extraction is unsuccessful, a thoracotomy may be required to remove the electrodes (code 33243).

When the "battery" of a pacemaker or pacing cardioverter-defibrillator is changed, it is actually the pulse generator that is changed. Replacement of a pulse generator should be reported with a code for removal of the pulse generator and another code for insertion of a pulse generator.

Repositioning of a pacemaker electrode, pacing cardioverter-defibrillator electrode(s), or a left ventricular pacing electrode is reported using 33215 or 33226, as appropriate. Replacement of a pacemaker electrode, pacing cardioverter-defibrillator electrode(s), or a left ventricular pacing electrode is reported using 33206-33208, 33210-33213, or 33224, as appropriate.

(For electronic, telephonic analysis of internal pacemaker system, see 93731-93736)

(For radiological supervision and interpretation with insertion of pacemaker, use 71090)

33200 Insertion of permanent pacemaker with epicardial electrode(s); by thoracotomy

33201 by xiphoid approach

⊙ **33206** Insertion or replacement of permanent pacemaker with transvenous electrode(s); atrial

⊙ **33207** ventricular

⊙ **33208** atrial and ventricular

(Codes 33206-33208 include subcutaneous insertion of the pulse generator and transvenous placement of electrode(s))

⊙ **33210** Insertion or replacement of temporary transvenous single chamber cardiac electrode or pacemaker catheter (separate procedure)

⊙ **33211** Insertion or replacement of temporary transvenous dual chamber pacing electrodes (separate procedure)

⊙ **33212** Insertion or replacement of pacemaker pulse generator only; single chamber, atrial or ventricular

⊙ **33213** dual chamber

⊙ **33214** Upgrade of implanted pacemaker system, conversion of single chamber system to dual chamber system (includes removal of previously placed pulse generator, testing of existing lead, insertion of new lead, insertion of new pulse generator)

33215 Repositioning of previously implanted transvenous pacemaker or pacing cardioverter-defibrillator (right atrial or right ventricular) electrode

⊙ **33216** Insertion of a transvenous electrode; single chamber (one electrode) permanent pacemaker or single chamber pacing cardioverter-defibrillator

⊙ **33217** dual chamber (two electrodes) permanent pacemaker or dual chamber pacing cardioverter-defibrillator

(Do not report 33216-33217 in conjunction with 33214)

⊙ **33218** Repair of single transvenous electrode for a single chamber, permanent pacemaker or single chamber pacing cardioverter-defibrillator

(For atrial or ventricular single chamber repair of pacemaker electrode(s) with replacement of pulse generator, see 33212 or 33213 and 33218 or 33220)

⊙ **33220** Repair of two transvenous electrodes for a dual chamber permanent pacemaker or dual chamber pacing cardioverter-defibrillator

⊙ **33222** Revision or relocation of skin pocket for pacemaker

⊙ **33223** Revision of skin pocket for single or dual chamber pacing cardioverter-defibrillator

33224 Insertion of pacing electrode, cardiac venous system, for left ventricular pacing, with attachment to previously placed pacemaker or pacing cardioverter-defibrillator pulse generator (including revision of pocket, removal, insertion and/or replacement of generator)

✚ **33225** Insertion of pacing electrode, cardiac venous system, for left ventricular pacing, at time of insertion of pacing cardioverter-defibrillator or pacemaker pulse generator (including upgrade to dual chamber system) (List separately in addition to code for primary procedure)

(Use 33225 in conjunction with 33206, 33207, 33208, 33212, 33213, 33214, 33216, 33217, 33222, 33233, 33234, 33235, 33240, 33249)

33226 Repositioning of previously implanted cardiac venous system (left ventricular) electrode (including removal, insertion and/or replacement of generator)

⊙ **33233** Removal of permanent pacemaker pulse generator

⊙ **33234** Removal of transvenous pacemaker electrode(s); single lead system, atrial or ventricular

⊙ **33235** dual lead system

33236 Removal of permanent epicardial pacemaker and electrodes by thoracotomy; single lead system, atrial or ventricular

33237 dual lead system

33238 Removal of permanent transvenous electrode(s) by thoracotomy

⊙ **33240** Insertion of single or dual chamber pacing cardioverter-defibrillator pulse generator

⊙ 33241   Subcutaneous removal of single or dual chamber pacing cardioverter-defibrillator pulse generator

(For removal of electrode(s) by thoracotomy, use 33243 in conjunction with 33241)

(For removal of electrode(s) by transvenous extraction, use 33244 in conjunction with 33241)

(For removal and reinsertion of a pacing cardioverter-defibrillator system (pulse generator and electrodes), report 33241 and 33243 or 33244 and 33249)

(For repair of implantable cardioverter-defibrillator pulse generator and/or leads, see 33218, 33220)

33243   Removal of single or dual chamber pacing cardioverter-defibrillator electrode(s); by thoracotomy

⊙ 33244   by transvenous extraction

(For subcutaneous removal of the pulse generator, use 33241 in conjunction with 33243 or 33244)

33245   Insertion of epicardial single or dual chamber pacing cardioverter-defibrillator electrodes by thoracotomy;

33246   with insertion of pulse generator

(For insertion of implantable cardioverter-defibrillator lead(s), without thoracotomy, use 33216)

⊙ 33249   Insertion or repositioning of electrode lead(s) for single or dual chamber pacing cardioverter-defibrillator and insertion of pulse generator

(For removal and reinsertion of a pacing cardioverter-defibrillator system (pulse generator and electrodes), report 33241 and 33243 or 33244 and 33249)

Electrophysiologic Operative Procedures

33250   Operative ablation of supraventricular arrhythmogenic focus or pathway (eg, Wolff-Parkinson-White, atrioventricular node re-entry), tract(s) and/or focus (foci); without cardiopulmonary bypass

33251   with cardiopulmonary bypass

33253   Operative incisions and reconstruction of atria for treatment of atrial fibrillation or atrial flutter (eg, maze procedure)

33261   Operative ablation of ventricular arrhythmogenic focus with cardiopulmonary bypass

Patient-Activated Event Recorder

33282   Implantation of patient-activated cardiac event recorder

(Initial implantation includes programming. For subsequent electronic analysis and/or reprogramming, use 93727)

33284   Removal of an implantable, patient-activated cardiac event recorder

Wounds of the Heart and Great Vessels

33300   Repair of cardiac wound; without bypass

33305   with cardiopulmonary bypass

33310   Cardiotomy, exploratory (includes removal of foreign body, atrial or ventricular thrombus); without bypass

33315   with cardiopulmonary bypass

(Do not report removal of thrombus (33310-33315) in conjunction with other cardiac procedures unless a separate incision in the heart is required to remove the atrial or ventricular thrombus)

(If removal of thrombus with coronary bypass (33315) is reported in conjunction with 33120, 33130, 33420-33430, 33460-33468, 33496, 33542, 33545, 33641-33647, 33670, 33681, 33975-33980 which requires a separate heart incision, report 33315 with modifier 59)

33320   Suture repair of aorta or great vessels; without shunt or cardiopulmonary bypass

33321   with shunt bypass

33322   with cardiopulmonary bypass

33330   Insertion of graft, aorta or great vessels; without shunt, or cardiopulmonary bypass

33332   with shunt bypass

33335   with cardiopulmonary bypass

Cardiac Valves

(For multiple valve procedures, see 33400-33478 and add modifier 51 to the secondary valve procedure code)

Aortic Valve

33400   Valvuloplasty, aortic valve; open, with cardiopulmonary bypass

33401   open, with inflow occlusion

33403   using transventricular dilation, with cardiopulmonary bypass

(Do not report modifier 63 in conjunction with 33401, 33403)

33404   Construction of apical-aortic conduit

33405   Replacement, aortic valve, with cardiopulmonary bypass; with prosthetic valve other than homograft or stentless valve

33406   with allograft valve (freehand)

(For aortic valve valvotomy, (commissurotomy) with inflow occlusion, use 33401)

(For aortic valve valvotomy, (commissurotomy) with cardiopulmonary bypass, use 33403)

33410   with stentless tissue valve

33411 Replacement, aortic valve; with aortic annulus enlargement, noncoronary cusp

33412 with transventricular aortic annulus enlargement (Konno procedure)

33413 by translocation of autologous pulmonary valve with allograft replacement of pulmonary valve (Ross procedure)

33414 Repair of left ventricular outflow tract obstruction by patch enlargement of the outflow tract

33415 Resection or incision of subvalvular tissue for discrete subvalvular aortic stenosis

33416 Ventriculomyotomy (-myectomy) for idiopathic hypertrophic subaortic stenosis (eg, asymmetric septal hypertrophy)

33417 Aortoplasty (gusset) for supravalvular stenosis

Mitral Valve

33420 Valvotomy, mitral valve; closed heart

33422 open heart, with cardiopulmonary bypass

33425 Valvuloplasty, mitral valve, with cardiopulmonary bypass;

33426 with prosthetic ring

33427 radical reconstruction, with or without ring

33430 Replacement, mitral valve, with cardiopulmonary bypass

Tricuspid Valve

33460 Valvectomy, tricuspid valve, with cardiopulmonary bypass

33463 Valvuloplasty, tricuspid valve; without ring insertion

33464 with ring insertion

33465 Replacement, tricuspid valve, with cardiopulmonary bypass

33468 Tricuspid valve repositioning and plication for Ebstein anomaly

Pulmonary Valve

33470 Valvotomy, pulmonary valve, closed heart; transventricular

(Do not report modifier 63 in conjunction with 33470)

33471 via pulmonary artery

(To report percutaneous valvuloplasty of pulmonary valve, use 92990)

33472 Valvotomy, pulmonary valve, open heart; with inflow occlusion

(Do not report modifier 63 in conjunction with 33472)

33474 with cardiopulmonary bypass

33475 Replacement, pulmonary valve

33476 Right ventricular resection for infundibular stenosis, with or without commissurotomy

33478 Outflow tract augmentation (gusset), with or without commissurotomy or infundibular resection

Other Valvular Procedures

33496 Repair of non-structural prosthetic valve dysfunction with cardiopulmonary bypass (separate procedure)

(For reoperation, use 33530 in addition to 33496)

Coronary Artery Anomalies

Basic procedures include endarterectomy or angioplasty.

33500 Repair of coronary arteriovenous or arteriocardiac chamber fistula; with cardiopulmonary bypass

33501 without cardiopulmonary bypass

33502 Repair of anomalous coronary artery; by ligation

33503 by graft, without cardiopulmonary bypass

(Do not report modifier 63 in conjunction with 33502, 33503)

33504 by graft, with cardiopulmonary bypass

33505 with construction of intrapulmonary artery tunnel (Takeuchi procedure)

33506 by translocation from pulmonary artery to aorta

(Do not report modifier 63 in conjunction with 33505, 33506)

Endoscopy

Surgical vascular endoscopy always includes diagnostic endoscopy.

+ 33508 Endoscopy, surgical, including video-assisted harvest of vein(s) for coronary artery bypass procedure (List separately in addition to code for primary procedure)

(Use 33508 in conjunction with 33510-33523)

(For open harvest of upper extremity vein procedure, use 35500)

Venous Grafting Only for Coronary Artery Bypass

The following codes are used to report coronary artery bypass procedures using venous grafts only. These codes should NOT be used to report the performance of coronary artery bypass procedures using arterial grafts and venous grafts during the same procedure. See 33517-33523 and 33533-33536 for reporting combined arterial-venous grafts.

Procurement of the saphenous vein graft is included in the description of the work for 33510-33516 and should not be reported as a separate service or co-surgery. To report harvesting of an upper extremity vein, use 35500 in addition to the bypass procedure. To report harvesting of a femoropopliteal vein segment, report 35572 in addition to the bypass procedure. When surgical assistant performs graft procurement, add modifier 80 to 33510-33516.

33510   Coronary artery bypass, vein only; single coronary venous graft

33511   two coronary venous grafts

33512   three coronary venous grafts

33513   four coronary venous grafts

33514   five coronary venous grafts

33516   six or more coronary venous grafts

Combined Arterial-Venous Grafting for Coronary Bypass

The following codes are used to report coronary artery bypass procedures using venous grafts and arterial grafts during the same procedure. These codes may NOT be used alone.

To report combined arterial-venous grafts it is necessary to report two codes: 1) the appropriate combined arterial-venous graft code (33517-33523); and 2) the appropriate arterial graft code (33533-33536).

Procurement of the saphenous vein graft is included in the description of the work for 33517-33523 and should not be reported as a separate service or co-surgery. Procurement of the artery for grafting is included in the description of the work for 33533-33536 and should not be reported as a separate service or co-surgery, except when an upper extremity artery (eg, radial artery) is procured. To report harvesting of an upper extremity artery, use 35600 in addition to the bypass procedure. To report harvesting of an upper extremity vein, use 35500 in addition to the bypass procedure. To report harvesting of a femoropopliteal vein segment, report 35572 in addition to the bypass procedure. When surgical assistant performs arterial and/or venous graft procurement, add modifier 80 to 33517-33523, 33533-33536, as appropriate.

⊘ **33517**   Coronary artery bypass, using venous graft(s) and arterial graft(s); single vein graft (List separately in addition to code for arterial graft)

⊘ **33518**   two venous grafts (List separately in addition to code for arterial graft)

⊘ **33519**   three venous grafts (List separately in addition to code for arterial graft)

⊘ **33521**   four venous grafts (List separately in addition to code for arterial graft)

⊘ **33522**   five venous grafts (List separately in addition to code for arterial graft)

⊘ **33523**   six or more venous grafts (List separately in addition to code for arterial graft)

+ **33530**   Reoperation, coronary artery bypass procedure or valve procedure, more than one month after original operation (List separately in addition to code for primary procedure)

(Use 33530 in conjunction with 33400-33496; 33510-33536, 33863)

Arterial Grafting for Coronary Artery Bypass

The following codes are used to report coronary artery bypass procedures using either arterial grafts only or a combination of arterial-venous grafts. The codes include the use of the internal mammary artery, gastroepiploic artery, epigastric artery, radial artery, and arterial conduits procured from other sites.

To report combined arterial-venous grafts it is necessary to report two codes: 1) the appropriate arterial graft code (33533-33536); and 2) the appropriate combined arterial-venous graft code (33517-33523).

Procurement of the artery for grafting is included in the description of the work for 33533-33536 and should not be reported as a separate service or co-surgery, except when an upper extremity artery (eg, radial artery) is procured. To report harvesting of an upper extremity artery, use 35600 in addition to the bypass procedure. To report harvesting of an upper extremity vein, use 35500 in addition to the bypass procedure. To report harvesting of a femoropopliteal vein segment, report 35572 in addition to the bypass procedure. When surgical assistant performs arterial and/or venous graft procurement, add modifier 80 to 33517-33523, 33533-33536, as appropriate.

33533   Coronary artery bypass, using arterial graft(s); single arterial graft

33534   two coronary arterial grafts

33535   three coronary arterial grafts

33536   four or more coronary arterial grafts

33542   Myocardial resection (eg, ventricular aneurysmectomy)

33545   Repair of postinfarction ventricular septal defect, with or without myocardial resection

Coronary Endarterectomy

+ **33572**   Coronary endarterectomy, open, any method, of left anterior descending, circumflex, or right coronary artery performed in conjunction with coronary artery bypass graft procedure, each vessel (List separately in addition to primary procedure)

(Use 33572 in conjunction with 33510-33516, 33533-33536)

Single Ventricle and Other Complex Cardiac Anomalies

33600 Closure of atrioventricular valve (mitral or tricuspid) by suture or patch

33602 Closure of semilunar valve (aortic or pulmonary) by suture or patch

33606 Anastomosis of pulmonary artery to aorta (Damus-Kaye-Stansel procedure)

33608 Repair of complex cardiac anomaly other than pulmonary atresia with ventricular septal defect by construction or replacement of conduit from right or left ventricle to pulmonary artery

(For repair of pulmonary atresia with ventricular septal defect, see 33918, 33919, 33920)

33610 Repair of complex cardiac anomalies (eg, single ventricle with subaortic obstruction) by surgical enlargement of ventricular septal defect

(Do not report modifier 63 in conjunction with 33610)

33611 Repair of double outlet right ventricle with intraventricular tunnel repair;

(Do not report modifier 63 in conjunction with 33611)

33612 with repair of right ventricular outflow tract obstruction

33615 Repair of complex cardiac anomalies (eg, tricuspid atresia) by closure of atrial septal defect and anastomosis of atria or vena cava to pulmonary artery (simple Fontan procedure)

33617 Repair of complex cardiac anomalies (eg, single ventricle) by modified Fontan procedure

33619 Repair of single ventricle with aortic outflow obstruction and aortic arch hypoplasia (hypoplastic left heart syndrome) (eg, Norwood procedure)

(Do not report modifier 63 in conjunction with 33619)

Septal Defect

33641 Repair atrial septal defect, secundum, with cardiopulmonary bypass, with or without patch

33645 Direct or patch closure, sinus venosus, with or without anomalous pulmonary venous drainage

33647 Repair of atrial septal defect and ventricular septal defect, with direct or patch closure

(Do not report modifier 63 in conjunction with 33647)

(For repair of tricuspid atresia (eg, Fontan, Gago procedures), use 33615)

33660 Repair of incomplete or partial atrioventricular canal (ostium primum atrial septal defect), with or without atrioventricular valve repair

33665 Repair of intermediate or transitional atrioventricular canal, with or without atrioventricular valve repair

33670 Repair of complete atrioventricular canal, with or without prosthetic valve

(Do not report modifier 63 in conjunction with 33670)

33681 Closure of ventricular septal defect, with or without patch;

33684 with pulmonary valvotomy or infundibular resection (acyanotic)

33688 with removal of pulmonary artery band, with or without gusset

33690 Banding of pulmonary artery

(Do not report modifier 63 in conjunction with 33690)

33692 Complete repair tetralogy of Fallot without pulmonary atresia;

33694 with transannular patch

(Do not report modifier 63 in conjunction with 33694)

(For ligation and takedown of a systemic-to-pulmonary artery shunt, performed in conjunction with a congenital heart procedure; see 33924)

33697 Complete repair tetralogy of Fallot with pulmonary atresia including construction of conduit from right ventricle to pulmonary artery and closure of ventricular septal defect

(For ligation and takedown of a systemic-to-pulmonary artery shunt, performed in conjunction with a congenital heart procedure; see 33924)

Sinus of Valsalva

33702 Repair sinus of Valsalva fistula, with cardiopulmonary bypass;

33710 with repair of ventricular septal defect

33720 Repair sinus of Valsalva aneurysm, with cardiopulmonary bypass

33722 Closure of aortico-left ventricular tunnel

Total Anomalous Pulmonary Venous Drainage

33730 Complete repair of anomalous venous return (supracardiac, intracardiac, or infracardiac types)

(Do not report modifier 63 in conjunction with 33730)

(For partial anomalous return, see atrial septal defect)

33732 Repair of cor triatriatum or supravalvular mitral ring by resection of left atrial membrane

(Do not report modifier 63 in conjunction with 33732)

Shunting Procedures

33735 Atrial septectomy or septostomy; closed heart (Blalock-Hanlon type operation)

33736   open heart with cardiopulmonary bypass

(Do not report modifier 63 in conjunction with 33735, 33736)

33737   open heart, with inflow occlusion

(For transvenous method cardiac catheterization balloon atrial septectomy or septostomy (Rashkind type), use 92992)

(For blade method cardiac catheterization atrial septectomy or septostomy (Sang-Park septostomy), use 92993)

33750 Shunt; subclavian to pulmonary artery (Blalock-Taussig type operation)

33755   ascending aorta to pulmonary artery (Waterston type operation)

33762   descending aorta to pulmonary artery (Potts-Smith type operation)

(Do not report modifier 63 in conjunction with 33750, 33755, 33762)

33764   central, with prosthetic graft

33766   superior vena cava to pulmonary artery for flow to one lung (classical Glenn procedure)

33767   superior vena cava to pulmonary artery for flow to both lungs (bidirectional Glenn procedure)

Transposition of the Great Vessels

33770 Repair of transposition of the great arteries with ventricular septal defect and subpulmonary stenosis; without surgical enlargement of ventricular septal defect

33771   with surgical enlargement of ventricular septal defect

33774 Repair of transposition of the great arteries, atrial baffle procedure (eg, Mustard or Senning type) with cardiopulmonary bypass;

33775   with removal of pulmonary band

33776   with closure of ventricular septal defect

33777   with repair of subpulmonic obstruction

33778 Repair of transposition of the great arteries, aortic pulmonary artery reconstruction (eg, Jatene type);

(Do not report modifier 63 in conjunction with 33778)

33779   with removal of pulmonary band

33780   with closure of ventricular septal defect

33781   with repair of subpulmonic obstruction

Truncus Arteriosus

33786 Total repair, truncus arteriosus (Rastelli type operation)

(Do not report modifier 63 in conjunction with 33786)

33788 Reimplantation of an anomalous pulmonary artery

(For pulmonary artery band, use 33690)

Aortic Anomalies

33800 Aortic suspension (aortopexy) for tracheal decompression (eg, for tracheomalacia) (separate procedure)

33802 Division of aberrant vessel (vascular ring);

33803   with reanastomosis

33813 Obliteration of aortopulmonary septal defect; without cardiopulmonary bypass

33814   with cardiopulmonary bypass

33820 Repair of patent ductus arteriosus; by ligation

33822   by division, under 18 years

33824   by division, 18 years and older

33840 Excision of coarctation of aorta, with or without associated patent ductus arteriosus; with direct anastomosis

33845   with graft

33851   repair using either left subclavian artery or prosthetic material as gusset for enlargement

33852 Repair of hypoplastic or interrupted aortic arch using autogenous or prosthetic material; without cardiopulmonary bypass

33853   with cardiopulmonary bypass

(For repair of hypoplastic left heart syndrome (eg, Norwood type), via excision of coarctation of aorta, use 33619)

Thoracic Aortic Aneurysm

33860 Ascending aorta graft, with cardiopulmonary bypass, with or without valve suspension;

33861   with coronary reconstruction

33863   with aortic root replacement using composite prosthesis and coronary reconstruction

(For graft of ascending aorta, with cardiopulmonary bypass and valve replacement, with or without coronary implant or valve suspension; use 33860 or 33861 and 33405 or 33406)

33870 Transverse arch graft, with cardiopulmonary bypass

33875 Descending thoracic aorta graft, with or without bypass

33877 Repair of thoracoabdominal aortic aneurysm with graft, with or without cardiopulmonary bypass

Surgery: Cardiovascular System

Pulmonary Artery

33910 Pulmonary artery embolectomy; with cardiopulmonary bypass

33915 without cardiopulmonary bypass

33916 Pulmonary endarterectomy, with or without embolectomy, with cardiopulmonary bypass

33917 Repair of pulmonary artery stenosis by reconstruction with patch or graft

33918 Repair of pulmonary atresia with ventricular septal defect, by unifocalization of pulmonary arteries; without cardiopulmonary bypass

33919 with cardiopulmonary bypass

(Do not report modifier 63 in conjunction with 33918, 33919)

33920 Repair of pulmonary atresia with ventricular septal defect, by construction or replacement of conduit from right or left ventricle to pulmonary artery

(For repair of other complex cardiac anomalies by construction or replacement of right or left ventricle to pulmonary artery conduit, use 33608)

33922 Transection of pulmonary artery with cardiopulmonary bypass

(Do not report modifier 63 in conjunction with 33922)

+ 33924 Ligation and takedown of a systemic-to-pulmonary artery shunt, performed in conjunction with a congenital heart procedure (List separately in addition to code for primary procedure)

(Use 33924 in conjunction with 33470-33475, 33600-33619, 33684-33688, 33692-33697, 33735-33767, 33770-33781, 33786, 33918-33922)

Heart/Lung Transplantation

►Heart with or without lung allotransplantation involves three distinct components of physician work:◄

►1) *Cadaver donor cardiectomy with or without pneumonectomy*, which includes harvesting the allograft and cold preservation of the allograft (perfusing with cold preservation solution and cold maintenance) (see 33930, 33940).◄

►2) *Backbench work*:◄

►Preparation of a cadaver donor heart and lung allograft prior to transplantation, including dissection of the allograft from surrounding soft tissues to prepare the aorta, superior vena cava, inferior vena cava, and trachea for implantation (use 33933).◄

►Preparation of a cadaver donor heart allograft prior to transplantation, including dissection of the allograft from surrounding soft tissues to prepare aorta, superior vena cava, inferior vena cava, pulmonary artery, and left atrium for implantation (use 33944).◄

►3) *Recipient heart with or without lung allotransplantation*, which includes transplantation of allograft and care of the recipient (see 33935, 33945).◄

(For implantation of a total replacement heart system (artificial heart) with recipient cardiectomy or heart replacement system components, see Category III codes 0051T-0053T)

▲ **33930** Donor cardiectomy-pneumonectomy (including cold preservation)

● **33933** Backbench standard preparation of cadaver donor heart/lung allograft prior to transplantation, including dissection of allograft from surrounding soft tissues to prepare aorta, superior vena cava, inferior vena cava, and trachea for implantation

33935 Heart-lung transplant with recipient cardiectomy-pneumonectomy

▲ **33940** Donor cardiectomy (including cold preservation)

● **33944** Backbench standard preparation of cadaver donor heart allograft prior to transplantation, including dissection of allograft from surrounding soft tissues to prepare aorta, superior vena cava, inferior vena cava, pulmonary artery, and left atrium for implantation

►(For repair or resection procedures on the donor heart, see 33300, 33310, 33320, 33400, 33463, 33464, 33510, 33641, 35216, 35276 or 35685)◄

33945 Heart transplant, with or without recipient cardiectomy

Cardiac Assist

(For percutaneous implantation of extracorporeal ventricular assist device or for removal of percutaneously implanted extracorporeal ventricular assist device, see Category III codes 0048T-0050T)

33960 Prolonged extracorporeal circulation for cardiopulmonary insufficiency; initial 24 hours

+ 33961 each additional 24 hours (List separately in addition to code for primary procedure)

(Do not report modifier 63 in conjunction with 33960, 33961)

(Use 33961 in conjunction with 33960)

(For insertion of cannula for prolonged extracorporeal circulation, use 36822)

33967 Insertion of intra-aortic balloon assist device, percutaneous

33968 Removal of intra-aortic balloon assist device, percutaneous

33970	Insertion of intra-aortic balloon assist device through the femoral artery, open approach
33971	Removal of intra-aortic balloon assist device including repair of femoral artery, with or without graft
33973	Insertion of intra-aortic balloon assist device through the ascending aorta
33974	Removal of intra-aortic balloon assist device from the ascending aorta, including repair of the ascending aorta, with or without graft
33975	Insertion of ventricular assist device; extracorporeal, single ventricle
33976	extracorporeal, biventricular
33977	Removal of ventricular assist device; extracorporeal, single ventricle
33978	extracorporeal, biventricular
33979	Insertion of ventricular assist device, implantable intracorporeal, single ventricle
33980	Removal of ventricular assist device, implantable intracorporeal, single ventricle

Other Procedures

33999	Unlisted procedure, cardiac surgery

Arteries and Veins

Primary vascular procedure listings include establishing both inflow and outflow by whatever procedures necessary. Also included is that portion of the operative arteriogram performed by the surgeon, as indicated. Sympathectomy, when done, is included in the listed aortic procedures. For unlisted vascular procedure, use 37799.

Embolectomy/Thrombectomy

Arterial, With or Without Catheter

34001	Embolectomy or thrombectomy, with or without catheter; carotid, subclavian or innominate artery, by neck incision
34051	innominate, subclavian artery, by thoracic incision
34101	axillary, brachial, innominate, subclavian artery, by arm incision
34111	radial or ulnar artery, by arm incision
34151	renal, celiac, mesentery, aortoiliac artery, by abdominal incision
34201	femoropopliteal, aortoiliac artery, by leg incision
34203	popliteal-tibio-peroneal artery, by leg incision

Venous, Direct or With Catheter

34401	Thrombectomy, direct or with catheter; vena cava, iliac vein, by abdominal incision
34421	vena cava, iliac, femoropopliteal vein, by leg incision
34451	vena cava, iliac, femoropopliteal vein, by abdominal and leg incision
34471	subclavian vein, by neck incision
34490	axillary and subclavian vein, by arm incision

Venous Reconstruction

34501	Valvuloplasty, femoral vein
34502	Reconstruction of vena cava, any method
34510	Venous valve transposition, any vein donor
34520	Cross-over vein graft to venous system
34530	Saphenopopliteal vein anastomosis

Endovascular Repair of Abdominal Aortic Aneurysm

Codes 34800-34826 represent a family of component procedures to report placement of an endovascular graft for abdominal aortic aneurysm repair. These codes describe open femoral or iliac artery exposure, device manipulation and deployment, and closure of the arteriotomy sites. Balloon angioplasty and/or stent deployment within the target treatment zone for the endoprosthesis, either before or after endograft deployment, are not separately reportable. Introduction of guidewires and catheters should be reported separately (eg, 36200, 36245-36248, 36140). Extensive repair or replacement of an artery should be additionally reported (eg, 35226 or 35286).

For fluoroscopic guidance in conjunction with endovascular aneurysm repair, see code 75952 or 75953, as appropriate. Code 75952 includes angiography of the aorta and its branches for diagnostic imaging prior to deployment of the endovascular device (including all routine components of modular devices), fluoroscopic guidance in the delivery of the endovascular components, and intraprocedural arterial angiography (eg, confirm position, detect endoleak, evaluate runoff). Code 75953 includes the analogous services for placement of additional extension prostheses (not for routine components of modular devices).

Other interventional procedures performed at the time of endovascular abdominal aortic aneurysm repair should be additionally reported (eg, renal transluminal angioplasty, arterial embolization, intravascular ultrasound, balloon angioplasty or stenting of native artery(s) outside the endoprosthesis target zone, when done before or after deployment of graft).

Surgery: Cardiovascular System

Surgery: Cardiovascular System

34800   Endovascular repair of infrarenal abdominal aortic aneurysm or dissection; using aorto-aortic tube prosthesis

34802   using modular bifurcated prosthesis (one docking limb)

● **34803**   using modular bifurcated prosthesis (two docking limbs)

▶(For endovascular repair of abdominal aortic aneurysm or dissection involving visceral vessels using a fenestrated modular bifurcated prosthesis (two docking limbs), use Category III codes 0078T, 0079T)◀

34804   using unibody bifurcated prosthesis

34805   using aorto-uniiliac or aorto-unifemoral prosthesis

✚ **34808**   Endovascular placement of iliac artery occlusion device (List separately in addition to code for primary procedure)

(Use 34808 in conjunction with 34800, 34805, 34813, 34825, 34826)

(For radiological supervision and interpretation, use 75952 in conjunction with ▶34800-34808◀)

(For open arterial exposure, report 34812, 34820, 34833, 34834 as appropriate, in addition to ▶34800-34808◀)

34812   Open femoral artery exposure for delivery of endovascular prosthesis, by groin incision, unilateral

(For bilateral procedure, use modifier 50)

✚ **34813**   Placement of femoral-femoral prosthetic graft during endovascular aortic aneurysm repair (List separately in addition to code for primary procedure)

(Use 34813 in conjunction with 34812)

(For femoral artery grafting, see 35521, 35533, 35546, 35551-35558, 35566, 35621, 35646, 35651-35661, 35666, 35700)

34820   Open iliac artery exposure for delivery of endovascular prosthesis or iliac occlusion during endovascular therapy, by abdominal or retroperitoneal incision, unilateral

(For bilateral procedure, use modifier 50)

34825   Placement of proximal or distal extension prosthesis for endovascular repair of infrarenal abdominal aortic or iliac aneurysm, false aneurysm, or dissection; initial vessel

✚ **34826**   each additional vessel (List separately in addition to code for primary procedure)

(Use 34826 in conjunction with 34825)

(Use 34825, 34826 in addition to 34800-34808, 34900 as appropriate)

(For staged procedure, use modifier 58)

(For radiological supervision and interpretation, use 75953)

34830   Open repair of infrarenal aortic aneurysm or dissection, plus repair of associated arterial trauma, following unsuccessful endovascular repair; tube prosthesis

34831   aorto-bi-iliac prosthesis

34832   aorto-bifemoral prosthesis

34833   Open iliac artery exposure with creation of conduit for delivery of infrarenal aortic or iliac endovascular prosthesis, by abdominal or retroperitoneal incision, unilateral

(For bilateral procedure, use modifier 50)

(Do not report 34833 in addition to 34820)

34834   Open brachial artery exposure to assist in the deployment of infrarenal aortic or iliac endovascular prosthesis by arm incision, unilateral

(For bilateral procedure, use modifier 50)

Endovascular Repair of Iliac Aneurysm

Code 34900 represents a procedure to report introduction, positioning, and deployment of an endovascular graft for treatment of aneurysm, pseudoaneurysm, or arteriovenous malformation or trauma of the iliac artery (common, hypogastric, external). All balloon angioplasty and/or stent deployments within the target treatment zone for the endoprosthesis, either before or after endograft deployment, are included in the work of 34900 and are not separately reportable. Open femoral or iliac artery exposure (eg, 34812, 34820), introduction of guidewires and catheters (eg, 36200, 36215-36218), and extensive repair or replacement of an artery (eg, 35206-35286) should be additionally reported.

For fluoroscopic guidance in conjunction with endovascular iliac aneurysm repair, see code 75954. Code 75954 includes angiography of the aorta and iliac arteries for diagnostic imaging prior to deployment of the endovascular device (including all routine components), fluoroscopic guidance in the delivery of the endovascular components, and intraprocedural arterial angiography to confirm appropriate position of the graft, detect endoleaks, and evaluate the status of the runoff vessels (eg, evaluation for dissection, stenosis, thrombosis, distal embolization, or iatrogenic injury).

Other interventional procedures performed at the time of endovascular aortic aneurysm repair should be additionally reported (eg, transluminal angioplasty outside the aneurysm target zone, arterial embolization, intravascular ultrasound).

34900   Endovascular graft placement for repair of iliac artery (eg, aneurysm, pseudoaneurysm, arteriovenous malformation, trauma)

(For radiological supervision and interpretation, use 75954)

(For placement of extension prosthesis during endovascular iliac artery repair, use 34825)

(For bilateral procedure, use modifier 50)

Direct Repair of Aneurysm or Excision (Partial or Total) and Graft Insertion for Aneurysm, Pseudoaneurysm, Ruptured Aneurysm, and Associated Occlusive Disease

Procedures 35001-▶35152◀ include preparation of artery for anastomosis including endarterectomy.

(For direct repairs associated with occlusive disease only, see 35201-35286)

(For intracranial aneurysm, see 61700 et seq)

(For endovascular repair of abdominal aortic aneurysm, see 34800-34826)

(For endovascular repair of iliac artery aneurysm, see 34900)

(For thoracic aortic aneurysm, see 33860-33875)

(For endovascular repair of thoracic aortic aneurysm, see Category III codes 0033T-0034T)

35001   Direct repair of aneurysm, pseudoaneurysm, or excision (partial or total) and graft insertion, with or without patch graft; for aneurysm and associated occlusive disease, carotid, subclavian artery, by neck incision

35002   for ruptured aneurysm, carotid, subclavian artery, by neck incision

35005   for aneurysm, pseudoaneurysm, and associated occlusive disease, vertebral artery

35011   for aneurysm and associated occlusive disease, axillary-brachial artery, by arm incision

35013   for ruptured aneurysm, axillary-brachial artery, by arm incision

35021   for aneurysm, pseudoaneurysm, and associated occlusive disease, innominate, subclavian artery, by thoracic incision

35022   for ruptured aneurysm, innominate, subclavian artery, by thoracic incision

35045   for aneurysm, pseudoaneurysm, and associated occlusive disease, radial or ulnar artery

35081   for aneurysm, pseudoaneurysm, and associated occlusive disease, abdominal aorta

35082   for ruptured aneurysm, abdominal aorta

35091   for aneurysm, pseudoaneurysm, and associated occlusive disease, abdominal aorta involving visceral vessels (mesenteric, celiac, renal)

35092   for ruptured aneurysm, abdominal aorta involving visceral vessels (mesenteric, celiac, renal)

35102   for aneurysm, pseudoaneurysm, and associated occlusive disease, abdominal aorta involving iliac vessels (common, hypogastric, external)

35103   for ruptured aneurysm, abdominal aorta involving iliac vessels (common, hypogastric, external)

35111   for aneurysm, pseudoaneurysm, and associated occlusive disease, splenic artery

35112   for ruptured aneurysm, splenic artery

35121   for aneurysm, pseudoaneurysm, and associated occlusive disease, hepatic, celiac, renal, or mesenteric artery

35122   for ruptured aneurysm, hepatic, celiac, renal, or mesenteric artery

35131   for aneurysm, pseudoaneurysm, and associated occlusive disease, iliac artery (common, hypogastric, external)

35132   for ruptured aneurysm, iliac artery (common, hypogastric, external)

35141   for aneurysm, pseudoaneurysm, and associated occlusive disease, common femoral artery (profunda femoris, superficial femoral)

35142   for ruptured aneurysm, common femoral artery (profunda femoris, superficial femoral)

35151   for aneurysm, pseudoaneurysm, and associated occlusive disease, popliteal artery

35152   for ruptured aneurysm, popliteal artery

▶(35161, 35162 have been deleted. To report, use 37799)◀

Repair Arteriovenous Fistula

35180   Repair, congenital arteriovenous fistula; head and neck

35182   thorax and abdomen

35184   extremities

35188   Repair, acquired or traumatic arteriovenous fistula; head and neck

35189   thorax and abdomen

35190   extremities

Repair Blood Vessel Other Than for Fistula, With or Without Patch Angioplasty

(For AV fistula repair, see 35180-35190)

35201   Repair blood vessel, direct; neck

35206   upper extremity

35207   hand, finger

35211   intrathoracic, with bypass

35216   intrathoracic, without bypass

35221   intra-abdominal

35226   lower extremity

Surgery: Cardiovascular System

Surgery: Cardiovascular System

35231	Repair blood vessel with vein graft; neck
35236	upper extremity
35241	intrathoracic, with bypass
35246	intrathoracic, without bypass
35251	intra-abdominal
35256	lower extremity
35261	Repair blood vessel with graft other than vein; neck
35266	upper extremity
35271	intrathoracic, with bypass
35276	intrathoracic, without bypass
35281	intra-abdominal
35286	lower extremity

Thromboendarterectomy

(For coronary artery, see 33510-33536 and 33572)

35301	Thromboendarterectomy, with or without patch graft; carotid, vertebral, subclavian, by neck incision
35311	subclavian, innominate, by thoracic incision
35321	axillary-brachial
35331	abdominal aorta
35341	mesenteric, celiac, or renal
35351	iliac
35355	iliofemoral
35361	combined aortoiliac
35363	combined aortoiliofemoral
35371	common femoral
35372	deep (profunda) femoral
35381	femoral and/or popliteal, and/or tibioperoneal
+ 35390	Reoperation, carotid, thromboendarterectomy, more than one month after original operation (List separately in addition to code for primary procedure)

(Use 35390 in conjunction with 35301)

Angioscopy

+ 35400	Angioscopy (non-coronary vessels or grafts) during therapeutic intervention (List separately in addition to code for primary procedure)

Transluminal Angioplasty

If done as part of another operation, use modifier 51 or use modifier 52.

(For radiological supervision and interpretation, see 75962-75968 and 75978)

Open

35450	Transluminal balloon angioplasty, open; renal or other visceral artery
35452	aortic
35454	iliac
35456	femoral-popliteal
35458	brachiocephalic trunk or branches, each vessel
35459	tibioperoneal trunk and branches
35460	venous

Percutaneous

Codes for catheter placement and the radiologic supervision and interpretation should also be reported, in addition to the code(s) for the therapeutic aspect of the procedure.

⊙ 35470	Transluminal balloon angioplasty, percutaneous; tibioperoneal trunk or branches, each vessel
⊙ 35471	renal or visceral artery
⊙ 35472	aortic
⊙ 35473	iliac
⊙ 35474	femoral-popliteal
⊙ 35475	brachiocephalic trunk or branches, each vessel
⊙ 35476	venous

(For radiological supervision and interpretation, use 75978)

Transluminal Atherectomy

If done as part of another operation, use modifier 51 or use modifier 52.

(For radiological supervision and interpretation, see 75992-75996)

Open

35480	Transluminal peripheral atherectomy, open; renal or other visceral artery
35481	aortic
35482	iliac
35483	femoral-popliteal
35484	brachiocephalic trunk or branches, each vessel
35485	tibioperoneal trunk and branches

Percutaneous

Codes for catheter placement and the radiologic supervision and interpretation should also be reported, in addition to the code(s) for the therapeutic aspect of the procedure.

35490   Transluminal peripheral atherectomy, percutaneous; renal or other visceral artery

35491   aortic

35492   iliac

35493   femoral-popliteal

35494   brachiocephalic trunk or branches, each vessel

35495   tibioperoneal trunk and branches

Bypass Graft

Vein

Procurement of the saphenous vein graft is included in the description of the work for 35501-35587 and should not be reported as a separate service or co-surgery. To report harvesting of an upper extremity vein, use 35500 in addition to the bypass procedure. To report harvesting of a femoropopliteal vein segment, use 35572 in addition to the bypass procedure. To report harvesting and construction of an autogenous composite graft of two segments from two distant locations, report 35682 in addition to the bypass procedure, for autogenous composite of three or more segments from distant sites, report 35683.

+ 35500   Harvest of upper extremity vein, one segment, for lower extremity or coronary artery bypass procedure (List separately in addition to code for primary procedure)

         (Use 35500 in conjunction with 33510-33536, 35556, 35566, 35571, 35583-35587)

         (For harvest of more than one vein segment, see 35682, 35683)

         (For endoscopic procedure, use 33508)

35501   Bypass graft, with vein; carotid

35506   carotid-subclavian

35507   subclavian-carotid

35508   carotid-vertebral

35509   carotid-carotid

35510   carotid-brachial

35511   subclavian-subclavian

35512   subclavian-brachial

35515   subclavian-vertebral

35516   subclavian-axillary

35518   axillary-axillary

35521   axillary-femoral

         (For bypass graft performed with synthetic graft, use 35621)

35522   axillary-brachial

35525   brachial-brachial

35526   aortosubclavian or carotid

         (For bypass graft performed with synthetic graft, use 35626)

35531   aortoceliac or aortomesenteric

35533   axillary-femoral-femoral

         (For bypass graft performed with synthetic graft, use 35654)

35536   splenorenal

35541   aortoiliac or bi-iliac

         (For bypass graft performed with synthetic graft, use 35641)

35546   aortofemoral or bifemoral

         (For bypass graft performed with synthetic graft, use 35646)

35548   aortoiliofemoral, unilateral

         (For bypass graft performed with synthetic graft, use 37799)

35549   aortoiliofemoral, bilateral

         (For bypass graft performed with synthetic graft, use 37799)

35551   aortofemoral-popliteal

35556   femoral-popliteal

35558   femoral-femoral

35560   aortorenal

35563   ilioiliac

35565   iliofemoral

35566   femoral-anterior tibial, posterior tibial, peroneal artery or other distal vessels

35571   popliteal-tibial, -peroneal artery or other distal vessels

+ 35572   Harvest of femoropopliteal vein, one segment, for vascular reconstruction procedure (eg, aortic, vena caval, coronary, peripheral artery) (List separately in addition to code for primary procedure)

         (Use 35572 in conjunction with 33510-33516, 33517-33523, 33533-33536, 34502, 34520, 35001, 35002, 35011-35022, 35102, 35103, 35121-35152, 35231-35256, 35501-35587, ▶35879◀-35907)

         (For bilateral procedure, use modifier 50)

Surgery: Cardiovascular System

In-Situ Vein

►(35582 has been deleted)◄

35583   In-situ vein bypass; femoral-popliteal

► (To report aortobifemoral bypass using synthetic conduit, and femoral-popliteal bypass with vein conduit in-situ, use 35646 and 35583. To report aorto(uni)femoral bypass with synthetic conduit, and femoral-popliteal bypass with vein conduit in-situ, use 35647 and 35583. To report aortofemoral bypass using vein conduit, and femoral-popliteal bypass with vein conduit in-situ, use 35546 and 35583)◄

35585   femoral-anterior tibial, posterior tibial, or peroneal artery

35587   popliteal-tibial, peroneal

Other Than Vein

(For arterial transposition and/or reimplantation, see 35691-35695)

⊘ 35600   Harvest of upper extremity artery, one segment, for coronary artery bypass procedure

35601   Bypass graft, with other than vein; carotid

35606   carotid-subclavian

(For open subclavian to carotid artery transposition performed in conjunction with endovascular thoracic aneurysm repair, use Category III code 0037T)

35612   subclavian-subclavian

35616   subclavian-axillary

35621   axillary-femoral

35623   axillary-popliteal or -tibial

35626   aortosubclavian or carotid

35631   aortoceliac, aortomesenteric, aortorenal

35636   splenorenal (splenic to renal arterial anastomosis)

35641   aortoiliac or bi-iliac

(For open placement of aorto-bi-iliac prosthesis following unsuccessful endovascular repair, use 34831)

35642   carotid-vertebral

35645   subclavian-vertebral

35646   aortobifemoral

(For open placement of aortobifemoral prosthesis following unsuccessful endovascular repair, use 34832)

35647   aortofemoral

35650   axillary-axillary

35651   aortofemoral-popliteal

35654   axillary-femoral-femoral

35656   femoral-popliteal

35661   femoral-femoral

35663   ilioiliac

35665   iliofemoral

35666   femoral-anterior tibial, posterior tibial, or peroneal artery

35671   popliteal-tibial or -peroneal artery

Composite Grafts

Codes 35682-35683 are used to report harvest and anastomosis of multiple vein segments from distant sites for use as arterial bypass graft conduits. These codes are intended for use when the two or more vein segments are harvested from a limb other than that undergoing bypass. Add-on codes 35682 and 35683 may be reported in addition to codes 35556, 35566, 35571, 35583-35587, as appropriate.

+ 35681   Bypass graft; composite, prosthetic and vein (List separately in addition to code for primary procedure)

(Do not report 35681 in addition to 35682, 35683)

+ 35682   autogenous composite, two segments of veins from two locations (List separately in addition to code for primary procedure)

(Do not report 35682 in addition to 35681, 35683)

+ 35683   autogenous composite, three or more segments of vein from two or more locations (List separately in addition to code for primary procedure)

(Do not report 35683 in addition to 35681, 35682)

Adjuvant Techniques

Adjuvant (additional) technique(s) may be required at the time a bypass graft is created to improve patency of the lower extremity autogenous or synthetic bypass graft (eg, femoral-popliteal, femoral-tibial, or popliteal-tibial arteries). Code 35685 should be reported in addition to the primary synthetic bypass graft procedure, when an interposition of venous tissue (vein patch or cuff) is placed at the anastomosis between the synthetic bypass conduit and the involved artery (includes harvest).

Code 35686 should be reported in addition to the primary bypass graft procedure, when autogenous vein is used to create a fistula between the tibial or peroneal artery and vein at or beyond the distal bypass anastomosis site of the involved artery.

(For composite graft(s), see 35681-35683)

+ 35685   Placement of vein patch or cuff at distal anastomosis of bypass graft, synthetic conduit (List separately in addition to code for primary procedure)

(Use 35685 in conjunction with 35656, 35666, or 35671)

+ 35686   Creation of distal arteriovenous fistula during lower extremity bypass surgery (non-hemodialysis) (List separately in addition to code for primary procedure)

(Use 35686 in conjunction with 35556, 35566, 35571, 35583-35587, 35623, 35656, 35666, 35671)

Arterial Transposition

35691   Transposition and/or reimplantation; vertebral to carotid artery

35693   vertebral to subclavian artery

35694   subclavian to carotid artery

(For open subclavian to carotid artery transposition performed in conjunction with endovascular thoracic aneurysm repair, use Category III code 0037T)

35695   carotid to subclavian artery

+ 35697   Reimplantation, visceral artery to infrarenal aortic prosthesis, each artery (List separately in addition to code for primary procedure)

(Do not report 35697 in conjunction with 33877)

Exploration/Revision

+ 35700   Reoperation, femoral-popliteal or femoral (popliteal)-anterior tibial, posterior tibial, peroneal artery or other distal vessels, more than one month after original operation (List separately in addition to code for primary procedure)

(Use 35700 in conjunction with 35556, 35566, 35571, 35583, 35585, 35587, 35656, 35666, 35671)

35701   Exploration (not followed by surgical repair), with or without lysis of artery; carotid artery

35721   femoral artery

35741   popliteal artery

35761   other vessels

35800   Exploration for postoperative hemorrhage, thrombosis or infection; neck

35820   chest

35840   abdomen

35860   extremity

35870   Repair of graft-enteric fistula

35875   Thrombectomy of arterial or venous graft (other than hemodialysis graft or fistula);

35876   with revision of arterial or venous graft

(For thrombectomy of hemodialysis graft or fistula, see 36831, 36833)

Codes 35879 and 35881 describe open revision of graft-threatening stenoses of lower extremity arterial bypass graft(s) (previously constructed with autogenous vein conduit) using vein patch angioplasty or segmental vein interposition techniques. For thrombectomy with revision of any non-coronary arterial or venous graft, including those of the lower extremity, (other than hemodialysis graft or fistula), use 35876. For direct repair (other than for fistula) of a lower extremity blood vessel

(with or without patch angioplasty), use 35226. For repair (other than for fistula) of a lower extremity blood vessel using a vein graft, use 35256.

35879   Revision, lower extremity arterial bypass, without thrombectomy, open; with vein patch angioplasty

35881   with segmental vein interposition

(For excision of infected graft, see 35901-35907 and appropriate revascularization code)

35901   Excision of infected graft; neck

35903   extremity

35905   thorax

35907   abdomen

Vascular Injection Procedures

Listed services for injection procedures include necessary local anesthesia, introduction of needles or catheter, injection of contrast media with or without automatic power injection, and/or necessary pre- and postinjection care specifically related to the injection procedure.

Catheters, drugs, and contrast media are not included in the listed service for the injection procedures.

Selective vascular catheterization should be coded to include introduction and all lesser order selective catheterization used in the approach (eg, the description for a selective right middle cerebral artery catheterization includes the introduction and placement catheterization of the right common and internal carotid arteries).

Additional second and/or third order arterial catheterization within the same family of arteries or veins supplied by a single first order vessel should be expressed by 36012, 36218 or 36248.

Additional first order or higher catheterization in vascular families supplied by a first order vessel different from a previously selected and coded family should be separately coded using the conventions described above.

(For radiological supervision and interpretation, see **Radiology**)

(For injection procedures in conjunction with cardiac catheterization, see 93541-93545)

(For chemotherapy of malignant disease, see 96400-96549)

Intravenous

An intracatheter is a sheathed combination of needle and short catheter.

36000   Introduction of needle or intracatheter, vein

36002   Injection procedures (eg, thrombin) for percutaneous treatment of extremity pseudoaneurysm

(For imaging guidance, see 76003, 76360, 76393, or 76942)

Surgery: Cardiovascular System

(For ultrasound guided compression repair of pseudoaneurysms, use 76936)

(Do not report 36002 for vascular sealant of an arteriotomy site)

36005 Injection procedure for extremity venography (including introduction of needle or intracatheter)

(For radiological supervision and interpretation, see 75820, 75822)

36010 Introduction of catheter, superior or inferior vena cava

36011 Selective catheter placement, venous system; first order branch (eg, renal vein, jugular vein)

36012 second order, or more selective, branch (eg, left adrenal vein, petrosal sinus)

36013 Introduction of catheter, right heart or main pulmonary artery

36014 Selective catheter placement, left or right pulmonary artery

36015 Selective catheter placement, segmental or subsegmental pulmonary artery

(For insertion of flow directed catheter (eg, Swan-Ganz), use 93503)

(For venous catheterization for selective organ blood sampling, use 36500)

Intra-Arterial—Intra-Aortic

(For radiological supervision and interpretation, see **Radiology**)

36100 Introduction of needle or intracatheter, carotid or vertebral artery

(For bilateral procedure, report 36100 with modifier 50)

36120 Introduction of needle or intracatheter; retrograde brachial artery

36140 extremity artery

36145 arteriovenous shunt created for dialysis (cannula, fistula, or graft)

(For insertion of arteriovenous cannula, see 36810-36821)

36160 Introduction of needle or intracatheter, aortic, translumbar

36200 Introduction of catheter, aorta

36215 Selective catheter placement, arterial system; each first order thoracic or brachiocephalic branch, within a vascular family

(For catheter placement for coronary angiography, use 93508)

36216 initial second order thoracic or brachiocephalic branch, within a vascular family

36217 initial third order or more selective thoracic or brachiocephalic branch, within a vascular family

+ 36218 additional second order, third order, and beyond, thoracic or brachiocephalic branch, within a vascular family (List in addition to code for initial second or third order vessel as appropriate)

(Use 36218 in conjunction with 36216, 36217)

(For angiography, see 75600-75790)

(For angioplasty, see 35470-35475)

(For transcatheter therapies, see 37200-37208, 61624, 61626)

(When coronary artery, arterial conduit (eg, internal mammary, inferior epigastric or free radical artery) or venous bypass graft angiography is performed in conjunction with cardiac catheterization, see the appropriate cardiac catheterization, injection procedure, and imaging supervision code(s) (93501-93556) in the **Medicine** section of *CPT*. When coronary artery, arterial coronary conduit or venous bypass graft angiography is performed without concomitant left heart cardiac catheterization, use 93508. When internal mammary artery angiography only is performed without a concomitant left heart cardiac catheterization, use 36216 or 36217 as appropriate.)

36245 Selective catheter placement, arterial system; each first order abdominal, pelvic, or lower extremity artery branch, within a vascular family

36246 initial second order abdominal, pelvic, or lower extremity artery branch, within a vascular family

36247 initial third order or more selective abdominal, pelvic, or lower extremity artery branch, within a vascular family

+ 36248 additional second order, third order, and beyond, abdominal, pelvic, or lower extremity artery branch, within a vascular family (List in addition to code for initial second or third order vessel as appropriate)

(Use 36248 in conjunction with 36246, 36247)

36260 Insertion of implantable intra-arterial infusion pump (eg, for chemotherapy of liver)

36261 Revision of implanted intra-arterial infusion pump

36262 Removal of implanted intra-arterial infusion pump

36299 Unlisted procedure, vascular injection

Venous

Venipuncture, needle or catheter for diagnostic study or intravenous therapy, percutaneous.

36400 Venipuncture, under age 3 years, necessitating physician's skill, not to be used for routine venipuncture; femoral or jugular vein

36405 scalp vein

36406 other vein

36410 Venipuncture, age 3 years or older, necessitating physician's skill (separate procedure), for diagnostic or therapeutic purposes (not to be used for routine venipuncture)

36415 Collection of venous blood by venipuncture

(Do not report modifier 63 in conjunction with 36415)

36416 Collection of capillary blood specimen (eg, finger, heel, ear stick)

36420 Venipuncture, cutdown; under age 1 year

(Do not report modifier 63 in conjunction with 36420)

36425 age 1 or over

36430 Transfusion, blood or blood components

36440 Push transfusion, blood, 2 years or under

36450 Exchange transfusion, blood; newborn

(Do not report modifier 63 in conjunction with 36450)

36455 other than newborn

36460 Transfusion, intrauterine, fetal

(Do not report modifier 63 in conjunction with 36460)

(For radiological supervision and interpretation, use 76941)

36468 Single or multiple injections of sclerosing solutions, spider veins (telangiectasia); limb or trunk

36469 face

36470 Injection of sclerosing solution; single vein

36471 multiple veins, same leg

● 36475 Endovenous ablation therapy of incompetent vein, extremity, inclusive of all imaging guidance and monitoring, percutaneous, radiofrequency; first vein treated

+● 36476 second and subsequent veins treated in a single extremity, each through separate access sites (List separately in addition to code for primary procedure)

►(Use 36476 in conjunction with 36475)◄

►(Do not report 36475, 36476 in conjunction with 36000-36005, 36410, 36425, 36478, 36479, 37204, 75894, 76000-76003, 76937, 76942, 93970, 93971)◄

● 36478 Endovenous ablation therapy of incompetent vein, extremity, inclusive of all imaging guidance and monitoring, percutaneous, laser; first vein treated

+● 36479 second and subsequent veins treated in a single extremity, each through separate access sites (List separately in addition to code for primary procedure)

►(Use 36479 in conjunction with 36478)◄

►(Do not report 36478, 36479 in conjunction with 36000-36005, 36410, 36425, 36475, 36476, 37204, 75894, 76000-76003, 76937, 76942, 93970, 93971)◄

36481 Percutaneous portal vein catheterization by any method

(For radiological supervision and interpretation, see 75885, 75887)

(36488-36491 have been deleted. To report, see 36555-36556, 36568-36569, 36580, 36584)

(36493 has been deleted. To report, use 36597)

36500 Venous catheterization for selective organ blood sampling

(For catheterization in superior or inferior vena cava, use 36010)

(For radiological supervision and interpretation, use 75893)

36510 Catheterization of umbilical vein for diagnosis or therapy, newborn

(Do not report modifier 63 in conjunction with 36510)

36511 Therapeutic apheresis; for white blood cells

36512 for red blood cells

36513 for platelets

36514 for plasma pheresis

36515 with extracorporeal immunoadsorption and plasma reinfusion

36516 with extracorporeal selective adsorption or selective filtration and plasma reinfusion

(For physician evaluation, use modifier 26)

(36520 has been deleted. To report, see 36511-36512)

(36521 has been deleted. To report, use 36515, 36516)

36522 Photopheresis, extracorporeal

(36530 has been deleted. To report, use 36563)

(36531 has been deleted. To report, see 36575-36576, 36578, 36581-36582, 36584-36585)

(36532 has been deleted. To report, use 36590)

(36533 has been deleted. To report, see 36557-36561, 36565-36566, 36570-36571)

(36534 has been deleted. To report, see 36575-36578, 36581-36583, 36585)

(36535 has been deleted. To report, use 36589)

(36536 has been deleted. To report, use 36595)

(36537 have been deleted. To report, use 36596)

36540 Collection of blood specimen from a completely implantable venous access device

(Do not report 36540 in conjunction with 36415, 36416)

(For collection of venous blood specimen by venipuncture, use 36415)

(For collection of capillary blood specimen, use 36416)

36550 Declotting by thrombolytic agent of implanted vascular access device or catheter

Surgery: Cardiovascular System

▲=Revised Code ●=New Code ►◄=New or Revised Text

Central Venous Access Procedures

To qualify as a central venous access catheter or device, the tip of the catheter/device must terminate in the subclavian, brachiocephalic (innominate) or iliac veins, the superior or inferior vena cava, or the right atrium. The venous access device may be either centrally inserted (jugular, subclavian, femoral vein or inferior vena cava catheter entry site) or peripherally inserted (eg, basilic or cephalic vein). The device may be accessed for use either via exposed catheter (external to the skin), via a subcutaneous port or via a subcutaneous pump.

The procedures involving these types of devices fall into five categories:

1) *Insertion* (placement of catheter through a newly established venous access)

2) *Repair* (fixing device without replacement of either catheter or port/pump, other than pharmacologic or mechanical correction of intracatheter or pericatheter occlusion (see 36595 or 36596))

3) *Partial replacement* of only the catheter component associated with a port/pump device, but not entire device

4) *Complete replacement* of entire device via same venous access site (complete exchange)

5) *Removal* of entire device.

There is no coding distinction between venous access achieved percutaneously versus by cutdown or based on catheter size.

For the repair, partial (catheter only) replacement, complete replacement, or removal of both catheters (placed from separate venous access sites) of a multi-catheter device, with or without subcutaneous ports/pumps, use the appropriate code describing the service with a frequency of two.

If an existing central venous access device is removed and a new one placed via a separate venous access site, appropriate codes for both procedures (removal of old, if code exists, and insertion of new device) should be reported.

When imaging is used for these procedures, either for gaining access to the venous entry site or for manipulating the catheter into final central position, use 76937, 75998.

> (For refilling and maintenance of an implantable pump or reservoir for intravenous or intra-arterial drug delivery, use 96530)

Insertion of Central Venous Access Device

⊙ **36555** Insertion of non-tunneled centrally inserted central venous catheter; under 5 years of age

> (For peripherally inserted non-tunneled central venous catheter, under 5 years of age, use 36568)

36556 age 5 years or older

> (For peripherally inserted non-tunneled central venous catheter, age 5 years or older, use 36569)

⊙ **36557** Insertion of tunneled centrally inserted central venous catheter, without subcutaneous port or pump; under 5 years of age

⊙ **36558** age 5 years or older

> (For peripherally inserted central venous catheter with port, 5 years or older, use 36571)

⊙ **36560** Insertion of tunneled centrally inserted central venous access device, with subcutaneous port; under 5 years of age

> (For peripherally inserted central venous access device with subcutaneous port, under 5 years of age, use 36570)

⊙ **36561** age 5 years or older

> (For peripherally inserted central venous catheter with subcutaneous port, 5 years or older, use 36571)

⊙ **36563** Insertion of tunneled centrally inserted central venous access device with subcutaneous pump

⊙ **36565** Insertion of tunneled centrally inserted central venous access device, requiring two catheters via two separate venous access sites; without subcutaneous port or pump (eg, Tesio type catheter)

⊙ **36566** with subcutaneous port(s)

⊙ **36568** Insertion of peripherally inserted central venous catheter (PICC), without subcutaneous port or pump; under 5 years of age

> (For placement of centrally inserted non-tunneled central venous catheter, without subcutaneous port or pump, under 5 years of age, use 36555)

36569 age 5 years or older

> (For placement of centrally inserted non-tunneled central venous catheter, without subcutaneous port or pump, age 5 years or older, use 36556)

⊙ **36570** Insertion of peripherally inserted central venous access device, with subcutaneous port; under 5 years of age

> (For insertion of tunneled centrally inserted central venous access device with subcutaneous port, under 5 years of age, use 36560)

⊙ **36571** age 5 years or older

> (For insertion of tunneled centrally inserted central venous access device with subcutaneous port, age 5 years or older, use 36561)

Surgery: Cardiovascular System

Repair of Central Venous Access Device

(For mechanical removal of pericatheter obstructive material, use 36595)

(For mechanical removal of intracatheter obstructive material, use 36596)

36575 Repair of tunneled or non-tunneled central venous access catheter, without subcutaneous port or pump, central or peripheral insertion site

⊙ **36576** Repair of central venous access device, with subcutaneous port or pump, central or peripheral insertion site

Partial Replacement of Central Venous Access Device (Catheter Only)

⊙ **36578** Replacement, catheter only, of central venous access device, with subcutaneous port or pump, central or peripheral insertion site

(For complete replacement of entire device through same venous access, use 36582 or 36583)

Complete Replacement of Central Venous Access Device Through Same Venous Access Site

36580 Replacement, complete, of a non-tunneled centrally inserted central venous catheter, without subcutaneous port or pump, through same venous access

⊙ **36581** Replacement, complete, of a tunneled centrally inserted central venous catheter, without subcutaneous port or pump, through same venous access

⊙ **36582** Replacement, complete, of a tunneled centrally inserted central venous access device, with subcutaneous port, through same venous access

⊙ **36583** Replacement, complete, of a tunneled centrally inserted central venous access device, with subcutaneous pump, through same venous access

36584 Replacement, complete, of a peripherally inserted central venous catheter (PICC), without subcutaneous port or pump, through same venous access

⊙ **36585** Replacement, complete, of a peripherally inserted central venous access device, with subcutaneous port, through same venous access

Removal of Central Venous Access Device

36589 Removal of tunneled central venous catheter, without subcutaneous port or pump

⊙ **36590** Removal of tunneled central venous access device, with subcutaneous port or pump, central or peripheral insertion

(Do not report 36589 or 36590 for removal of non-tunneled central venous catheters)

Mechanical Removal of Obstructive Material

36595 Mechanical removal of pericatheter obstructive material (eg, fibrin sheath) from central venous device via separate venous access

(Do not report 36550 in addition to 36595)

(For venous catheterization, see 36010-36012)

(For radiological supervision and interpretation, use 75901)

36596 Mechanical removal of intraluminal (intracatheter) obstructive material from central venous device through device lumen

(Do not report 36550 in addition to 36596)

(For venous catheterization, see 36010-36012)

(For radiological supervision and interpretation, use 75902)

Other Central Venous Access Procedures

36597 Repositioning of previously placed central venous catheter under fluoroscopic guidance

(For fluoroscopic guidance, use 76000)

Arterial

36600 Arterial puncture, withdrawal of blood for diagnosis

⊘ **36620** Arterial catheterization or cannulation for sampling, monitoring or transfusion (separate procedure); percutaneous

36625   cutdown

36640 Arterial catheterization for prolonged infusion therapy (chemotherapy), cutdown

(See also 96420-96425)

(For arterial catheterization for occlusion therapy, see 75894)

⊘ **36660** Catheterization, umbilical artery, newborn, for diagnosis or therapy

(Do not report modifier 63 in conjunction with 36660)

Intraosseous

36680 Placement of needle for intraosseous infusion

Hemodialysis Access, Intervascular Cannulation for Extracorporeal Circulation, or Shunt Insertion

36800 Insertion of cannula for hemodialysis, other purpose (separate procedure); vein to vein

36810   arteriovenous, external (Scribner type)

36815   arteriovenous, external revision, or closure

● **36818** Arteriovenous anastomosis, open; by upper arm cephalic vein transposition

▶(Do not report 36818 in conjunction with 36819, 36820, 36821, 36830 during a unilateral upper extremity procedure. For bilateral upper extremity open arteriovenous anastomoses performed at the same operative session, use modifier 50 or 59 as appropriate)◀

36819 by upper arm basilic vein transposition

▶(Do not report 36819 in conjunction with 36818, 36820, 36821, 36830 during a unilateral upper extremity procedure. For bilateral upper extremity open arteriovenous anastomoses performed at the same operative session, use modifier 50 or 59 as appropriate)◀

36820 by forearm vein transposition

36821 direct, any site (eg, Cimino type) (separate procedure)

36822 Insertion of cannula(s) for prolonged extracorporeal circulation for cardiopulmonary insufficiency (ECMO) (separate procedure)

(For maintenance of prolonged extracorporeal circulation, see 33960, 33961)

36823 Insertion of arterial and venous cannula(s) for isolated extracorporeal circulation including regional chemotherapy perfusion to an extremity, with or without hyperthermia, with removal of cannula(s) and repair of arteriotomy and venotomy sites

(36823 includes chemotherapy perfusion supported by a membrane oxygenator/perfusion pump. Do not report 96408-96425 in conjunction with 36823)

36825 Creation of arteriovenous fistula by other than direct arteriovenous anastomosis (separate procedure); autogenous graft

(For direct arteriovenous anastomosis, use 36821)

36830 nonautogenous graft (eg, biological collagen, thermoplastic graft)

(For direct arteriovenous anastomosis, use 36821)

36831 Thrombectomy, open, arteriovenous fistula without revision, autogenous or nonautogenous dialysis graft (separate procedure)

36832 Revision, open, arteriovenous fistula; without thrombectomy, autogenous or nonautogenous dialysis graft (separate procedure)

36833 with thrombectomy, autogenous or nonautogenous dialysis graft (separate procedure)

36834 Plastic repair of arteriovenous aneurysm (separate procedure)

36835 Insertion of Thomas shunt (separate procedure)

36838 Distal revascularization and interval ligation (DRIL), upper extremity hemodialysis access (steal syndrome)

(Do not report 36838 in conjunction with 35512, 35522, 36832, 37607, 37618)

36860 External cannula declotting (separate procedure); without balloon catheter

36861 with balloon catheter

(If imaging guidance is performed, use 76000)

⊙ **36870** Thrombectomy, percutaneous, arteriovenous fistula, autogenous or nonautogenous graft (includes mechanical thrombus extraction and intra-graft thrombolysis)

(Do not report 36550 in conjunction with 36870)

(For catheterization, use 36145)

(For radiological supervision and interpretation, use 75790)

Portal Decompression Procedures

37140 Venous anastomosis, open; portocaval

(For peritoneal-venous shunt, use 49425)

37145 renoportal

37160 caval-mesenteric

37180 splenorenal, proximal

37181 splenorenal, distal (selective decompression of esophagogastric varices, any technique)

(For percutaneous procedure, use 37182)

37182 Insertion of transvenous intrahepatic portosystemic shunt(s) (TIPS) (includes venous access, hepatic and portal vein catheterization, portography with hemodynamic evaluation, intrahepatic tract formation/dilatation, stent placement and all associated imaging guidance and documentation)

(Do not report 75885 or 75887 in conjunction with 37182)

(For open procedure, use 37140)

37183 Revision of transvenous intrahepatic portosystemic shunt(s) (TIPS) (includes venous access, hepatic and portal vein catheterization, portography with hemodynamic evaluation, intrahepatic tract recanulization/dilatation, stent placement and all associated imaging guidance and documentation)

(Do not report 75885 or 75887 in conjunction with 37183)

(For repair of arteriovenous aneurysm, use 36834)

Transcatheter Procedures

Codes for catheter placement and the radiologic supervision and interpretation should also be reported, in addition to the code(s) for the therapeutic aspect of the procedure.

37195 Thrombolysis, cerebral, by intravenous infusion

37200 Transcatheter biopsy

(For radiological supervision and interpretation, use 75970)

⊘ = Modifier 51 Exempt   ⊙ = Conscious Sedation   ✦ = Add-on Code

37201   Transcatheter therapy, infusion for thrombolysis other than coronary

(For radiological supervision and interpretation, use 75896)

37202   Transcatheter therapy, infusion other than for thrombolysis, any type (eg, spasmolytic, vasoconstrictive)

(For thrombolysis of coronary vessels, see 92975, 92977)

(For radiological supervision and interpretation, use 75896)

⊙ **37203**   Transcatheter retrieval, percutaneous, of intravascular foreign body (eg, fractured venous or arterial catheter)

(For radiological supervision and interpretation, use 75961)

37204   Transcatheter occlusion or embolization (eg, for tumor destruction, to achieve hemostasis, to occlude a vascular malformation), percutaneous, any method, non-central nervous system, non-head or neck

(See also 61624, 61626)

(For radiological supervision and interpretation, use 75894)

▲ **37205**   Transcatheter placement of an intravascular stent(s), (except coronary, carotid, and vertebral vessel), percutaneous; initial vessel

(For radiological supervision and interpretation, use 75960)

▶(For coronary stent placement, see 92980, 92981)◀

+ **37206**   each additional vessel (List separately in addition to code for primary procedure)

(Use 37206 in conjunction with 37205)

(For transcatheter placement of ▶intravascular cervical carotid◀ artery stent(s), see ▶37215, 37216◀)

▶(For transcatheter placement of extracranial vertebral or intrathoracic carotid artery stent(s), see Category III codes 0075T, 0076T)◀

(For radiological supervision and interpretation, use 75960)

37207   Transcatheter placement of an intravascular stent(s), (non-coronary vessel), open; initial vessel

+ **37208**   each additional vessel (List separately in addition to code for primary procedure)

(Use 37208 in conjunction with 37207)

(For radiological supervision and interpretation, use 75960)

(For catheterizations, see 36215-36248)

(For transcatheter placement of intracoronary stent(s), see 92980, 92981)

37209   Exchange of a previously placed arterial catheter during thrombolytic therapy

(For radiological supervision and interpretation, use 75900)

⊙● **37215**   Transcatheter placement of intravascular stent(s), cervical carotid artery, percutaneous; with distal embolic protection

⊙● **37216**   without distal embolic protection

▶(37215 and 37216 include all ipsilateral selective carotid catheterization, all diagnostic imaging for ipsilateral, cervical and cerebral carotid arteriography, and all related radiological supervision and interpretation. When ipsilateral carotid arteriogram (including imaging and selective catheterization) confirms the need for carotid stenting, 37215 and 37216 are inclusive of these services. If carotid stenting is not indicated, then the appropriate codes for carotid catheterization and imaging should be reported in lieu of 37215 and 37216)◀

▶(Do not report 37215, 37216 in conjunction with 75671, 75680)◀

▶(For transcatheter placement of extracranial vertebral or intrathoracic carotid artery stent(s), see Category III codes 0075T, 0076T)◀

▶(For percutaneous transcatheter placement of intravascular stents other than coronary, carotid, or vertebral, see 37205, 37206)◀

Intravascular Ultrasound Services

Intravascular ultrasound services include all transducer manipulations and repositioning within the specific vessel being examined, both before and after therapeutic intervention (eg, stent placement).

Vascular access for intravascular ultrasound performed during a therapeutic intervention is not reported separately.

+ **37250**   Intravascular ultrasound (non-coronary vessel) during diagnostic evaluation and/or therapeutic intervention; initial vessel (List separately in addition to code for primary procedure)

+ **37251**   each additional vessel (List separately in addition to code for primary procedure)

(Use 37251 in conjunction with 37250)

(For catheterizations, see 36215-36248)

(For transcatheter therapies, see 37200-37208, 61624, 61626)

(For radiological supervision and interpretation see 75945, 75946)

Surgery: Cardiovascular System

Surgery: Cardiovascular System

Endoscopy

Surgical vascular endoscopy always includes diagnostic endoscopy.

37500 Vascular endoscopy, surgical, with ligation of perforator veins, subfascial (SEPS)

(For open procedure, use 37760)

37501 Unlisted vascular endoscopy procedure

Ligation

(For phleborraphy and arteriorraphy, see 35201-35286)

37565 Ligation, internal jugular vein

37600 Ligation; external carotid artery

37605 internal or common carotid artery

37606 internal or common carotid artery, with gradual occlusion, as with Selverstone or Crutchfield clamp

(For transcatheter permanent arterial occlusion or embolization, see 61624-61626)

(For endovascular temporary arterial balloon occlusion, use 61623)

(For ligation treatment of intracranial aneurysm, use 61703)

37607 Ligation or banding of angioaccess arteriovenous fistula

37609 Ligation or biopsy, temporal artery

37615 Ligation, major artery (eg, post-traumatic, rupture); neck

37616 chest

37617 abdomen

37618 extremity

37620 Interruption, partial or complete, of inferior vena cava by suture, ligation, plication, clip, extravascular, intravascular (umbrella device)

(For radiological supervision and interpretation, use 75940)

37650 Ligation of femoral vein

(For bilateral procedure, report 37650 with modifier 50)

37660 Ligation of common iliac vein

37700 Ligation and division of long saphenous vein at saphenofemoral junction, or distal interruptions

(For bilateral procedure, report 37700 with modifier 50)

37720 Ligation and division and complete stripping of long or short saphenous veins

(For bilateral procedure, report 37720 with modifier 50)

37730 Ligation and division and complete stripping of long and short saphenous veins

(For bilateral procedure, report 37730 with modifier 50)

37735 Ligation and division and complete stripping of long or short saphenous veins with radical excision of ulcer and skin graft and/or interruption of communicating veins of lower leg, with excision of deep fascia

(For bilateral procedure, report 37735 with modifier 50)

37760 Ligation of perforator veins, subfascial, radical (Linton type), with or without skin graft, open

(For endoscopic procedure, use 37500)

37765 Stab phlebectomy of varicose veins, one extremity; 10-20 stab incisions

(For less than 10 incisions, use 37799)

(For more than 20 incisions, use 37766)

37766 more than 20 incisions

37780 Ligation and division of short saphenous vein at saphenopopliteal junction (separate procedure)

(For bilateral procedure, report 37780 with modifier 50)

37785 Ligation, division, and/or excision of varicose vein cluster(s), one leg

(For bilateral procedure, report 37785 with modifier 50)

Other Procedures

37788 Penile revascularization, artery, with or without vein graft

37790 Penile venous occlusive procedure

37799 Unlisted procedure, vascular surgery

Hemic and Lymphatic Systems

Spleen

Excision

38100 Splenectomy; total (separate procedure)

38101 partial (separate procedure)

+ 38102 total, en bloc for extensive disease, in conjunction with other procedure (List in addition to code for primary procedure)

Repair

38115 Repair of ruptured spleen (splenorrhaphy) with or without partial splenectomy

Laparoscopy

Surgical laparoscopy always includes diagnostic laparoscopy. To report a diagnostic laparoscopy (peritoneoscopy) (separate procedure), use 49320.

38120 Laparoscopy, surgical, splenectomy

38129 Unlisted laparoscopy procedure, spleen

Introduction

38200   Injection procedure for splenoportography

(For radiological supervision and interpretation, use 75810)

General

Bone Marrow or Stem Cell Services/Procedures

Codes 38207-38215 describe various steps used to preserve, prepare and purify bone marrow/stem cells prior to transplantation or reinfusion. Each code may be reported only once per day regardless of the quantity of bone marrow/stem cells manipulated.

38204   Management of recipient hematopoietic progenitor cell donor search and cell acquisition

38205   Blood-derived hematopoietic progenitor cell harvesting for transplantation, per collection; allogenic

38206   autologous

38207   Transplant preparation of hematopoietic progenitor cells; cryopreservation and storage

(For diagnostic cryopreservation and storage, see 88240)

38208   thawing of previously frozen harvest, without washing

(For diagnostic thawing and expansion of frozen cells, see 88241)

38209   thawing of previously frozen harvest, with washing

38210   specific cell depletion within harvest, T-cell depletion

38211   tumor cell depletion

38212   red blood cell removal

38213   platelet depletion

38214   plasma (volume) depletion

38215   cell concentration in plasma, mononuclear, or buffy coat layer

(Do not report 38207-38215 in conjunction with ▶88182, 88184-88189◄)

38220   Bone marrow; aspiration only

38221   biopsy, needle or trocar

(For bone marrow biopsy interpretation, use 88305)

38230   Bone marrow harvesting for transplantation

(For autologous and allogenic blood-derived peripheral stem cell harvesting for transplantation, see 38205-38206)

(38231 has been deleted. To report, use 38205-38206)

38240   Bone marrow or blood-derived peripheral stem cell transplantation; allogenic

38241   autologous

38242   allogeneic donor lymphocyte infusions

(For bone marrow aspiration, use 38220)

(For modification, treatment, and processing of bone marrow or blood-derived stem cell specimens for transplantation, use 38210-38213)

(For cryopreservation, freezing and storage of blood-derived stem cells for transplantation, use 88240)

(For thawing and expansion of blood-derived stem cells for transplantation, use 88241)

(For compatibility studies, see 86812-86822)

Lymph Nodes and Lymphatic Channels

Incision

38300   Drainage of lymph node abscess or lymphadenitis; simple

38305   extensive

38308   Lymphangiotomy or other operations on lymphatic channels

38380   Suture and/or ligation of thoracic duct; cervical approach

38381   thoracic approach

38382   abdominal approach

Excision

(For injection for sentinel node identification, use 38792)

38500   Biopsy or excision of lymph node(s); open, superficial

(Do not report 38500 with 38700-38780)

38505   by needle, superficial (eg, cervical, inguinal, axillary)

(If imaging guidance is performed, see 76360, 76393, 76942)

(For fine needle aspiration, use 10021 or 10022)

(For evaluation of fine needle aspirate, see 88172, 88173)

38510   open, deep cervical node(s)

38520   open, deep cervical node(s) with excision scalene fat pad

38525   open, deep axillary node(s)

38530   open, internal mammary node(s)

(Do not report 38530 with 38720-38746)

(For percutaneous needle biopsy, retroperitoneal lymph node or mass, use 49180. For fine needle aspiration, use 10022)

38542   Dissection, deep jugular node(s)

(For radical cervical neck dissection, use 38720)

38550   Excision of cystic hygroma, axillary or cervical; without deep neurovascular dissection

38555   with deep neurovascular dissection

Surgery: Cardiovascular System

Surgery: Cardiovascular System

Limited Lymphadenectomy for Staging

38562   Limited lymphadenectomy for staging (separate procedure); pelvic and para-aortic

(When combined with prostatectomy, use 55812 or 55842)

(When combined with insertion of radioactive substance into prostate, use 55862)

38564   retroperitoneal (aortic and/or splenic)

Laparoscopy

Surgical laparoscopy always includes diagnostic laparoscopy. To report a diagnostic laparoscopy (peritoneoscopy) (separate procedure), use 49320.

38570   Laparoscopy, surgical; with retroperitoneal lymph node sampling (biopsy), single or multiple

38571   with bilateral total pelvic lymphadenectomy

38572   with bilateral total pelvic lymphadenectomy and peri-aortic lymph node sampling (biopsy), single or multiple

(For drainage of lymphocele to peritoneal cavity, use 49323)

38589   Unlisted laparoscopy procedure, lymphatic system

Radical Lymphadenectomy (Radical Resection of Lymph Nodes)

(For limited pelvic and retroperitoneal lymphadenectomies, see 38562, 38564)

38700   Suprahyoid lymphadenectomy

(For bilateral procedure, report 38700 with modifier 50)

38720   Cervical lymphadenectomy (complete)

(For bilateral procedure, report 38720 with modifier 50)

38724   Cervical lymphadenectomy (modified radical neck dissection)

38740   Axillary lymphadenectomy; superficial

38745   complete

+ 38746   Thoracic lymphadenectomy, regional, including mediastinal and peritracheal nodes (List separately in addition to code for primary procedure)

+ 38747   Abdominal lymphadenectomy, regional, including celiac, gastric, portal, peripancreatic, with or without para-aortic and vena caval nodes (List separately in addition to code for primary procedure)

38760   Inguinofemoral lymphadenectomy, superficial, including Cloquets node (separate procedure)

(For bilateral procedure, report 38760 with modifier 50

38765   Inguinofemoral lymphadenectomy, superficial, in continuity with pelvic lymphadenectomy, including external iliac, hypogastric, and obturator nodes (separate procedure)

(For bilateral procedure, report 38765 with modifier 50)

38770   Pelvic lymphadenectomy, including external iliac, hypogastric, and obturator nodes (separate procedure)

(For bilateral procedure, report 38770 with modifier 50)

38780   Retroperitoneal transabdominal lymphadenectomy, extensive, including pelvic, aortic, and renal nodes (separate procedure)

(For excision and repair of lymphedematous skin and subcutaneous tissue, see 15000, 15570-15650)

Introduction

38790   Injection procedure; lymphangiography

(For bilateral procedure, report 38790 with modifier 50)

(For radiological supervision and interpretation, see 75801-75807)

⊘ 38792   for identification of sentinel node

(For excision of sentinel node, see 38500-38542)

(For nuclear medicine lymphatics and lymph gland imaging, use 78195)

38794   Cannulation, thoracic duct

Other Procedures

38999   Unlisted procedure, hemic or lymphatic system

Mediastinum and Diaphragm

Mediastinum

Incision

39000   Mediastinotomy with exploration, drainage, removal of foreign body, or biopsy; cervical approach

39010   transthoracic approach, including either transthoracic or median sternotomy

Excision

39200   Excision of mediastinal cyst

39220   Excision of mediastinal tumor

(For substernal thyroidectomy, use 60270)

(For thymectomy, use 60520)

Endoscopy

39400   Mediastinoscopy, with or without biopsy

Other Procedures

39499   Unlisted procedure, mediastinum

Diaphragm

Repair

(For transabdominal repair of diaphragmatic (esophageal hiatal) hernia, see 43324, 43325)

39501   Repair, laceration of diaphragm, any approach

39502   Repair, paraesophageal hiatus hernia, transabdominal, with or without fundoplasty, vagotomy, and/or pyloroplasty, except neonatal

39503   Repair, neonatal diaphragmatic hernia, with or without chest tube insertion and with or without creation of ventral hernia

(Do not report modifier 63 in conjunction with 39503)

39520   Repair, diaphragmatic hernia (esophageal hiatal); transthoracic

39530   combined, thoracoabdominal

39531   combined, thoracoabdominal, with dilation of stricture (with or without gastroplasty)

39540   Repair, diaphragmatic hernia (other than neonatal), traumatic; acute

39541   chronic

39545   Imbrication of diaphragm for eventration, transthoracic or transabdominal, paralytic or nonparalytic

39560   Resection, diaphragm; with simple repair (eg, primary suture)

39561   with complex repair (eg, prosthetic material, local muscle flap)

Other Procedures

39599   Unlisted procedure, diaphragm

Notes

Digestive System

Lips

(For procedures on skin of lips, see 10040 et seq)

Excision

40490   Biopsy of lip

40500   Vermilionectomy (lip shave), with mucosal advancement

40510   Excision of lip; transverse wedge excision with primary closure

40520   V-excision with primary direct linear closure

(For excision of mucous lesions, see 40810-40816)

40525   full thickness, reconstruction with local flap (eg, Estlander or fan)

40527   full thickness, reconstruction with cross lip flap (Abbe-Estlander)

40530   Resection of lip, more than one-fourth, without reconstruction

(For reconstruction, see 13131 et seq)

Repair (Cheiloplasty)

40650   Repair lip, full thickness; vermilion only

40652   up to half vertical height

40654   over one-half vertical height, or complex

40700   Plastic repair of cleft lip/nasal deformity; primary, partial or complete, unilateral

40701   primary bilateral, one stage procedure

40702   primary bilateral, one of two stages

40720   secondary, by recreation of defect and reclosure

(For bilateral procedure, report 40720 with modifier 50)

(To report rhinoplasty only for nasal deformity secondary to congenital cleft lip, see 30460, 30462)

(For repair of cleft lip, with cross lip pedicle flap (Abbe-Estlander type), use 40527)

40761   with cross lip pedicle flap (Abbe-Estlander type), including sectioning and inserting of pedicle

(For repair cleft palate, see 42200 et seq)

(For other reconstructive procedures, see 14060, 14061, 15120-15261, 15574, 15576, 15630)

Other Procedures

40799   Unlisted procedure, lips

Vestibule of Mouth

The vestibule is the part of the oral cavity outside the dentoalveolar structures; it includes the mucosal and submucosal tissue of lips and cheeks.

Incision

40800   Drainage of abscess, cyst, hematoma, vestibule of mouth; simple

40801   complicated

40804   Removal of embedded foreign body, vestibule of mouth; simple

40805   complicated

40806   Incision of labial frenum (frenotomy)

Excision, Destruction

40808   Biopsy, vestibule of mouth

40810   Excision of lesion of mucosa and submucosa, vestibule of mouth; without repair

40812   with simple repair

40814   with complex repair

40816   complex, with excision of underlying muscle

40818   Excision of mucosa of vestibule of mouth as donor graft

40819   Excision of frenum, labial or buccal (frenumectomy, frenulectomy, frenectomy)

40820   Destruction of lesion or scar of vestibule of mouth by physical methods (eg, laser, thermal, cryo, chemical)

Repair

40830   Closure of laceration, vestibule of mouth; 2.5 cm or less

40831   over 2.5 cm or complex

40840   Vestibuloplasty; anterior

40842   posterior, unilateral

40843   posterior, bilateral

40844   entire arch

40845   complex (including ridge extension, muscle repositioning)

(For skin grafts, see 15000 et seq)

Other Procedures

40899   Unlisted procedure, vestibule of mouth

Surgery: Digestive System

Tongue and Floor of Mouth

Incision

41000   Intraoral incision and drainage of abscess, cyst, or hematoma of tongue or floor of mouth; lingual

41005   sublingual, superficial

41006   sublingual, deep, supramylohyoid

41007   submental space

41008   submandibular space

41009   masticator space

41010   Incision of lingual frenum (frenotomy)

41015   Extraoral incision and drainage of abscess, cyst, or hematoma of floor of mouth; sublingual

41016   submental

41017   submandibular

41018   masticator space

(For frenoplasty, use 41520)

Excision

41100   Biopsy of tongue; anterior two-thirds

41105   posterior one-third

41108   Biopsy of floor of mouth

41110   Excision of lesion of tongue without closure

41112   Excision of lesion of tongue with closure; anterior two-thirds

41113   posterior one-third

41114   with local tongue flap

(List 41114 in addition to code 41112 or 41113)

41115   Excision of lingual frenum (frenectomy)

41116   Excision, lesion of floor of mouth

41120   Glossectomy; less than one-half tongue

41130   hemiglossectomy

41135   partial, with unilateral radical neck dissection

41140   complete or total, with or without tracheostomy, without radical neck dissection

41145   complete or total, with or without tracheostomy, with unilateral radical neck dissection

41150   composite procedure with resection floor of mouth and mandibular resection, without radical neck dissection

41153   composite procedure with resection floor of mouth, with suprahyoid neck dissection

41155   composite procedure with resection floor of mouth, mandibular resection, and radical neck dissection (Commando type)

Repair

41250   Repair of laceration 2.5 cm or less; floor of mouth and/or anterior two-thirds of tongue

41251   posterior one-third of tongue

41252   Repair of laceration of tongue, floor of mouth, over 2.6 cm or complex

Other Procedures

41500   Fixation of tongue, mechanical, other than suture (eg, K-wire)

41510   Suture of tongue to lip for micrognathia (Douglas type procedure)

41520   Frenoplasty (surgical revision of frenum, eg, with Z-plasty)

(For frenotomy, see 40806, 41010)

41599   Unlisted procedure, tongue, floor of mouth

Dentoalveolar Structures

Incision

41800   Drainage of abscess, cyst, hematoma from dentoalveolar structures

41805   Removal of embedded foreign body from dentoalveolar structures; soft tissues

41806   bone

Excision, Destruction

41820   Gingivectomy, excision gingiva, each quadrant

41821   Operculectomy, excision pericoronal tissues

41822   Excision of fibrous tuberosities, dentoalveolar structures

41823   Excision of osseous tuberosities, dentoalveolar structures

41825   Excision of lesion or tumor (except listed above), dentoalveolar structures; without repair

41826   with simple repair

41827   with complex repair

(For nonexcisional destruction, use 41850)

41828   Excision of hyperplastic alveolar mucosa, each quadrant (specify)

41830   Alveolectomy, including curettage of osteitis or sequestrectomy

41850   Destruction of lesion (except excision), dentoalveolar structures

Other Procedures

41870   Periodontal mucosal grafting

41872   Gingivoplasty, each quadrant (specify)

41874   Alveoloplasty, each quadrant (specify)

(For closure of lacerations, see 40830, 40831)

(For segmental osteotomy, use 21206)

(For reduction of fractures, see 21421-21490)

41899   Unlisted procedure, dentoalveolar structures

Palate and Uvula

Incision

42000   Drainage of abscess of palate, uvula

Excision, Destruction

42100   Biopsy of palate, uvula

42104   Excision, lesion of palate, uvula; without closure

42106   with simple primary closure

42107   with local flap closure

(For skin graft, see 14040-14300)

(For mucosal graft, use 40818)

42120   Resection of palate or extensive resection of lesion

(For reconstruction of palate with extraoral tissue, see 14040-14300, 15050, 15120, 15240, 15576)

42140   Uvulectomy, excision of uvula

42145   Palatopharyngoplasty (eg, uvulopalatopharyngoplasty, uvulopharyngoplasty)

(For removal of exostosis of the bony palate, see 21031, 21032)

42160   Destruction of lesion, palate or uvula (thermal, cryo or chemical)

Repair

42180   Repair, laceration of palate; up to 2 cm

42182   over 2 cm or complex

42200   Palatoplasty for cleft palate, soft and/or hard palate only

42205   Palatoplasty for cleft palate, with closure of alveolar ridge; soft tissue only

42210   with bone graft to alveolar ridge (includes obtaining graft)

42215   Palatoplasty for cleft palate; major revision

42220   secondary lengthening procedure

42225   attachment pharyngeal flap

42226   Lengthening of palate, and pharyngeal flap

42227   Lengthening of palate, with island flap

42235   Repair of anterior palate, including vomer flap

(For repair of oronasal fistula, use 30600)

42260   Repair of nasolabial fistula

(For repair of cleft lip, see 40700 et seq)

42280   Maxillary impression for palatal prosthesis

42281   Insertion of pin-retained palatal prosthesis

Other Procedures

42299   Unlisted procedure, palate, uvula

Salivary Gland and Ducts

Incision

42300   Drainage of abscess; parotid, simple

42305   parotid, complicated

42310   Drainage of abscess; submaxillary or sublingual, intraoral

42320   submaxillary, external

42325   Fistulization of sublingual salivary cyst (ranula);

42326   with prosthesis

42330   Sialolithotomy; submandibular (submaxillary), sublingual or parotid, uncomplicated, intraoral

42335   submandibular (submaxillary), complicated, intraoral

42340   parotid, extraoral or complicated intraoral

Excision

42400   Biopsy of salivary gland; needle

(For fine needle aspiration, see 10021, 10022)

(For evaluation of fine needle aspirate, see 88172, 88173)

(If imaging guidance is performed, see 76003, 76360, 76393, 76942)

42405   incisional

(If imaging guidance is performed, see 76003, 76360, 76393, 76942)

42408   Excision of sublingual salivary cyst (ranula)

42409   Marsupialization of sublingual salivary cyst (ranula)

(For fistulization of sublingual salivary cyst, use 42325)

42410   Excision of parotid tumor or parotid gland; lateral lobe, without nerve dissection

42415   lateral lobe, with dissection and preservation of facial nerve

42420   total, with dissection and preservation of facial nerve

42425   total, en bloc removal with sacrifice of facial nerve

42426   total, with unilateral radical neck dissection

(For suture or grafting of facial nerve, see 64864, 64865, 69740, 69745)

Surgery: Digestive System

42440	Excision of submandibular (submaxillary) gland
42450	Excision of sublingual gland

Repair

42500	Plastic repair of salivary duct, sialodochoplasty; primary or simple
42505	secondary or complicated
42507	Parotid duct diversion, bilateral (Wilke type procedure);
42508	with excision of one submandibular gland
42509	with excision of both submandibular glands
42510	with ligation of both submandibular (Wharton's) ducts

Other Procedures

42550	Injection procedure for sialography
	(For radiological supervision and interpretation, use 70390)
42600	Closure salivary fistula
42650	Dilation salivary duct
42660	Dilation and catheterization of salivary duct, with or without injection
42665	Ligation salivary duct, intraoral
42699	Unlisted procedure, salivary glands or ducts

Pharynx, Adenoids, and Tonsils

Incision

42700	Incision and drainage abscess; peritonsillar
42720	retropharyngeal or parapharyngeal, intraoral approach
42725	retropharyngeal or parapharyngeal, external approach

Excision, Destruction

42800	Biopsy; oropharynx
42802	hypopharynx
42804	nasopharynx, visible lesion, simple
42806	nasopharynx, survey for unknown primary lesion
	(For laryngoscopic biopsy, see 31510, 31535, 31536)
42808	Excision or destruction of lesion of pharynx, any method
42809	Removal of foreign body from pharynx
42810	Excision branchial cleft cyst or vestige, confined to skin and subcutaneous tissues
42815	Excision branchial cleft cyst, vestige, or fistula, extending beneath subcutaneous tissues and/or into pharynx

42820	Tonsillectomy and adenoidectomy; under age 12
42821	age 12 or over
42825	Tonsillectomy, primary or secondary; under age 12
42826	age 12 or over
42830	Adenoidectomy, primary; under age 12
42831	age 12 or over
42835	Adenoidectomy, secondary; under age 12
42836	age 12 or over
42842	Radical resection of tonsil, tonsillar pillars, and/or retromolar trigone; without closure
42844	closure with local flap (eg, tongue, buccal)
42845	closure with other flap
	(For closure with other flap(s), use appropriate number for flap(s))
	(When combined with radical neck dissection, use also 38720)
42860	Excision of tonsil tags
42870	Excision or destruction lingual tonsil, any method (separate procedure)
	(For resection of the nasopharynx (eg, juvenile angiofibroma) by bicoronal and/or transzygomatic approach, see 61586 and 61600)
42890	Limited pharyngectomy
42892	Resection of lateral pharyngeal wall or pyriform sinus, direct closure by advancement of lateral and posterior pharyngeal walls
	(When combined with radical neck dissection, use also 38720)
42894	Resection of pharyngeal wall requiring closure with myocutaneous flap
	(When combined with radical neck dissection, use also 38720)
	(For limited pharyngectomy with radical neck dissection, use 38720 with 42890)

Repair

42900	Suture pharynx for wound or injury
42950	Pharyngoplasty (plastic or reconstructive operation on pharynx)
	(For pharyngeal flap, use 42225)
42953	Pharyngoesophageal repair
	(For closure with myocutaneous or other flap, use appropriate number in addition)

Surgery: Digestive System

Other Procedures

42955   Pharyngostomy (fistulization of pharynx, external for feeding)

42960   Control oropharyngeal hemorrhage, primary or secondary (eg, post-tonsillectomy); simple

42961   complicated, requiring hospitalization

42962   with secondary surgical intervention

42970   Control of nasopharyngeal hemorrhage, primary or secondary (eg, postadenoidectomy); simple, with posterior nasal packs, with or without anterior packs and/or cautery

42971   complicated, requiring hospitalization

42972   with secondary surgical intervention

42999   Unlisted procedure, pharynx, adenoids, or tonsils

Esophagus

Incision

     (For esophageal intubation with laparotomy, use 43510)

43020   Esophagotomy, cervical approach, with removal of foreign body

43030   Cricopharyngeal myotomy

43045   Esophagotomy, thoracic approach, with removal of foreign body

Excision

     (For gastrointestinal reconstruction for previous esophagectomy, see 43360, 43361)

43100   Excision of lesion, esophagus, with primary repair; cervical approach

43101   thoracic or abdominal approach

     (For wide excision of malignant lesion of cervical esophagus, with total laryngectomy without radical neck dissection, see 43107, 43116, 43124, and 31360)

     (For wide excision of malignant lesion of cervical esophagus, with total laryngectomy with radical neck dissection, see 43107, 43116, 43124, and 31365)

43107   Total or near total esophagectomy, without thoracotomy; with pharyngogastrostomy or cervical esophagogastrostomy, with or without pyloroplasty (transhiatal)

43108   with colon interposition or small intestine reconstruction, including intestine mobilization, preparation and anastomosis(es)

43112   Total or near total esophagectomy, with thoracotomy; with pharyngogastrostomy or cervical esophagogastrostomy, with or without pyloroplasty

43113   with colon interposition or small intestine reconstruction, including intestine mobilization, preparation, and anastomosis(es)

43116   Partial esophagectomy, cervical, with free intestinal graft, including microvascular anastomosis, obtaining the graft and intestinal reconstruction

     (Do not report code 69990 in addition to code 43116)

     (Report 43116 with the modifier 52 appended if intestinal or free jejunal graft with microvascular anastomosis is performed by another physician)

     (For free jejunal graft with microvascular anastomosis performed by another physician, use 43496)

43117   Partial esophagectomy, distal two-thirds, with thoracotomy and separate abdominal incision, with or without proximal gastrectomy; with thoracic esophagogastrostomy, with or without pyloroplasty (Ivor Lewis)

43118   with colon interposition or small intestine reconstruction, including intestine mobilization, preparation, and anastomosis(es)

     (For total esophagectomy with gastropharyngostomy, see 43107, 43124)

     (For esophagogastrectomy (lower third) and vagotomy, use 43122)

43121   Partial esophagectomy, distal two-thirds, with thoracotomy only, with or without proximal gastrectomy, with thoracic esophagogastrostomy, with or without pyloroplasty

43122   Partial esophagectomy, thoracoabdominal or abdominal approach, with or without proximal gastrectomy; with esophagogastrostomy, with or without pyloroplasty

43123   with colon interposition or small intestine reconstruction, including intestine mobilization, preparation, and anastomosis(es)

43124   Total or partial esophagectomy, without reconstruction (any approach), with cervical esophagostomy

43130   Diverticulectomy of hypopharynx or esophagus, with or without myotomy; cervical approach

43135   thoracic approach

Endoscopy

For endoscopic procedures, code appropriate endoscopy of each anatomic site examined.

Surgical endoscopy always includes diagnostic endoscopy.

     (For upper gastrointestinal endoscopy with suturing of the esophagogastric junction, use Category III code 0008T)

⊙ **43200**   Esophagoscopy, rigid or flexible; diagnostic, with or without collection of specimen(s) by brushing or washing (separate procedure)

⊙ **43201**   with directed submucosal injection(s), any substance

     (For injection sclerosis of esophageal varices, use 43204)

⊙ **43202**   with biopsy, single or multiple

⊙ **43204**   with injection sclerosis of esophageal varices

▲=Revised Code   ●=New Code   ▶◀=New or Revised Text

Surgery: Digestive System

⊙ **43205**   with band ligation of esophageal varices

⊙ **43215**   with removal of foreign body

(For radiological supervision and interpretation, use 74235)

⊙ **43216**   with removal of tumor(s), polyp(s), or other lesion(s) by hot biopsy forceps or bipolar cautery

⊙ **43217**   with removal of tumor(s), polyp(s), or other lesion(s) by snare technique

⊙ **43219**   with insertion of plastic tube or stent

⊙ **43220**   with balloon dilation (less than 30 mm diameter)

(If imaging guidance is performed, use 74360)

(For endoscopic dilation with balloon 30 mm diameter or larger, use 43458)

(For dilation without visualization, use 43450-43453)

(For diagnostic fiberoptic esophagogastroscopy, use 43200, 43235)

(For fiberoptic esophagogastroscopy with biopsy or collection of specimen, use 43200, 43202, 43235, 43239)

(For fiberoptic esophagogastroscopy with removal of foreign body, use 43215, 43247)

(For fiberoptic esophagogastroscopy with removal of polyp(s), use 43217, 43251)

⊙ **43226**   with insertion of guide wire followed by dilation over guide wire

(For radiological supervision and interpretation, use 74360)

⊙ **43227**   with control of bleeding (eg, injection, bipolar cautery, unipolar cautery, laser, heater probe, stapler, plasma coagulator)

⊙ **43228**   with ablation of tumor(s), polyp(s), or other lesion(s), not amenable to removal by hot biopsy forceps, bipolar cautery or snare technique

(For esophagoscopic photodynamic therapy, report 43228 in addition to 96570, 96571 as appropriate)

⊙ **43231**   with endoscopic ultrasound examination

(Do not report 43231 in conjunction with 76975)

⊙ **43232**   with transendoscopic ultrasound-guided intramural or transmural fine needle aspiration/biopsy(s)

(Do not report 43232 in conjunction with 76942, 76975)

(For interpretation of specimen, see 88172-88173)

⊙ **43234**   Upper gastrointestinal endoscopy, simple primary examination (eg, with small diameter flexible endoscope) (separate procedure)

⊙ **43235**   Upper gastrointestinal endoscopy including esophagus, stomach, and either the duodenum and/or jejunum as appropriate; diagnostic, with or without collection of specimen(s) by brushing or washing (separate procedure)

⊙ **43236**   with directed submucosal injection(s), any substance

(For injection sclerosis of esophageal and/or gastric varices, use 43243)

43237   with endoscopic ultrasound examination limited to the esophagus

(Do not report 43237 in conjunction with 76942, 76975)

43238   with transendoscopic ultrasound-guided intramural or transmural fine needle aspiration/biopsy(s), esophagus (includes endoscopic ultrasound examination limited to the esophagus)

(Do not report 43238 in conjunction with 76942 or 76975)

⊙ **43239**   with biopsy, single or multiple

(For upper gastrointestinal endoscopy with suturing of the esophagogastric junction, use Category III code 0008T)

⊙ **43240**   with transmural drainage of pseudocyst

⊙ **43241**   with transendoscopic intraluminal tube or catheter placement

⊙ **43242**   with transendoscopic ultrasound-guided intramural or transmural fine needle aspiration/biopsy(s) (includes endoscopic ultrasound examination of the esophagus, stomach, and either the duodenum and/or jejunum as appropriate)

(Do not report 43242 in conjunction with 76942, 76975)

(For transendoscopic fine needle aspiration/biopsy limited to esophagus, use 43238)

(For interpretation of specimen, see 88172-88173)

⊙ **43243**   with injection sclerosis of esophageal and/or gastric varices

⊙ **43244**   with band ligation of esophageal and/or gastric varices

⊙ **43245**   with dilation of gastric outlet for obstruction (eg, balloon, guide wire, bougie)

(Do not report 43245 in conjunction with 43256)

⊙ **43246**   with directed placement of percutaneous gastrostomy tube

(For radiological supervision and interpretation, use 74350)

⊙ **43247**   with removal of foreign body

(For radiological supervision and interpretation, use 74235)

⊙ **43248**   with insertion of guide wire followed by dilation of esophagus over guide wire

⊙ **43249**   with balloon dilation of esophagus (less than 30 mm diameter)

⊙ **43250**   with removal of tumor(s), polyp(s), or other lesion(s) by hot biopsy forceps or bipolar cautery

⊙ **43251**   with removal of tumor(s), polyp(s), or other lesion(s) by snare technique

⊙ **43255**   with control of bleeding, any method

⊙ **43256**　　　with transendoscopic stent placement (includes predilation)

⊙● **43257**　　　with delivery of thermal energy to the muscle of lower esophageal sphincter and/or gastric cardia, for treatment of gastroesophageal reflux disease

⊙ **43258**　　　with ablation of tumor(s), polyp(s), or other lesion(s) not amenable to removal by hot biopsy forceps, bipolar cautery or snare technique

（For injection sclerosis of esophageal varices, use 43204, 43243）

⊙ **43259**　　　with endoscopic ultrasound examination, including the esophagus, stomach, and either the duodenum and/or jejunum as appropriate

（Do not report 43259 in conjunction with 76975）

⊙ **43260**　　　Endoscopic retrograde cholangiopancreatography (ERCP); diagnostic, with or without collection of specimen(s) by brushing or washing (separate procedure)

（For radiological supervision and interpretation, see 74328, 74329, 74330）

⊙ **43261**　　　with biopsy, single or multiple

（For radiological supervision and interpretation, see 74328, 74329, 74330）

⊙ **43262**　　　with sphincterotomy/papillotomy

（For radiological supervision and interpretation, see 74328, 74329, 74330）

⊙ **43263**　　　with pressure measurement of sphincter of Oddi (pancreatic duct or common bile duct)

（For radiological supervision and interpretation, see 74328, 74329, 74330）

⊙ **43264**　　　with endoscopic retrograde removal of calculus/calculi from biliary and/or pancreatic ducts

（When done with sphincterotomy, also use 43262）

（For radiological supervision and interpretation, see 74328, 74329, 74330）

⊙ **43265**　　　with endoscopic retrograde destruction, lithotripsy of calculus/calculi, any method

（When done with sphincterotomy, also use 43262）

（For radiological supervision and interpretation, see 74328, 74329, 74330）

⊙ **43267**　　　with endoscopic retrograde insertion of nasobiliary or nasopancreatic drainage tube

（When done with sphincterotomy, also use 43262）

（For radiological supervision and interpretation, see 74328, 74329, 74330）

⊙ **43268**　　　with endoscopic retrograde insertion of tube or stent into bile or pancreatic duct

（When done with sphincterotomy, also use 43262）

（For radiological supervision and interpretation, see 74328, 74329, 74330）

⊙ **43269**　　　with endoscopic retrograde removal of foreign body and/or change of tube or stent

（When done with sphincterotomy, also use 43262）

（For radiological supervision and interpretation, see 74328, 74329, 74330）

⊙ **43271**　　　with endoscopic retrograde balloon dilation of ampulla, biliary and/or pancreatic duct(s)

（When done with sphincterotomy, also use 43262）

（For radiological supervision and interpretation, see 74328, 74329, 74330）

⊙ **43272**　　　with ablation of tumor(s), polyp(s), or other lesion(s) not amenable to removal by hot biopsy forceps, bipolar cautery or snare technique

（For radiological supervision and interpretation, see 74328, 74329, 74330）

Laparoscopy

Surgical laparoscopy always includes diagnostic laparoscopy. To report a diagnostic laparoscopy (peritoneoscopy) (separate procedure), use 49320.

43280　　Laparoscopy, surgical, esophagogastric fundoplasty (eg, Nissen, Toupet procedures)

（For open approach, use 43324）

43289　　Unlisted laparoscopy procedure, esophagus

Repair

43300　　Esophagoplasty (plastic repair or reconstruction), cervical approach; without repair of tracheoesophageal fistula

43305　　　with repair of tracheoesophageal fistula

43310　　Esophagoplasty (plastic repair or reconstruction), thoracic approach; without repair of tracheoesophageal fistula

43312　　　with repair of tracheoesophageal fistula

43313　　Esophagoplasty for congenital defect (plastic repair or reconstruction), thoracic approach; without repair of congenital tracheoesophageal fistula

43314　　　with repair of congenital tracheoesophageal fistula

（Do not report modifier 63 in conjunction with 43313, 43314）

43320　　Esophagogastrostomy (cardioplasty), with or without vagotomy and pyloroplasty, transabdominal or transthoracic approach

43324　　Esophagogastric fundoplasty (eg, Nissen, Belsey IV, Hill procedures)

（For laparoscopic procedure, use 43280）

43325　　Esophagogastric fundoplasty; with fundic patch (Thal-Nissen procedure)

（For cricopharyngeal myotomy, use 43030）

43326　　　with gastroplasty (eg, Collis)

▲=Revised Code　　●=New Code　　▶ ◀=New or Revised Text

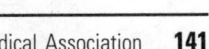

Surgery: Digestive System

43330 Esophagomyotomy (Heller type); abdominal approach

43331 thoracic approach

(For thoracoscopic esophagomyotomy, use 32665)

43340 Esophagojejunostomy (without total gastrectomy); abdominal approach

43341 thoracic approach

43350 Esophagostomy, fistulization of esophagus, external; abdominal approach

43351 thoracic approach

43352 cervical approach

43360 Gastrointestinal reconstruction for previous esophagectomy, for obstructing esophageal lesion or fistula, or for previous esophageal exclusion; with stomach, with or without pyloroplasty

43361 with colon interposition or small intestine reconstruction, including intestine mobilization, preparation, and anastomosis(es)

43400 Ligation, direct, esophageal varices

43401 Transection of esophagus with repair, for esophageal varices

43405 Ligation or stapling at gastroesophageal junction for pre-existing esophageal perforation

43410 Suture of esophageal wound or injury; cervical approach

43415 transthoracic or transabdominal approach

43420 Closure of esophagostomy or fistula; cervical approach

43425 transthoracic or transabdominal approach

(For repair of esophageal hiatal hernia, see 39520 et seq)

Manipulation

(For associated esophagogram, use 74220)

43450 Dilation of esophagus, by unguided sound or bougie, single or multiple passes

⊙ **43453** Dilation of esophagus, over guide wire

(For dilation with direct visualization, use 43220)

(For dilation of esophagus, by balloon or dilator, see 43220, 43458, and 74360)

⊙ **43456** Dilation of esophagus, by balloon or dilator, retrograde

⊙ **43458** Dilation of esophagus with balloon (30 mm diameter or larger) for achalasia

(For dilation with balloon less than 30 mm diameter, use 43220)

(For radiological supervision and interpretation, use 74360)

43460 Esophagogastric tamponade, with balloon (Sengstaaken type)

(For removal of esophageal foreign body by balloon catheter, see 43215, 43247, 74235)

Other Procedures

43496 Free jejunum transfer with microvascular anastomosis

(Do not report code 69990 in addition to code 43496)

43499 Unlisted procedure, esophagus

Stomach

Incision

43500 Gastrotomy; with exploration or foreign body removal

43501 with suture repair of bleeding ulcer

43502 with suture repair of pre-existing esophagogastric laceration (eg, Mallory-Weiss)

43510 with esophageal dilation and insertion of permanent intraluminal tube (eg, Celestin or Mousseaux-Barbin)

43520 Pyloromyotomy, cutting of pyloric muscle (Fredet-Ramstedt type operation)

(Do not report modifier 63 in conjunction with 43520)

Excision

43600 Biopsy of stomach; by capsule, tube, peroral (one or more specimens)

43605 by laparotomy

43610 Excision, local; ulcer or benign tumor of stomach

43611 malignant tumor of stomach

43620 Gastrectomy, total; with esophagoenterostomy

43621 with Roux-en-Y reconstruction

43622 with formation of intestinal pouch, any type

43631 Gastrectomy, partial, distal; with gastroduodenostomy

43632 with gastrojejunostomy

43633 with Roux-en-Y reconstruction

43634 with formation of intestinal pouch

✛ **43635** Vagotomy when performed with partial distal gastrectomy (List separately in addition to code(s) for primary procedure)

(Use 43635 in conjunction with 43631, 43632, 43633, 43634)

43638 Gastrectomy, partial, proximal, thoracic or abdominal approach including esophagogastrostomy, with vagotomy;

43639 with pyloroplasty or pyloromyotomy

(For regional thoracic lymphadenectomy, use 38746)

(For regional abdominal lymphadenectomy, use 38747)

Surgery: Digestive System

43640   Vagotomy including pyloroplasty, with or without gastrostomy; truncal or selective

(For pyloroplasty, use 43800)

(For vagotomy, see 64752-64760)

43641   parietal cell (highly selective)

(For upper gastrointestinal endoscopy, see 43234-43259)

Laparoscopy

Surgical laparoscopy always includes diagnostic laparoscopy. To report a diagnostic laparoscopy (peritoneoscopy) (separate procedure), use 49320.

(For upper gastrointestinal endoscopy including esophagus, stomach, and either the duodenum and/or jejunum, see 43235-43259)

● **43644**   Laparoscopy, surgical, gastric restrictive procedure; with gastric bypass and Roux-en-Y gastroenterostomy (roux limb 150 cm or less)

►(Do not report 43644 in conjunction with 43846, 49320)◄

►(Esophagogastroduodenoscopy (EGD) performed for a separate condition should be reported with modifier 59)◄

● **43645**   with gastric bypass and small intestine reconstruction to limit absorption

►(Do not report 43645 in conjunction with 49320, 43847)◄

43651   Laparoscopy, surgical; transection of vagus nerves, truncal

43652   transection of vagus nerves, selective or highly selective

43653   gastrostomy, without construction of gastric tube (eg, Stamm procedure) (separate procedure)

43659   Unlisted laparoscopy procedure, stomach

Introduction

43750   Percutaneous placement of gastrostomy tube

(For radiological supervision and interpretation, use 74350)

43752   Naso- or oro-gastric tube placement, requiring physician's skill and fluoroscopic guidance (includes fluoroscopy, image documentation and report)

(For enteric tube placement, see 44500, 74340)

(Do not report 43752 in conjunction with critical care codes 99291-99292, neonatal critical care codes 99295-99296, pediatric critical care codes 99293-99294 or low birth weight intensive care service codes 99298-99299)

43760   Change of gastrostomy tube

(For endoscopic placement of gastrostomy tube, use 43246)

(For radiological supervision and interpretation, use 75984)

43761   Repositioning of the gastric feeding tube, any method, through the duodenum for enteric nutrition

(If imaging guidance is performed, use 75984)

Other Procedures

43800   Pyloroplasty

(For pyloroplasty and vagotomy, use 43640)

43810   Gastroduodenostomy

43820   Gastrojejunostomy; without vagotomy

43825   with vagotomy, any type

43830   Gastrostomy, open; without construction of gastric tube (eg, Stamm procedure) (separate procedure)

43831   neonatal, for feeding

(For change of gastrostomy tube, use 43760)

(Do not report modifier 63 in conjunction with 43831)

43832   with construction of gastric tube (eg, Janeway procedure)

(For percutaneous endoscopic gastrostomy, use 43246)

43840   Gastrorrhaphy, suture of perforated duodenal or gastric ulcer, wound, or injury

43842   Gastric restrictive procedure, without gastric bypass, for morbid obesity; vertical-banded gastroplasty

43843   other than vertical-banded gastroplasty

● **43845**   Gastric restrictive procedure with partial gastrectomy, pylorus-preserving duodenoileostomy and ileoileostomy (50 to 100 cm common channel) to limit absorption (biliopancreatic diversion with duodenal switch)

►(Do not report 43845 in conjunction with 43633, 43847, 44130, 49000)◄

▲ **43846**   Gastric restrictive procedure, with gastric bypass for morbid obesity; with short limb (150 cm or less) Roux-en-Y gastroenterostomy

►(For greater than 150 cm, use 43847)◄

►(For laparoscopic procedure, use 43644)◄

43847   with small intestine reconstruction to limit absorption

43848   Revision of gastric restrictive procedure for morbid obesity (separate procedure)

43850   Revision of gastroduodenal anastomosis (gastroduodenostomy) with reconstruction; without vagotomy

43855   with vagotomy

▲=Revised Code   ●=New Code   ► ◄=New or Revised Text

43860   Revision of gastrojejunal anastomosis (gastrojejunostomy) with reconstruction, with or without partial gastrectomy or intestine resection; without vagotomy

43865   with vagotomy

43870   Closure of gastrostomy, surgical

43880   Closure of gastrocolic fistula

43999   Unlisted procedure, stomach

Intestines (Except Rectum)

Incision

44005   Enterolysis (freeing of intestinal adhesion) (separate procedure)

   (Do not report 44005 in addition to 45136)

   (For laparoscopic approach, use 44200)

44010   Duodenotomy, for exploration, biopsy(s), or foreign body removal

+ **44015**   Tube or needle catheter jejunostomy for enteral alimentation, intraoperative, any method (List separately in addition to primary procedure)

44020   Enterotomy, small intestine, other than duodenum; for exploration, biopsy(s), or foreign body removal

44021   for decompression (eg, Baker tube)

44025   Colotomy, for exploration, biopsy(s), or foreign body removal

   (For exteriorization of intestine (Mikulicz resection with crushing of spur), see 44602-44605)

44050   Reduction of volvulus, intussusception, internal hernia, by laparotomy

44055   Correction of malrotation by lysis of duodenal bands and/or reduction of midgut volvulus (eg, Ladd procedure)

   (Do not report modifier 63 in conjunction with 44055)

Excision

▶Intestinal allotransplantation involves three distinct components of physician work:◀

▶1) *Cadaver donor enterectomy*, which includes harvesting the intestine graft and cold preservation of the graft (perfusing with cold preservation solution and cold maintenance) (use 44132). *Living donor enterectomy*, which includes harvesting the intestine graft, cold preservation of the graft (perfusing with cold preservation solution and cold maintenance), and care of the donor (use 44133).◀

▶2) *Backbench work*:◀

▶Standard preparation of an intestine allograft prior to transplantation includes mobilization and fashioning of the superior mesenteric artery and vein (see 44715).◀

▶Additional reconstruction of an intestine allograft prior to transplantation may include venous and/or arterial anastomosis(es) (see 44720-44721).◀

▶3) *Recipient intestinal allotransplantation with or without recipient enterectomy*, which includes transplantation of allograft and care of the recipient (see 44135, 44136).◀

44100   Biopsy of intestine by capsule, tube, peroral (one or more specimens)

44110   Excision of one or more lesions of small or large intestine not requiring anastomosis, exteriorization, or fistulization; single enterotomy

44111   multiple enterotomies

44120   Enterectomy, resection of small intestine; single resection and anastomosis

   (Do not report 44120 in addition to 45136)

+ **44121**   each additional resection and anastomosis (List separately in addition to code for primary procedure)

   (Use 44121 in conjunction with 44120)

44125   with enterostomy

44126   Enterectomy, resection of small intestine for congenital atresia, single resection and anastomosis of proximal segment of intestine; without tapering

44127   with tapering

+ **44128**   each additional resection and anastomosis (List separately in addition to code for primary procedure)

   (Use 44128 in conjunction with 44126, 44127)

   (Do not report modifier 63 in conjunction with 44126, 44127, 44128)

44130   Enteroenterostomy, anastomosis of intestine, with or without cutaneous enterostomy (separate procedure)

▲ **44132**   Donor enterectomy (including cold preservation), open; from cadaver donor

44133   partial, from living donor

   ▶(For backbench intestinal graft preparation or reconstruction, see 44715, 44720, 44721)◀

44135   Intestinal allotransplantation; from cadaver donor

44136   from living donor

● **44137**   Removal of transplanted intestinal allograft, complete

   ▶(For partial removal of transplant allograft, see 44120, 44121, 44140)◀

+ **44139**   Mobilization (take-down) of splenic flexure performed in conjunction with partial colectomy (List separately in addition to primary procedure)

   (Use 44139 in conjunction with 44140-44147)

44140   Colectomy, partial; with anastomosis

   (For laparoscopic procedure, use 44204)

44141   with skin level cecostomy or colostomy

44143	with end colostomy and closure of distal segment (Hartmann type procedure)
	(For laparoscopic procedure, use 44206)
44144	with resection, with colostomy or ileostomy and creation of mucofistula
44145	with coloproctostomy (low pelvic anastomosis)
	(For laparoscopic procedure, use 44207)
44146	with coloproctostomy (low pelvic anastomosis), with colostomy
	(For laparoscopic procedure, use 44208)
44147	abdominal and transanal approach
44150	Colectomy, total, abdominal, without proctectomy; with ileostomy or ileoproctostomy
	(For laparoscopic procedure, use 44210)
44151	with continent ileostomy
44152	with rectal mucosectomy, ileoanal anastomosis, with or without loop ileostomy
	(For laparoscopic procedure, use 44211)
44153	with rectal mucosectomy, ileoanal anastomosis, creation of ileal reservoir (S or J), with or without loop ileostomy
	(For laparoscopic procedure, use 44211)
44155	Colectomy, total, abdominal, with proctectomy; with ileostomy
	(For laparoscopic procedure, use 44212)
44156	with continent ileostomy
44160	Colectomy, partial, with removal of terminal ileum with ileocolostomy
	(For laparoscopic procedure, use 44205)

Laparoscopy

Surgical laparoscopy always includes diagnostic laparoscopy. To report a diagnostic laparoscopy (peritoneoscopy) (separate procedure), use 49320.

44200	Laparoscopy, surgical; enterolysis (freeing of intestinal adhesion) (separate procedure)
	(For laparoscopy with salpingolysis, ovariolysis, use 58660)
44201	jejunostomy (eg, for decompression or feeding)
44202	enterectomy, resection of small intestine, single resection and anastomosis
+ 44203	each additional small intestine resection and anastomosis (List separately in addition to code for primary procedure)
	(Use 44203 in conjunction with 44202)
	(For open procedure, see 44120, 44121)
44204	colectomy, partial, with anastomosis

	(For open procedure, use 44140)
44205	colectomy, partial, with removal of terminal ileum with ileocolostomy
	(For open procedure, use 44160)
44206	colectomy, partial, with end colostomy and closure of distal segment (Hartmann type procedure)
	(For open procedure, use 44143)
44207	colectomy, partial, with anastomosis, with coloproctostomy (low pelvic anastomosis)
	(For open procedure, use 44145)
44208	colectomy, partial, with anastomosis, with coloproctostomy (low pelvic anastomosis) with colostomy
	(For open procedure, use 44146)
	(44209 has been deleted. To report, use 44238)
44210	colectomy, total, abdominal, without proctectomy, with ileostomy or ileoproctostomy
	(For open procedure, use 44150)
44211	colectomy, total, abdominal, with proctectomy, with ileoanal anastomosis, creation of ileal reservoir (S or J), with loop ileostomy, with or without rectal mucosectomy
	(For open procedure, see 44152, 44153)
44212	colectomy, total, abdominal, with proctectomy, with ileostomy
	(For open procedure, use 44155)
44238	Unlisted laparoscopy procedure, intestine (except rectum)
44239	Unlisted laparoscopy procedure, rectum

Enterostomy—External Fistulization of Intestines

44300	Enterostomy or cecostomy, tube (eg, for decompression or feeding) (separate procedure)
44310	Ileostomy or jejunostomy, non-tube (separate procedure)
	(Do not report 44310 in addition to 45136)
44312	Revision of ileostomy; simple (release of superficial scar) (separate procedure)
44314	complicated (reconstruction in-depth) (separate procedure)
44316	Continent ileostomy (Kock procedure) (separate procedure)
	(For fiberoptic evaluation, use 44385)
44320	Colostomy or skin level cecostomy; (separate procedure)
44322	with multiple biopsies (eg, for congenital megacolon) (separate procedure)

Surgery: Digestive System

44340 Revision of colostomy; simple (release of superficial scar) (separate procedure)

44345 complicated (reconstruction in-depth) (separate procedure)

44346 with repair of paracolostomy hernia (separate procedure)

Endoscopy, Small Intestine and Stomal

Surgical endoscopy always includes diagnostic endoscopy.

(For upper gastrointestinal endoscopy, see 43234-43258)

⊙ **44360** Small intestinal endoscopy, enteroscopy beyond second portion of duodenum, not including ileum; diagnostic, with or without collection of specimen(s) by brushing or washing (separate procedure)

⊙ **44361** with biopsy, single or multiple

⊙ **44363** with removal of foreign body

⊙ **44364** with removal of tumor(s), polyp(s), or other lesion(s) by snare technique

⊙ **44365** with removal of tumor(s), polyp(s), or other lesion(s) by hot biopsy forceps or bipolar cautery

⊙ **44366** with control of bleeding (eg, injection, bipolar cautery, unipolar cautery, laser, heater probe, stapler, plasma coagulator)

⊙ **44369** with ablation of tumor(s), polyp(s), or other lesion(s) not amenable to removal by hot biopsy forceps, bipolar cautery or snare technique

⊙ **44370** with transendoscopic stent placement (includes predilation)

⊙ **44372** with placement of percutaneous jejunostomy tube

⊙ **44373** with conversion of percutaneous gastrostomy tube to percutaneous jejunostomy tube

(For fiberoptic jejunostomy through stoma, use 43235)

⊙ **44376** Small intestinal endoscopy, enteroscopy beyond second portion of duodenum, including ileum; diagnostic, with or without collection of specimen(s) by brushing or washing (separate procedure)

⊙ **44377** with biopsy, single or multiple

⊙ **44378** with control of bleeding (eg, injection, bipolar cautery, unipolar cautery, laser, heater probe, stapler, plasma coagulator)

⊙ **44379** with transendoscopic stent placement (includes predilation)

⊙ **44380** Ileoscopy, through stoma; diagnostic, with or without collection of specimen(s) by brushing or washing (separate procedure)

⊙ **44382** with biopsy, single or multiple

⊙ **44383** with transendoscopic stent placement (includes predilation)

⊙ **44385** Endoscopic evaluation of small intestinal (abdominal or pelvic) pouch; diagnostic, with or without collection of specimen(s) by brushing or washing (separate procedure)

⊙ **44386** with biopsy, single or multiple

⊙ **44388** Colonoscopy through stoma; diagnostic, with or without collection of specimen(s) by brushing or washing (separate procedure)

⊙ **44389** with biopsy, single or multiple

⊙ **44390** with removal of foreign body

⊙ **44391** with control of bleeding (eg, injection, bipolar cautery, unipolar cautery, laser, heater probe, stapler, plasma coagulator)

⊙ **44392** with removal of tumor(s), polyp(s), or other lesion(s) by hot biopsy forceps or bipolar cautery

⊙ **44393** with ablation of tumor(s), polyp(s), or other lesion(s) not amenable to removal by hot biopsy forceps, bipolar cautery or snare technique

⊙ **44394** with removal of tumor(s), polyp(s), or other lesion(s) by snare technique

(For colonoscopy per rectum, see 45330-45385)

⊙ **44397** with transendoscopic stent placement (includes predilation)

Introduction

⊙⊘ **44500** Introduction of long gastrointestinal tube (eg, Miller-Abbott) (separate procedure)

(For radiological supervision and interpretation, use 74340)

(For naso- or oro-gastric tube placement, use 43752)

Repair

44602 Suture of small intestine (enterorrhaphy) for perforated ulcer, diverticulum, wound, injury or rupture; single perforation

44603 multiple perforations

44604 Suture of large intestine (colorrhaphy) for perforated ulcer, diverticulum, wound, injury or rupture (single or multiple perforations); without colostomy

44605 with colostomy

44615 Intestinal stricturoplasty (enterotomy and enterorrhaphy) with or without dilation, for intestinal obstruction

44620 Closure of enterostomy, large or small intestine;

44625 with resection and anastomosis other than colorectal

44626 with resection and colorectal anastomosis (eg, closure of Hartmann type procedure)

44640 Closure of intestinal cutaneous fistula

44650 Closure of enteroenteric or enterocolic fistula

44660   Closure of enterovesical fistula; without intestinal or bladder resection

44661   with intestine and/or bladder resection

(For closure of renocolic fistula, see 50525, 50526)

(For closure of gastrocolic fistula, use 43880)

(For closure of rectovesical fistula, see 45800, 45805)

44680   Intestinal plication (separate procedure)

Other Procedures

44700   Exclusion of small intestine from pelvis by mesh or other prosthesis, or native tissue (eg, bladder or omentum)

(For therapeutic radiation clinical treatment, see **Radiation Oncology** section)

+ 44701 Intraoperative colonic lavage (List separately in addition to code for primary procedure)

(Use 44701 in conjunction with 44140, 44145, 44150, or 44604 as appropriate)

(Do not report 44701 in conjunction with 44300, 44950-44960)

● 44715 Backbench standard preparation of cadaver or living donor intestine allograft prior to transplantation, including mobilization and fashioning of the superior mesenteric artery and vein

● 44720 Backbench reconstruction of cadaver or living donor intestine allograft prior to transplantation; venous anastomosis, each

● 44721   arterial anastomosis, each

44799   Unlisted procedure, intestine

(For unlisted laparoscopic procedure, intestine except rectum, use 44238)

Meckel's Diverticulum and the Mesentery

Excision

44800   Excision of Meckel's diverticulum (diverticulectomy) or omphalomesenteric duct

44820   Excision of lesion of mesentery (separate procedure)

(With intestine resection, see 44120 or 44140 et seq)

Suture

44850   Suture of mesentery (separate procedure)

(For reduction and repair of internal hernia, use 44050)

Other Procedures

44899   Unlisted procedure, Meckel's diverticulum and the mesentery

Appendix

Incision

44900   Incision and drainage of appendiceal abscess; open

⊙ 44901   percutaneous

(For radiological supervision and interpretation, use 75989)

Excision

44950   Appendectomy;

(Incidental appendectomy during intra-abdominal surgery does not usually warrant a separate identification. If necessary to report, add modifier 52)

+ 44955   when done for indicated purpose at time of other major procedure (not as separate procedure) (List separately in addition to code for primary procedure)

44960   for ruptured appendix with abscess or generalized peritonitis

Laparoscopy

Surgical laparoscopy always includes diagnostic laparoscopy. To report a diagnostic laparoscopy (peritoneoscopy) (separate procedure), use 49320.

44970   Laparoscopy, surgical, appendectomy

44979   Unlisted laparoscopy procedure, appendix

Rectum

Incision

45000   Transrectal drainage of pelvic abscess

45005   Incision and drainage of submucosal abscess, rectum

45020   Incision and drainage of deep supralevator, pelvirectal, or retrorectal abscess

(See also 46050, 46060)

Excision

45100   Biopsy of anorectal wall, anal approach (eg, congenital megacolon)

(For endoscopic biopsy, use 45305)

45108   Anorectal myomectomy

45110   Proctectomy; complete, combined abdominoperineal, with colostomy

45111   partial resection of rectum, transabdominal approach

45112   Proctectomy, combined abdominoperineal, pull-through procedure (eg, colo-anal anastomosis)

(For colo-anal anastomosis with colonic reservoir or pouch, use 45119)

Surgery: Digestive System

45113   Proctectomy, partial, with rectal mucosectomy, ileoanal anastomosis, creation of ileal reservoir (S or J), with or without loop ileostomy

45114   Proctectomy, partial, with anastomosis; abdominal and transsacral approach

45116   transsacral approach only (Kraske type)

45119   Proctectomy, combined abdominoperineal pull-through procedure (eg, colo-anal anastomosis), with creation of colonic reservoir (eg, J-pouch), with or without proximal diverting ostomy

45120   Proctectomy, complete (for congenital megacolon), abdominal and perineal approach; with pull-through procedure and anastomosis (eg, Swenson, Duhamel, or Soave type operation)

45121   with subtotal or total colectomy, with multiple biopsies

45123   Proctectomy, partial, without anastomosis, perineal approach

45126   Pelvic exenteration for colorectal malignancy, with proctectomy (with or without colostomy), with removal of bladder and ureteral transplantations, and/or hysterectomy, or cervicectomy, with or without removal of tube(s), with or without removal of ovary(s), or any combination thereof

45130   Excision of rectal procidentia, with anastomosis; perineal approach

45135   abdominal and perineal approach

45136   Excision of ileoanal reservoir with ileostomy

        (Do not report 45136 in addition to 44005, 44120, 44310)

45150   Division of stricture of rectum

45160   Excision of rectal tumor by proctotomy, transsacral or transcoccygeal approach

45170   Excision of rectal tumor, transanal approach

Destruction

45190   Destruction of rectal tumor (eg, electrodessication, electrosurgery, laser ablation, laser resection, cryosurgery) transanal approach

Endoscopy

Definitions

Proctosigmoidoscopy is the examination of the rectum and sigmoid colon.

Sigmoidoscopy is the examination of the entire rectum, sigmoid colon and may include examination of a portion of the descending colon.

Colonoscopy is the examination of the entire colon, from the rectum to the cecum, and may include the examination of the terminal ileum.

For an incomplete colonoscopy, with full preparation for a colonoscopy, use a colonoscopy code with the modifier 52 and provide documentation.

Surgical endoscopy always includes diagnostic endoscopy.

45300   Proctosigmoidoscopy, rigid; diagnostic, with or without collection of specimen(s) by brushing or washing (separate procedure)

⊙ **45303**   with dilation (eg, balloon, guide wire, bougie)

        (For radiological supervision and interpretation, use 74360)

⊙ **45305**   with biopsy, single or multiple

⊙ **45307**   with removal of foreign body

⊙ **45308**   with removal of single tumor, polyp, or other lesion by hot biopsy forceps or bipolar cautery

⊙ **45309**   with removal of single tumor, polyp, or other lesion by snare technique

⊙ **45315**   with removal of multiple tumors, polyps, or other lesions by hot biopsy forceps, bipolar cautery or snare technique

⊙ **45317**   with control of bleeding (eg, injection, bipolar cautery, unipolar cautery, laser, heater probe, stapler, plasma coagulator)

⊙ **45320**   with ablation of tumor(s), polyp(s), or other lesion(s) not amenable to removal by hot biopsy forceps, bipolar cautery or snare technique (eg, laser)

45321   with decompression of volvulus

⊙ **45327**   with transendoscopic stent placement (includes predilation)

45330   Sigmoidoscopy, flexible; diagnostic, with or without collection of specimen(s) by brushing or washing (separate procedure)

45331   with biopsy, single or multiple

⊙ **45332**   with removal of foreign body

⊙ **45333**   with removal of tumor(s), polyp(s), or other lesion(s) by hot biopsy forceps or bipolar cautery

⊙ **45334**   with control of bleeding (eg, injection, bipolar cautery, unipolar cautery, laser, heater probe, stapler, plasma coagulator)

45335   with directed submucosal injection(s), any substance

⊙ **45337**   with decompression of volvulus, any method

⊙ **45338**   with removal of tumor(s), polyp(s), or other lesion(s) by snare technique

⊙ **45339**   with ablation of tumor(s), polyp(s), or other lesion(s) not amenable to removal by hot biopsy forceps, bipolar cautery or snare technique

⊙ **45340**   with dilation by balloon, 1 or more strictures

        (Do not report 45340 in conjunction with 45345)

⊙ **45341**   with endoscopic ultrasound examination

⊙ **45342**   with transendoscopic ultrasound guided intramural or transmural fine needle aspiration/biopsy(s)

(Do not report 45341, 45342 in conjunction with 76942)

(Do not report 45341, 45342 in conjunction with 76975)

(For interpretation of specimen, see 88172-88173)

(For transrectal ultrasound utilizing rigid probe device, use 76872)

⊙ **45345**   with transendoscopic stent placement (includes predilation)

⊙ **45355**   Colonoscopy, rigid or flexible, transabdominal via colotomy, single or multiple

(For fiberoptic colonoscopy beyond 25cm to splenic flexure, see 45330-45345)

⊙ **45378**   Colonoscopy, flexible, proximal to splenic flexure; diagnostic, with or without collection of specimen(s) by brushing or washing, with or without colon decompression (separate procedure)

⊙ **45379**   with removal of foreign body

⊙ **45380**   with biopsy, single or multiple

⊙ **45381**   with directed submucosal injection(s), any substance

⊙ **45382**   with control of bleeding (eg, injection, bipolar cautery, unipolar cautery, laser, heater probe, stapler, plasma coagulator)

⊙ **45383**   with ablation of tumor(s), polyp(s), or other lesion(s) not amenable to removal by hot biopsy forceps, bipolar cautery or snare technique

⊙ **45384**   with removal of tumor(s), polyp(s), or other lesion(s) by hot biopsy forceps or bipolar cautery

⊙ **45385**   with removal of tumor(s), polyp(s), or other lesion(s) by snare technique

(For small intestine and stomal endoscopy, see 44360-44393)

⊙ **45386**   with dilation by balloon, 1 or more strictures

(Do not report 45386 in conjunction with 45387)

⊙ **45387**   with transendoscopic stent placement (includes predilation)

⊙● **45391**   with endoscopic ultrasound examination

▶(Do not report 45391 in conjunction with 45330, 45341, 45342, 45378, 76872)◀

⊙● **45392**   with transendoscopic ultrasound guided intramural or transmural fine needle aspiration/biopsy(s)

▶(Do not report 45392 in conjunction with 45330, 45341, 45342, 45378, 76872)◀

Repair

45500   Proctoplasty; for stenosis

45505   for prolapse of mucous membrane

45520   Perirectal injection of sclerosing solution for prolapse

45540   Proctopexy for prolapse; abdominal approach

45541   perineal approach

45550   Proctopexy combined with sigmoid resection, abdominal approach

45560   Repair of rectocele (separate procedure)

(For repair of rectocele with posterior colporrhaphy, use 57250)

45562   Exploration, repair, and presacral drainage for rectal injury;

45563   with colostomy

45800   Closure of rectovesical fistula;

45805   with colostomy

45820   Closure of rectourethral fistula;

45825   with colostomy

(For rectovaginal fistula closure, see 57300-57308)

Manipulation

45900   Reduction of procidentia (separate procedure) under anesthesia

45905   Dilation of anal sphincter (separate procedure) under anesthesia other than local

45910   Dilation of rectal stricture (separate procedure) under anesthesia other than local

45915   Removal of fecal impaction or foreign body (separate procedure) under anesthesia

Other Procedures

45999   Unlisted procedure, rectum

(For unlisted laparoscopic procedure, rectum, use 44239)

Anus

Incision

(For subcutaneous fistulotomy, use 46270)

46020   Placement of seton

(Do not report 46020 in addition to 46060, 46280, 46600)

46030   Removal of anal seton, other marker

46040   Incision and drainage of ischiorectal and/or perirectal abscess (separate procedure)

46045   Incision and drainage of intramural, intramuscular, or submucosal abscess, transanal, under anesthesia

46050   Incision and drainage, perianal abscess, superficial

(See also 45020, 46060)

▲=Revised Code   ●=New Code   ►◄=New or Revised Text

46060 Incision and drainage of ischiorectal or intramural abscess, with fistulectomy or fistulotomy, submuscular, with or without placement of seton

(Do not report 46060 in addition to 46020)

(See also 45020)

46070 Incision, anal septum (infant)

(For anoplasty, see 46700-46705)

(Do not report modifier 63 in conjunction with 46070)

46080 Sphincterotomy, anal, division of sphincter (separate procedure)

46083 Incision of thrombosed hemorrhoid, external

Excision

46200 Fissurectomy, with or without sphincterotomy

46210 Cryptectomy; single

46211   multiple (separate procedure)

46220 Papillectomy or excision of single tag, anus (separate procedure)

46221 Hemorrhoidectomy, by simple ligature (eg, rubber band)

46230 Excision of external hemorrhoid tags and/or multiple papillae

46250 Hemorrhoidectomy, external, complete

46255 Hemorrhoidectomy, internal and external, simple;

46257   with fissurectomy

46258   with fistulectomy, with or without fissurectomy

46260 Hemorrhoidectomy, internal and external, complex or extensive;

46261   with fissurectomy

46262   with fistulectomy, with or without fissurectomy

▶(For injection of hemorrhoids, use 46500; for destruction, see 46934-46936; for ligation, see 46945, 46946; for hemorrhoidopexy, use 46947)◀

46270 Surgical treatment of anal fistula (fistulectomy/fistulotomy); subcutaneous

46275   submuscular

46280   complex or multiple, with or without placement of seton

(Do not report 46280 in addition to 46020)

46285   second stage

46288 Closure of anal fistula with rectal advancement flap

46320 Enucleation or excision of external thrombotic hemorrhoid

Introduction

46500 Injection of sclerosing solution, hemorrhoids

▶(For excision of hemorrhoids, see 46250-46262; for destruction, see 46934-46936; for ligation, see 46945, 46946; for hemorrhoidopexy, use 46947)◀

Endoscopy

Surgical endoscopy always includes diagnostic endoscopy.

46600 Anoscopy; diagnostic, with or without collection of specimen(s) by brushing or washing (separate procedure)

(Do not report 46600 in addition to 46020)

46604   with dilation (eg, balloon, guide wire, bougie)

46606   with biopsy, single or multiple

46608   with removal of foreign body

46610   with removal of single tumor, polyp, or other lesion by hot biopsy forceps or bipolar cautery

46611   with removal of single tumor, polyp, or other lesion by snare technique

46612   with removal of multiple tumors, polyps, or other lesions by hot biopsy forceps, bipolar cautery or snare technique

46614   with control of bleeding (eg, injection, bipolar cautery, unipolar cautery, laser, heater probe, stapler, plasma coagulator)

46615   with ablation of tumor(s), polyp(s), or other lesion(s) not amenable to removal by hot biopsy forceps, bipolar cautery or snare technique

Repair

46700 Anoplasty, plastic operation for stricture; adult

46705   infant

(For simple incision of anal septum, use 46070)

(Do not report modifier 63 in conjunction with 46705)

46706 Repair of anal fistula with fibrin glue

46715 Repair of low imperforate anus; with anoperineal fistula (cut-back procedure)

46716   with transposition of anoperineal or anovestibular fistula

(Do not report modifier 63 in conjunction with 46715, 46716)

46730 Repair of high imperforate anus without fistula; perineal or sacroperineal approach

46735   combined transabdominal and sacroperineal approaches

(Do not report modifier 63 in conjunction with 46730, 46735)

Surgery: Digestive System

46740   Repair of high imperforate anus with rectourethral or rectovaginal fistula; perineal or sacroperineal approach

46742   combined transabdominal and sacroperineal approaches

(Do not report modifier 63 in conjunction with 46740, 46742)

46744   Repair of cloacal anomaly by anorectovaginoplasty and urethroplasty, sacroperineal approach

(Do not report modifier 63 in conjunction with 46744)

46746   Repair of cloacal anomaly by anorectovaginoplasty and urethroplasty, combined abdominal and sacroperineal approach;

46748   with vaginal lengthening by intestinal graft or pedicle flaps

46750   Sphincteroplasty, anal, for incontinence or prolapse; adult

46751   child

46753   Graft (Thiersch operation) for rectal incontinence and/or prolapse

46754   Removal of Thiersch wire or suture, anal canal

46760   Sphincteroplasty, anal, for incontinence, adult; muscle transplant

46761   levator muscle imbrication (Park posterior anal repair)

46762   implantation artificial sphincter

Destruction

46900   Destruction of lesion(s), anus (eg, condyloma, papilloma, molluscum contagiosum, herpetic vesicle), simple; chemical

46910   electrodesiccation

46916   cryosurgery

46917   laser surgery

46922   surgical excision

46924   Destruction of lesion(s), anus (eg, condyloma, papilloma, molluscum contagiosum, herpetic vesicle), extensive (eg, laser surgery, electrosurgery, cryosurgery, chemosurgery)

46934   Destruction of hemorrhoids, any method; internal

46935   external

46936   internal and external

▶(For excision of hemorrhoids, see 46250-46262; for injection, use 46500; for ligation, see 46945, 46946; for hemorrhoidopexy, use 46947)◀

46937   Cryosurgery of rectal tumor; benign

46938   malignant

46940   Curettage or cautery of anal fissure, including dilation of anal sphincter (separate procedure); initial

46942   subsequent

Suture

46945   Ligation of internal hemorrhoids; single procedure

46946   multiple procedures

● **46947**   Hemorrhoidopexy (eg, for prolapsing internal hemorrhoids) by stapling

▶(For excision of hemorrhoids, see 46250-46262; for injection, use 46500; for destruction, see 46934-46936)◀

Other Procedures

46999   Unlisted procedure, anus

Liver

Incision

47000   Biopsy of liver, needle; percutaneous

(If imaging guidance is performed, see 76003, 76360, 76393, 76942)

+ **47001**   when done for indicated purpose at time of other major procedure (List separately in addition to code for primary procedure)

(If imaging guidance is performed, see 76003, 76942)

(For fine needle aspiration in conjunction with 47000, 47001, see 10021, 10022)

(For evaluation of fine needle aspirate in conjunction with 47000, 47001, see 88172, 88173)

47010   Hepatotomy; for open drainage of abscess or cyst, one or two stages

⊙ **47011**   for percutaneous drainage of abscess or cyst, one or two stages

(For radiological supervision and interpretation, use 75989)

47015   Laparotomy, with aspiration and/or injection of hepatic parasitic (eg, amoebic or echinococcal) cyst(s) or abscess(es)

Excision

47100   Biopsy of liver, wedge

47120   Hepatectomy, resection of liver; partial lobectomy

47122   trisegmentectomy

47125   total left lobectomy

47130   total right lobectomy

Surgery: Digestive System

►Liver Transplantation◄

►Liver allotransplantation involves three distinct components of physician work:◄

►1) *Cadaver donor hepatectomy*, which includes harvesting the graft and cold preservation of the graft (perfusing with cold preservation solution and cold maintenance) (use 47133). *Living donor hepatectomy*, which includes harvesting the graft, cold preservation of the graft (perfusing with cold preservation solution and cold maintenance), and care of the donor (see 47140-47142).◄

►2) *Backbench work*:◄

►Standard preparation of the whole liver graft will include one of the following:◄

►Preparation of whole liver graft (including cholecystectomy, if necessary, and dissection and removal of surrounding soft tissues to prepare vena cava, portal vein, hepatic artery, and common bile duct for implantation) (use 47143).◄

►Preparation as described for whole liver graft, plus trisegment split into two partial grafts (use 47144).◄

►Preparation as described for whole liver graft, plus lobe split into two partial grafts (use 47145).◄

►Additional reconstruction of the liver graft may include venous and/or arterial anastomosis(es) (see 47146, 47147).◄

►3) *Recipient liver allotransplantation*, which includes recipient hepatectomy (partial or whole), transplantation of the allograft (partial or whole), and care of the recipient (see 47135, 47136).◄

▲ **47133**   Donor hepatectomy (including cold preservation), from cadaver donor

(47134 has been deleted. To report, use 47140)

47135   Liver allotransplantation; orthotopic, partial or whole, from cadaver or living donor, any age

47136   heterotopic, partial or whole, from cadaver or living donor, any age

▲ **47140**   Donor hepatectomy (including cold preservation), from living donor; left lateral segment only (segments II and III)

47141   total left lobectomy (segments II, III and IV)

47142   total right lobectomy (segments V, VI, VII and VIII)

● **47143**   Backbench standard preparation of cadaver donor whole liver graft prior to allotransplantation, including cholecystectomy, if necessary, and dissection and removal of surrounding soft tissues to prepare the vena cava, portal vein, hepatic artery, and common bile duct for implantation; without trisegment or lobe split

● **47144**   with trisegment split of whole liver graft into two partial liver grafts (ie, left lateral segment (segments II and III) and right trisegment (segments I and IV through VIII))

● **47145**   with lobe split of whole liver graft into two partial liver grafts (ie, left lobe (segments II, III, and IV) and right lobe (segments I and V through VIII))

● **47146**   Backbench reconstruction of cadaver or living donor liver graft prior to allotransplantation; venous anastomosis, each

● **47147**   arterial anastomosis, each

►(Do not report 47143-47147 in conjunction with 47120-47125, 47600, 47610)◄

Repair

47300   Marsupialization of cyst or abscess of liver

47350   Management of liver hemorrhage; simple suture of liver wound or injury

47360   complex suture of liver wound or injury, with or without hepatic artery ligation

47361   exploration of hepatic wound, extensive debridement, coagulation and/or suture, with or without packing of liver

47362   re-exploration of hepatic wound for removal of packing

Laparoscopy

Surgical laparoscopy always includes diagnostic laparoscopy. To report a diagnostic laparoscopy (peritoneoscopy) (separate procedure), use 49320.

47370   Laparoscopy, surgical, ablation of one or more liver tumor(s); radiofrequency

(For imaging guidance, use 76940)

47371   cryosurgical

(For imaging guidance, use 76940)

47379   Unlisted laparoscopic procedure, liver

Other Procedures

47380   Ablation, open, of one or more liver tumor(s); radiofrequency

(For imaging guidance, use 76940)

47381   cryosurgical

(For imaging guidance, use 76940)

47382   Ablation, one or more liver tumor(s), percutaneous, radiofrequency

(For imaging guidance and monitoring, see code 76362, 76394, or 76940)

47399   Unlisted procedure, liver

Biliary Tract

Incision

47400 Hepaticotomy or hepaticostomy with exploration, drainage, or removal of calculus

47420 Choledochotomy or choledochostomy with exploration, drainage, or removal of calculus, with or without cholecystotomy; without transduodenal sphincterotomy or sphincteroplasty

47425   with transduodenal sphincterotomy or sphincteroplasty

47460 Transduodenal sphincterotomy or sphincteroplasty, with or without transduodenal extraction of calculus (separate procedure)

47480 Cholecystotomy or cholecystostomy with exploration, drainage, or removal of calculus (separate procedure)

47490 Percutaneous cholecystostomy

(For radiological supervision and interpretation, use 75989)

Introduction

47500 Injection procedure for percutaneous transhepatic cholangiography

(For radiological supervision and interpretation, use 74320)

47505 Injection procedure for cholangiography through an existing catheter (eg, percutaneous transhepatic or T-tube)

(For radiological supervision and interpretation, use 74305)

47510 Introduction of percutaneous transhepatic catheter for biliary drainage

(For radiological supervision and interpretation, use 75980)

47511 Introduction of percutaneous transhepatic stent for internal and external biliary drainage

(For radiological supervision and interpretation, use 75982)

47525 Change of percutaneous biliary drainage catheter

(For radiological supervision and interpretation, use 75984)

47530 Revision and/or reinsertion of transhepatic tube

(For radiological supervision and interpretation, use 75984)

Endoscopy

Surgical endoscopy always includes diagnostic endoscopy.

+ 47550 Biliary endoscopy, intraoperative (choledochoscopy) (List separately in addition to code for primary procedure)

47552 Biliary endoscopy, percutaneous via T-tube or other tract; diagnostic, with or without collection of specimen(s) by brushing and/or washing (separate procedure)

47553   with biopsy, single or multiple

47554   with removal of calculus/calculi

47555   with dilation of biliary duct stricture(s) without stent

(For ERCP, see 43260-43272, 74363)

(If imaging guidance is performed, see 74363, 75982)

47556   with dilation of biliary duct stricture(s) with stent

(If imaging guidance is performed, see 74363, 75982)

Laparoscopy

Surgical laparoscopy always includes diagnostic laparoscopy. To report a diagnostic laparoscopy (peritoneoscopy) (separate procedure), use 49320.

47560 Laparoscopy, surgical; with guided transhepatic cholangiography, without biopsy

47561   with guided transhepatic cholangiography with biopsy

47562   cholecystectomy

47563   cholecystectomy with cholangiography

47564   cholecystectomy with exploration of common duct

47570   cholecystoenterostomy

47579 Unlisted laparoscopy procedure, biliary tract

Excision

47600 Cholecystectomy;

47605   with cholangiography

(For laparoscopic approach, see 47562-47564)

47610 Cholecystectomy with exploration of common duct;

(For cholecystectomy with exploration of common duct with biliary endoscopy, use 47610 with 47550)

47612   with choledochoenterostomy

47620   with transduodenal sphincterotomy or sphincteroplasty, with or without cholangiography

47630 Biliary duct stone extraction, percutaneous via T-tube tract, basket, or snare (eg, Burhenne technique)

(For radiological supervision and interpretation, use 74327)

Surgery: Digestive System

47700 Exploration for congenital atresia of bile ducts, without repair, with or without liver biopsy, with or without cholangiography

(Do not report modifier 63 in conjunction with 47700)

47701 Portoenterostomy (eg, Kasai procedure)

(Do not report modifier 63 in conjunction with 47701)

47711 Excision of bile duct tumor, with or without primary repair of bile duct; extrahepatic

47712 intrahepatic

(For anastomosis, see 47760-47800)

47715 Excision of choledochal cyst

47716 Anastomosis, choledochal cyst, without excision

Repair

47720 Cholecystoenterostomy; direct

(For laparoscopic approach, use 47570)

47721 with gastroenterostomy

47740 Roux-en-Y

47741 Roux-en-Y with gastroenterostomy

47760 Anastomosis, of extrahepatic biliary ducts and gastrointestinal tract

47765 Anastomosis, of intrahepatic ducts and gastrointestinal tract

47780 Anastomosis, Roux-en-Y, of extrahepatic biliary ducts and gastrointestinal tract

47785 Anastomosis, Roux-en-Y, of intrahepatic biliary ducts and gastrointestinal tract

47800 Reconstruction, plastic, of extrahepatic biliary ducts with end-to-end anastomosis

47801 Placement of choledochal stent

47802 U-tube hepaticoenterostomy

47900 Suture of extrahepatic biliary duct for pre-existing injury (separate procedure)

Other Procedures

47999 Unlisted procedure, biliary tract

Pancreas

(For peroral pancreatic endoscopic procedures, see 43260-43272)

Incision

48000 Placement of drains, peripancreatic, for acute pancreatitis;

48001 with cholecystostomy, gastrostomy, and jejunostomy

48005 Resection or debridement of pancreas and peripancreatic tissue for acute necrotizing pancreatitis

48020 Removal of pancreatic calculus

Excision

48100 Biopsy of pancreas, open (eg, fine needle aspiration, needle core biopsy, wedge biopsy)

48102 Biopsy of pancreas, percutaneous needle

(For radiological supervision and interpretation, see 76003, 76360, 76393, 76942)

(For fine needle aspiration, use 10022)

(For evaluation of fine needle aspirate, see 88172, 88173)

48120 Excision of lesion of pancreas (eg, cyst, adenoma)

48140 Pancreatectomy, distal subtotal, with or without splenectomy; without pancreaticojejunostomy

48145 with pancreaticojejunostomy

48146 Pancreatectomy, distal, near-total with preservation of duodenum (Child-type procedure)

48148 Excision of ampulla of Vater

48150 Pancreatectomy, proximal subtotal with total duodenectomy, partial gastrectomy, choledochoenterostomy and gastrojejunostomy (Whipple-type procedure); with pancreatojejunostomy

48152 without pancreatojejunostomy

48153 Pancreatectomy, proximal subtotal with near-total duodenectomy, choledochoenterostomy and duodenojejunostomy (pylorus-sparing, Whipple-type procedure); with pancreatojejunostomy

48154 without pancreatojejunostomy

48155 Pancreatectomy, total

48160 Pancreatectomy, total or subtotal, with autologous transplantation of pancreas or pancreatic islet cells

48180 Pancreaticojejunostomy, side-to-side anastomosis (Puestow-type operation)

Introduction

+ 48400 Injection procedure for intraoperative pancreatography (List separately in addition to code for primary procedure)

(For radiological supervision and interpretation, see 74300-74305)

Repair

48500 Marsupialization of pancreatic cyst

48510 External drainage, pseudocyst of pancreas; open

⊙ **48511** percutaneous

(For radiological supervision and interpretation, use 75989)

48520	Internal anastomosis of pancreatic cyst to gastrointestinal tract; direct
48540	Roux-en-Y
48545	Pancreatorrhaphy for injury
48547	Duodenal exclusion with gastrojejunostomy for pancreatic injury

Pancreas Transplantation

▶Pancreas allotransplantation involves three distinct components of physician work:◀

▶1) *Cadaver donor pancreatectomy*, which includes harvesting the pancreas graft, with or without duodenal segment, and cold preservation of the graft (perfusing with cold preservation solution and cold maintenance) (use 48550).◀

▶2) *Backbench work*:◀

▶Standard preparation of a cadaver donor pancreas allograft prior to transplantation includes dissection of the allograft from surrounding soft tissues, splenectomy, duodenotomy, ligation of bile duct, ligation of mesenteric vessels, and Y-graft arterial anastomoses from the iliac artery to the superior mesenteric artery and to the splenic artery (use 48551).◀

▶Additional reconstruction of a cadaver donor pancreas allograft prior to transplantation may include venous anastomosis(es) (use 48552).◀

▶3) *Recipient pancreas allotransplantation*, which includes transplantation of allograft, and care of the recipient (use 48554).◀

▲ 48550	Donor pancreatectomy (including cold preservation), with or without duodenal segment for transplantation
● 48551	Backbench standard preparation of cadaver donor pancreas allograft prior to transplantation, including dissection of allograft from surrounding soft tissues, splenectomy, duodenotomy, ligation of bile duct, ligation of mesenteric vessels, and Y-graft arterial anastomoses from iliac artery to superior mesenteric artery and to splenic artery
● 48552	Backbench reconstruction of cadaver donor pancreas allograft prior to transplantation, venous anastomosis, each

▶(Do not report 48551 and 48552 in conjunction with 35531, 35563, 35685, 38100-38102, 44010, 44820, 44850, 47460, 47505-47525, 47550-47556, 48100-48120, 48545)◀

| 48554 | Transplantation of pancreatic allograft |
| 48556 | Removal of transplanted pancreatic allograft |

Other Procedures

| 48999 | Unlisted procedure, pancreas |

Abdomen, Peritoneum, and Omentum

Incision

| 49000 | Exploratory laparotomy, exploratory celiotomy with or without biopsy(s) (separate procedure) |

(To report wound exploration due to penetrating trauma without laparotomy, use 20102)

| 49002 | Reopening of recent laparotomy |

(To report re-exploration of hepatic wound for removal of packing, use 47362)

| 49010 | Exploration, retroperitoneal area with or without biopsy(s) (separate procedure) |

(To report wound exploration due to penetrating trauma without laparotomy, use 20102)

| 49020 | Drainage of peritoneal abscess or localized peritonitis, exclusive of appendiceal abscess; open |

(For appendiceal abscess, use 44900)

| ⊙ 49021 | percutaneous |

(For radiological supervision and interpretation, use 75989)

| 49040 | Drainage of subdiaphragmatic or subphrenic abscess; open |
| ⊙ 49041 | percutaneous |

(For radiological supervision and interpretation, use 75989)

| 49060 | Drainage of retroperitoneal abscess; open |
| ⊙ 49061 | percutaneous |

(For laparoscopic drainage, use 49323)

(For radiological supervision and interpretation, use 75989)

49062	Drainage of extraperitoneal lymphocele to peritoneal cavity, open
49080	Peritoneocentesis, abdominal paracentesis, or peritoneal lavage (diagnostic or therapeutic); initial
49081	subsequent

(If imaging guidance is performed, see 76360, 76942)

| 49085 | Removal of peritoneal foreign body from peritoneal cavity |

(For lysis of intestinal adhesions, use 44005)

Surgery: Digestive System

Excision, Destruction

49180 Biopsy, abdominal or retroperitoneal mass, percutaneous needle

(If imaging guidance is performed, see 76003, 76360, 76393, 76942)

(For fine needle aspiration, use 10021 or 10022)

(For evaluation of fine needle aspirate, see 88172, 88173)

49200 Excision or destruction, open, intra-abdominal or retroperitoneal tumors or cysts or endometriomas;

49201 extensive

49215 Excision of presacral or sacrococcygeal tumor

(Do not report modifier 63 in conjunction with 49215)

49220 Staging laparotomy for Hodgkins disease or lymphoma (includes splenectomy, needle or open biopsies of both liver lobes, possibly also removal of abdominal nodes, abdominal node and/or bone marrow biopsies, ovarian repositioning)

49250 Umbilectomy, omphalectomy, excision of umbilicus (separate procedure)

49255 Omentectomy, epiploectomy, resection of omentum (separate procedure)

Laparoscopy

Surgical laparoscopy always includes diagnostic laparoscopy. To report a diagnostic laparoscopy (peritoneoscopy), (separate procedure), use 49320.

For laparoscopic fulguration or excision of lesions of the ovary, pelvic viscera, or peritoneal surface use 58662.

49320 Laparoscopy, abdomen, peritoneum, and omentum, diagnostic, with or without collection of specimen(s) by brushing or washing (separate procedure)

49321 Laparoscopy, surgical; with biopsy (single or multiple)

49322 with aspiration of cavity or cyst (eg, ovarian cyst) (single or multiple)

49323 with drainage of lymphocele to peritoneal cavity

(For percutaneous or open drainage, see 49060, 49061)

49329 Unlisted laparoscopy procedure, abdomen, peritoneum and omentum

Introduction, Revision, and/or Removal

49400 Injection of air or contrast into peritoneal cavity (separate procedure)

(For radiological supervision and interpretation, use 74190)

49419 Insertion of intraperitoneal cannula or catheter, with subcutaneous reservoir, permanent (ie, totally implantable)

(For removal, use 49422)

49420 Insertion of intraperitoneal cannula or catheter for drainage or dialysis; temporary

49421 permanent

49422 Removal of permanent intraperitoneal cannula or catheter

(For removal of a temporary catheter/cannula, use appropriate E/M code)

49423 Exchange of previously placed abscess or cyst drainage catheter under radiological guidance (separate procedure)

(For radiological supervision and interpretation, use 75984)

49424 Contrast injection for assessment of abscess or cyst via previously placed drainage catheter or tube (separate procedure)

(For radiological supervision and interpretation, use 76080)

49425 Insertion of peritoneal-venous shunt

49426 Revision of peritoneal-venous shunt

(For shunt patency test, use 78291)

49427 Injection procedure (eg, contrast media) for evaluation of previously placed peritoneal-venous shunt

(For radiological supervision and interpretation, see 75809, 78291)

49428 Ligation of peritoneal-venous shunt

49429 Removal of peritoneal-venous shunt

Repair

Hernioplasty, Herniorrhaphy, Herniotomy

The hernia repair codes in this section are categorized primarily by the type of hernia (inguinal, femoral, incisional, etc.).

Some types of hernias are further categorized as "initial" or "recurrent" based on whether or not the hernia has required previous repair(s).

Additional variables accounted for by some of the codes include patient age and clinical presentation (reducible vs. incarcerated or strangulated).

With the exception of the incisional hernia repairs (see 49560-49566) the use of mesh or other prostheses is not separately reported.

The excision/repair of strangulated organs or structures such as testicle(s), intestine, ovaries are reported by using the appropriate code for the excision/repair (eg, 44120, 54520, and 58940) in addition to the appropriate code for the repair of the strangulated hernia.

Surgery: Digestive System

(For reduction and repair of intra-abdominal hernia, use 44050)

(For debridement of abdominal wall, see 11042, 11043)

(Codes 49491-49651 are unilateral procedures. To report bilateral procedures, report modifier 50 with the appropriate procedure code)

49491   Repair, initial inguinal hernia, preterm infant (less than 37 weeks gestation at birth), performed from birth up to 50 weeks postconception age, with or without hydrocelectomy; reducible

49492   incarcerated or strangulated

(Do not report modifier 63 in conjunction with 49491, 49492)

(Postconception age equals gestational age at birth plus age of infant in weeks at the time of the hernia repair. Initial inguinal hernia repairs that are performed on preterm infants who are over 50 weeks postconception age and under age 6 months at the time of surgery, should be reported using codes 49495, 49496)

49495   Repair, initial inguinal hernia, full term infant under age 6 months, or preterm infant over 50 weeks postconception age and under age 6 months at the time of surgery, with or without hydrocelectomy; reducible

49496   incarcerated or strangulated

(Do not report modifier 63 in conjunction with 49495, 49496)

(Postconception age equals gestational age at birth plus age in weeks at the time of the hernia repair. Initial inguinal hernia repairs that are performed on preterm infants who are under or up to 50 weeks postconception age but under 6 months of age since birth, should be reported using codes 49491, 49492. Inguinal hernia repairs on infants age 6 months to under 5 years should be reported using codes 49500-49501)

49500   Repair initial inguinal hernia, age 6 months to under 5 years, with or without hydrocelectomy; reducible

49501   incarcerated or strangulated

49505   Repair initial inguinal hernia, age 5 years or over; reducible

49507   incarcerated or strangulated

(For inguinal hernia repair, with simple orchiectomy, see 49505 or 49507 and 54520)

(For inguinal hernia repair, with excision of hydrocele or spermatocele, see 49505 or 49507 and 54840 or 55040)

49520   Repair recurrent inguinal hernia, any age; reducible

49521   incarcerated or strangulated

49525   Repair inguinal hernia, sliding, any age

(For incarcerated or strangulated inguinal hernia repair, see 49496, 49501, 49507, 49521)

49540   Repair lumbar hernia

49550   Repair initial femoral hernia, any age; reducible

49553   incarcerated or strangulated

49555   Repair recurrent femoral hernia; reducible

49557   incarcerated or strangulated

49560   Repair initial incisional or ventral hernia; reducible

49561   incarcerated or strangulated

49565   Repair recurrent incisional or ventral hernia; reducible

49566   incarcerated or strangulated

+ 49568 Implantation of mesh or other prosthesis for incisional or ventral hernia repair (List separately in addition to code for the incisional or ventral hernia repair)

49570   Repair epigastric hernia (eg, preperitoneal fat); reducible (separate procedure)

49572   incarcerated or strangulated

49580   Repair umbilical hernia, under age 5 years; reducible

49582   incarcerated or strangulated

49585   Repair umbilical hernia, age 5 years or over; reducible

49587   incarcerated or strangulated

49590   Repair spigelian hernia

49600   Repair of small omphalocele, with primary closure

(Do not report modifier 63 in conjunction with 49600)

49605   Repair of large omphalocele or gastroschisis; with or without prosthesis

49606   with removal of prosthesis, final reduction and closure, in operating room

(Do not report modifier 63 in conjunction with 49605, 49606)

49610   Repair of omphalocele (Gross type operation); first stage

49611   second stage

(Do not report modifier 63 in conjunction with 49610, 49611)

(For diaphragmatic or hiatal hernia repair, see 39502-39541)

(For surgical repair of omentum, use 49999)

Laparoscopy

Surgical laparoscopy always includes diagnostic laparoscopy. To report a diagnostic laparoscopy (peritoneoscopy) (separate procedure), use 49320.

49650   Laparoscopy, surgical; repair initial inguinal hernia

49651   repair recurrent inguinal hernia

49659   Unlisted laparoscopy procedure, hernioplasty, herniorrhaphy, herniotomy

Surgery: Digestive System

Suture

49900   Suture, secondary, of abdominal wall for evisceration or dehiscence

(For suture of ruptured diaphragm, see 39540, 39541)

(For debridement of abdominal wall, see 11042, 11043)

Other Procedures

49904   Omental flap, extra-abdominal (eg, for reconstruction of sternal and chest wall defects)

(Code 49904 includes harvest and transfer. If a second surgeon harvests the omental flap, then the two surgeons should code 49904 as co-surgeons, using modifier 62)

✛ 49905   Omental flap, intra-abdominal (List separately in addition to code for primary procedure)

(Do not report 49905 in conjunction with 44700)

49906   Free omental flap with microvascular anastomosis

(Do not report code 69990 in addition to 49906)

49999   Unlisted procedure, abdomen, peritoneum and omentum

Surgery: Digestive System

Urinary System

(For provision of chemotherapeutic agents, use 96545 in addition to code for primary procedure)

Kidney

Incision

(For retroperitoneal exploration, abscess, tumor, or cyst, see 49010, 49060, 49200, 49201)

50010   Renal exploration, not necessitating other specific procedures

(For laparoscopic ablation of renal mass lesion(s), use 50542)

50020   Drainage of perirenal or renal abscess; open

⊙ **50021**   percutaneous

(For radiological supervision and interpretation, use 75989)

50040   Nephrostomy, nephrotomy with drainage

50045   Nephrotomy, with exploration

(For renal endoscopy performed in conjunction with this procedure, see 50570-50580)

50060   Nephrolithotomy; removal of calculus

50065   secondary surgical operation for calculus

50070   complicated by congenital kidney abnormality

50075   removal of large staghorn calculus filling renal pelvis and calyces (including anatrophic pyelolithotomy)

50080   Percutaneous nephrostolithotomy or pyelostolithotomy, with or without dilation, endoscopy, lithotripsy, stenting, or basket extraction; up to 2 cm

50081   over 2 cm

(For establishment of nephrostomy without nephrostolithotomy, see 50040, 50395, 52334)

(For fluoroscopic guidance, see 76000, 76001)

50100   Transection or repositioning of aberrant renal vessels (separate procedure)

50120   Pyelotomy; with exploration

(For renal endoscopy performed in conjunction with this procedure, see 50570-50580)

50125   with drainage, pyelostomy

50130   with removal of calculus (pyelolithotomy, pelviolithotomy, including coagulum pyelolithotomy)

50135   complicated (eg, secondary operation, congenital kidney abnormality)

(For supply of anticarcinogenic agents, use 99070 in addition to code for primary procedure)

Excision

(For excision of retroperitoneal tumor or cyst, see 49200, 49201)

(For laparoscopic ablation of renal mass lesion(s), use 50542)

50200   Renal biopsy; percutaneous, by trocar or needle

(For radiological supervision and interpretation, see 76003, 76360, 76393, 76942)

(For fine needle aspiration, use 10022)

(For evaluation of fine needle aspirate, see 88172, 88173)

50205   by surgical exposure of kidney

50220   Nephrectomy, including partial ureterectomy, any open approach including rib resection;

50225   complicated because of previous surgery on same kidney

50230   radical, with regional lymphadenectomy and/or vena caval thrombectomy

(When vena caval resection with reconstruction is necessary, use 37799)

50234   Nephrectomy with total ureterectomy and bladder cuff; through same incision

50236   through separate incision

50240   Nephrectomy, partial

(For laparoscopic partial nephrectomy, use 50543)

50280   Excision or unroofing of cyst(s) of kidney

(For laparoscopic ablation of renal cysts, use 50541)

50290   Excision of perinephric cyst

Renal Transplantation

▶Renal *auto*transplantation includes reimplantation of the autograft as the primary procedure, along with secondary extra-corporeal procedure(s) (eg, partial nephrectomy, nephrolithotomy) reported with modifier 51 (see 50380 and applicable secondary procedure(s)).◀

▶Renal *allo*transplantation involves three distinct components of physician work:◀

▶1) *Cadaver donor nephrectomy, unilateral or bilateral*, which includes harvesting the graft(s) and cold preservation of the graft(s) (perfusing with cold preservation solution and cold maintenance) (use 50300). *Living donor nephrectomy*, which includes harvesting the graft, cold preservation of the graft (perfusing with cold preservation solution and cold maintenance), and care of the donor (see 50320, 50547).◀

▶2) *Backbench work:*◀

▶Standard preparation of a cadaver donor renal allograft prior to transplantation including dissection and removal of perinephric fat, diaphragmatic and retroperitoneal attachments; excision of adrenal gland; and preparation of ureter(s), renal vein(s), and renal artery(s), ligating branches, as necessary (use 50323).◀

▶Standard preparation of a living donor renal allograft (open or laparoscopic) prior to transplantation including dissection and removal of perinephric fat and preparation of ureter(s), renal vein(s), and renal artery(s), ligating branches, as necessary (use 50325).◀

▶Additional reconstruction of a cadaver or living donor renal allograft prior to transplantation may include venous, arterial, and/or ureteral anastomosis(es) necessary for implantation (see 50327-50329).◀

▶3) *Recipient renal allotransplantation*, which includes transplantation of the allograft (with or without recipient nephrectomy) and care of the recipient (see 50360, 50365).◀

(For dialysis, see 90935-90999)

(For laparoscopic donor nephrectomy, use 50547)

(For laparoscopic drainage of lymphocele to peritoneal cavity, use 49323)

▲ **50300** Donor nephrectomy (including cold preservation); from cadaver donor, unilateral or bilateral

▲ **50320** open, from living donor

● **50323** Backbench standard preparation of cadaver donor renal allograft prior to transplantation, including dissection and removal of perinephric fat, diaphragmatic and retroperitoneal attachments, excision of adrenal gland, and preparation of ureter(s), renal vein(s), and renal artery(s), ligating branches, as necessary

▶(Do not report 50323 in conjunction with 60540, 60545)◀

● **50325** Backbench standard preparation of living donor renal allograft (open or laparoscopic) prior to transplantation, including dissection and removal of perinephric fat and preparation of ureter(s), renal vein(s), and renal artery(s), ligating branches, as necessary

● **50327** Backbench reconstruction of cadaver or living donor renal allograft prior to transplantation; venous anastomosis, each

● **50328** arterial anastomosis, each

● **50329** ureteral anastomosis, each

50340 Recipient nephrectomy (separate procedure)

(For bilateral procedure, report 50340 with modifier 50)

▲ **50360** Renal allotransplantation, implantation of graft; without recipient nephrectomy

50365 with recipient nephrectomy

(For bilateral procedure, report 50365 with modifier 50)

50370 Removal of transplanted renal allograft

50380 Renal autotransplantation, reimplantation of kidney

(For ▶renal autotransplantation◀ extra-corporeal ▶(bench)◀ surgery, use autotransplantation as the primary procedure and report secondary procedure▶(s)◀ (eg, partial nephrectomy, nephrolithotomy) ▶with◀ modifier 51)

Introduction

50390 Aspiration and/or injection of renal cyst or pelvis by needle, percutaneous

(For radiological supervision and interpretation, see 74425, 74470, 76003, 76360, 76393, 76942)

(For evaluation of fine needle aspirate, see 88172, 88173)

● **50391** Instillation(s) of therapeutic agent into renal pelvis and/or ureter through established nephrostomy, pyelostomy or ureterostomy tube (eg, anticarcinogenic or antifungal agent)

50392 Introduction of intracatheter or catheter into renal pelvis for drainage and/or injection, percutaneous

(For radiological supervision and interpretation, see 74475, 76360, 76942)

50393 Introduction of ureteral catheter or stent into ureter through renal pelvis for drainage and/or injection, percutaneous

(For radiological supervision and interpretation, see 74480, 76003, 76360, 76942)

50394 Injection procedure for pyelography (as nephrostogram, pyelostogram, antegrade pyeloureterograms) through nephrostomy or pyelostomy tube, or indwelling ureteral catheter

(For radiological supervision and interpretation, use 74425)

50395 Introduction of guide into renal pelvis and/or ureter with dilation to establish nephrostomy tract, percutaneous

(For radiological supervision and interpretation, see 74475, 74480, 74485)

(For nephrostolithotomy, see 50080, 50081)

(For retrograde percutaneous nephrostomy, use 52334)

(For endoscopic surgery, see 50551-50561)

50396 Manometric studies through nephrostomy or pyelostomy tube, or indwelling ureteral catheter

(For radiological supervision and interpretation, see 74425, 74475, 74480)

⊘ =Modifier 51 Exempt   ⊙ =Conscious Sedation   ✚ =Add-on Code

50398 Change of nephrostomy or pyelostomy tube

(For radiological supervision and interpretation, use 75984)

Repair

50400 Pyeloplasty (Foley Y-pyeloplasty), plastic operation on renal pelvis, with or without plastic operation on ureter, nephropexy, nephrostomy, pyelostomy, or ureteral splinting; simple

50405 complicated (congenital kidney abnormality, secondary pyeloplasty, solitary kidney, calycoplasty)

(For laparoscopic approach, use 50544)

50500 Nephrorrhaphy, suture of kidney wound or injury

50520 Closure of nephrocutaneous or pyelocutaneous fistula

50525 Closure of nephrovisceral fistula (eg, renocolic), including visceral repair; abdominal approach

50526 thoracic approach

50540 Symphysiotomy for horseshoe kidney with or without pyeloplasty and/or other plastic procedure, unilateral or bilateral (one operation)

Laparoscopy

Surgical laparoscopy always includes diagnostic laparoscopy. To report a diagnostic laparoscopy (peritoneoscopy) (separate procedure), use 49320.

50541 Laparoscopy, surgical; ablation of renal cysts

50542 ablation of renal mass lesion(s)

(For open procedure, see 50220-50240)

50543 partial nephrectomy

(For open procedure, use 50240)

50544 pyeloplasty

50545 radical nephrectomy (includes removal of Gerota's fascia and surrounding fatty tissue, removal of regional lymph nodes, and adrenalectomy)

(For open procedure, use 50230)

50546 nephrectomy, including partial ureterectomy

▲ **50547** donor nephrectomy (including cold preservation), from living donor

(For open procedure, use 50320)

►(For backbench renal allograft standard preparation prior to transplantation, use 50325)◄

►(For backbench renal allograft reconstruction prior to transplantation, see 50327-50329)◄

50548 nephrectomy with total ureterectomy

(For open procedure, see 50234, 50236)

50549 Unlisted laparoscopy procedure, renal

(For laparoscopic drainage of lymphocele to peritoneal cavity, use 49323)

Endoscopy

(For supplies and materials, use 99070)

50551 Renal endoscopy through established nephrostomy or pyelostomy, with or without irrigation, instillation, or ureteropyelography, exclusive of radiologic service;

50553 with ureteral catheterization, with or without dilation of ureter

50555 with biopsy

50557 with fulguration and/or incision, with or without biopsy

►(50559 has been deleted)◄

50561 with removal of foreign body or calculus

50562 with resection of tumor

(When procedures 50570-50580 provide a significant identifiable service, they may be added to 50045 and 50120)

50570 Renal endoscopy through nephrotomy or pyelotomy, with or without irrigation, instillation, or ureteropyelography, exclusive of radiologic service;

(For nephrotomy, use 50045)

(For pyelotomy, use 50120)

50572 with ureteral catheterization, with or without dilation of ureter

50574 with biopsy

50575 with endopyelotomy (includes cystoscopy, ureteroscopy, dilation of ureter and ureteral pelvic junction, incision of ureteral pelvic junction and insertion of endopyelotomy stent)

50576 with fulguration and/or incision, with or without biopsy

►(50578 has been deleted)◄

50580 with removal of foreign body or calculus

Other Procedures

50590 Lithotripsy, extracorporeal shock wave

Ureter

Incision

50600 Ureterotomy with exploration or drainage (separate procedure)

(For ureteral endoscopy performed in conjunction with this procedure, see 50970-50980)

Surgery: Urinary System

50605   Ureterotomy for insertion of indwelling stent, all types

50610   Ureterolithotomy; upper one-third of ureter

50620   middle one-third of ureter

50630   lower one-third of ureter

(For laparoscopic approach, use 50945)

(For transvesical ureterolithotomy, use 51060)

(For cystotomy with stone basket extraction of ureteral calculus, use 51065)

(For endoscopic extraction or manipulation of ureteral calculus, see 50080, 50081, 50561, 50961, 50980, 52320-52330, 52352, 52353)

Excision

(For ureterocele, see 51535, 52300)

50650   Ureterectomy, with bladder cuff (separate procedure)

50660   Ureterectomy, total, ectopic ureter, combination abdominal, vaginal and/or perineal approach

Introduction

50684   Injection procedure for ureterography or ureteropyelography through ureterostomy or indwelling ureteral catheter

(For radiological supervision and interpretation, use 74425)

50686   Manometric studies through ureterostomy or indwelling ureteral catheter

50688   Change of ureterostomy tube

(If imaging guidance is performed, use 75984)

50690   Injection procedure for visualization of ileal conduit and/or ureteropyelography, exclusive of radiologic service

(For radiological supervision and interpretation, use 74425)

Repair

50700   Ureteroplasty, plastic operation on ureter (eg, stricture)

50715   Ureterolysis, with or without repositioning of ureter for retroperitoneal fibrosis

(For bilateral procedure, report 50715 with modifier 50)

50722   Ureterolysis for ovarian vein syndrome

50725   Ureterolysis for retrocaval ureter, with reanastomosis of upper urinary tract or vena cava

50727   Revision of urinary-cutaneous anastomosis (any type urostomy);

50728   with repair of fascial defect and hernia

50740   Ureteropyelostomy, anastomosis of ureter and renal pelvis

50750   Ureterocalycostomy, anastomosis of ureter to renal calyx

50760   Ureteroureterostomy

50770   Transureteroureterostomy, anastomosis of ureter to contralateral ureter

(Codes 50780-50785 include minor procedures to prevent vesicoureteral reflux)

50780   Ureteroneocystostomy; anastomosis of single ureter to bladder

(For bilateral procedure, report 50780 with modifier 50)

(When combined with cystourethroplasty or vesical neck revision, use 51820)

50782   anastomosis of duplicated ureter to bladder

50783   with extensive ureteral tailoring

50785   with vesico-psoas hitch or bladder flap

(For bilateral procedure, report 50785 with modifier 50)

50800   Ureteroenterostomy, direct anastomosis of ureter to intestine

(For bilateral procedure, report 50800 with modifier 50)

50810   Ureterosigmoidostomy, with creation of sigmoid bladder and establishment of abdominal or perineal colostomy, including intestine anastomosis

50815   Ureterocolon conduit, including intestine anastomosis

(For bilateral procedure, report 50815 with modifier 50)

50820   Ureteroileal conduit (ileal bladder), including intestine anastomosis (Bricker operation)

(For bilateral procedure, report 50820 with modifier 50)

(For combination of 50800-50820 with cystectomy, see 51580-51595)

50825   Continent diversion, including intestine anastomosis using any segment of small and/or large intestine (Kock pouch or Camey enterocystoplasty)

50830   Urinary undiversion (eg, taking down of ureteroileal conduit, ureterosigmoidostomy or ureteroenterostomy with ureteroureterostomy or ureteroneocystostomy)

50840   Replacement of all or part of ureter by intestine segment, including intestine anastomosis

(For bilateral procedure, report 50840 with modifier 50)

50845   Cutaneous appendico-vesicostomy

50860   Ureterostomy, transplantation of ureter to skin

(For bilateral procedure, report 50860 with modifier 50)

50900   Ureterorrhaphy, suture of ureter (separate procedure)

50920   Closure of ureterocutaneous fistula

50930   Closure of ureterovisceral fistula (including visceral repair)

50940   Deligation of ureter

(For ureteroplasty, ureterolysis, see 50700-50860)

Laparoscopy

Surgical laparoscopy always includes diagnostic laparoscopy. To report a diagnostic laparoscopy (peritoneoscopy) (separate procedure), use 49320.

50945 Laparoscopy, surgical; ureterolithotomy

50947 ureteroneocystostomy with cystoscopy and ureteral stent placement

50948 ureteroneocystostomy without cystoscopy and ureteral stent placement

(For open ureteroneocystostomy, see 50780-50785)

50949 Unlisted laparoscopy procedure, ureter

Endoscopy

50951 Ureteral endoscopy through established ureterostomy, with or without irrigation, instillation, or ureteropyelography, exclusive of radiologic service;

50953 with ureteral catheterization, with or without dilation of ureter

50955 with biopsy

50957 with fulguration and/or incision, with or without biopsy

►(50959 has been deleted)◄

50961 with removal of foreign body or calculus

(When procedures 50970-50980 provide a significant identifiable service, they may be added to 50600)

50970 Ureteral endoscopy through ureterotomy, with or without irrigation, instillation, or ureteropyelography, exclusive of radiologic service;

(For ureterotomy, use 50600)

50972 with ureteral catheterization, with or without dilation of ureter

50974 with biopsy

50976 with fulguration and/or incision, with or without biopsy

►(50978 has been deleted)◄

50980 with removal of foreign body or calculus

Bladder

Incision

51000 Aspiration of bladder by needle

51005 Aspiration of bladder; by trocar or intracatheter

51010 with insertion of suprapubic catheter

(If imaging guidance is performed, see 76003, 76360, 76942)

51020 Cystotomy or cystostomy; with fulguration and/or insertion of radioactive material

51030 with cryosurgical destruction of intravesical lesion

51040 Cystostomy, cystotomy with drainage

51045 Cystotomy, with insertion of ureteral catheter or stent (separate procedure)

51050 Cystolithotomy, cystotomy with removal of calculus, without vesical neck resection

51060 Transvesical ureterolithotomy

51065 Cystotomy, with calculus basket extraction and/or ultrasonic or electrohydraulic fragmentation of ureteral calculus

51080 Drainage of perivesical or prevesical space abscess

Excision

51500 Excision of urachal cyst or sinus, with or without umbilical hernia repair

51520 Cystotomy; for simple excision of vesical neck (separate procedure)

51525 for excision of bladder diverticulum, single or multiple (separate procedure)

51530 for excision of bladder tumor

(For transurethral resection, see 52234-52240, 52305)

51535 Cystotomy for excision, incision, or repair of ureterocele

(For bilateral procedure, report 51535 with modifier 50)

(For transurethral excision, use 52300)

51550 Cystectomy, partial; simple

51555 complicated (eg, postradiation, previous surgery, difficult location)

51565 Cystectomy, partial, with reimplantation of ureter(s) into bladder (ureteroneocystostomy)

51570 Cystectomy, complete; (separate procedure)

51575 with bilateral pelvic lymphadenectomy, including external iliac, hypogastric, and obturator nodes

51580 Cystectomy, complete, with ureterosigmoidostomy or ureterocutaneous transplantations;

51585 with bilateral pelvic lymphadenectomy, including external iliac, hypogastric, and obturator nodes

51590 Cystectomy, complete, with ureteroileal conduit or sigmoid bladder, including intestine anastomosis;

51595 with bilateral pelvic lymphadenectomy, including external iliac, hypogastric, and obturator nodes

51596 Cystectomy, complete, with continent diversion, any open technique, using any segment of small and/or large intestine to construct neobladder

Surgery: Urinary System

51597   Pelvic exenteration, complete, for vesical, prostatic or urethral malignancy, with removal of bladder and ureteral transplantations, with or without hysterectomy and/or abdominoperineal resection of rectum and colon and colostomy, or any combination thereof

(For pelvic exenteration for gynecologic malignancy, use 58240)

Introduction

51600   Injection procedure for cystography or voiding urethrocystography

(For radiological supervision and interpretation, see 74430, 74455)

51605   Injection procedure and placement of chain for contrast and/or chain urethrocystography

(For radiological supervision and interpretation, use 74430)

51610   Injection procedure for retrograde urethrocystography

(For radiological supervision and interpretation, use 74450)

51700   Bladder irrigation, simple, lavage and/or instillation

(Codes 51701-51702 are reported only when performed independently. Do not report 51701-51702 when catheter insertion is an inclusive component of another procedure.)

51701   Insertion of non-indwelling bladder catheter (eg, straight catheterization for residual urine)

51702   Insertion of temporary indwelling bladder catheter; simple (eg, Foley)

51703   complicated (eg, altered anatomy, fractured catheter/balloon)

51705   Change of cystostomy tube; simple

51710   complicated

(If imaging guidance is performed, use 75984)

51715   Endoscopic injection of implant material into the submucosal tissues of the urethra and/or bladder neck

51720   Bladder instillation of anticarcinogenic agent (including detention time)

Urodynamics

The following section (51725-51797) lists procedures that may be used separately or in many and varied combinations.

When multiple procedures are performed in the same investigative session, modifier 51 should be employed.

All procedures in this section imply that these services are performed by, or are under the direct supervision of, a physician and that all instruments, equipment, fluids, gases, probes, catheters, technician's fees, medications, gloves, trays, tubing and other sterile supplies be provided by the physician. When the physician only interprets the results and/or operates the equipment, a professional component, modifier 26, should be used to identify physicians' services.

51725   Simple cystometrogram (CMG) (eg, spinal manometer)

51726   Complex cystometrogram (eg, calibrated electronic equipment)

51736   Simple uroflowmetry (UFR) (eg, stop-watch flow rate, mechanical uroflowmeter)

51741   Complex uroflowmetry (eg, calibrated electronic equipment)

51772   Urethral pressure profile studies (UPP) (urethral closure pressure profile), any technique

51784   Electromyography studies (EMG) of anal or urethral sphincter, other than needle, any technique

51785   Needle electromyography studies (EMG) of anal or urethral sphincter, any technique

51792   Stimulus evoked response (eg, measurement of bulbocavernosus reflex latency time)

51795   Voiding pressure studies (VP); bladder voiding pressure, any technique

51797   intra-abdominal voiding pressure (AP) (rectal, gastric, intraperitoneal)

51798   Measurement of post-voiding residual urine and/or bladder capacity by ultrasound, non-imaging

Repair

51800   Cystoplasty or cystourethroplasty, plastic operation on bladder and/or vesical neck (anterior Y-plasty, vesical fundus resection), any procedure, with or without wedge resection of posterior vesical neck

51820   Cystourethroplasty with unilateral or bilateral ureteroneocystostomy

51840   Anterior vesicourethropexy, or urethropexy (eg, Marshall-Marchetti-Krantz, Burch); simple

51841   complicated (eg, secondary repair)

(For urethropexy (Pereyra type), use 57289)

51845   Abdomino-vaginal vesical neck suspension, with or without endoscopic control (eg, Stamey, Raz, modified Pereyra)

51860   Cystorrhaphy, suture of bladder wound, injury or rupture; simple

51865   complicated

51880   Closure of cystostomy (separate procedure)

51900   Closure of vesicovaginal fistula, abdominal approach

(For vaginal approach, see 57320-57330)

51920   Closure of vesicouterine fistula;

51925   with hysterectomy

(For closure of vesicoenteric fistula, see 44660, 44661)

(For closure of rectovesical fistula, see 45800-45805)

51940   Closure, exstrophy of bladder

(See also 54390)

51960   Enterocystoplasty, including intestinal anastomosis

51980   Cutaneous vesicostomy

Laparoscopy

Surgical laparoscopy always includes diagnostic laparoscopy. To report a diagnostic laparoscopy (peritoneoscopy) (separate procedure), use 49320.

51990   Laparoscopy, surgical; urethral suspension for stress incontinence

51992   sling operation for stress incontinence (eg, fascia or synthetic)

(For open sling operation for stress incontinence, use 57288)

(For reversal or removal of sling operation for stress incontinence, use 57287)

Endoscopy—Cystoscopy, Urethroscopy, Cystourethroscopy

Endoscopic descriptions are listed so that the main procedure can be identified without having to list all the minor related functions performed at the same time. For example: meatotomy, urethral calibration and/or dilation, urethro-scopy, and cystoscopy prior to a transurethral resection of prostate; ureteral catheterization following extraction of ureteral calculus; internal urethrotomy and bladder neck fulguration when performing a cystourethroscopy for the female urethral syndrome. When the secondary procedure requires significant additional time and effort, it may be identified by the addition of modifier 22.

For example: urethrotomy performed for a documented pre-existing stricture or bladder neck contracture.

52000   Cystourethroscopy (separate procedure)

52001   Cystourethroscopy with irrigation and evacuation of multiple obstructing clots

(Do not report 52001 in addition to 52000)

52005   Cystourethroscopy, with ureteral catheterization, with or without irrigation, instillation, or ureteropyelography, exclusive of radiologic service;

52007   with brush biopsy of ureter and/or renal pelvis

52010   Cystourethroscopy, with ejaculatory duct catheterization, with or without irrigation, instillation, or duct radiography, exclusive of radiologic service

(For radiological supervision and interpretation, use 74440)

Transurethral Surgery

Urethra and Bladder

52204   Cystourethroscopy, with biopsy

52214   Cystourethroscopy, with fulguration (including cryosurgery or laser surgery) of trigone, bladder neck, prostatic fossa, urethra, or periurethral glands

52224   Cystourethroscopy, with fulguration (including cryosurgery or laser surgery) or treatment of MINOR (less than 0.5 cm) lesion(s) with or without biopsy

▲ **52234**   Cystourethroscopy, with fulguration (including cryosurgery or laser surgery) and/or resection of; SMALL bladder tumor(s) (0.5 up to 2.0 cm)

52235   MEDIUM bladder tumor(s) (2.0 to 5.0 cm)

52240   LARGE bladder tumor(s)

52250   Cystourethroscopy with insertion of radioactive substance, with or without biopsy or fulguration

52260   Cystourethroscopy, with dilation of bladder for interstitial cystitis; general or conduction (spinal) anesthesia

52265   local anesthesia

52270   Cystourethroscopy, with internal urethrotomy; female

52275   male

52276   Cystourethroscopy with direct vision internal urethrotomy

52277   Cystourethroscopy, with resection of external sphincter (sphincterotomy)

52281   Cystourethroscopy, with calibration and/or dilation of urethral stricture or stenosis, with or without meatotomy, with or without injection procedure for cystography, male or female

52282   Cystourethroscopy, with insertion of urethral stent

52283   Cystourethroscopy, with steroid injection into stricture

52285   Cystourethroscopy for treatment of the female urethral syndrome with any or all of the following: urethral meatotomy, urethral dilation, internal urethrotomy, lysis of urethrovaginal septal fibrosis, lateral incisions of the bladder neck, and fulguration of polyp(s) of urethra, bladder neck, and/or trigone

Surgery: Urinary System

52290   Cystourethroscopy; with ureteral meatotomy, unilateral or bilateral

52300   with resection or fulguration of orthotopic ureterocele(s), unilateral or bilateral

52301   with resection or fulguration of ectopic ureterocele(s), unilateral or bilateral

52305   with incision or resection of orifice of bladder diverticulum, single or multiple

52310   Cystourethroscopy, with removal of foreign body, calculus, or ureteral stent from urethra or bladder (separate procedure); simple

52315   complicated

52317   Litholapaxy: crushing or fragmentation of calculus by any means in bladder and removal of fragments; simple or small (less than 2.5 cm)

52318   complicated or large (over 2.5 cm)

Ureter and Pelvis

Surgical cystourethroscopy always includes diagnostic cystourethroscopy. To report a diagnostic cystourethroscopy, use 52351.

Do not report 52351 in conjunction with 52341-52346, 52352-52355.

The insertion and removal of a temporary stent during diagnostic or therapeutic cystourethroscopic intervention(s) is included in 52320-52355 and should not be reported separately.

To report insertion of a self-retaining, indwelling stent performed during cystourethroscopic diagnostic or therapeutic intervention(s), report 52332, in addition to primary procedure(s) performed, and append modifier 51. 52332 is used to report a unilateral procedure unless otherwise specified.

For bilateral insertion of self-retaining, indwelling ureteral stents, use code 52332, and append modifier 50.

To report cystourethroscopic removal of a self-retaining, indwelling ureteral stent, see 52310, 52315, and append modifier 58.

52320   Cystourethroscopy (including ureteral catheterization); with removal of ureteral calculus

52325   with fragmentation of ureteral calculus (eg, ultrasonic or electro-hydraulic technique)

52327   with subureteric injection of implant material

52330   with manipulation, without removal of ureteral calculus

52332   Cystourethroscopy, with insertion of indwelling ureteral stent (eg, Gibbons or double-J type)

52334   Cystourethroscopy with insertion of ureteral guide wire through kidney to establish a percutaneous nephrostomy, retrograde

(For percutaneous nephrostolithotomy, see 50080, 50081; for establishment of nephrostomy tract only, use 50395)

(For cystourethroscopy, with ureteroscopy and/or pyeloscopy, see 52351-52355)

(For cystourethroscopy with incision, fulguration, or resection of congenital posterior urethral valves or obstructive hypertrophic mucosal folds, use 52400)

52341   Cystourethroscopy; with treatment of ureteral stricture (eg, balloon dilation, laser, electrocautery, and incision)

52342   with treatment of ureteropelvic junction stricture (eg, balloon dilation, laser, electrocautery, and incision)

52343   with treatment of intra-renal stricture (eg, balloon dilation, laser, electrocautery, and incision)

52344   Cystourethroscopy with ureteroscopy; with treatment of ureteral stricture (eg, balloon dilation, laser, electrocautery, and incision)

52345   with treatment of ureteropelvic junction stricture (eg, balloon dilation, laser, electrocautery, and incision)

52346   with treatment of intra-renal stricture (eg, balloon dilation, laser, electrocautery, and incision)

►(52347 has been deleted)◄

►(For transurethral resection or incision of ejaculatory ducts, use 52402)◄

52351   Cystourethroscopy, with ureteroscopy and/or pyeloscopy; diagnostic

(For radiological supervision and interpretation, use 74485)

(Do not report 52351 in conjunction with 52341-52346, 52352-52355)

52352   with removal or manipulation of calculus (ureteral catheterization is included)

52353   with lithotripsy (ureteral catheterization is included)

52354   with biopsy and/or fulguration of ureteral or renal pelvic lesion

52355   with resection of ureteral or renal pelvic tumor

Vesical Neck and Prostate

52400   Cystourethroscopy with incision, fulguration, or resection of congenital posterior urethral valves, or congenital obstructive hypertrophic mucosal folds

● **52402**   Cystourethroscopy with transurethral resection or incision of ejaculatory ducts

52450   Transurethral incision of prostate

52500   Transurethral resection of bladder neck (separate procedure)

52510   Transurethral balloon dilation of the prostatic urethra

52601   Transurethral electrosurgical resection of prostate, including control of postoperative bleeding, complete (vasectomy, meatotomy, cystourethroscopy, urethral calibration and/or dilation, and internal urethrotomy are included)

      (For other approaches, see 55801-55845)

52606   Transurethral fulguration for postoperative bleeding occurring after the usual follow-up time

52612   Transurethral resection of prostate; first stage of two-stage resection (partial resection)

52614   second stage of two-stage resection (resection completed)

52620   Transurethral resection; of residual obstructive tissue after 90 days postoperative

52630   of regrowth of obstructive tissue longer than one year postoperative

52640   of postoperative bladder neck contracture

52647   Non-contact laser coagulation of prostate, including control of postoperative bleeding, complete (vasectomy, meatotomy, cystourethroscopy, urethral calibration and/or dilation, and internal urethrotomy are included)

52648   Contact laser vaporization with or without transurethral resection of prostate, including control of postoperative bleeding, complete (vasectomy, meatotomy, cystourethroscopy, urethral calibration and/or dilation, and internal urethrotomy are included)

52700   Transurethral drainage of prostatic abscess

      (For litholapaxy, use 52317, 52318)

Urethra

(For endoscopy, see cystoscopy, urethroscopy, cystourethroscopy, 52000-52700)

(For injection procedure for urethrocystography, see 51600-51610)

Incision

53000   Urethrotomy or urethrostomy, external (separate procedure); pendulous urethra

53010   perineal urethra, external

53020   Meatotomy, cutting of meatus (separate procedure); except infant

53025   infant

      (Do not report modifier 63 in conjunction with 53025)

53040   Drainage of deep periurethral abscess

      (For subcutaneous abscess, see 10060, 10061)

53060   Drainage of Skene's gland abscess or cyst

53080   Drainage of perineal urinary extravasation; uncomplicated (separate procedure)

53085   complicated

Excision

53200   Biopsy of urethra

53210   Urethrectomy, total, including cystostomy; female

53215   male

53220   Excision or fulguration of carcinoma of urethra

53230   Excision of urethral diverticulum (separate procedure); female

53235   male

53240   Marsupialization of urethral diverticulum, male or female

53250   Excision of bulbourethral gland (Cowper's gland)

53260   Excision or fulguration; urethral polyp(s), distal urethra

      (For endoscopic approach, see 52214, 52224)

53265   urethral caruncle

53270   Skene's glands

53275   urethral prolapse

Repair

(For hypospadias, see 54300-54352)

53400   Urethroplasty; first stage, for fistula, diverticulum, or stricture (eg, Johannsen type)

53405   second stage (formation of urethra), including urinary diversion

53410   Urethroplasty, one-stage reconstruction of male anterior urethra

53415   Urethroplasty, transpubic or perineal, one stage, for reconstruction or repair of prostatic or membranous urethra

53420   Urethroplasty, two-stage reconstruction or repair of prostatic or membranous urethra; first stage

53425   second stage

53430   Urethroplasty, reconstruction of female urethra

53431   Urethroplasty with tubularization of posterior urethra and/or lower bladder for incontinence (eg, Tenago, Leadbetter procedure)

53440   Sling operation for correction of male urinary incontinence (eg, fascia or synthetic)

53442   Removal or revision of sling for male urinary incontinence (eg, fascia or synthetic)

53444   Insertion of tandem cuff (dual cuff)

53445   Insertion of inflatable urethral/bladder neck sphincter, including placement of pump, reservoir, and cuff

53446   Removal of inflatable urethral/bladder neck sphincter, including pump, reservoir, and cuff

53447   Removal and replacement of inflatable urethral/bladder neck sphincter including pump, reservoir, and cuff at the same operative session

Surgery: Urinary System

▲=Revised Code   ●=New Code   ▶◀=New or Revised Text

53448 Removal and replacement of inflatable urethral/bladder neck sphincter including pump, reservoir, and cuff through an infected field at the same operative session including irrigation and debridement of infected tissue

(Do not report 11040-11043 in addition to 53448)

53449 Repair of inflatable urethral/bladder neck sphincter, including pump, reservoir, and cuff

53450 Urethromeatoplasty, with mucosal advancement

(For meatotomy, see 53020, 53025)

53460 Urethromeatoplasty, with partial excision of distal urethral segment (Richardson type procedure)

53500 Urethrolysis, transvaginal, secondary, open, including cystourethroscopy (eg, postsurgical obstruction, scarring)

(For urethrolysis by retropubic approach, use 53899)

(Do not report 53500 in conjunction with 52000)

53502 Urethrorrhaphy, suture of urethral wound or injury, female

53505 Urethrorrhaphy, suture of urethral wound or injury; penile

53510 perineal

53515 prostatomembranous

53520 Closure of urethrostomy or urethrocutaneous fistula, male (separate procedure)

(For closure of urethrovaginal fistula, use 57310)

(For closure of urethrorectal fistula, see 45820, 45825)

Manipulation

(For radiological supervision and interpretation, use 74485)

53600 Dilation of urethral stricture by passage of sound or urethral dilator, male; initial

53601 subsequent

53605 Dilation of urethral stricture or vesical neck by passage of sound or urethral dilator, male, general or conduction (spinal) anesthesia

53620 Dilation of urethral stricture by passage of filiform and follower, male; initial

53621 subsequent

53660 Dilation of female urethra including suppository and/or instillation; initial

53661 subsequent

53665 Dilation of female urethra, general or conduction (spinal) anesthesia

(For urethral catheterization, see 51701-51703)

(53670 has been deleted. To report, see 51701, 51702)

(53675 has been deleted. To report, use 51703)

Other Procedures

(For two or three glass urinalysis, use 81020)

53850 Transurethral destruction of prostate tissue; by microwave thermotherapy

53852 by radiofrequency thermotherapy

53853 by water-induced thermotherapy

53899 Unlisted procedure, urinary system

Surgery: Urinary System

Male Genital System

Penis

Incision

▶(For abdominal perineal gangrene debridement, see 11004-11006)◀

54000 Slitting of prepuce, dorsal or lateral (separate procedure); newborn

(Do not report modifier 63 in conjunction with 54000)

54001 except newborn

54015 Incision and drainage of penis, deep

(For skin and subcutaneous abscess, see 10060-10160)

Destruction

54050 Destruction of lesion(s), penis (eg, condyloma, papilloma, molluscum contagiosum, herpetic vesicle), simple; chemical

54055 electrodesiccation

54056 cryosurgery

54057 laser surgery

54060 surgical excision

54065 Destruction of lesion(s), penis (eg, condyloma, papilloma, molluscum contagiosum, herpetic vesicle), extensive (eg, laser surgery, electrosurgery, cryosurgery, chemosurgery)

(For destruction or excision of other lesions, see **Integumentary System**)

Excision

54100 Biopsy of penis; (separate procedure)

54105 deep structures

54110 Excision of penile plaque (Peyronie disease);

54111 with graft to 5 cm in length

54112 with graft greater than 5 cm in length

54115 Removal foreign body from deep penile tissue (eg, plastic implant)

54120 Amputation of penis; partial

54125 complete

54130 Amputation of penis, radical; with bilateral inguinofemoral lymphadenectomy

54135 in continuity with bilateral pelvic lymphadenectomy, including external iliac, hypogastric and obturator nodes

(For lymphadenectomy (separate procedure), see 38760-38770)

54150 Circumcision, using clamp or other device; newborn

(Do not report modifier 63 in conjunction with 54150)

54152 except newborn

54160 Circumcision, surgical excision other than clamp, device or dorsal slit; newborn

(Do not report modifier 63 in conjunction with 54160)

54161 except newborn

54162 Lysis or excision of penile post-circumcision adhesions

54163 Repair incomplete circumcision

54164 Frenulotomy of penis

(Do not report 54164 with circumcision codes 54150-54161, 54162, 54163)

Introduction

54200 Injection procedure for Peyronie disease;

54205 with surgical exposure of plaque

54220 Irrigation of corpora cavernosa for priapism

54230 Injection procedure for corpora cavernosography

(For radiological supervision and interpretation, use 74445)

54231 Dynamic cavernosometry, including intracavernosal injection of vasoactive drugs (eg, papaverine, phentolamine)

54235 Injection of corpora cavernosa with pharmacologic agent(s) (eg, papaverine, phentolamine)

54240 Penile plethysmography

54250 Nocturnal penile tumescence and/or rigidity test

Repair

(For other urethroplasties, see 53400-53430)

(For penile revascularization, use 37788)

54300 Plastic operation of penis for straightening of chordee (eg, hypospadias), with or without mobilization of urethra

54304 Plastic operation on penis for correction of chordee or for first stage hypospadias repair with or without transplantation of prepuce and/or skin flaps

54308 Urethroplasty for second stage hypospadias repair (including urinary diversion); less than 3 cm

54312 greater than 3 cm

54316 Urethroplasty for second stage hypospadias repair (including urinary diversion) with free skin graft obtained from site other than genitalia

54318 Urethroplasty for third stage hypospadias repair to release penis from scrotum (eg, third stage Cecil repair)

Surgery: Male/Female Genital System

54322 One stage distal hypospadias repair (with or without chordee or circumcision); with simple meatal advancement (eg, Magpi, V-flap)

54324 with urethroplasty by local skin flaps (eg, flip-flap, prepucial flap)

54326 with urethroplasty by local skin flaps and mobilization of urethra

54328 with extensive dissection to correct chordee and urethroplasty with local skin flaps, skin graft patch, and/or island flap

(For urethroplasty and straightening of chordee, use 54308)

54332 One stage proximal penile or penoscrotal hypospadias repair requiring extensive dissection to correct chordee and urethroplasty by use of skin graft tube and/or island flap

54336 One stage perineal hypospadias repair requiring extensive dissection to correct chordee and urethroplasty by use of skin graft tube and/or island flap

54340 Repair of hypospadias complications (ie, fistula, stricture, diverticula); by closure, incision, or excision, simple

54344 requiring mobilization of skin flaps and urethroplasty with flap or patch graft

54348 requiring extensive dissection and urethroplasty with flap, patch or tubed graft (includes urinary diversion)

54352 Repair of hypospadias cripple requiring extensive dissection and excision of previously constructed structures including re-release of chordee and reconstruction of urethra and penis by use of local skin as grafts and island flaps and skin brought in as flaps or grafts

54360 Plastic operation on penis to correct angulation

54380 Plastic operation on penis for epispadias distal to external sphincter;

54385 with incontinence

54390 with exstrophy of bladder

54400 Insertion of penile prosthesis; non-inflatable (semi-rigid)

54401 inflatable (self-contained)

(For removal or replacement of penile prosthesis, see 54415, 54416)

54405 Insertion of multi-component, inflatable penile prosthesis, including placement of pump, cylinders, and reservoir

(For reduced services, report 54405 with modifier 52)

54406 Removal of all components of a multi-component, inflatable penile prosthesis without replacement of prosthesis

(For reduced services, report 54406 with modifier 52)

54408 Repair of component(s) of a multi-component, inflatable penile prosthesis

54410 Removal and replacement of all component(s) of a multi-component, inflatable penile prosthesis at the same operative session

54411 Removal and replacement of all components of a multi-component inflatable penile prosthesis through an infected field at the same operative session, including irrigation and debridement of infected tissue

(For reduced services, report 54411 with modifier 52)

(Do not report 11040-11043 in addition to 54411)

54415 Removal of non-inflatable (semi-rigid) or inflatable (self-contained) penile prosthesis, without replacement of prosthesis

54416 Removal and replacement of non-inflatable (semi-rigid) or inflatable (self-contained) penile prosthesis at the same operative session

54417 Removal and replacement of non-inflatable (semi-rigid) or inflatable (self-contained) penile prosthesis through an infected field at the same operative session, including irrigation and debridement of infected tissue

(Do not report 11040-11043 in addition to 54417)

54420 Corpora cavernosa-saphenous vein shunt (priapism operation), unilateral or bilateral

54430 Corpora cavernosa-corpus spongiosum shunt (priapism operation), unilateral or bilateral

54435 Corpora cavernosa-glans penis fistulization (eg, biopsy needle, Winter procedure, rongeur, or punch) for priapism

54440 Plastic operation of penis for injury

Manipulation

54450 Foreskin manipulation including lysis of preputial adhesions and stretching

Testis

Excision

▶(For abdominal perineal gangrene debridement, see 11004-11006)◀

54500 Biopsy of testis, needle (separate procedure)

(For fine needle aspiration, see 10021, 10022)

(For evaluation of fine needle aspirate, see 88172, 88173)

54505 Biopsy of testis, incisional (separate procedure)

(For bilateral procedure, report 54505 with modifier 50)

(When combined with vasogram, seminal vesiculogram, or epididymogram, use 55300)

54512 Excision of extraparenchymal lesion of testis

54520 Orchiectomy, simple (including subcapsular), with or without testicular prosthesis, scrotal or inguinal approach

(For bilateral procedure, report 54520 with modifier 50)

Surgery: Male/Female Genital System

54522   Orchiectomy, partial

54530   Orchiectomy, radical, for tumor; inguinal approach

54535   with abdominal exploration

(For orchiectomy with repair of hernia, see 49505 or 49507 and 54520)

(For radical retroperitoneal lymphadenectomy, use 38780)

54550   Exploration for undescended testis (inguinal or scrotal area)

(For bilateral procedure, report 54550 with modifier 50)

54560   Exploration for undescended testis with abdominal exploration

(For bilateral procedure, report 54560 with modifier 50)

Repair

54600   Reduction of torsion of testis, surgical, with or without fixation of contralateral testis

54620   Fixation of contralateral testis (separate procedure)

54640   Orchiopexy, inguinal approach, with or without hernia repair

(For bilateral procedure, report 54640 with modifier 50

(For inguinal hernia repair performed in conjunction with inguinal orchiopexy, see 49495-49525)

54650   Orchiopexy, abdominal approach, for intra-abdominal testis (eg, Fowler-Stephens)

(For laparoscopic approach, use 54692)

54660   Insertion of testicular prosthesis (separate procedure)

(For bilateral procedure, report 54660 with modifier 50)

54670   Suture or repair of testicular injury

54680   Transplantation of testis(es) to thigh (because of scrotal destruction)

Laparoscopy

Surgical laparoscopy always includes diagnostic laparoscopy. To report a diagnostic laparoscopy (peritoneoscopy) (separate procedure), use 49320.

54690   Laparoscopy, surgical; orchiectomy

54692   orchiopexy for intra-abdominal testis

54699   Unlisted laparoscopy procedure, testis

Epididymis

Incision

54700   Incision and drainage of epididymis, testis and/or scrotal space (eg, abscess or hematoma)

Excision

54800   Biopsy of epididymis, needle

(For fine needle aspiration, see 10021, 10022)

(For evaluation of fine needle aspirate, see 88172, 88173)

54820   Exploration of epididymis, with or without biopsy

54830   Excision of local lesion of epididymis

54840   Excision of spermatocele, with or without epididymectomy

54860   Epididymectomy; unilateral

54861   bilateral

Repair

54900   Epididymovasostomy, anastomosis of epididymis to vas deferens; unilateral

54901   bilateral

(For operating microscope, use 69990)

Tunica Vaginalis

Incision

55000   Puncture aspiration of hydrocele, tunica vaginalis, with or without injection of medication

Excision

55040   Excision of hydrocele; unilateral

55041   bilateral

(With hernia repair, see 49495-49501)

Repair

55060   Repair of tunica vaginalis hydrocele (Bottle type)

Scrotum

Incision

55100   Drainage of scrotal wall abscess

(See also 54700)

55110   Scrotal exploration

55120   Removal of foreign body in scrotum

Excision

(For excision of local lesion of skin of scrotum, see **Integumentary System**)

55150   Resection of scrotum

Surgery: Male/Female Genital System

Surgery: Male/Female Genital System

Repair

55175   Scrotoplasty; simple

55180   complicated

Vas Deferens

Incision

55200   Vasotomy, cannulization with or without incision of vas, unilateral or bilateral (separate procedure)

Excision

55250   Vasectomy, unilateral or bilateral (separate procedure), including postoperative semen examination(s)

Introduction

55300   Vasotomy for vasograms, seminal vesiculograms, or epididymograms, unilateral or bilateral

(For radiological supervision and interpretation, use 74440)

(When combined with biopsy of testis, see 54505 and use modifier 51)

Repair

55400   Vasovasostomy, vasovasorrhaphy

(For bilateral procedure, report 55400 with modifier 50)

(For operating microscope, use 69990)

Suture

55450   Ligation (percutaneous) of vas deferens, unilateral or bilateral (separate procedure)

Spermatic Cord

Excision

55500   Excision of hydrocele of spermatic cord, unilateral (separate procedure)

55520   Excision of lesion of spermatic cord (separate procedure)

55530   Excision of varicocele or ligation of spermatic veins for varicocele; (separate procedure)

55535   abdominal approach

55540   with hernia repair

Laparoscopy

Surgical laparoscopy always includes diagnostic laparoscopy. To report a diagnostic laparoscopy (peritoneoscopy) (separate procedure), use 49320.

55550   Laparoscopy, surgical, with ligation of spermatic veins for varicocele

55559   Unlisted laparoscopy procedure, spermatic cord

Seminal Vesicles

Incision

55600   Vesiculotomy;

(For bilateral procedure, report 55600 with modifier 50)

55605   complicated

Excision

55650   Vesiculectomy, any approach

(For bilateral procedure, report 55650 with modifier 50)

55680   Excision of Mullerian duct cyst

(For injection procedure, see 52010, 55300)

Prostate

Incision

55700   Biopsy, prostate; needle or punch, single or multiple, any approach

(If imaging guidance is performed, use 76942)

(For fine needle aspiration, see 10021, 10022)

(For evaluation of fine needle aspirate, see 88172, 88173)

55705   incisional, any approach

55720   Prostatotomy, external drainage of prostatic abscess, any approach; simple

55725   complicated

(For transurethral drainage, use 52700)

Excision

(For transurethral removal of prostate, see 52601-52640)

(For transurethral destruction of prostate, see 53850-53852)

(For limited pelvic lymphadenectomy for staging (separate procedure), use 38562)

(For independent node dissection, see 38770-38780)

55801   Prostatectomy, perineal, subtotal (including control of postoperative bleeding, vasectomy, meatotomy, urethral calibration and/or dilation, and internal urethrotomy)

55810   Prostatectomy, perineal radical;

55812   with lymph node biopsy(s) (limited pelvic lymphadenectomy)

55815   with bilateral pelvic lymphadenectomy, including external iliac, hypogastric and obturator nodes

            (If 55815 is carried out on separate days, use 38770 with modifier 50 and 55810)

55821   Prostatectomy (including control of postoperative bleeding, vasectomy, meatotomy, urethral calibration and/or dilation, and internal urethrotomy); suprapubic, subtotal, one or two stages

55831   retropubic, subtotal

55840   Prostatectomy, retropubic radical, with or without nerve sparing;

55842   with lymph node biopsy(s) (limited pelvic lymphadenectomy)

55845   with bilateral pelvic lymphadenectomy, including external iliac, hypogastric, and obturator nodes

            (If 55845 is carried out on separate days, use 38770 with modifier 50 and 55840)

            (For laparoscopic retropubic radical prostatectomy, use 55866)

55859   Transperineal placement of needles or catheters into prostate for interstitial radioelement application, with or without cystoscopy

            (For interstitial radioelement application, see 77776-►77784◄)

            (For ultrasonic guidance for interstitial radioelement application, use 76965)

55860   Exposure of prostate, any approach, for insertion of radioactive substance;

            (For application of interstitial radioelement, see 77776-77778)

55862   with lymph node biopsy(s) (limited pelvic lymphadenectomy)

55865   with bilateral pelvic lymphadenectomy, including external iliac, hypogastric and obturator nodes

Laparoscopy

Surgical laparoscopy always includes diagnostic laparoscopy. To report a diagnostic laparoscopy (peritoneoscopy) (separate procedure), use 49320.

55866   Laparoscopy, surgical prostatectomy, retropubic radical, including nerve sparing

            (For open procedure, use 55840)

Other Procedures

            (For artificial insemination, see 58321, 58322)

55870   Electroejaculation

55873   Cryosurgical ablation of the prostate (includes ultrasonic guidance for interstitial cryosurgical probe placement)

55899   Unlisted procedure, male genital system

Intersex Surgery

55970   Intersex surgery; male to female

55980   female to male

Notes

⊘ =Modifier 51 Exempt   ⊙ =Conscious Sedation   ✚ =Add-on Code

Female Genital System

(For pelvic laparotomy, use 49000)

(For excision or destruction of endometriomas, open method, see 49200, 49201)

(For paracentesis, see 49080, 49081)

(For secondary closure of abdominal wall evisceration or disruption, use 49900)

(For fulguration or excision of lesions, laparoscopic approach, use 58662)

(For chemotherapy, see 96400-96549)

Vulva, Perineum and Introitus

Definitions

The following definitions apply to the vulvectomy codes (56620-56640).

A *simple* procedure is the removal of skin and superficial subcutaneous tissues.

A *radical* procedure is the removal of skin and deep subcutaneous tissue.

A *partial* procedure is the removal of less than 80% of the vulvar area.

A *complete* procedure is the removal of greater than 80% of the vulvar area.

Incision

(For incision and drainage of sebaceous cyst, furuncle, or abscess, see 10040, 10060, 10061)

56405	Incision and drainage of vulva or perineal abscess
56420	Incision and drainage of Bartholin's gland abscess

(For incision and drainage of Skene's gland abscess or cyst, use 53060)

56440	Marsupialization of Bartholin's gland cyst
56441	Lysis of labial adhesions

Destruction

56501	Destruction of lesion(s), vulva; simple (eg, laser surgery, electrosurgery, cryosurgery, chemosurgery)
56515	extensive (eg, laser surgery, electrosurgery, cryosurgery, chemosurgery)

(For destruction of Skene's gland cyst or abscess, use 53270)

(For cautery destruction of urethral caruncle, use 53265)

Excision

56605	Biopsy of vulva or perineum (separate procedure); one lesion
+ 56606	each separate additional lesion (List separately in addition to code for primary procedure)

(Use 56606 in conjunction with 56605)

(For excision of local lesion, see 11420-11426, 11620-11626)

56620	Vulvectomy simple; partial
56625	complete

(For skin graft, see 15000 et seq)

56630	Vulvectomy, radical, partial;

(For skin graft, if used, see 15000, 15120, 15121, 15240, 15241)

56631	with unilateral inguinofemoral lymphadenectomy
56632	with bilateral inguinofemoral lymphadenectomy
56633	Vulvectomy, radical, complete;
56634	with unilateral inguinofemoral lymphadenectomy
56637	with bilateral inguinofemoral lymphadenectomy
56640	Vulvectomy, radical, complete, with inguinofemoral, iliac, and pelvic lymphadenectomy

(For bilateral procedure, report 56640 with modifier 50)

(For lymphadenectomy, see 38760-38780)

56700	Partial hymenectomy or revision of hymenal ring
56720	Hymenotomy, simple incision
56740	Excision of Bartholin's gland or cyst

(For excision of Skene's gland, use 53270)

(For excision of urethral caruncle, use 53265)

(For excision or fulguration of urethral carcinoma, use 53220)

(For excision or marsupialization of urethral diverticulum, see 53230, 53240)

Repair

(For repair of urethra for mucosal prolapse, use 53275)

56800	Plastic repair of introitus
56805	Clitoroplasty for intersex state
56810	Perineoplasty, repair of perineum, nonobstetrical (separate procedure)

(See also 56800)

(For repair of wounds to genitalia, see 12001-12007, 12041-12047, 13131-13133)

(For repair of recent injury of vagina and perineum, nonobstetrical, use 57210)

Surgery: Male/Female Genital System

(For anal sphincteroplasty, see 46750, 46751)

(For episiorrhaphy, episioperineorrhaphy for recent injury of vulva and/or perineum, nonobstetrical, use 57210)

Endoscopy

56820 Colposcopy of the vulva;

56821   with biopsy(s)

(For colposcopic examinations/procedures involving the vagina, see 57420, 57421; cervix, see 57452-57461)

Vagina

Incision

57000 Colpotomy; with exploration

57010   with drainage of pelvic abscess

57020 Colpocentesis (separate procedure)

57022 Incision and drainage of vaginal hematoma; obstetrical/postpartum

57023   non-obstetrical (eg, post-trauma, spontaneous bleeding)

Destruction

57061 Destruction of vaginal lesion(s); simple (eg, laser surgery, electrosurgery, cryosurgery, chemosurgery)

57065   extensive (eg, laser surgery, electrosurgery, cryosurgery, chemosurgery)

Excision

57100 Biopsy of vaginal mucosa; simple (separate procedure)

57105   extensive, requiring suture (including cysts)

57106 Vaginectomy, partial removal of vaginal wall;

57107   with removal of paravaginal tissue (radical vaginectomy)

57109   with removal of paravaginal tissue (radical vaginectomy) with bilateral total pelvic lymphadenectomy and para-aortic lymph node sampling (biopsy)

57110 Vaginectomy, complete removal of vaginal wall;

57111   with removal of paravaginal tissue (radical vaginectomy)

57112   with removal of paravaginal tissue (radical vaginectomy) with bilateral total pelvic lymphadenectomy and para-aortic lymph node sampling (biopsy)

57120 Colpocleisis (Le Fort type)

57130 Excision of vaginal septum

57135 Excision of vaginal cyst or tumor

Introduction

57150 Irrigation of vagina and/or application of medicament for treatment of bacterial, parasitic, or fungoid disease

57155 Insertion of uterine tandems and/or vaginal ovoids for clinical brachytherapy

(For insertion of radioelement sources or ribbons, see 77761-77763, 77781-77784)

57160 Fitting and insertion of pessary or other intravaginal support device

57170 Diaphragm or cervical cap fitting with instructions

57180 Introduction of any hemostatic agent or pack for spontaneous or traumatic nonobstetrical vaginal hemorrhage (separate procedure)

Repair

(For urethral suspension, Marshall-Marchetti-Krantz type, abdominal approach, see 51840, 51841)

(For laparoscopic suspension, use 51990)

57200 Colporrhaphy, suture of injury of vagina (nonobstetrical)

57210 Colpoperineorrhaphy, suture of injury of vagina and/or perineum (nonobstetrical)

57220 Plastic operation on urethral sphincter, vaginal approach (eg, Kelly urethral plication)

57230 Plastic repair of urethrocele

57240 Anterior colporrhaphy, repair of cystocele with or without repair of urethrocele

57250 Posterior colporrhaphy, repair of rectocele with or without perineorrhaphy

(For repair of rectocele (separate procedure) without posterior colporrhaphy, use 45560)

57260 Combined anteroposterior colporrhaphy;

57265   with enterocele repair

+● 57267 Insertion of mesh or other prosthesis for repair of pelvic floor defect, each site (anterior, posterior compartment), vaginal approach (List separately in addition to code for primary procedure)

►(Use 57267 in addition to 45560, 57240-57265)◄

57268 Repair of enterocele, vaginal approach (separate procedure)

57270 Repair of enterocele, abdominal approach (separate procedure)

57280 Colpopexy, abdominal approach

▲ 57282 Colpopexy, vaginal; extra-peritoneal approach (sacrospinous, iliococcygeus)

● 57283   intra-peritoneal approach (uterosacral, levator myorrhaphy)

Surgery: Male/Female Genital System

57284   Paravaginal defect repair (including repair of cystocele, stress urinary incontinence, and/or incomplete vaginal prolapse)

57287   Removal or revision of sling for stress incontinence (eg, fascia or synthetic)

57288   Sling operation for stress incontinence (eg, fascia or synthetic)

(For laparoscopic approach, use 51992)

57289   Pereyra procedure, including anterior colporrhaphy

57291   Construction of artificial vagina; without graft

57292   with graft

57300   Closure of rectovaginal fistula; vaginal or transanal approach

57305   abdominal approach

57307   abdominal approach, with concomitant colostomy

57308   transperineal approach, with perineal body reconstruction, with or without levator plication

57310   Closure of urethrovaginal fistula;

57311   with bulbocavernosus transplant

57320   Closure of vesicovaginal fistula; vaginal approach

(For concomitant cystostomy, see 51005-51040)

57330   transvesical and vaginal approach

(For abdominal approach, use 51900)

57335   Vaginoplasty for intersex state

Manipulation

57400   Dilation of vagina under anesthesia

57410   Pelvic examination under anesthesia

57415   Removal of impacted vaginal foreign body (separate procedure) under anesthesia

(For removal without anesthesia of an impacted vaginal foreign body, use the appropriate E/M code)

Endoscopy

(For speculoscopy, see Category III codes 0031T, 0032T)

57420   Colposcopy of the entire vagina, with cervix if present;

57421   with biopsy(s)

(For colposcopic visualization of cervix and adjacent upper vagina, use 57452)

(When reporting colposcopies of multiple sites, use modifier 51 as appropriate. For colposcopic examinations/procedures involving the vulva, see 56820, 56821; cervix, see 57452-57461)

(57450, 57451 have been deleted)

57425   Laparoscopy, surgical, colpopexy (suspension of vaginal apex)

Cervix Uteri

(For cervicography, see Category III code 0003T)

Endoscopy

(For colposcopic examinations/procedures involving the vulva, see 56820, 56821; vagina, see 57420, 57421)

57452   Colposcopy of the cervix including upper/adjacent vagina;

(Do not report 57452 in addition to 57454-57461)

57454   with biopsy(s) of the cervix and endocervical curettage

57455   with biopsy(s) of the cervix

57456   with endocervical curettage

57460   with loop electrode biopsy(s) of the cervix

57461   with loop electrode conization of the cervix

(Do not report 57456 in addition to 57461)

Excision

(For radical surgical procedures, see 58200-58240)

57500   Biopsy, single or multiple, or local excision of lesion, with or without fulguration (separate procedure)

57505   Endocervical curettage (not done as part of a dilation and curettage)

57510   Cautery of cervix; electro or thermal

57511   cryocautery, initial or repeat

57513   laser ablation

57520   Conization of cervix, with or without fulguration, with or without dilation and curettage, with or without repair; cold knife or laser

(See also 58120)

57522   loop electrode excision

57530   Trachelectomy (cervicectomy), amputation of cervix (separate procedure)

57531   Radical trachelectomy, with bilateral total pelvic lymphadenectomy and para-aortic lymph node sampling biopsy, with or without removal of tube(s), with or without removal of ovary(s)

(For radical abdominal hysterectomy, use 58210)

57540   Excision of cervical stump, abdominal approach;

57545   with pelvic floor repair

57550   Excision of cervical stump, vaginal approach;

57555   with anterior and/or posterior repair

57556   with repair of enterocele

(For insertion of intrauterine device, use 58300)

(For insertion of any hemostatic agent or pack for control of spontaneous non-obstetrical hemorrhage, see 57180)

Surgery: Male/Female Genital System

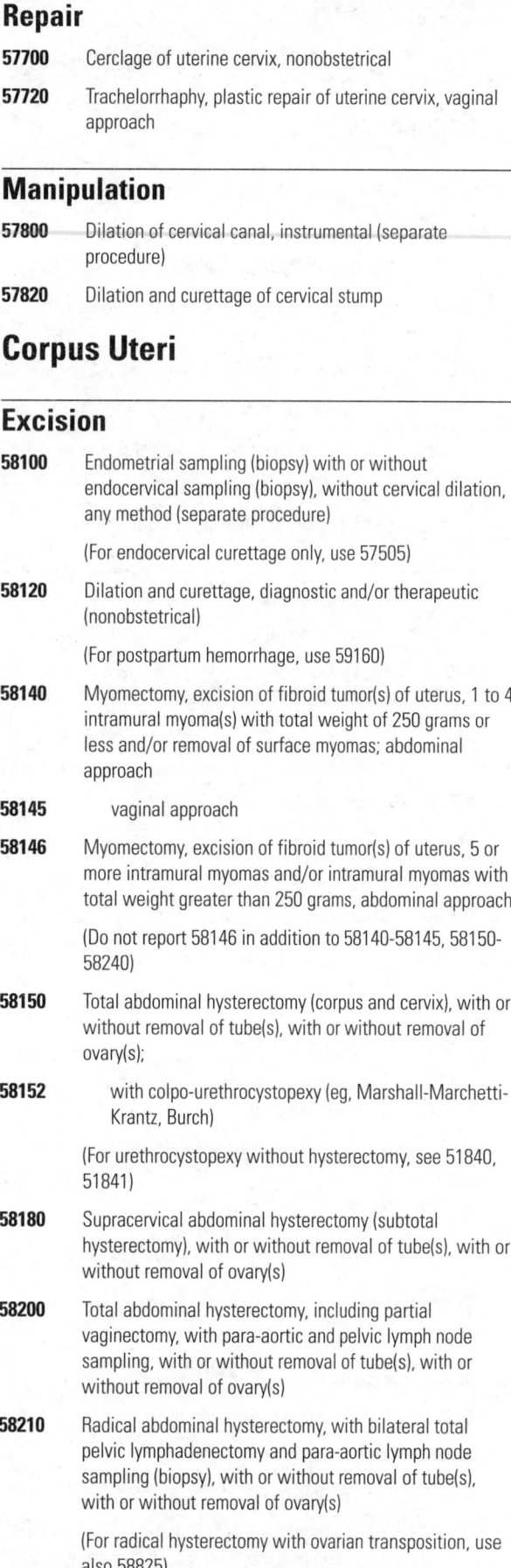

Repair

57700 Cerclage of uterine cervix, nonobstetrical

57720 Trachelorrhaphy, plastic repair of uterine cervix, vaginal approach

Manipulation

57800 Dilation of cervical canal, instrumental (separate procedure)

57820 Dilation and curettage of cervical stump

Corpus Uteri

Excision

58100 Endometrial sampling (biopsy) with or without endocervical sampling (biopsy), without cervical dilation, any method (separate procedure)

(For endocervical curettage only, use 57505)

58120 Dilation and curettage, diagnostic and/or therapeutic (nonobstetrical)

(For postpartum hemorrhage, use 59160)

58140 Myomectomy, excision of fibroid tumor(s) of uterus, 1 to 4 intramural myoma(s) with total weight of 250 grams or less and/or removal of surface myomas; abdominal approach

58145   vaginal approach

58146 Myomectomy, excision of fibroid tumor(s) of uterus, 5 or more intramural myomas and/or intramural myomas with total weight greater than 250 grams, abdominal approach

(Do not report 58146 in addition to 58140-58145, 58150-58240)

58150 Total abdominal hysterectomy (corpus and cervix), with or without removal of tube(s), with or without removal of ovary(s);

58152   with colpo-urethrocystopexy (eg, Marshall-Marchetti-Krantz, Burch)

(For urethrocystopexy without hysterectomy, see 51840, 51841)

58180 Supracervical abdominal hysterectomy (subtotal hysterectomy), with or without removal of tube(s), with or without removal of ovary(s)

58200 Total abdominal hysterectomy, including partial vaginectomy, with para-aortic and pelvic lymph node sampling, with or without removal of tube(s), with or without removal of ovary(s)

58210 Radical abdominal hysterectomy, with bilateral total pelvic lymphadenectomy and para-aortic lymph node sampling (biopsy), with or without removal of tube(s), with or without removal of ovary(s)

(For radical hysterectomy with ovarian transposition, use also 58825)

58240 Pelvic exenteration for gynecologic malignancy, with total abdominal hysterectomy or cervicectomy, with or without removal of tube(s), with or without removal of ovary(s), with removal of bladder and ureteral transplantations, and/or abdominoperineal resection of rectum and colon and colostomy, or any combination thereof

(For pelvic exenteration for lower urinary tract or male genital malignancy, use 51597)

58260 Vaginal hysterectomy, for uterus 250 grams or less;

58262   with removal of tube(s), and/or ovary(s)

58263   with removal of tube(s), and/or ovary(s), with repair of enterocele

▶(Do not report 58263 in addition to 57283)◀

58267   with colpo-urethrocystopexy (Marshall-Marchetti-Krantz type, Pereyra type) with or without endoscopic control

58270   with repair of enterocele

(For repair of enterocele with removal of tubes and/or ovaries, use 58263)

58275 Vaginal hysterectomy, with total or partial vaginectomy;

58280   with repair of enterocele

58285 Vaginal hysterectomy, radical (Schauta type operation)

58290 Vaginal hysterectomy, for uterus greater than 250 grams;

58291   with removal of tube(s) and/or ovary(s)

58292   with removal of tube(s) and/or ovary(s), with repair of enterocele

58293   with colpo-urethrocystopexy (Marshall-Marchetti-Krantz type, Pereyra type) with or without endoscopic control

58294   with repair of enterocele

Introduction

(For insertion/removal of implantable contraceptive capsules, see 11975, 11976, 11977)

58300 Insertion of intrauterine device (IUD)

58301 Removal of intrauterine device (IUD)

58321 Artificial insemination; intra-cervical

58322   intra-uterine

58323 Sperm washing for artificial insemination

58340 Catheterization and introduction of saline or contrast material for saline infusion sonohysterography (SIS) or hysterosalpingography

(For radiological supervision and interpretation of saline infusion sonohysterography, use 76831)

(For radiological supervision and interpretation of hysterosalpingography, use 74740)

Surgery: Male/Female Genital System

58345   Transcervical introduction of fallopian tube catheter for diagnosis and/or re-establishing patency (any method), with or without hysterosalpingography

(For radiological supervision and interpretation, use 74742)

58346   Insertion of Heyman capsules for clinical brachytherapy

(For insertion of radioelement sources or ribbons, see 77761-77763, 77781-77784)

58350   Chromotubation of oviduct, including materials

(For materials supplied by physician, use 99070)

58353   Endometrial ablation, thermal, without hysteroscopic guidance

(For hysteroscopic procedure, use 58563)

● **58356**   Endometrial cryoablation with ultrasonic guidance, including endometrial curettage, when performed

►(Do not report 58356 in conjunction with 58100, 58120, 58340, 76700, 76856)◄

Repair

58400   Uterine suspension, with or without shortening of round ligaments, with or without shortening of sacrouterine ligaments; (separate procedure)

58410   with presacral sympathectomy

(For anastomosis of tubes to uterus, use 58752)

58520   Hysterorrhaphy, repair of ruptured uterus (nonobstetrical)

58540   Hysteroplasty, repair of uterine anomaly (Strassman type)

(For closure of vesicouterine fistula, use 51920)

Laparoscopy/Hysteroscopy

Surgical laparoscopy always includes diagnostic laparoscopy. To report a diagnostic laparoscopy (peritoneoscopy) (separate procedure), use 49320. To report a diagnostic hysteroscopy (separate procedure), use 58555.

58545   Laparoscopy, surgical, myomectomy, excision; 1 to 4 intramural myomas with total weight of 250 grams or less and/or removal of surface myomas

58546   5 or more intramural myomas and/or intramural myomas with total weight greater than 250 grams

58550   Laparoscopy surgical, with vaginal hysterectomy, for uterus 250 grams or less;

(58551 has been deleted. To report see 58545, 58546)

58552   with removal of tube(s) and/or ovary(s)

58553   Laparoscopy, surgical, with vaginal hysterectomy, for uterus greater than 250 grams;

58554   with removal of tube(s) and/or ovary(s)

58555   Hysteroscopy, diagnostic (separate procedure)

58558   Hysteroscopy, surgical; with sampling (biopsy) of endometrium and/or polypectomy, with or without D & C

58559   with lysis of intrauterine adhesions (any method)

58560   with division or resection of intrauterine septum (any method)

58561   with removal of leiomyomata

58562   with removal of impacted foreign body

58563   with endometrial ablation (eg, endometrial resection, electrosurgical ablation, thermoablation)

● **58565**   with bilateral fallopian tube cannulation to induce occlusion by placement of permanent implants

►(Do not report 58565 in conjunction with 58555 or 57800)◄

►(For unilateral procedure, use modifier 52)◄

58578   Unlisted laparoscopy procedure, uterus

58579   Unlisted hysteroscopy procedure, uterus

Oviduct/Ovary

Incision

58600   Ligation or transection of fallopian tube(s), abdominal or vaginal approach, unilateral or bilateral

58605   Ligation or transection of fallopian tube(s), abdominal or vaginal approach, postpartum, unilateral or bilateral, during same hospitalization (separate procedure)

(For laparoscopic procedures, use 58670, 58671)

+ **58611**   Ligation or transection of fallopian tube(s) when done at the time of cesarean delivery or intra-abdominal surgery (not a separate procedure) (List separately in addition to code for primary procedure)

58615   Occlusion of fallopian tube(s) by device (eg, band, clip, Falope ring) vaginal or suprapubic approach

(For laparoscopic approach, use 58671)

(For lysis of adnexal adhesions, use 58740)

Laparoscopy

Surgical laparoscopy always includes diagnostic laparoscopy. To report a diagnostic laparoscopy (peritoneoscopy) (separate procedure), use 49320.

(For laparoscopic biopsy of the ovary or fallopian tube, use 49321)

58660   Laparoscopy, surgical; with lysis of adhesions (salpingolysis, ovariolysis) (separate procedure)

58661   with removal of adnexal structures (partial or total oophorectomy and/or salpingectomy)

58662   with fulguration or excision of lesions of the ovary, pelvic viscera, or peritoneal surface by any method

Surgery: Male/Female Genital System

58670   with fulguration of oviducts (with or without transection)

58671   with occlusion of oviducts by device (eg, band, clip, or Falope ring)

58672   with fimbrioplasty

58673   with salpingostomy (salpingoneostomy)

(Codes 58672 and 58673 are used to report unilateral procedures. For bilateral procedure, use modifier 50)

58679   Unlisted laparoscopy procedure, oviduct, ovary

Excision

58700   Salpingectomy, complete or partial, unilateral or bilateral (separate procedure)

58720   Salpingo-oophorectomy, complete or partial, unilateral or bilateral (separate procedure)

Repair

58740   Lysis of adhesions (salpingolysis, ovariolysis)

(For laparoscopic approach, use 58660)

(For excision or destruction of endometriomas, open method, see 49200, 49201)

(For fulguration or excision of lesions, laparoscopic approach, use 58662)

58750   Tubotubal anastomosis

58752   Tubouterine implantation

58760   Fimbrioplasty

(For laparoscopic approach, use 58672)

58770   Salpingostomy (salpingoneostomy)

(For laparoscopic approach, use 58673)

Ovary

Incision

58800   Drainage of ovarian cyst(s), unilateral or bilateral, (separate procedure); vaginal approach

58805   abdominal approach

58820   Drainage of ovarian abscess; vaginal approach, open

58822   abdominal approach

⊙ 58823   Drainage of pelvic abscess, transvaginal or transrectal approach, percutaneous (eg, ovarian, pericolic)

(For radiological supervision and interpretation, use 75989)

58825   Transposition, ovary(s)

Excision

58900   Biopsy of ovary, unilateral or bilateral (separate procedure)

(For laparoscopic biopsy of the ovary or fallopian tube, use 49321)

58920   Wedge resection or bisection of ovary, unilateral or bilateral

58925   Ovarian cystectomy, unilateral or bilateral

58940   Oophorectomy, partial or total, unilateral or bilateral;

(For oophorectomy with concomitant debulking for ovarian malignancy, use 58952)

58943   for ovarian, tubal or primary peritoneal malignancy, with para-aortic and pelvic lymph node biopsies, peritoneal washings, peritoneal biopsies, diaphragmatic assessments, with or without salpingectomy(s), with or without omentectomy

58950   Resection of ovarian, tubal or primary peritoneal malignancy with bilateral salpingo-oophorectomy and omentectomy;

58951   with total abdominal hysterectomy, pelvic and limited para-aortic lymphadenectomy

58952   with radical dissection for debulking (ie, radical excision or destruction, intra-abdominal or retroperitoneal tumors)

58953   Bilateral salpingo-oophorectomy with omentectomy, total abdominal hysterectomy and radical dissection for debulking;

58954   with pelvic lymphadenectomy and limited para-aortic lymphadenectomy

● 58956   Bilateral salpingo-oophorectomy with total omentectomy, total abdominal hysterectomy for malignancy

▶(Do not report 58956 in conjunction with 49255, 58150, 58180, 58262, 58263, 58550, 58661, 58700, 58720, 58900, 58925, 58940)◀

58960   Laparotomy, for staging or restaging of ovarian, tubal or primary peritoneal malignancy (second look), with or without omentectomy, peritoneal washing, biopsy of abdominal and pelvic peritoneum, diaphragmatic assessment with pelvic and limited para-aortic lymphadenectomy

In Vitro Fertilization

58970   Follicle puncture for oocyte retrieval, any method

(For radiological supervision and interpretation, use 76948)

58974   Embryo transfer, intrauterine

58976   Gamete, zygote, or embryo intrafallopian transfer, any method

(For laparoscopic adnexal procedures, see 58660-58673)

Other Procedures

58999   Unlisted procedure, female genital system
(nonobstetrical)

Maternity Care and Delivery

The services normally provided in uncomplicated
maternity cases include antepartum care, delivery, and
postpartum care.

Antepartum care includes the initial and subsequent
history, physical examinations, recording of weight, blood
pressures, fetal heart tones, routine chemical urinalysis,
and monthly visits up to 28 weeks gestation, biweekly
visits to 36 weeks gestation, and weekly visits until
delivery. Any other visits or services within this time
period should be coded separately.

Delivery services include admission to the hospital, the
admission history and physical examination, management
of uncomplicated labor, vaginal delivery (with or without
episiotomy, with or without forceps), or cesarean delivery.
Medical problems complicating labor and delivery
management may require additional resources and should
be identified by utilizing the codes in the **Medicine** and
Evaluation and Management Services section in addition
to codes for maternity care.

Postpartum care includes hospital and office visits
following vaginal or cesarean section delivery.

For medical complications of pregnancy (eg, cardiac
problems, neurological problems, diabetes, hypertension,
toxemia, hyperemesis, pre-term labor, premature rupture
of membranes), see services in the **Medicine** and
Evaluation and Management Services section.

For surgical complications of pregnancy (eg,
appendectomy, hernia, ovarian cyst, Bartholin cyst), see
services in the **Surgery** section.

If a physician provides all or part of the antepartum
and/or postpartum patient care but does not perform
delivery due to termination of pregnancy by abortion or
referral to another physician for delivery, see the
antepartum and postpartum care codes 59425-59426 and
59430.

(For circumcision of newborn, see 54150, 54160)

Antepartum Services

(For insertion of transcervical or transvaginal fetal
oximetry sensor, use Category III code 0021T)

59000   Amniocentesis; diagnostic

(For radiological supervision and interpretation, use
76946)

59001   therapeutic amniotic fluid reduction (includes
ultrasound guidance)

59012   Cordocentesis (intrauterine), any method

(For radiological supervision and interpretation, use
76941)

59015   Chorionic villus sampling, any method

(For radiological supervision and interpretation, use
76945)

59020   Fetal contraction stress test

59025   Fetal non-stress test

59030   Fetal scalp blood sampling

(For repeat fetal scalp blood sampling, use 59030 and see
modifiers 76 and 77)

59050   Fetal monitoring during labor by consulting physician (ie,
non-attending physician) with written report; supervision
and interpretation

59051   interpretation only

59070   Transabdominal amnioinfusion, including ultrasound
guidance

59072   Fetal umbilical cord occlusion, including ultrasound
guidance

59074   Fetal fluid drainage (eg, vesicocentesis, thoracocentesis,
paracentesis), including ultrasound guidance

59076   Fetal shunt placement, including ultrasound guidance

(For unlisted fetal invasive procedure, use 59897)

Excision

59100   Hysterotomy, abdominal (eg, for hydatidiform mole,
abortion)

(When tubal ligation is performed at the same time as
hysterotomy, use 58611 in addition to 59100)

59120   Surgical treatment of ectopic pregnancy; tubal or ovarian,
requiring salpingectomy and/or oophorectomy, abdominal
or vaginal approach

59121   tubal or ovarian, without salpingectomy and/or
oophorectomy

59130   abdominal pregnancy

59135   interstitial, uterine pregnancy requiring total
hysterectomy

59136   interstitial, uterine pregnancy with partial resection
of uterus

59140   cervical, with evacuation

59150   Laparoscopic treatment of ectopic pregnancy; without
salpingectomy and/or oophorectomy

59151   with salpingectomy and/or oophorectomy

59160   Curettage, postpartum

Surgery: Male/Female Genital System

Introduction

(For intrauterine fetal transfusion, use 36460)

(For introduction of hypertonic solution and/or prostaglandins to initiate labor, see 59850-59857)

59200 Insertion of cervical dilator (eg, laminaria, prostaglandin) (separate procedure)

Repair

(For tracheloplasty, use 57700)

59300 Episiotomy or vaginal repair, by other than attending physician

59320 Cerclage of cervix, during pregnancy; vaginal

59325 abdominal

59350 Hysterorrhaphy of ruptured uterus

Vaginal Delivery, Antepartum and Postpartum Care

(For insertion of transcervical or transvaginal fetal oximetry sensor, use Category III code 0021T)

59400 Routine obstetric care including antepartum care, vaginal delivery (with or without episiotomy, and/or forceps) and postpartum care

59409 Vaginal delivery only (with or without episiotomy and/or forceps);

59410 including postpartum care

59412 External cephalic version, with or without tocolysis

(Use 59412 in addition to code(s) for delivery)

59414 Delivery of placenta (separate procedure)

(For antepartum care only, see 59425, 59426 or appropriate E/M code(s))

(For 1-3 antepartum care visits, see appropriate E/M code(s))

59425 Antepartum care only; 4-6 visits

59426 7 or more visits

59430 Postpartum care only (separate procedure)

Cesarean Delivery

(For insertion of transcervical or transvaginal fetal oximetry sensor, use Category III code 0021T)

(For standby attendance for infant, use 99360)

(For low cervical Cesarean section, see 59510, 59515, 59525)

59510 Routine obstetric care including antepartum care, cesarean delivery, and postpartum care

59514 Cesarean delivery only;

59515 including postpartum care

(For classic Cesarean section, see 59510, 59515, 59525)

✦ 59525 Subtotal or total hysterectomy after cesarean delivery (List separately in addition to code for primary procedure)

(Use 59525 in conjunction with 59510, 59514, 59515, 59618, 59620, 59622)

(For extraperitoneal Cesarean section, or Cesarean section with subtotal or total hysterectomy, see 59510, 59515, 59525)

Delivery After Previous Cesarean Delivery

Patients who have had a previous cesarean delivery and now present with the expectation of a vaginal delivery are coded using codes 59610-59622. If the patient has a successful vaginal delivery after a previous cesarean delivery (VBAC), use codes 59610-59614. If the attempt is unsuccessful and another cesarean delivery is carried out, use codes 59618-59622. To report elective cesarean deliveries use code 59510, 59514 or 59515.

(For insertion of transcervical or transvaginal fetal oximetry sensor, use Category III code 0021T)

59610 Routine obstetric care including antepartum care, vaginal delivery (with or without episiotomy, and/or forceps) and postpartum care, after previous cesarean delivery

59612 Vaginal delivery only, after previous cesarean delivery (with or without episiotomy and/or forceps);

59614 including postpartum care

59618 Routine obstetric care including antepartum care, cesarean delivery, and postpartum care, following attempted vaginal delivery after previous cesarean delivery

59620 Cesarean delivery only, following attempted vaginal delivery after previous cesarean delivery;

59622 including postpartum care

Abortion

(For medical treatment of spontaneous complete abortion, any trimester, use E/M codes 99201-99233)

(For surgical treatment of spontaneous abortion, use 59812)

59812 Treatment of incomplete abortion, any trimester, completed surgically

59820 Treatment of missed abortion, completed surgically; first trimester

59821 second trimester

59830 Treatment of septic abortion, completed surgically

59840	Induced abortion, by dilation and curettage
59841	Induced abortion, by dilation and evacuation
59850	Induced abortion, by one or more intra-amniotic injections (amniocentesis-injections), including hospital admission and visits, delivery of fetus and secundines;
59851	with dilation and curettage and/or evacuation
59852	with hysterotomy (failed intra-amniotic injection)
	(For insertion of cervical dilator, use 59200)
59855	Induced abortion, by one or more vaginal suppositories (eg, prostaglandin) with or without cervical dilation (eg, laminaria), including hospital admission and visits, delivery of fetus and secundines;
59856	with dilation and curettage and/or evacuation
59857	with hysterotomy (failed medical evacuation)

Other Procedures

59866	Multifetal pregnancy reduction(s) (MPR)
59870	Uterine evacuation and curettage for hydatidiform mole
59871	Removal of cerclage suture under anesthesia (other than local)
59897	Unlisted fetal invasive procedure, including ultrasound guidance
59898	Unlisted laparoscopy procedure, maternity care and delivery
59899	Unlisted procedure, maternity care and delivery

Surgery: Male/Female Genital System

Notes

⊘ =Modifier 51 Exempt   ⊙ =Conscious Sedation   ✚ =Add-on Code

Endocrine System

(For pituitary and pineal surgery, see **Nervous System**)

Thyroid Gland

Incision

60000   Incision and drainage of thyroglossal duct cyst, infected

Excision

60001   Aspiration and/or injection, thyroid cyst

             (For fine needle aspiration, see 10021, 10022)

             (If imaging guidance is performed, see 76360, 76942)

60100   Biopsy thyroid, percutaneous core needle

             (If imaging guidance is performed, see 76003, 76360, 76393, 76942)

             (For fine needle aspiration, use 10021 or 10022)

             (For evaluation of fine needle aspirate, see 88172, 88173)

60200   Excision of cyst or adenoma of thyroid, or transection of isthmus

60210   Partial thyroid lobectomy, unilateral; with or without isthmusectomy

60212   with contralateral subtotal lobectomy, including isthmusectomy

60220   Total thyroid lobectomy, unilateral; with or without isthmusectomy

60225   with contralateral subtotal lobectomy, including isthmusectomy

60240   Thyroidectomy, total or complete

             (For thyroidectomy, subtotal or partial, use 60271)

60252   Thyroidectomy, total or subtotal for malignancy; with limited neck dissection

60254   with radical neck dissection

60260   Thyroidectomy, removal of all remaining thyroid tissue following previous removal of a portion of thyroid

             (For bilateral procedure, report 60260 with modifier 50)

60270   Thyroidectomy, including substernal thyroid; sternal split or transthoracic approach

60271   cervical approach

60280   Excision of thyroglossal duct cyst or sinus;

60281   recurrent

             (For thyroid ultrasonography, use 76536)

Parathyroid, Thymus, Adrenal Glands, Pancreas, and Carotid Body

Excision

(For pituitary and pineal surgery, see **Nervous System**)

60500   Parathyroidectomy or exploration of parathyroid(s);

60502   re-exploration

60505   with mediastinal exploration, sternal split or transthoracic approach

+ 60512   Parathyroid autotransplantation (List separately in addition to code for primary procedure)

             (Use 60512 in conjunction with 60500, 60502, 60505, 60212, 60225, 60240, 60252, 60254, 60260, 60270, 60271)

60520   Thymectomy, partial or total; transcervical approach (separate procedure)

60521   sternal split or transthoracic approach, without radical mediastinal dissection (separate procedure)

60522   sternal split or transthoracic approach, with radical mediastinal dissection (separate procedure)

60540   Adrenalectomy, partial or complete, or exploration of adrenal gland with or without biopsy, transabdominal, lumbar or dorsal (separate procedure);

60545   with excision of adjacent retroperitoneal tumor

             ▶(Do not report 60540, 60545 in conjunction with 50323)◀

             (For bilateral procedure, report 60540 with modifier 50)

             (For excision of remote or disseminated pheochromocytoma, see 49200, 49201)

             (For laparoscopic approach, use 60650)

60600   Excision of carotid body tumor; without excision of carotid artery

60605   with excision of carotid artery

Laparoscopy

Surgical laparoscopy always includes diagnostic laparoscopy. To report a diagnostic laparoscopy (peritoneoscopy) (separate procedure), use 49320.

60650   Laparoscopy, surgical, with adrenalectomy, partial or complete, or exploration of adrenal gland with or without biopsy, transabdominal, lumbar or dorsal

60659   Unlisted laparoscopy procedure, endocrine system

Other Procedures

60699   Unlisted procedure, endocrine system

Surgery: Nervous System

Notes

⃠ =Modifier 51 Exempt   ⊙ =Conscious Sedation   ✚ =Add-on Code

Nervous System

Skull, Meninges, and Brain

(For injection procedure for cerebral angiography, see 36100-36218)

(For injection procedure for ventriculography, see 61026, 61120)

(For injection procedure for pneumoencephalography, use 61055)

Injection, Drainage, or Aspiration

61000   Subdural tap through fontanelle, or suture, infant, unilateral or bilateral; initial

61001   subsequent taps

61020   Ventricular puncture through previous burr hole, fontanelle, suture, or implanted ventricular catheter/reservoir; without injection

61026   with injection of medication or other substance for diagnosis or treatment

61050   Cisternal or lateral cervical (C1-C2) puncture; without injection (separate procedure)

61055   with injection of medication or other substance for diagnosis or treatment (eg, C1-C2)

(For radiological supervision and interpretation, see **Radiology**)

61070   Puncture of shunt tubing or reservoir for aspiration or injection procedure

(For radiological supervision and interpretation, use 75809)

Twist Drill, Burr Hole(s), or Trephine

61105   Twist drill hole for subdural or ventricular puncture;

⊘ **61107**   for implanting ventricular catheter or pressure recording device

(For intracranial neuroendoscopic ventricular catheter placement, use 62160)

►(For twist drill or burr hole performed to place thermal perfusion probe, use Category III code 0077T)◄

61108   for evacuation and/or drainage of subdural hematoma

61120   Burr hole(s) for ventricular puncture (including injection of gas, contrast media, dye, or radioactive material)

61140   Burr hole(s) or trephine; with biopsy of brain or intracranial lesion

61150   with drainage of brain abscess or cyst

61151   with subsequent tapping (aspiration) of intracranial abscess or cyst

61154   Burr hole(s) with evacuation and/or drainage of hematoma, extradural or subdural

(For bilateral procedure, report 61154 with modifier 50)

61156   Burr hole(s); with aspiration of hematoma or cyst, intracerebral

⊘ **61210**   for implanting ventricular catheter, reservoir, EEG electrode(s) or pressure recording device (separate procedure)

(For intracranial neuroendoscopic ventricular catheter placement, use 62160)

61215   Insertion of subcutaneous reservoir, pump or continuous infusion system for connection to ventricular catheter

(For refilling and maintenance of an implantable infusion pump for spinal or brain drug therapy, use 95990)

(For chemotherapy, use 96450)

61250   Burr hole(s) or trephine, supratentorial, exploratory, not followed by other surgery

(For bilateral procedure, report 61250 with modifier 50)

61253   Burr hole(s) or trephine, infratentorial, unilateral or bilateral

(If burr hole(s) or trephine are followed by craniotomy at same operative session, use 61304-61321; do not use 61250 or 61253)

Craniectomy or Craniotomy

61304   Craniectomy or craniotomy, exploratory; supratentorial

61305   infratentorial (posterior fossa)

61312   Craniectomy or craniotomy for evacuation of hematoma, supratentorial; extradural or subdural

61313   intracerebral

61314   Craniectomy or craniotomy for evacuation of hematoma, infratentorial; extradural or subdural

61315   intracerebellar

+ **61316**   Incision and subcutaneous placement of cranial bone graft (List separately in addition to code for primary procedure)

(Use 61316 in conjunction with 61304, 61312, 61313, 61322, 61323, 61340, 61570, 61571, 61680-61705)

61320   Craniectomy or craniotomy, drainage of intracranial abscess; supratentorial

61321   infratentorial

61322   Craniectomy or craniotomy, decompressive, with or without duraplasty, for treatment of intracranial hypertension, without evacuation of associated intraparenchymal hematoma; without lobectomy

(Do not report 61313 in addition to 61322)

(For subtemporal decompression, use 61340)

Surgery: Nervous System

61323   with lobectomy

(Do not report 61313 in addition to 61323)

(For subtemporal decompression, use 61340)

61330   Decompression of orbit only, transcranial approach

(For bilateral procedure, report 61330 with modifier 50)

61332   Exploration of orbit (transcranial approach); with biopsy

61333   with removal of lesion

61334   with removal of foreign body

61340   Subtemporal cranial decompression (pseudotumor cerebri, slit ventricle syndrome)

(For bilateral procedure, report 61340 with modifier 50)

(For decompressive craniotomy or craniectomy for intracranial hypertension, without hematoma evacuation, see 61322, 61323)

61343   Craniectomy, suboccipital with cervical laminectomy for decompression of medulla and spinal cord, with or without dural graft (eg, Arnold-Chiari malformation)

61345   Other cranial decompression, posterior fossa

(For orbital decompression by lateral wall approach, Kroenlein type, use 67445)

61440   Craniotomy for section of tentorium cerebelli (separate procedure)

61450   Craniectomy, subtemporal, for section, compression, or decompression of sensory root of gasserian ganglion

61458   Craniectomy, suboccipital; for exploration or decompression of cranial nerves

61460   for section of one or more cranial nerves

61470   for medullary tractotomy

61480   for mesencephalic tractotomy or pedunculotomy

61490   Craniotomy for lobotomy, including cingulotomy

(For bilateral procedure, report 61490 with modifier 50)

61500   Craniectomy; with excision of tumor or other bone lesion of skull

61501   for osteomyelitis

61510   Craniectomy, trephination, bone flap craniotomy; for excision of brain tumor, supratentorial, except meningioma

61512   for excision of meningioma, supratentorial

61514   for excision of brain abscess, supratentorial

61516   for excision or fenestration of cyst, supratentorial

(For excision of pituitary tumor or craniopharyngioma, see 61545, 61546, 61548)

+ 61517   Implantation of brain intracavitary chemotherapy agent (List separately in addition to code for primary procedure)

(Use 61517 only in conjunction with 61510 or 61518)

(Do not report 61517 for brachytherapy insertion. For intracavitary insertion of radioelement sources or ribbons, see 77781-77784)

61518   Craniectomy for excision of brain tumor, infratentorial or posterior fossa; except meningioma, cerebellopontine angle tumor, or midline tumor at base of skull

61519   meningioma

61520   cerebellopontine angle tumor

61521   midline tumor at base of skull

61522   Craniectomy, infratentorial or posterior fossa; for excision of brain abscess

61524   for excision or fenestration of cyst

61526   Craniectomy, bone flap craniotomy, transtemporal (mastoid) for excision of cerebellopontine angle tumor;

61530   combined with middle/posterior fossa craniotomy/craniectomy

61531   Subdural implantation of strip electrodes through one or more burr or trephine hole(s) for long term seizure monitoring

(For stereotactic implantation of electrodes, use 61760)

(For craniotomy for excision of intracranial arteriovenous malformation, see 61680-61692)

61533   Craniotomy with elevation of bone flap; for subdural implantation of an electrode array, for long term seizure monitoring

(For continuous EEG monitoring, see 95950-95954)

61534   for excision of epileptogenic focus without electrocorticography during surgery

61535   for removal of epidural or subdural electrode array, without excision of cerebral tissue (separate procedure)

61536   for excision of cerebral epileptogenic focus, with electrocorticography during surgery (includes removal of electrode array)

61537   for lobectomy, temporal lobe, without electrocorticography during surgery

61538   for lobectomy, temporal lobe, with electrocorticography during surgery

61539   for lobectomy, other than temporal lobe, partial or total, with electrocorticography during surgery

61540   for lobectomy, other than temporal lobe, partial or total, without electrocorticography during surgery

61541   for transection of corpus callosum

61542   for total hemispherectomy

Surgery: Nervous System

61543   for partial or subtotal (functional) hemispherectomy

61544   for excision or coagulation of choroid plexus

61545   for excision of craniopharyngioma

(For craniotomy for selective amygdalohippocampectomy, use 61566)

(For craniotomy for multiple subpial transections during surgery, use 61567)

61546   Craniotomy for hypophysectomy or excision of pituitary tumor, intracranial approach

61548   Hypophysectomy or excision of pituitary tumor, transnasal or transseptal approach, nonstereotactic

(Do not report code 69990 in addition to code 61548)

61550   Craniectomy for craniosynostosis; single cranial suture

61552   multiple cranial sutures

(For cranial reconstruction for orbital hypertelorism, see 21260-21263)

(For reconstruction, see 21172-21180)

61556   Craniotomy for craniosynostosis; frontal or parietal bone flap

61557   bifrontal bone flap

61558   Extensive craniectomy for multiple cranial suture craniosynostosis (eg, cloverleaf skull); not requiring bone grafts

61559   recontouring with multiple osteotomies and bone autografts (eg, barrel-stave procedure) (includes obtaining grafts)

(For reconstruction, see 21172-21180)

61563   Excision, intra and extracranial, benign tumor of cranial bone (eg, fibrous dysplasia); without optic nerve decompression

61564   with optic nerve decompression

(For reconstruction, see 21181-21183)

61566   Craniotomy with elevation of bone flap; for selective amygdalohippocampectomy

61567   for multiple subpial transections, with electrocorticography during surgery

61570   Craniectomy or craniotomy; with excision of foreign body from brain

61571   with treatment of penetrating wound of brain

(For sequestrectomy for osteomyelitis, use 61501)

61575   Transoral approach to skull base, brain stem or upper spinal cord for biopsy, decompression or excision of lesion;

61576   requiring splitting of tongue and/or mandible (including tracheostomy)

(For arthrodesis, use 22548)

Surgery of Skull Base

The surgical management of lesions involving the skull base (base of anterior, middle, and posterior cranial fossae) often requires the skills of several surgeons of different surgical specialties working together or in tandem during the operative session. These operations are usually not staged because of the need for definitive closure of dura, subcutaneous tissues, and skin to avoid serious infections such as osteomyelitis and/or meningitis.

The procedures are categorized according to: 1) *approach procedure* necessary to obtain adequate exposure to the lesion (pathologic entity), 2) *definitive procedure(s)* necessary to biopsy, excise or otherwise treat the lesion, and 3) *repair/reconstruction* of the defect present following the definitive procedure(s).

The *approach procedure* is described according to anatomical area involved, ie, anterior cranial fossa, middle cranial fossa, posterior cranial fossa, and brain stem or upper spinal cord.

The *definitive procedure(s)* describes the repair, biopsy, resection, or excision of various lesions of the skull base and, when appropriate, primary closure of the dura, mucous membranes, and skin.

The *repair/reconstruction procedure(s)* is reported separately if extensive dural grafting, cranioplasty, local or regional myocutaneous pedicle flaps, or extensive skin grafts are required.

For primary closure, see the appropriate codes, ie, 15732, 15756-15758.

When one surgeon performs the approach procedure, another surgeon performs the definitive procedure, and another surgeon performs the repair/reconstruction procedure, each surgeon reports only the code for the specific procedure performed.

If one surgeon performs more than one procedure (ie, approach procedure and definitive procedure), then both codes are reported, adding modifier 51 to the secondary, additional procedure(s).

Approach Procedures

Anterior Cranial Fossa

61580   Craniofacial approach to anterior cranial fossa; extradural, including lateral rhinotomy, ethmoidectomy, sphenoidectomy, without maxillectomy or orbital exenteration

61581   extradural, including lateral rhinotomy, orbital exenteration, ethmoidectomy, sphenoidectomy and/or maxillectomy

Surgery: Nervous System

61582   extradural, including unilateral or bifrontal craniotomy, elevation of frontal lobe(s), osteotomy of base of anterior cranial fossa

61583   intradural, including unilateral or bifrontal craniotomy, elevation or resection of frontal lobe, osteotomy of base of anterior cranial fossa

61584   Orbitocranial approach to anterior cranial fossa, extradural, including supraorbital ridge osteotomy and elevation of frontal and/or temporal lobe(s); without orbital exenteration

61585   with orbital exenteration

61586   Bicoronal, transzygomatic and/or LeFort I osteotomy approach to anterior cranial fossa with or without internal fixation, without bone graft

Middle Cranial Fossa

61590   Infratemporal pre-auricular approach to middle cranial fossa (parapharyngeal space, infratemporal and midline skull base, nasopharynx), with or without disarticulation of the mandible, including parotidectomy, craniotomy, decompression and/or mobilization of the facial nerve and/or petrous carotid artery

61591   Infratemporal post-auricular approach to middle cranial fossa (internal auditory meatus, petrous apex, tentorium, cavernous sinus, parasellar area, infratemporal fossa) including mastoidectomy, resection of sigmoid sinus, with or without decompression and/or mobilization of contents of auditory canal or petrous carotid artery

61592   Orbitocranial zygomatic approach to middle cranial fossa (cavernous sinus and carotid artery, clivus, basilar artery or petrous apex) including osteotomy of zygoma, craniotomy, extra- or intradural elevation of temporal lobe

Posterior Cranial Fossa

61595   Transtemporal approach to posterior cranial fossa, jugular foramen or midline skull base, including mastoidectomy, decompression of sigmoid sinus and/or facial nerve, with or without mobilization

61596   Transcochlear approach to posterior cranial fossa, jugular foramen or midline skull base, including labyrinthectomy, decompression, with or without mobilization of facial nerve and/or petrous carotid artery

61597   Transcondylar (far lateral) approach to posterior cranial fossa, jugular foramen or midline skull base, including occipital condylectomy, mastoidectomy, resection of C1-C3 vertebral body(s), decompression of vertebral artery, with or without mobilization

61598   Transpetrosal approach to posterior cranial fossa, clivus or foramen magnum, including ligation of superior petrosal sinus and/or sigmoid sinus

Definitive Procedures

Base of Anterior Cranial Fossa

61600   Resection or excision of neoplastic, vascular or infectious lesion of base of anterior cranial fossa; extradural

61601   intradural, including dural repair, with or without graft

Base of Middle Cranial Fossa

61605   Resection or excision of neoplastic, vascular or infectious lesion of infratemporal fossa, parapharyngeal space, petrous apex; extradural

61606   intradural, including dural repair, with or without graft

61607   Resection or excision of neoplastic, vascular or infectious lesion of parasellar area, cavernous sinus, clivus or midline skull base; extradural

61608   intradural, including dural repair, with or without graft

Codes 61609-61612 are reported in addition to code(s) for primary procedure(s) 61605-61608. Report only one transection or ligation of carotid artery code per operative session.

+ 61609   Transection or ligation, carotid artery in cavernous sinus; without repair (List separately in addition to code for primary procedure)

+ 61610   with repair by anastomosis or graft (List separately in addition to code for primary procedure)

+ 61611   Transection or ligation, carotid artery in petrous canal; without repair (List separately in addition to code for primary procedure)

+ 61612   with repair by anastomosis or graft (List separately in addition to code for primary procedure)

61613   Obliteration of carotid aneurysm, arteriovenous malformation, or carotid-cavernous fistula by dissection within cavernous sinus

Base of Posterior Cranial Fossa

61615   Resection or excision of neoplastic, vascular or infectious lesion of base of posterior cranial fossa, jugular foramen, foramen magnum, or C1-C3 vertebral bodies; extradural

61616   intradural, including dural repair, with or without graft

Repair and/or Reconstruction of Surgical Defects of Skull Base

61618   Secondary repair of dura for cerebrospinal fluid leak, anterior, middle or posterior cranial fossa following surgery of the skull base; by free tissue graft (eg, pericranium, fascia, tensor fascia lata, adipose tissue, homologous or synthetic grafts)

61619   by local or regionalized vascularized pedicle flap or myocutaneous flap (including galea, temporalis, frontalis or occipitalis muscle)

Surgery: Nervous System

Endovascular Therapy

61623   Endovascular temporary balloon arterial occlusion, head or neck (extracranial/intracranial) including selective catheterization of vessel to be occluded, positioning and inflation of occlusion balloon, concomitant neurological monitoring, and radiologic supervision and interpretation of all angiography required for balloon occlusion and to exclude vascular injury post occlusion

(If selective catheterization and angiography of arteries other than artery to be occluded is performed, use appropriate catheterization and radiologic supervision and interpretation codes)

(If complete diagnostic angiography of the artery to be occluded is performed immediately prior to temporary occlusion, use appropriate radiologic supervision and interpretation codes only)

61624   Transcatheter permanent occlusion or embolization (eg, for tumor destruction, to achieve hemostasis, to occlude a vascular malformation), percutaneous, any method; central nervous system (intracranial, spinal cord)

(See also 37204)

(For radiological supervision and interpretation, use 75894)

61626   non-central nervous system, head or neck (extracranial, brachiocephalic branch)

(See also 37204)

(For radiological supervision and interpretation, use 75894)

Surgery for Aneurysm, Arteriovenous Malformation or Vascular Disease

Includes craniotomy when appropriate for procedure.

61680   Surgery of intracranial arteriovenous malformation; supratentorial, simple

61682   supratentorial, complex

61684   infratentorial, simple

61686   infratentorial, complex

61690   dural, simple

61692   dural, complex

61697   Surgery of complex intracranial aneurysm, intracranial approach; carotid circulation

61698   vertebrobasilar circulation

(61697, 61698 involve aneurysms that are larger than 15 mm or with calcification of the aneurysm neck, or with incorporation of normal vessels into the aneurysm neck, or a procedure requiring temporary vessel occlusion, trapping or cardiopulmonary bypass to successfully treat the aneurysm)

61700   Surgery of simple intracranial aneurysm, intracranial approach; carotid circulation

61702   vertebrobasilar circulation

61703   Surgery of intracranial aneurysm, cervical approach by application of occluding clamp to cervical carotid artery (Selverstone-Crutchfield type)

(For cervical approach for direct ligation of carotid artery, see 37600-37606)

61705   Surgery of aneurysm, vascular malformation or carotid-cavernous fistula; by intracranial and cervical occlusion of carotid artery

61708   by intracranial electrothrombosis

(For ligation or gradual occlusion of internal/common carotid artery, see 37605, 37606)

61710   by intra-arterial embolization, injection procedure, or balloon catheter

61711   Anastomosis, arterial, extracranial-intracranial (eg, middle cerebral/cortical) arteries

(For carotid or vertebral thromboendarterectomy, use 35301)

(Use 69990 when the surgical microscope is employed for the microsurgical procedure. Do not use 69990 for visualization with magnifying loupes or corrected vision)

Stereotaxis

61720   Creation of lesion by stereotactic method, including burr hole(s) and localizing and recording techniques, single or multiple stages; globus pallidus or thalamus

61735   subcortical structure(s) other than globus pallidus or thalamus

61750   Stereotactic biopsy, aspiration, or excision, including burr hole(s), for intracranial lesion;

61751   with computed tomography and/or magnetic resonance guidance

(For radiological supervision and interpretation of computerized tomography, see 70450, 70460, or 70470 as appropriate)

(For radiological supervision and interpretation of magnetic resonance imaging, see 70551, 70552, or 70553 as appropriate)

61760   Stereotactic implantation of depth electrodes into the cerebrum for long term seizure monitoring

61770   Stereotactic localization, including burr hole(s), with insertion of catheter(s) or probe(s) for placement of radiation source

61790   Creation of lesion by stereotactic method, percutaneous, by neurolytic agent (eg, alcohol, thermal, electrical, radiofrequency); gasserian ganglion

61791   trigeminal medullary tract

Surgery: Nervous System

61793 Stereotactic radiosurgery (particle beam, gamma ray or linear accelerator), one or more sessions

(For intensity modulated beam delivery plan and treatment, see 77301, 77418)

+ 61795 Stereotactic computer assisted volumetric (navigational) procedure, intracranial, extracranial, or spinal (List separately in addition to code for primary procedure)

Neurostimulators (Intracranial)

Codes 61850-61888 apply to both simple and complex neurostimulators. For initial or subsequent electronic analysis and programming of neurostimulator pulse generators, see codes 95970-95975.

Microelectrode recording, when performed by the operating surgeon in association with implantation of neurostimulator electrode arrays, is an inclusive service and should not be reported separately. If another physician participates in neurophysiological mapping during a deep brain stimulator implantation procedure, this service may be reported by the other physician with codes 95961-95962.

61850 Twist drill or burr hole(s) for implantation of neurostimulator electrodes, cortical

61860 Craniectomy or craniotomy for implantation of neurostimulator electrodes, cerebral, cortical

(61862 has been deleted. To report, see 61867, 61868)

61863 Twist drill, burr hole, craniotomy, or craniectomy with stereotactic implantation of neurostimulator electrode array in subcortical site (eg, thalamus, globus pallidus, subthalamic nucleus, periventricular, periaqueductal gray), without use of intraoperative microelectrode recording; first array

+ 61864 each additional array (List separately in addition to primary procedure)

(Use 61864 in conjunction with 61863)

(61865 has been deleted. To report, use 61867, 61868)

61867 Twist drill, burr hole, craniotomy, or craniectomy with stereotactic implantation of neurostimulator electrode array in subcortical site (eg, thalamus, globus pallidus, subthalamic nucleus, periventricular, periaqueductal gray), with use of intraoperative microelectrode recording; first array

+ 61868 each additional array (List separately in addition to primary procedure)

(Use 61868 in conjunction with 61867)

61870 Craniectomy for implantation of neurostimulator electrodes, cerebellar; cortical

61875 subcortical

61880 Revision or removal of intracranial neurostimulator electrodes

▲ 61885 Insertion or replacement of cranial neurostimulator pulse generator or receiver, direct or inductive coupling; with connection to a single electrode array

61886 with connection to two or more electrode arrays

(For open placement of cranial nerve (eg, vagal, trigeminal) neurostimulator electrode(s), use 64573)

(For percutaneous placement of cranial nerve (eg, vagal, trigeminal) neurostimulator electrode(s), use 64553)

(For revision or removal of cranial nerve (eg, vagal, trigeminal) neurostimulator electrode(s), use 64585)

61888 Revision or removal of cranial neurostimulator pulse generator or receiver

▶(Do not report 61888 in conjunction with 61885 or 61886 for the same pulse generator)◀

Repair

62000 Elevation of depressed skull fracture; simple, extradural

62005 compound or comminuted, extradural

62010 with repair of dura and/or debridement of brain

62100 Craniotomy for repair of dural/cerebrospinal fluid leak, including surgery for rhinorrhea/otorrhea

(For repair of spinal dural/CSF leak, see 63707, 63709)

62115 Reduction of craniomegalic skull (eg, treated hydrocephalus); not requiring bone grafts or cranioplasty

62116 with simple cranioplasty

62117 requiring craniotomy and reconstruction with or without bone graft (includes obtaining grafts)

62120 Repair of encephalocele, skull vault, including cranioplasty

62121 Craniotomy for repair of encephalocele, skull base

62140 Cranioplasty for skull defect; up to 5 cm diameter

62141 larger than 5 cm diameter

62142 Removal of bone flap or prosthetic plate of skull

62143 Replacement of bone flap or prosthetic plate of skull

62145 Cranioplasty for skull defect with reparative brain surgery

62146 Cranioplasty with autograft (includes obtaining bone grafts); up to 5 cm diameter

62147 larger than 5 cm diameter

+ 62148 Incision and retrieval of subcutaneous cranial bone graft for cranioplasty (List separately in addition to code for primary procedure)

(Use 62148 in conjunction with 62140-62147)

Surgery: Nervous System

Neuroendoscopy

Surgical endoscopy always includes diagnostic endoscopy.

+ 62160   Neuroendoscopy, intracranial, for placement or replacement of ventricular catheter and attachment to shunt system or external drainage (List separately in addition to code for primary procedure)

(Use 62160 only in conjunction with 61107, 61210, 62220, 62223, 62225, or 62230)

62161   Neuroendoscopy, intracranial; with dissection of adhesions, fenestration of septum pellucidum or intraventricular cysts (including placement, replacement, or removal of ventricular catheter)

62162   with fenestration or excision of colloid cyst, including placement of external ventricular catheter for drainage

62163   with retrieval of foreign body

62164   with excision of brain tumor, including placement of external ventricular catheter for drainage

62165   with excision of pituitary tumor, transnasal or transsphenoidal approach

Cerebrospinal Fluid (CSF) Shunt

62180   Ventriculocisternostomy (Torkildsen type operation)

62190   Creation of shunt; subarachnoid/subdural-atrial, -jugular, -auricular

62192   subarachnoid/subdural-peritoneal, -pleural, other terminus

62194   Replacement or irrigation, subarachnoid/subdural catheter

62200   Ventriculocisternostomy, third ventricle;

62201   stereotactic, neuroendoscopic method

(For intracranial neuroendoscopic procedures, see 62161-62165)

62220   Creation of shunt; ventriculo-atrial, -jugular, -auricular

(For intracranial neuroendoscopic ventricular catheter placement, use 62160)

62223   ventriculo-peritoneal, -pleural, other terminus

(For intracranial neuroendoscopic ventricular catheter placement, use 62160)

62225   Replacement or irrigation, ventricular catheter

(For intracranial neuroendoscopic ventricular catheter placement, use 62160)

62230   Replacement or revision of cerebrospinal fluid shunt, obstructed valve, or distal catheter in shunt system

(For intracranial neuroendoscopic ventricular catheter placement, use 62160)

62252   Reprogramming of programmable cerebrospinal shunt

62256   Removal of complete cerebrospinal fluid shunt system; without replacement

62258   with replacement by similar or other shunt at same operation

(For percutaneous irrigation or aspiration of shunt reservoir, use 61070)

(For reprogramming of programmable CSF shunt, use 62252)

Spine and Spinal Cord

(For application of caliper or tongs, use 20660)

(For treatment of fracture or dislocation of spine, see 22305-22327)

Injection, Drainage, or Aspiration

Injection of contrast during fluoroscopic guidance and localization is an inclusive component of codes 62263-62264, 62270-62273, 62280-62282, 62310-62319, 0027T. Fluoroscopic guidance and localization is reported by code 76005, unless a formal contrast study (myelography, epidurography, or arthrography) is performed, in which case the use of fluoroscopy is included in the supervision and interpretation codes.

For radiologic supervision and interpretation of epidurography, use 72275. Code 72275 is only to be used when an epidurogram is performed, images documented, and a formal radiologic report is issued.

Code 62263 describes a catheter-based treatment involving targeted injection of various substances (eg, hypertonic saline, steroid, anesthetic) via an indwelling epidural catheter. Code 62263 includes percutaneous insertion and removal of an epidural catheter (remaining in place over a several-day period), for the administration of multiple injections of a neurolytic agent(s) performed during serial treatment sessions (ie, spanning two or more treatment days). If required, adhesions or scarring may also be lysed by mechanical means. Code 62263 is NOT reported for each adhesiolysis treatment, but should be reported ONCE to describe the entire series of injections/infusions spanning two or more treatment days. For endoscopic lysis of adhesions, use 0027T.

Code 62264 describes multiple adhesiolysis treatment sessions performed on the same day. Adhesions or scarring may be lysed by injections of neurolytic agent(s). If required, adhesions or scarring may also be lysed mechanically using a percutaneously-deployed catheter.

Codes 62263 and 62264 include the procedure of injections of contrast for epidurography (72275) and fluoroscopic guidance and localization (76005) during initial or subsequent sessions.

Surgery: Nervous System

(Report 01996 for daily hospital management of continuous epidural or subarachnoid drug administration performed in conjunction with 62318-62319)

(For endoscopic lysis of epidural adhesions, use Category III code 0027T)

62263 Percutaneous lysis of epidural adhesions using solution injection (eg, hypertonic saline, enzyme) or mechanical means (eg, catheter) including radiologic localization (includes contrast when administered), multiple adhesiolysis sessions; 2 or more days

(62263 includes codes 76005 and 72275)

62264 1 day

(Do not report 62264 with 62263)

(62264 includes codes 76005 and 72275)

62268 Percutaneous aspiration, spinal cord cyst or syrinx

(For radiological supervision and interpretation, see 76003, 76360, 76942)

62269 Biopsy of spinal cord, percutaneous needle

(For radiological supervision and interpretation, see 76003, 76360, 76942)

(For fine needle aspiration, see 10021, 10022)

(For evaluation of fine needle aspirate, see 88172, 88173)

62270 Spinal puncture, lumbar, diagnostic

62272 Spinal puncture, therapeutic, for drainage of cerebrospinal fluid (by needle or catheter)

62273 Injection, epidural, of blood or clot patch

(For injection of diagnostic or therapeutic substance(s), see 62310, 62311, 62318, 62319)

62280 Injection/infusion of neurolytic substance (eg, alcohol, phenol, iced saline solutions), with or without other therapeutic substance; subarachnoid

62281 epidural, cervical or thoracic

62282 epidural, lumbar, sacral (caudal)

⊘ **62284** Injection procedure for myelography and/or computed tomography, spinal (other than C1-C2 and posterior fossa)

(For injection procedure at C1-C2, use 61055)

(For radiological supervision and interpretation, see **Radiology**)

62287 Aspiration or decompression procedure, percutaneous, of nucleus pulposus of intervertebral disk, any method, single or multiple levels, lumbar (eg, manual or automated percutaneous diskectomy, percutaneous laser diskectomy)

(For fluoroscopic guidance, use 76003)

(For injection of non-neurolytic diagnostic or therapeutic substance(s), see 62310, 62311)

62290 Injection procedure for diskography, each level; lumbar

62291 cervical or thoracic

(For radiological supervision and interpretation, see 72285, 72295)

62292 Injection procedure for chemonucleolysis, including diskography, intervertebral disk, single or multiple levels, lumbar

62294 Injection procedure, arterial, for occlusion of arteriovenous malformation, spinal

62310 Injection, single (not via indwelling catheter), not including neurolytic substances, with or without contrast (for either localization or epidurography), of diagnostic or therapeutic substance(s) (including anesthetic, antispasmodic, opioid, steroid, other solution), epidural or subarachnoid; cervical or thoracic

62311 lumbar, sacral (caudal)

62318 Injection, including catheter placement, continuous infusion or intermittent bolus, not including neurolytic substances, with or without contrast (for either localization or epidurography), of diagnostic or therapeutic substance(s) (including anesthetic, antispasmodic, opioid, steroid, other solution), epidural or subarachnoid; cervical or thoracic

62319 lumbar, sacral (caudal)

(For transforaminal epidural injection, see 64479-64484)

(Report 01996 for daily hospital management of continuous epidural or subarachnoid drug administration performed in conjunction with 62318-62319)

Catheter Implantation

(For percutaneous placement of intrathecal or epidural catheter, see codes 62270-62273, 62280-62284, 62310-62319)

62350 Implantation, revision or repositioning of tunneled intrathecal or epidural catheter, for long-term medication administration via an external pump or implantable reservoir/infusion pump; without laminectomy

62351 with laminectomy

(For refilling and maintenance of an implantable infusion pump for spinal or brain drug therapy, use 95990)

62355 Removal of previously implanted intrathecal or epidural catheter

Reservoir/Pump Implantation

62360 Implantation or replacement of device for intrathecal or epidural drug infusion; subcutaneous reservoir

62361 non-programmable pump

62362 programmable pump, including preparation of pump, with or without programming

62365   Removal of subcutaneous reservoir or pump, previously implanted for intrathecal or epidural infusion

62367   Electronic analysis of programmable, implanted pump for intrathecal or epidural drug infusion (includes evaluation of reservoir status, alarm status, drug prescription status); without reprogramming

62368   with reprogramming

(For refilling and maintenance of an implantable infusion pump for spinal or brain drug therapy, use 95990-95991)

Posterior Extradural Laminotomy or Laminectomy for Exploration/ Decompression of Neural Elements or Excision of Herniated Intervertebral Disks

(When 63001-63048 are followed by arthrodesis, see 22590-22614)

63001   Laminectomy with exploration and/or decompression of spinal cord and/or cauda equina, without facetectomy, foraminotomy or diskectomy, (eg, spinal stenosis), one or two vertebral segments; cervical

63003   thoracic

63005   lumbar, except for spondylolisthesis

63011   sacral

63012   Laminectomy with removal of abnormal facets and/or pars inter-articularis with decompression of cauda equina and nerve roots for spondylolisthesis, lumbar (Gill type procedure)

63015   Laminectomy with exploration and/or decompression of spinal cord and/or cauda equina, without facetectomy, foraminotomy or diskectomy, (eg, spinal stenosis), more than 2 vertebral segments; cervical

63016   thoracic

63017   lumbar

63020   Laminotomy (hemilaminectomy), with decompression of nerve root(s), including partial facetectomy, foraminotomy and/or excision of herniated intervertebral disk; one interspace, cervical

(For bilateral procedure, report 63020 with modifier 50)

63030   one interspace, lumbar (including open or endoscopically-assisted approach)

(For bilateral procedure, report 63030 with modifier 50)

+ 63035   each additional interspace, cervical or lumbar (List separately in addition to code for primary procedure)

(Use 63035 in conjunction with 63020-63030)

(For bilateral procedure, report 63035 with modifier 50)

63040   Laminotomy (hemilaminectomy), with decompression of nerve root(s), including partial facetectomy, foraminotomy and/or excision of herniated intervertebral disk, reexploration, single interspace; cervical

(For bilateral procedure, report 63040 with modifier 50)

63042   lumbar

(For bilateral procedure, report 63042 with modifier 50)

+ 63043   each additional cervical interspace (List separately in addition to code for primary procedure)

(Use 63043 in conjunction with 63040)

(For bilateral procedure, report 63043 with modifier 50)

+ 63044   each additional lumbar interspace (List separately in addition to code for primary procedure)

(Use 63044 in conjunction with 63042)

(For bilateral procedure, report 63044 with modifier 50)

63045   Laminectomy, facetectomy and foraminotomy (unilateral or bilateral with decompression of spinal cord, cauda equina and/or nerve root(s), (eg, spinal or lateral recess stenosis)), single vertebral segment; cervical

63046   thoracic

63047   lumbar

+ 63048   each additional segment, cervical, thoracic, or lumbar (List separately in addition to code for primary procedure)

(Use 63048 in conjunction with 63045-63047)

● 63050   Laminoplasty, cervical, with decompression of the spinal cord, two or more vertebral segments;

● 63051   with reconstruction of the posterior bony elements (including the application of bridging bone graft and non-segmental fixation devices (eg, wire, suture, mini-plates), when performed)

▶(Do not report 63050 or 63051 in conjunction with 22600, 22614, 22840-22842, 63001, 63015, 63045, 63048, 63295 for the same vertebral segment(s))◀

Transpedicular or Costovertebral Approach for Posterolateral Extradural Exploration/Decompression

63055   Transpedicular approach with decompression of spinal cord, equina and/or nerve root(s) (eg, herniated intervertebral disk), single segment; thoracic

63056   lumbar (including transfacet, or lateral extraforaminal approach) (eg, far lateral herniated intervertebral disk)

+ 63057   each additional segment, thoracic or lumbar (List separately in addition to code for primary procedure)

(Use 63057 in conjunction with 63055, 63056)

Surgery: Nervous System

63064 Costovertebral approach with decompression of spinal cord or nerve root(s), (eg, herniated intervertebral disk), thoracic; single segment

+ **63066** each additional segment (List separately in addition to code for primary procedure)

(Use 63066 in conjunction with 63064)

(For excision of thoracic intraspinal lesions by laminectomy, see 63266, 63271, 63276, 63281, 63286)

Anterior or Anterolateral Approach for Extradural Exploration/Decompression

For the following codes, when two surgeons work together as primary surgeons performing distinct part(s) of spinal cord exploration/decompression operation, each surgeon should report his/her distinct operative work by appending modifier 62 to the procedure code (and any associated add-on codes for that procedure code as long as both surgeons continue to work together as primary surgeons). In this situation, modifier 62 may be appended to the definitive procedure code(s) 63075, 63077, 63081, 63085, 63087, 63090 and, as appropriate, to associated additional interspace add-on code(s) 63076, 63078 or additional segment add-on code(s) 63082, 63086, 63088, 63091 as long as both surgeons continue to work together as primary surgeons.

63075 Diskectomy, anterior, with decompression of spinal cord and/or nerve root(s), including osteophytectomy; cervical, single interspace

+ **63076** cervical, each additional interspace (List separately in addition to code for primary procedure)

(Use 63076 in conjunction with 63075)

63077 thoracic, single interspace

+ **63078** thoracic, each additional interspace (List separately in addition to code for primary procedure)

(Use 63078 in conjunction with 63077)

(Do not report code 69990 in addition to codes 63075-63078)

63081 Vertebral corpectomy (vertebral body resection), partial or complete, anterior approach with decompression of spinal cord and/or nerve root(s); cervical, single segment

+ **63082** cervical, each additional segment (List separately in addition to code for primary procedure)

(Use 63082 in conjunction with 63081)

(For transoral approach, see 61575, 61576)

63085 Vertebral corpectomy (vertebral body resection), partial or complete, transthoracic approach with decompression of spinal cord and/or nerve root(s); thoracic, single segment

+ **63086** thoracic, each additional segment (List separately in addition to code for primary procedure)

(Use 63086 in conjunction with 63085)

63087 Vertebral corpectomy (vertebral body resection), partial or complete, combined thoracolumbar approach with decompression of spinal cord, cauda equina or nerve root(s), lower thoracic or lumbar; single segment

+ **63088** each additional segment (List separately in addition to code for primary procedure)

(Use 63088 in conjunction with 63087)

63090 Vertebral corpectomy (vertebral body resection), partial or complete, transperitoneal or retroperitoneal approach with decompression of spinal cord, cauda equina or nerve root(s), lower thoracic, lumbar, or sacral; single segment

+ **63091** each additional segment (List separately in addition to code for primary procedure)

(Use 63091 in conjunction with 63090)

(Procedures 63081-63091 include diskectomy above and/or below vertebral segment)

(If followed by arthrodesis, see 22548-22812)

(For reconstruction of spine, use appropriate vertebral corpectomy codes 63081-63091, bone graft codes 20930-20938, arthrodesis codes 22548-22812, and spinal instrumentation codes 22840-22855)

Lateral Extracavitary Approach for Extradural Exploration/Decompression

63101 Vertebral corpectomy (vertebral body resection), partial or complete, lateral extracavitary approach with decompression of spinal cord and/or nerve root(s) (eg, for tumor or retropulsed bone fragments); thoracic, single segment

63102 lumbar, single segment

+ **63103** thoracic or lumbar, each additional segment (List separately in addition to code for primary procedure)

(Use 63103 in conjunction with 63101 and 63102)

Incision

63170 Laminectomy with myelotomy (eg, Bischof or DREZ type), cervical, thoracic, or thoracolumbar

63172 Laminectomy with drainage of intramedullary cyst/syrinx; to subarachnoid space

63173 to peritoneal or pleural space

63180 Laminectomy and section of dentate ligaments, with or without dural graft, cervical; one or two segments

63182 more than two segments

63185 Laminectomy with rhizotomy; one or two segments

63190 more than two segments

63191 Laminectomy with section of spinal accessory nerve

(For bilateral procedure, report 63191 with modifier 50)

(For resection of sternocleidomastoid muscle, use 21720)

Surgery: Nervous System

63194   Laminectomy with cordotomy, with section of one spinothalamic tract, one stage; cervical

63195   thoracic

63196   Laminectomy with cordotomy, with section of both spinothalamic tracts, one stage; cervical

63197   thoracic

63198   Laminectomy with cordotomy with section of both spinothalamic tracts, two stages within 14 days; cervical

63199   thoracic

63200   Laminectomy, with release of tethered spinal cord, lumbar

Excision by Laminectomy of Lesion Other Than Herniated Disk

63250   Laminectomy for excision or occlusion of arteriovenous malformation of spinal cord; cervical

63251   thoracic

63252   thoracolumbar

63265   Laminectomy for excision or evacuation of intraspinal lesion other than neoplasm, extradural; cervical

63266   thoracic

63267   lumbar

63268   sacral

63270   Laminectomy for excision of intraspinal lesion other than neoplasm, intradural; cervical

63271   thoracic

63272   lumbar

63273   sacral

63275   Laminectomy for biopsy/excision of intraspinal neoplasm; extradural, cervical

63276   extradural, thoracic

63277   extradural, lumbar

63278   extradural, sacral

63280   intradural, extramedullary, cervical

63281   intradural, extramedullary, thoracic

63282   intradural, extramedullary, lumbar

63283   intradural, sacral

63285   intradural, intramedullary, cervical

63286   intradural, intramedullary, thoracic

63287   intradural, intramedullary, thoracolumbar

63290   combined extradural-intradural lesion, any level

        (For drainage of intramedullary cyst/syrinx, use 63172, 63173)

+● 63295   Osteoplastic reconstruction of dorsal spinal elements, following primary intraspinal procedure (List separately in addition to code for primary procedure)

        ►(Use 63295 in conjunction with 63172, 63173, 63185, 63190, 63200-63290)◄

        ►(Do not report 63295 in conjunction with 22590-22614, 22840-22844, 63050, 63051 for the same vertebral segment(s))◄

Excision, Anterior or Anterolateral Approach, Intraspinal Lesion

For the following codes, when two surgeons work together as primary surgeons performing distinct part(s) of an anterior approach for an intraspinal excision, each surgeon should report his/her distinct operative work by appending modifier 62 to the single definitive procedure code. In this situation, modifier 62 may be appended to the definitive procedure code(s) 63300-63307 and, as appropriate, to the associated additional segment add-on code 63308 as long as both surgeons continue to work together as primary surgeons.

        (For arthrodesis, see 22548-22585)

        (For reconstruction of spine, see 20930-20938)

63300   Vertebral corpectomy (vertebral body resection), partial or complete, for excision of intraspinal lesion, single segment; extradural, cervical

63301   extradural, thoracic by transthoracic approach

63302   extradural, thoracic by thoracolumbar approach

63303   extradural, lumbar or sacral by transperitoneal or retroperitoneal approach

63304   intradural, cervical

63305   intradural, thoracic by transthoracic approach

63306   intradural, thoracic by thoracolumbar approach

63307   intradural, lumbar or sacral by transperitoneal or retroperitoneal approach

+ 63308   each additional segment (List separately in addition to codes for single segment)

        (Use 63308 in conjunction with 63300-63307)

Stereotaxis

63600   Creation of lesion of spinal cord by stereotactic method, percutaneous, any modality (including stimulation and/or recording)

63610   Stereotactic stimulation of spinal cord, percutaneous, separate procedure not followed by other surgery

63615   Stereotactic biopsy, aspiration, or excision of lesion, spinal cord

Surgery: Nervous System

Neurostimulators (Spinal)

Codes 63650-63688 apply to both simple and complex neurostimulators. For initial or subsequent electronic analysis and programming of neurostimulator pulse generators, see codes 95970-95975.

Codes 63650, 63655, and 63660 describe the operative placement, revision, or removal of the spinal neurostimulator system components to provide spinal electrical stimulation. A neurostimulator system includes an implanted neurostimulator, external controller, extension, and collection of contacts. Multiple contacts or electrodes (4 or more) provide the actual electrical stimulation in the epidural space.

For percutaneously placed neurostimulator systems (63650, 63660), the contacts are on a catheter-like lead. An array defines the collection of contacts that are on one catheter.

For systems placed via an open surgical exposure (63655, 63660), the contacts are on a plate or paddle-shaped surface.

63650   Percutaneous implantation of neurostimulator electrode array, epidural

63655   Laminectomy for implantation of neurostimulator electrodes, plate/paddle, epidural

63660   Revision or removal of spinal neurostimulator electrode percutaneous array(s) or plate/paddle(s)

▲ **63685**   Insertion or replacement of spinal neurostimulator pulse generator or receiver, direct or inductive coupling

►(Do not report 63685 in conjunction with 63688 for the same pulse generator or receiver)◄

63688   Revision or removal of implanted spinal neurostimulator pulse generator or receiver

(For electronic analysis of implanted neurostimulator pulse generator system, see 95970-95975)

Repair

63700   Repair of meningocele; less than 5 cm diameter

63702   larger than 5 cm diameter

(Do not use modifier 63 in conjunction with 63700, 63702)

63704   Repair of myelomeningocele; less than 5 cm diameter

63706   larger than 5 cm diameter

(Do not use modifier 63 in conjunction with 63704, 63706)

(For complex skin closure, see **Integumentary System**)

63707   Repair of dural/cerebrospinal fluid leak, not requiring laminectomy

63709   Repair of dural/cerebrospinal fluid leak or pseudomeningocele, with laminectomy

63710   Dural graft, spinal

(For laminectomy and section of dentate ligaments, with or without dural graft, cervical, see 63180, 63182)

Shunt, Spinal CSF

63740   Creation of shunt, lumbar, subarachnoid-peritoneal, -pleural, or other; including laminectomy

63741   percutaneous, not requiring laminectomy

63744   Replacement, irrigation or revision of lumbosubarachnoid shunt

63746   Removal of entire lumbosubarachnoid shunt system without replacement

(For insertion of subarachnoid catheter with reservoir and/or pump for intermittent or continuous infusion of drug including laminectomy, see 62351 and 62360, 62361 or 62362)

(For insertion or replacement of subarachnoid or epidural catheter, with reservoir and/or pump for drug infusion without laminectomy, see 62350 and 62360, 62361 or 62362)

Extracranial Nerves, Peripheral Nerves, and Autonomic Nervous System

(For intracranial surgery on cranial nerves, see 61450, 61460, 61790)

Introduction/Injection of Anesthetic Agent (Nerve Block), Diagnostic or Therapeutic

Somatic Nerves

64400   Injection, anesthetic agent; trigeminal nerve, any division or branch

64402   facial nerve

64405   greater occipital nerve

64408   vagus nerve

64410   phrenic nerve

64412   spinal accessory nerve

64413   cervical plexus

64415   brachial plexus, single

64416   brachial plexus, continuous infusion by catheter (including catheter placement) including daily management for anesthetic agent administration

(Do not report 01996 in addition to 64416)

64417   axillary nerve

64418   suprascapular nerve

64420   intercostal nerve, single

Surgery: Nervous System

64421	intercostal nerves, multiple, regional block
64425	ilioinguinal, iliohypogastric nerves
64430	pudendal nerve
64435	paracervical (uterine) nerve
64445	sciatic nerve, single
64446	sciatic nerve, continuous infusion by catheter, (including catheter placement) including daily management for anesthetic agent administration

(Do not report 01996 in addition to 64446)

64447	femoral nerve, single

(Do not report 01996 in addition to 64447)

64448	femoral nerve, continuous infusion by catheter (including catheter placement) including daily management for anesthetic agent administration

(Do not report 01996 in addition to 64448)

64449	lumbar plexus, posterior approach, continuous infusion by catheter (including catheter placement) including daily management for anesthetic agent administration

(Do not report 01996 in conjunction with 64449)

64450	other peripheral nerve or branch

(For phenol destruction, see 64622-64627)

(For subarachnoid or subdural injection, see 62280, 62310-62319)

(For epidural or caudal injection, see 62273, 62281-62282, 62310-62319)

(Codes 64470-64484 are unilateral procedures. For bilateral procedures, use modifier 50)

(For fluoroscopic guidance and localization for needle placement and injection in conjunction with 64470-64484, use code 76005)

64470	Injection, anesthetic agent and/or steroid, paravertebral facet joint or facet joint nerve; cervical or thoracic, single level
+ 64472	cervical or thoracic, each additional level (List separately in addition to code for primary procedure)

(Use 64472 in conjunction with 64470)

64475	lumbar or sacral, single level
+ 64476	lumbar or sacral, each additional level (List separately in addition to code for primary procedure)

(Use 64476 in conjunction with 64475)

64479	Injection, anesthetic agent and/or steroid, transforaminal epidural; cervical or thoracic, single level
+ 64480	cervical or thoracic, each additional level (List separately in addition to code for primary procedure)

(Use 64480 in conjunction with 64479)

64483	lumbar or sacral, single level
+ 64484	lumbar or sacral, each additional level (List separately in addition to code for primary procedure)

(Use 64484 in conjunction with 64483)

Sympathetic Nerves

64505	Injection, anesthetic agent; sphenopalatine ganglion
64508	carotid sinus (separate procedure)
64510	stellate ganglion (cervical sympathetic)
64517	superior hypogastric plexus
64520	lumbar or thoracic (paravertebral sympathetic)
64530	celiac plexus, with or without radiologic monitoring

Neurostimulators (Peripheral Nerve)

Codes 64553-64595 apply to both simple and complex neurostimulators. For initial or subsequent electronic analysis and programming of neurostimulator pulse generators, see codes 95970-95975.

64550	Application of surface (transcutaneous) neurostimulator
64553	Percutaneous implantation of neurostimulator electrodes; cranial nerve

(For open placement of cranial nerve (eg, vagal, trigeminal) neurostimulator pulse generator or receiver, see 61885, 61886, as appropriate)

64555	peripheral nerve (excludes sacral nerve)
64560	autonomic nerve
64561	sacral nerve (transforaminal placement)
64565	neuromuscular
64573	Incision for implantation of neurostimulator electrodes; cranial nerve

(For open placement of cranial nerve (eg, vagal, trigeminal) neurostimulator pulse generator or receiver, see 61885, 61886, as appropriate)

(For revision or removal of cranial nerve (eg, vagal, trigeminal) neurostimulator pulse generator or receiver, use 61888)

64575	peripheral nerve (excludes sacral nerve)
64577	autonomic nerve
64580	neuromuscular
64581	sacral nerve (transforaminal placement)
64585	Revision or removal of peripheral neurostimulator electrodes
▲ **64590**	Insertion or replacement of peripheral neurostimulator pulse generator or receiver, direct or inductive coupling

►(Do not report 64590 in conjunction with 64595)◄

64595	Revision or removal of peripheral neurostimulator pulse generator or receiver

Surgery: Nervous System

Destruction by Neurolytic Agent (eg, Chemical, Thermal, Electrical or Radiofrequency)

(Codes 64600-64681 include the injection of other therapeutic agents (eg, corticosteroids).

Somatic Nerves

64600 Destruction by neurolytic agent, trigeminal nerve; supraorbital, infraorbital, mental, or inferior alveolar branch

64605 second and third division branches at foramen ovale

64610 second and third division branches at foramen ovale under radiologic monitoring

64612 Chemodenervation of muscle(s); muscle(s) innervated by facial nerve (eg, for blepharospasm, hemifacial spasm)

64613 cervical spinal muscle(s) (eg, for spasmodic torticollis)

64614 extremity(s) and/or trunk muscle(s) (eg, for dystonia, cerebral palsy, multiple sclerosis)

(For chemodenervation for strabismus involving the extraocular muscles, use 67345)

64620 Destruction by neurolytic agent, intercostal nerve

(For fluoroscopic guidance and localization for needle placement and neurolysis in conjunction with 64622-64627, use 76005)

64622 Destruction by neurolytic agent, paravertebral facet joint nerve; lumbar or sacral, single level

(For bilateral procedure, report 64622 with modifier 50)

+ 64623 lumbar or sacral, each additional level (List separately in addition to code for primary procedure)

(Use 64623 in conjunction with 64622)

(For bilateral procedure, report 64623 with modifier 50)

64626 cervical or thoracic, single level

(For bilateral procedure, report 64626 with modifier 50)

+ 64627 cervical or thoracic, each additional level (List separately in addition to code for primary procedure)

(Use 64627 in conjunction with 64626)

(For bilateral procedure, report 64627 with modifier 50)

64630 Destruction by neurolytic agent; pudendal nerve

64640 other peripheral nerve or branch

Sympathetic Nerves

64680 Destruction by neurolytic agent, with or without radiologic monitoring; celiac plexus

64681 superior hypogastric plexus

Neuroplasty (Exploration, Neurolysis or Nerve Decompression)

Neuroplasty is the decompression or freeing of intact nerve from scar tissue, including external neurolysis and/or transposition.

(For internal neurolysis requiring use of operating microscope, use 64727)

(For facial nerve decompression, use 69720)

64702 Neuroplasty; digital, one or both, same digit

64704 nerve of hand or foot

64708 Neuroplasty, major peripheral nerve, arm or leg; other than specified

64712 sciatic nerve

64713 brachial plexus

64714 lumbar plexus

64716 Neuroplasty and/or transposition; cranial nerve (specify)

64718 ulnar nerve at elbow

64719 ulnar nerve at wrist

64721 median nerve at carpal tunnel

(For arthroscopic procedure, use 29848)

64722 Decompression; unspecified nerve(s) (specify)

64726 plantar digital nerve

+ 64727 Internal neurolysis, requiring use of operating microscope (List separately in addition to code for neuroplasty) (Neuroplasty includes external neurolysis)

(Do not report code 69990 in addition to code 64727)

Transection or Avulsion

(For stereotactic lesion of gasserian ganglion, use 61790)

64732 Transection or avulsion of; supraorbital nerve

64734 infraorbital nerve

64736 mental nerve

64738 inferior alveolar nerve by osteotomy

64740 lingual nerve

64742 facial nerve, differential or complete

64744 greater occipital nerve

64746 phrenic nerve

(For section of recurrent laryngeal nerve, use 31595)

64752 vagus nerve (vagotomy), transthoracic

64755 vagus nerves limited to proximal stomach (selective proximal vagotomy, proximal gastric vagotomy, parietal cell vagotomy, supra- or highly selective vagotomy)

(For laparoscopic approach, use 43652)

64760   vagus nerve (vagotomy), abdominal

(For laparoscopic approach, use 43651)

64761   pudendal nerve

(For bilateral procedure, report 64761 with modifier 50)

64763   Transection or avulsion of obturator nerve, extrapelvic, with or without adductor tenotomy

(For bilateral procedure, report 64763 with modifier 50)

64766   Transection or avulsion of obturator nerve, intrapelvic, with or without adductor tenotomy

(For bilateral procedure, report 64766 with modifier 50)

64771   Transection or avulsion of other cranial nerve, extradural

64772   Transection or avulsion of other spinal nerve, extradural

(For excision of tender scar, skin and subcutaneous tissue, with or without tiny neuroma, see 11400-11446, 13100-13153)

Excision

Somatic Nerves

(For Morton neurectomy, use 28080)

64774   Excision of neuroma; cutaneous nerve, surgically identifiable

64776   digital nerve, one or both, same digit

+ 64778   digital nerve, each additional digit (List separately in addition to code for primary procedure)

(Use 64778 in conjunction with 64776)

64782   hand or foot, except digital nerve

+ 64783   hand or foot, each additional nerve, except same digit (List separately in addition to code for primary procedure)

(Use 64783 in conjunction with 64782)

64784   major peripheral nerve, except sciatic

64786   sciatic nerve

+ 64787   Implantation of nerve end into bone or muscle (List separately in addition to neuroma excision)

(Use 64787 in conjunction with 64774-64786)

64788   Excision of neurofibroma or neurolemmoma; cutaneous nerve

64790   major peripheral nerve

64792   extensive (including malignant type)

64795   Biopsy of nerve

Sympathetic Nerves

64802   Sympathectomy, cervical

(For bilateral procedure, report 64802 with modifier 50)

64804   Sympathectomy, cervicothoracic

(For bilateral procedure, report 64804 with modifier 50)

64809   Sympathectomy, thoracolumbar

(For bilateral procedure, report 64809 with modifier 50)

64818   Sympathectomy, lumbar

(For bilateral procedure, report 64818 with modifier 50)

64820   Sympathectomy; digital arteries, each digit

(Do not report 69990 in addition to code 64820)

64821   radial artery

(Do not report 69990 in addition to code 64821)

64822   ulnar artery

(Do not report 69990 in addition to code 64822)

64823   superficial palmar arch

(Do not report 69990 in addition to code 64823)

Neurorrhaphy

64831   Suture of digital nerve, hand or foot; one nerve

+ 64832   each additional digital nerve (List separately in addition to code for primary procedure)

(Use 64832 in conjunction with 64831)

64834   Suture of one nerve, hand or foot; common sensory nerve

64835   median motor thenar

64836   ulnar motor

+ 64837   Suture of each additional nerve, hand or foot (List separately in addition to code for primary procedure)

(Use 64837 in conjunction with 64834-64836)

64840   Suture of posterior tibial nerve

64856   Suture of major peripheral nerve, arm or leg, except sciatic; including transposition

64857   without transposition

64858   Suture of sciatic nerve

+ 64859   Suture of each additional major peripheral nerve (List separately in addition to code for primary procedure)

(Use 64859 in conjunction with 64856, 64857)

64861   Suture of; brachial plexus

64862   lumbar plexus

64864   Suture of facial nerve; extracranial

64865   infratemporal, with or without grafting

Surgery: Nervous System

64866	Anastomosis; facial-spinal accessory
64868	facial-hypoglossal
64870	facial-phrenic
+ 64872	Suture of nerve; requiring secondary or delayed suture (List separately in addition to code for primary neurorrhaphy)

(Use 64872 in conjunction with 64831-64865)

| + 64874 | requiring extensive mobilization, or transposition of nerve (List separately in addition to code for nerve suture) |

(Use 64874 in conjunction with 64831-64865)

| + 64876 | requiring shortening of bone of extremity (List separately in addition to code for nerve suture) |

(Use 64876 in conjunction with 64831-64865)

Neurorrhaphy With Nerve Graft

64885	Nerve graft (includes obtaining graft), head or neck; up to 4 cm in length
64886	more than 4 cm length
64890	Nerve graft (includes obtaining graft), single strand, hand or foot; up to 4 cm length
64891	more than 4 cm length
64892	Nerve graft (includes obtaining graft), single strand, arm or leg; up to 4 cm length
64893	more than 4 cm length
64895	Nerve graft (includes obtaining graft), multiple strands (cable), hand or foot; up to 4 cm length
64896	more than 4 cm length
64897	Nerve graft (includes obtaining graft), multiple strands (cable), arm or leg; up to 4 cm length
64898	more than 4 cm length
+ 64901	Nerve graft, each additional nerve; single strand (List separately in addition to code for primary procedure)

(Use 64901 in conjunction with 64885-64893)

| + 64902 | multiple strands (cable) (List separately in addition to code for primary procedure) |

(Use 64902 in conjunction with 64885, 64886, 64895-64898)

| 64905 | Nerve pedicle transfer; first stage |
| 64907 | second stage |

Other Procedures

| 64999 | Unlisted procedure, nervous system |

Eye and Ocular Adnexa

(For diagnostic and treatment ophthalmological services, see **Medicine, Ophthalmology,** and 92002 et seq)

(Do not report code 69990 in addition to codes 65091-68850)

Eyeball

Removal of Eye

65091   Evisceration of ocular contents; without implant

65093   with implant

65101   Enucleation of eye; without implant

65103   with implant, muscles not attached to implant

65105   with implant, muscles attached to implant

(For conjunctivoplasty after enucleation, see 68320 et seq)

65110   Exenteration of orbit (does not include skin graft), removal of orbital contents; only

65112   with therapeutic removal of bone

65114   with muscle or myocutaneous flap

(For skin graft to orbit (split skin), see 15120, 15121; free, full thickness, see 15260, 15261)

(For eyelid repair involving more than skin, see 67930 et seq)

Secondary Implant(s) Procedures

An ocular implant is an implant inside muscular cone; an orbital implant is an implant outside muscular cone.

65125   Modification of ocular implant with placement or replacement of pegs (eg, drilling receptacle for prosthesis appendage) (separate procedure)

65130   Insertion of ocular implant secondary; after evisceration, in scleral shell

65135   after enucleation, muscles not attached to implant

65140   after enucleation, muscles attached to implant

65150   Reinsertion of ocular implant; with or without conjunctival graft

65155   with use of foreign material for reinforcement and/or attachment of muscles to implant

65175   Removal of ocular implant

(For orbital implant (implant outside muscle cone) insertion, use 67550; removal, use 67560)

Removal of Foreign Body

(For removal of implanted material: ocular implant, use 65175; anterior segment implant, use 65920; posterior segment implant, use 67120; orbital implant, use 67560)

(For diagnostic x-ray for foreign body, use 70030)

(For diagnostic echography for foreign body, use 76529)

(For removal of foreign body from orbit: frontal approach, use 67413; lateral approach, use 67430; transcranial approach, use 61334)

(For removal of foreign body from eyelid, embedded, use 67938)

(For removal of foreign body from lacrimal system, use 68530)

65205   Removal of foreign body, external eye; conjunctival superficial

65210   conjunctival embedded (includes concretions), subconjunctival, or scleral nonperforating

65220   corneal, without slit lamp

65222   corneal, with slit lamp

(For repair of corneal laceration with foreign body, use 65275)

65235   Removal of foreign body, intraocular; from anterior chamber of eye or lens

(For removal of implanted material from anterior segment, use 65920)

65260   from posterior segment, magnetic extraction, anterior or posterior route

65265   from posterior segment, nonmagnetic extraction

(For removal of implanted material from posterior segment, use 67120)

Repair of Laceration

(For fracture of orbit, see 21385 et seq)

(For repair of wound of eyelid, skin, linear, simple, see 12011-12018; intermediate, layered closure, see 12051-12057; linear, complex, see 13150-13160; other, see 67930, 67935)

(For repair of wound of lacrimal system, use 68700)

(For repair of operative wound, use 66250)

65270   Repair of laceration; conjunctiva, with or without nonperforating laceration sclera, direct closure

65272   conjunctiva, by mobilization and rearrangement, without hospitalization

65273   conjunctiva, by mobilization and rearrangement, with hospitalization

Surgery: Ocular/Auditory System

65275	cornea, nonperforating, with or without removal foreign body
65280	cornea and/or sclera, perforating, not involving uveal tissue
65285	cornea and/or sclera, perforating, with reposition or resection of uveal tissue
65286	application of tissue glue, wounds of cornea and/or sclera

(Repair of laceration includes use of conjunctival flap and restoration of anterior chamber, by air or saline injection when indicated)

(For repair of iris or ciliary body, use 66680)

65290	Repair of wound, extraocular muscle, tendon and/or Tenon's capsule

Anterior Segment

Cornea

Excision

65400	Excision of lesion, cornea (keratectomy, lamellar, partial), except pterygium
65410	Biopsy of cornea
65420	Excision or transposition of pterygium; without graft
65426	with graft

Removal or Destruction

65430	Scraping of cornea, diagnostic, for smear and/or culture
65435	Removal of corneal epithelium; with or without chemocauterization (abrasion, curettage)
65436	with application of chelating agent (eg, EDTA)
65450	Destruction of lesion of cornea by cryotherapy, photocoagulation or thermocauterization
65600	Multiple punctures of anterior cornea (eg, for corneal erosion, tattoo)

Keratoplasty

Corneal transplant includes use of fresh or preserved grafts, and preparation of donor material.

(Keratoplasty excludes refractive keratoplasty procedures, 65760, 65765, and 65767)

65710	Keratoplasty (corneal transplant); lamellar
65730	penetrating (except in aphakia)
65750	penetrating (in aphakia)
65755	penetrating (in pseudophakia)

Other Procedures

65760	Keratomileusis
65765	Keratophakia
65767	Epikeratoplasty
65770	Keratoprosthesis
65771	Radial keratotomy
65772	Corneal relaxing incision for correction of surgically induced astigmatism
65775	Corneal wedge resection for correction of surgically induced astigmatism

(For fitting of contact lens for treatment of disease, use 92070)

(For unlisted procedures on cornea, use 66999)

65780	Ocular surface reconstruction; amniotic membrane transplantation
65781	limbal stem cell allograft (eg, cadaveric or living donor)
65782	limbal conjunctival autograft (includes obtaining graft)

(For harvesting conjunctival allograft, living donor, use 68371)

Anterior Chamber

Incision

65800	Paracentesis of anterior chamber of eye (separate procedure); with diagnostic aspiration of aqueous
65805	with therapeutic release of aqueous
65810	with removal of vitreous and/or discission of anterior hyaloid membrane, with or without air injection
65815	with removal of blood, with or without irrigation and/or air injection

(For injection, see 66020-66030)

(For removal of blood clot, use 65930)

65820	Goniotomy

(Do not report modifier 63 in conjunction with 65820)

65850	Trabeculotomy ab externo
65855	Trabeculoplasty by laser surgery, one or more sessions (defined treatment series)

(If re-treatment is necessary after several months because of disease progression, a new treatment or treatment series should be reported with a modifier, if necessary, to indicate lesser or greater complexity)

(For trabeculectomy, use 66170)

65860	Severing adhesions of anterior segment, laser technique (separate procedure)

Other Procedures

65865   Severing adhesions of anterior segment of eye, incisional technique (with or without injection of air or liquid) (separate procedure); goniosynechiae

(For trabeculoplasty by laser surgery, use 65855)

65870   anterior synechiae, except goniosynechiae

65875   posterior synechiae

65880   corneovitreal adhesions

(For laser surgery, use 66821)

65900   Removal of epithelial downgrowth, anterior chamber of eye

65920   Removal of implanted material, anterior segment of eye

65930   Removal of blood clot, anterior segment of eye

66020   Injection, anterior chamber of eye (separate procedure); air or liquid

66030   medication

(For unlisted procedures on anterior segment, use 66999)

Anterior Sclera

Excision

(For removal of intraocular foreign body, use 65235)

(For operations on posterior sclera, use 67250, 67255)

66130   Excision of lesion, sclera

66150   Fistulization of sclera for glaucoma; trephination with iridectomy

66155   thermocauterization with iridectomy

66160   sclerectomy with punch or scissors, with iridectomy

66165   iridencleisis or iridotasis

66170   trabeculectomy ab externo in absence of previous surgery

(For trabeculotomy ab externo, use 65850)

(For repair of operative wound, use 66250)

66172   trabeculectomy ab externo with scarring from previous ocular surgery or trauma (includes injection of antifibrotic agents)

66180   Aqueous shunt to extraocular reservoir (eg, Molteno, Schocket, Denver-Krupin)

66185   Revision of aqueous shunt to extraocular reservoir

(For removal of implanted shunt, use 67120)

Repair or Revision

(For scleral procedures in retinal surgery, see 67101 et seq)

66220   Repair of scleral staphyloma; without graft

66225   with graft

(For scleral reinforcement, see 67250, 67255)

66250   Revision or repair of operative wound of anterior segment, any type, early or late, major or minor procedure

(For unlisted procedures on anterior sclera, use 66999)

Iris, Ciliary Body

Incision

66500   Iridotomy by stab incision (separate procedure); except transfixion

66505   with transfixion as for iris bombe

(For iridotomy by photocoagulation, use 66761)

Excision

66600   Iridectomy, with corneoscleral or corneal section; for removal of lesion

66605   with cyclectomy

66625   peripheral for glaucoma (separate procedure)

66630   sector for glaucoma (separate procedure)

66635   optical (separate procedure)

(For coreoplasty by photocoagulation, use 66762)

Repair

66680   Repair of iris, ciliary body (as for iridodialysis)

(For reposition or resection of uveal tissue with perforating wound of cornea or sclera, use 65285)

66682   Suture of iris, ciliary body (separate procedure) with retrieval of suture through small incision (eg, McCannel suture)

Destruction

66700   Ciliary body destruction; diathermy

▲ **66710**   cyclophotocoagulation, transscleral

● **66711**   cyclophotocoagulation, endoscopic

►(Do not report 66711 in conjunction with 66990)◄

☉ **66720**   cryotherapy

66740   cyclodialysis

66761   Iridotomy/iridectomy by laser surgery (eg, for glaucoma) (one or more sessions)

Surgery: Ocular/Auditory System

66762   Iridoplasty by photocoagulation (one or more sessions) (eg, for improvement of vision, for widening of anterior chamber angle)

66770   Destruction of cyst or lesion iris or ciliary body (nonexcisional procedure)

(For excision lesion iris, ciliary body, see 66600, 66605; for removal of epithelial downgrowth, use 65900)

(For unlisted procedures on iris, ciliary body, use 66999)

Lens

Incision

66820   Discission of secondary membranous cataract (opacified posterior lens capsule and/or anterior hyaloid); stab incision technique (Ziegler or Wheeler knife)

66821   laser surgery (eg, YAG laser) (one or more stages)

66825   Repositioning of intraocular lens prosthesis, requiring an incision (separate procedure)

Removal Cataract

Lateral canthotomy, iridectomy, iridotomy, anterior capsulotomy, posterior capsulotomy, the use of viscoelastic agents, enzymatic zonulysis, use of other pharmacologic agents, and subconjunctival or sub-tenon injections are included as part of the code for the extraction of lens.

66830   Removal of secondary membranous cataract (opacified posterior lens capsule and/or anterior hyaloid) with corneo-scleral section, with or without iridectomy (iridocapsulotomy, iridocapsulectomy)

66840   Removal of lens material; aspiration technique, one or more stages

66850   phacofragmentation technique (mechanical or ultrasonic) (eg, phacoemulsification), with aspiration

66852   pars plana approach, with or without vitrectomy

66920   intracapsular

66930   intracapsular, for dislocated lens

66940   extracapsular (other than 66840, 66850, 66852)

(For removal of intralenticular foreign body without lens extraction, use 65235)

(For repair of operative wound, use 66250)

66982   Extracapsular cataract removal with insertion of intraocular lens prosthesis (one stage procedure), manual or mechanical technique (eg, irrigation and aspiration or phacoemulsification), complex, requiring devices or techniques not generally used in routine cataract surgery (eg, iris expansion device, suture support for intraocular lens, or primary posterior capsulorrhexis) or performed on patients in the amblyogenic developmental stage

66983   Intracapsular cataract extraction with insertion of intraocular lens prosthesis (one stage procedure)

66984   Extracapsular cataract removal with insertion of intraocular lens prosthesis (one stage procedure), manual or mechanical technique (eg, irrigation and aspiration or phacoemulsification)

(For complex extracapsular cataract removal, use 66982)

66985   Insertion of intraocular lens prosthesis (secondary implant), not associated with concurrent cataract removal

(To code implant at time of concurrent cataract surgery, see 66982, 66983, 66984)

(For intraocular lens prosthesis supplied by physician, use 99070)

(For ultrasonic determination of intraocular lens power, use 76519)

(For removal of implanted material from anterior segment, use 65920)

(For secondary fixation (separate procedure), use 66682)

66986   Exchange of intraocular lens

+ 66990   Use of ophthalmic endoscope (List separately in addition to code for primary procedure)

(66990 may be used only with codes 65820, 65875, 65920, 66985, 66986, 67038, 67039, 67040)

Other Procedures

66999   Unlisted procedure, anterior segment of eye

Posterior Segment

Vitreous

67005   Removal of vitreous, anterior approach (open sky technique or limbal incision); partial removal

67010   subtotal removal with mechanical vitrectomy

(For removal of vitreous by paracentesis of anterior chamber, use 65810)

(For removal of corneovitreal adhesions, use 65880)

67015   Aspiration or release of vitreous, subretinal or choroidal fluid, pars plana approach (posterior sclerotomy)

67025   Injection of vitreous substitute, pars plana or limbal approach, (fluid-gas exchange), with or without aspiration (separate procedure)

67027   Implantation of intravitreal drug delivery system (eg, ganciclovir implant), includes concomitant removal of vitreous

(For removal, use 67121)

Surgery: Ocular/Auditory System

67028   Intravitreal injection of a pharmacologic agent (separate procedure)

67030   Discission of vitreous strands (without removal), pars plana approach

67031   Severing of vitreous strands, vitreous face adhesions, sheets, membranes or opacities, laser surgery (one or more stages)

67036   Vitrectomy, mechanical, pars plana approach;

67038   with epiretinal membrane stripping

67039   with focal endolaser photocoagulation

67040   with endolaser panretinal photocoagulation

(For use of ophthalmic endoscope with 67038, 67039, 67040, use 66990)

(For associated lensectomy, use 66850)

(For use of vitrectomy in retinal detachment surgery, use 67108)

(For associated removal of foreign body, see 65260, 65265)

(For unlisted procedures on vitreous, use 67299)

Retina or Choroid

Repair

(If diathermy, cryotherapy and/or photocoagulation are combined, report under principal modality used)

67101   Repair of retinal detachment, one or more sessions; cryotherapy or diathermy, with or without drainage of subretinal fluid

67105   photocoagulation, with or without drainage of subretinal fluid

67107   Repair of retinal detachment; scleral buckling (such as lamellar scleral dissection, imbrication or encircling procedure), with or without implant, with or without cryotherapy, photocoagulation, and drainage of subretinal fluid

67108   with vitrectomy, any method, with or without air or gas tamponade, focal endolaser photocoagulation, cryotherapy, drainage of subretinal fluid, scleral buckling, and/or removal of lens by same technique

67110   by injection of air or other gas (eg, pneumatic retinopexy)

67112   by scleral buckling or vitrectomy, on patient having previous ipsilateral retinal detachment repair(s) using scleral buckling or vitrectomy techniques

(For aspiration or drainage of subretinal or subchoroidal fluid, use 67015)

67115   Release of encircling material (posterior segment)

67120   Removal of implanted material, posterior segment; extraocular

67121   intraocular

(For removal from anterior segment, use 65920)

(For removal of foreign body, see 65260, 65265)

Prophylaxis

Repetitive services. The services listed below are often performed in multiple sessions or groups of sessions. The methods of reporting vary.

The following descriptors are intended to include all sessions in a defined treatment period.

67141   Prophylaxis of retinal detachment (eg, retinal break, lattice degeneration) without drainage, one or more sessions; cryotherapy, diathermy

67145   photocoagulation (laser or xenon arc)

Destruction

67208   Destruction of localized lesion of retina (eg, macular edema, tumors), one or more sessions; cryotherapy, diathermy

67210   photocoagulation

67218   radiation by implantation of source (includes removal of source)

67220   Destruction of localized lesion of choroid (eg, choroidal neovascularization); photocoagulation (eg, laser), one or more sessions

(For destruction of macular drusen, photocoagulation, use Category III code 0017T)

(For destruction of localized lesion of choroid by transpupillary thermotherapy, use Category III code 0016T)

67221   photodynamic therapy (includes intravenous infusion)

+ **67225**   photodynamic therapy, second eye, at single session (List separately in addition to code for primary eye treatment)

(Use 67225 in conjunction with 67221)

67227   Destruction of extensive or progressive retinopathy (eg, diabetic retinopathy), one or more sessions; cryotherapy, diathermy

67228   photocoagulation (laser or xenon arc)

(For unlisted procedures on retina, use 67299)

Surgery: Ocular/Auditory System

Sclera

Repair

(For excision lesion sclera, use 66130)

67250 Scleral reinforcement (separate procedure); without graft

67255 with graft

(For repair scleral staphyloma, see 66220, 66225)

Other Procedures

67299 Unlisted procedure, posterior segment

Ocular Adnexa

Extraocular Muscles

67311 Strabismus surgery, recession or resection procedure; one horizontal muscle

67312 two horizontal muscles

67314 one vertical muscle (excluding superior oblique)

67316 two or more vertical muscles (excluding superior oblique)

(For adjustable sutures, use 67335 in addition to codes 67311-67334 for primary procedure reflecting number of muscles operated on)

67318 Strabismus surgery, any procedure, superior oblique muscle

+ 67320 Transposition procedure (eg, for paretic extraocular muscle), any extraocular muscle (specify) (List separately in addition to code for primary procedure)

(Use 67320 in conjunction with 67311-67318)

+ 67331 Strabismus surgery on patient with previous eye surgery or injury that did not involve the extraocular muscles (List separately in addition to code for primary procedure)

(Use 67331 in conjunction with 67311-67318)

+ 67332 Strabismus surgery on patient with scarring of extraocular muscles (eg, prior ocular injury, strabismus or retinal detachment surgery) or restrictive myopathy (eg, dysthyroid ophthalmopathy) (List separately in addition to code for primary procedure)

(Use 67332 in conjunction with 67311-67318)

+ 67334 Strabismus surgery by posterior fixation suture technique, with or without muscle recession (List separately in addition to code for primary procedure)

(Use 67334 in conjunction with 67311-67318)

+ 67335 Placement of adjustable suture(s) during strabismus surgery, including postoperative adjustment(s) of suture(s) (List separately in addition to code for specific strabismus surgery)

(Use 67335 in conjunction with 67311-67334)

+ 67340 Strabismus surgery involving exploration and/or repair of detached extraocular muscle(s) (List separately in addition to code for primary procedure)

(Use 67340 in conjunction with 67311-67334)

67343 Release of extensive scar tissue without detaching extraocular muscle (separate procedure)

(Use 67343 in conjunction with 67311-67340, when such procedures are performed other than on the affected muscle)

67345 Chemodenervation of extraocular muscle

(For chemodenervation for blepharospasm and other neurological disorders, see 64612 and 64613)

Other Procedures

67350 Biopsy of extraocular muscle

(For repair of wound, extraocular muscle, tendon or Tenon's capsule, use 65290)

67399 Unlisted procedure, ocular muscle

Orbit

Exploration, Excision, Decompression

67400 Orbitotomy without bone flap (frontal or transconjunctival approach); for exploration, with or without biopsy

67405 with drainage only

67412 with removal of lesion

67413 with removal of foreign body

67414 with removal of bone for decompression

67415 Fine needle aspiration of orbital contents

(For exenteration, enucleation, and repair, see 65101 et seq; for optic nerve decompression, use 67570)

67420 Orbitotomy with bone flap or window, lateral approach (eg, Kroenlein); with removal of lesion

67430 with removal of foreign body

67440 with drainage

67445 with removal of bone for decompression

(For optic nerve sheath decompression, use 67570)

67450 for exploration, with or without biopsy

(For orbitotomy, transcranial approach, see 61330-61334)

(For orbital implant, see 67550, 67560)

(For removal of eyeball or for repair after removal, see 65091-65175)

Other Procedures

67500 Retrobulbar injection; medication (separate procedure, does not include supply of medication)

67505   alcohol

67515 Injection of medication or other substance into Tenon's capsule

(For subconjunctival injection, use 68200)

67550 Orbital implant (implant outside muscle cone); insertion

67560   removal or revision

(For ocular implant (implant inside muscle cone), see 65093-65105, 65130-65175)

(For treatment of fractures of malar area, orbit, see 21355 et seq)

67570 Optic nerve decompression (eg, incision or fenestration of optic nerve sheath)

67599 Unlisted procedure, orbit

Eyelids

Incision

67700 Blepharotomy, drainage of abscess, eyelid

67710 Severing of tarsorrhaphy

67715 Canthotomy (separate procedure)

(For canthoplasty, use 67950)

(For division of symblepharon, use 68340)

Excision

Codes for removal of lesion include more than skin (ie, involving lid margin, tarsus, and/or palpebral conjunctiva).

(For removal of lesion, involving mainly skin of eyelid, see 11310-11313; 11440-11446; 11640-11646; 17000-17004)

(For repair of wounds, blepharoplasty, grafts, reconstructive surgery, see 67930-67975)

67800 Excision of chalazion; single

67801   multiple, same lid

67805   multiple, different lids

67808   under general anesthesia and/or requiring hospitalization, single or multiple

67810 Biopsy of eyelid

67820 Correction of trichiasis; epilation, by forceps only

67825   epilation by other than forceps (eg, by electrosurgery, cryotherapy, laser surgery)

67830   incision of lid margin

67835   incision of lid margin, with free mucous membrane graft

67840 Excision of lesion of eyelid (except chalazion) without closure or with simple direct closure

(For excision and repair of eyelid by reconstructive surgery, see 67961, 67966)

67850 Destruction of lesion of lid margin (up to 1 cm)

(For Mohs micrographic surgery, see 17304-17310)

(For initiation or follow-up care of topical chemotherapy (eg, 5-FU or similar agents), see appropriate office visits)

Tarsorrhaphy

67875 Temporary closure of eyelids by suture (eg, Frost suture)

67880 Construction of intermarginal adhesions, median tarsorrhaphy, or canthorrhaphy;

67882   with transposition of tarsal plate

(For severing of tarsorrhaphy, use 67710)

(For canthoplasty, reconstruction canthus, use 67950)

(For canthotomy, use 67715)

Repair (Brow Ptosis, Blepharoptosis, Lid Retraction, Ectropion, Entropion)

67900 Repair of brow ptosis (supraciliary, mid-forehead or coronal approach)

(For forehead rhytidectomy, use 15824)

67901 Repair of blepharoptosis; frontalis muscle technique with suture or other material

67902   frontalis muscle technique with fascial sling (includes obtaining fascia)

67903   (tarso) levator resection or advancement, internal approach

67904   (tarso) levator resection or advancement, external approach

67906   superior rectus technique with fascial sling (includes obtaining fascia)

67908   conjunctivo-tarso-Muller's muscle-levator resection (eg, Fasanella-Servat type)

67909 Reduction of overcorrection of ptosis

67911 Correction of lid retraction

(For obtaining autogenous graft materials, see 20920, 20922 or 20926)

(For correction of trichiasis by mucous membrane graft, use 67835)

67912 Correction of lagophthalmos, with implantation of upper eyelid lid load (eg, gold weight)

Surgery: Ocular/Auditory System

67914	Repair of ectropion; suture
67915	thermocauterization
67916	excision tarsal wedge
67917	extensive (eg, tarsal strip operations)

(For correction of everted punctum, use 68705)

67921	Repair of entropion; suture
67922	thermocauterization
67923	excision tarsal wedge
67924	extensive (eg, tarsal strip or capsulopalpebral fascia repairs operation)

(For repair of cicatricial ectropion or entropion requiring scar excision or skin graft, see also 67961 et seq)

Reconstruction

Codes for blepharoplasty involve more than skin (ie, involving lid margin, tarsus, and/or palpebral conjunctiva).

67930	Suture of recent wound, eyelid, involving lid margin, tarsus, and/or palpebral conjunctiva direct closure; partial thickness
67935	full thickness
67938	Removal of embedded foreign body, eyelid

(For repair of skin of eyelid, see 12011-12018; 12051-12057; 13150-13153)

(For tarsorrhaphy, canthorrhaphy, see 67880, 67882)

(For repair of blepharoptosis and lid retraction, see 67901-67911)

(For blepharoplasty for entropion, ectropion, see 67916, 67917, 67923, 67924)

(For correction of blepharochalasis (blepharorhytidectomy), see 15820-15823)

(For repair of skin of eyelid, adjacent tissue transfer, see 14060, 14061; preparation for graft, use 15000; free graft, see 15120, 15121, 15260, 15261)

(For excision of lesion of eyelid, use 67800 et seq)

(For repair of lacrimal canaliculi, use 68700)

67950	Canthoplasty (reconstruction of canthus)
67961	Excision and repair of eyelid, involving lid margin, tarsus, conjunctiva, canthus, or full thickness, may include preparation for skin graft or pedicle flap with adjacent tissue transfer or rearrangement; up to one-fourth of lid margin
67966	over one-fourth of lid margin

(For canthoplasty, use 67950)

(For free skin grafts, see 15120, 15121, 15260, 15261)

(For tubed pedicle flap preparation, use 15576; for delay, use 15630; for attachment, use 15650)

67971	Reconstruction of eyelid, full thickness by transfer of tarsoconjunctival flap from opposing eyelid; up to two-thirds of eyelid, one stage or first stage
67973	total eyelid, lower, one stage or first stage
67974	total eyelid, upper, one stage or first stage
67975	second stage

Other Procedures

67999	Unlisted procedure, eyelids

Conjunctiva

(For removal of foreign body, see 65205 et seq)

Incision and Drainage

68020	Incision of conjunctiva, drainage of cyst
68040	Expression of conjunctival follicles (eg, for trachoma)

Excision and/or Destruction

68100	Biopsy of conjunctiva
68110	Excision of lesion, conjunctiva; up to 1 cm
68115	over 1 cm
68130	with adjacent sclera
68135	Destruction of lesion, conjunctiva

Injection

(For injection into Tenon's capsule or retrobulbar injection, see 67500-67515)

68200	Subconjunctival injection

Conjunctivoplasty

(For wound repair, see 65270-65273)

68320	Conjunctivoplasty; with conjunctival graft or extensive rearrangement
68325	with buccal mucous membrane graft (includes obtaining graft)
68326	Conjunctivoplasty, reconstruction cul-de-sac; with conjunctival graft or extensive rearrangement
68328	with buccal mucous membrane graft (includes obtaining graft)
68330	Repair of symblepharon; conjunctivoplasty, without graft
68335	with free graft conjunctiva or buccal mucous membrane (includes obtaining graft)
68340	division of symblepharon, with or without insertion of conformer or contact lens

Other Procedures

68360   Conjunctival flap; bridge or partial (separate procedure)

68362   total (such as Gunderson thin flap or purse string flap)

(For conjunctival flap for perforating injury, see 65280, 65285)

(For repair of operative wound, use 66250)

(For removal of conjunctival foreign body, see 65205, 65210)

68371   Harvesting conjunctival allograft, living donor

68399   Unlisted procedure, conjunctiva

Lacrimal System

Incision

68400   Incision, drainage of lacrimal gland

68420   Incision, drainage of lacrimal sac (dacryocystotomy or dacryocystostomy)

68440   Snip incision of lacrimal punctum

Excision

68500   Excision of lacrimal gland (dacryoadenectomy), except for tumor; total

68505   partial

68510   Biopsy of lacrimal gland

68520   Excision of lacrimal sac (dacryocystectomy)

68525   Biopsy of lacrimal sac

68530   Removal of foreign body or dacryolith, lacrimal passages

68540   Excision of lacrimal gland tumor; frontal approach

68550   involving osteotomy

Repair

68700   Plastic repair of canaliculi

68705   Correction of everted punctum, cautery

68720   Dacryocystorhinostomy (fistulization of lacrimal sac to nasal cavity)

68745   Conjunctivorhinostomy (fistulization of conjunctiva to nasal cavity); without tube

68750   with insertion of tube or stent

68760   Closure of the lacrimal punctum; by thermocauterization, ligation, or laser surgery

68761   by plug, each

68770   Closure of lacrimal fistula (separate procedure)

Probing and/or Related Procedures

68801   Dilation of lacrimal punctum, with or without irrigation

(To report a bilateral procedure, use 68801 with modifier 50)

68810   Probing of nasolacrimal duct, with or without irrigation;

(For bilateral procedure, report 68810 with modifier 50)

68811   requiring general anesthesia

(For bilateral procedure, report 68811 with modifier 50)

68815   with insertion of tube or stent

(See also 92018)

(For bilateral procedure, report 68815 with modifier 50)

68840   Probing of lacrimal canaliculi, with or without irrigation

68850   Injection of contrast medium for dacryocystography

(For radiological supervision and interpretation, see 70170, 78660)

Other Procedures

68899   Unlisted procedure, lacrimal system

Surgery: Ocular/Auditory System

Notes

Auditory System

(For diagnostic services (eg, audiometry, vestibular tests), see 92502 et seq)

External Ear

Incision

69000   Drainage external ear, abscess or hematoma; simple

69005   complicated

69020   Drainage external auditory canal, abscess

69090   Ear piercing

Excision

69100   Biopsy external ear

69105   Biopsy external auditory canal

69110   Excision external ear; partial, simple repair

69120   complete amputation

(For reconstruction of ear, see 15120 et seq)

69140   Excision exostosis(es), external auditory canal

69145   Excision soft tissue lesion, external auditory canal

69150   Radical excision external auditory canal lesion; without neck dissection

69155   with neck dissection

(For resection of temporal bone, use 69535)

(For skin grafting, see 15000-15261)

Removal of Foreign Body

69200   Removal foreign body from external auditory canal; without general anesthesia

69205   with general anesthesia

69210   Removal impacted cerumen (separate procedure), one or both ears

69220   Debridement, mastoidectomy cavity, simple (eg, routine cleaning)

(For bilateral procedure, report 69220 with modifier 50)

69222   Debridement, mastoidectomy cavity, complex (eg, with anesthesia or more than routine cleaning)

(For bilateral procedure, report 69222 with modifier 50)

Repair

(For suture of wound or injury of external ear, see 12011-14300)

69300   Otoplasty, protruding ear, with or without size reduction

(For bilateral procedure, report 69300 with modifier 50)

69310   Reconstruction of external auditory canal (meatoplasty) (eg, for stenosis due to injury, infection) (separate procedure)

69320   Reconstruction external auditory canal for congenital atresia, single stage

(For combination with middle ear reconstruction, see 69631, 69641)

(For other reconstructive procedures with grafts (eg, skin, cartilage, bone), see 13150-15760, 21230-21235)

Other Procedures

(For otoscopy under general anesthesia, use 92502)

69399   Unlisted procedure, external ear

Middle Ear

Introduction

69400   Eustachian tube inflation, transnasal; with catheterization

69401   without catheterization

69405   Eustachian tube catheterization, transtympanic

69410   Focal application of phase control substance, middle ear (baffle technique)

Incision

69420   Myringotomy including aspiration and/or eustachian tube inflation

69421   Myringotomy including aspiration and/or eustachian tube inflation requiring general anesthesia

69424   Ventilating tube removal requiring general anesthesia

(For bilateral procedure, report 69424 with modifier 50)

(Do not report code 69424 in conjunction with 69205, 69210, 69420, 69421, 69433-69676, 69710-69745, 69801-69930)

69433   Tympanostomy (requiring insertion of ventilating tube), local or topical anesthesia

(For bilateral procedure, report 69433 with modifier 50)

69436   Tympanostomy (requiring insertion of ventilating tube), general anesthesia

(For bilateral procedure, report 69436 with modifier 50)

69440   Middle ear exploration through postauricular or ear canal incision

(For atticotomy, see 69601 et seq)

69450   Tympanolysis, transcanal

Excision

69501 Transmastoid antrotomy (simple mastoidectomy)

69502 Mastoidectomy; complete

69505   modified radical

69511   radical

    (For skin graft, see 15000 et seq)

    (For mastoidectomy cavity debridement, see 69220, 69222)

69530 Petrous apicectomy including radical mastoidectomy

69535 Resection temporal bone, external approach

    (For middle fossa approach, see 69950-69970)

69540 Excision aural polyp

69550 Excision aural glomus tumor; transcanal

69552   transmastoid

69554   extended (extratemporal)

Repair

69601 Revision mastoidectomy; resulting in complete mastoidectomy

69602   resulting in modified radical mastoidectomy

69603   resulting in radical mastoidectomy

69604   resulting in tympanoplasty

    (For planned secondary tympanoplasty after mastoidectomy, see 69631, 69632)

69605   with apicectomy

    (For skin graft, see 15120, 15121, 15260, 15261)

69610 Tympanic membrane repair, with or without site preparation of perforation for closure, with or without patch

69620 Myringoplasty (surgery confined to drumhead and donor area)

69631 Tympanoplasty without mastoidectomy (including canalplasty, atticotomy and/or middle ear surgery), initial or revision; without ossicular chain reconstruction

69632   with ossicular chain reconstruction (eg, postfenestration)

69633   with ossicular chain reconstruction and synthetic prosthesis (eg, partial ossicular replacement prosthesis (PORP), total ossicular replacement prosthesis (TORP))

69635 Tympanoplasty with antrotomy or mastoidotomy (including canalplasty, atticotomy, middle ear surgery, and/or tympanic membrane repair); without ossicular chain reconstruction

69636   with ossicular chain reconstruction

69637   with ossicular chain reconstruction and synthetic prosthesis (eg, partial ossicular replacement prosthesis (PORP), total ossicular replacement prosthesis (TORP))

69641 Tympanoplasty with mastoidectomy (including canalplasty, middle ear surgery, tympanic membrane repair); without ossicular chain reconstruction

69642   with ossicular chain reconstruction

69643   with intact or reconstructed wall, without ossicular chain reconstruction

69644   with intact or reconstructed canal wall, with ossicular chain reconstruction

69645   radical or complete, without ossicular chain reconstruction

69646   radical or complete, with ossicular chain reconstruction

69650 Stapes mobilization

69660 Stapedectomy or stapedotomy with reestablishment of ossicular continuity, with or without use of foreign material;

69661   with footplate drill out

69662 Revision of stapedectomy or stapedotomy

69666 Repair oval window fistula

69667 Repair round window fistula

69670 Mastoid obliteration (separate procedure)

69676 Tympanic neurectomy

    (For bilateral procedure, report 69676 with modifier 50)

Other Procedures

69700 Closure postauricular fistula, mastoid (separate procedure)

69710 Implantation or replacement of electromagnetic bone conduction hearing device in temporal bone

    (Replacement procedure includes removal of old device)

69711 Removal or repair of electromagnetic bone conduction hearing device in temporal bone

69714 Implantation, osseointegrated implant, temporal bone, with percutaneous attachment to external speech processor/cochlear stimulator; without mastoidectomy

69715   with mastoidectomy

69717 Replacement (including removal of existing device), osseointegrated implant, temporal bone, with percutaneous attachment to external speech processor/cochlear stimulator; without mastoidectomy

69718   with mastoidectomy

Surgery: Ocular/Auditory System

69720   Decompression facial nerve, intratemporal; lateral to geniculate ganglion

69725   including medial to geniculate ganglion

69740   Suture facial nerve, intratemporal, with or without graft or decompression; lateral to geniculate ganglion

69745   including medial to geniculate ganglion

        (For extracranial suture of facial nerve, use 64864)

69799   Unlisted procedure, middle ear

Inner Ear

Incision and/or Destruction

69801   Labyrinthotomy, with or without cryosurgery including other nonexcisional destructive procedures or perfusion of vestibuloactive drugs (single or multiple perfusions); transcanal

        (69801 includes all required infusions performed on initial and subsequent days of treatment)

69802   with mastoidectomy

69805   Endolymphatic sac operation; without shunt

69806   with shunt

69820   Fenestration semicircular canal

69840   Revision fenestration operation

Excision

69905   Labyrinthectomy; transcanal

69910   with mastoidectomy

69915   Vestibular nerve section, translabyrinthine approach

        (For transcranial approach, use 69950)

Introduction

69930   Cochlear device implantation, with or without mastoidectomy

Other Procedures

69949   Unlisted procedure, inner ear

Temporal Bone, Middle Fossa Approach

        (For external approach, use 69535)

69950   Vestibular nerve section, transcranial approach

69955   Total facial nerve decompression and/or repair (may include graft)

69960   Decompression internal auditory canal

69970   Removal of tumor, temporal bone

Other Procedures

69979   Unlisted procedure, temporal bone, middle fossa approach

Operating Microscope

The surgical microscope is employed when the surgical services are performed using the techniques of microsurgery. Code 69990 should be reported (without modifier 51 appended) in addition to the code for the primary procedure performed. Do not use 69990 for visualization with magnifying loupes or corrected vision. Do not report code 69990 in addition to procedures where use of the operating microscope is an inclusive component (15756-15758, 15842, 19364, 19368, 20955-20962, 20969-20973, 26551-26554, 26556, 31526, 31531, 31536, 31541, 31561, 31571, 43116, 43496, 49906, 61548, 63075-63078, 64727, 64820-64823, 65091-68850).

+ 69990   Microsurgical techniques, requiring use of operating microscope (List separately in addition to code for primary procedure)

Surgery: Ocular/Auditory System

Notes

Surgery: Ocular/Auditory System

Radiology Guidelines (Including Nuclear Medicine and Diagnostic Ultrasound)

Items used by all physicians in reporting their services are presented in the **Introduction.** Some of the commonalities are repeated here for the convenience of those physicians referring to this section on **Radiology (Including Nuclear Medicine and Diagnostic Ultrasound).** Other definitions and items unique to Radiology are also listed.

Subject Listings

Subject listings apply when radiological services are performed by or under the responsible supervision of a physician.

Separate Procedures

Some of the procedures or services listed in *CPT* that are commonly carried out as an integral component of a total service or procedure have been identified by the inclusion of the term "separate procedure." The codes designated as "separate procedure" should not be reported in addition to the code for the total procedure or service of which it is considered an integral component.

However, when a procedure or service that is designated as a "separate procedure" is carried out independently or considered to be unrelated or distinct from other procedures/services provided at that time, it may be reported by itself, or in addition to other procedures/services by appending modifier 59 to the specific "separate procedure" code to indicate that the procedure is not considered to be a component of another procedure, but is a distinct, independent procedure. This may represent a different session or patient encounter, different procedure or surgery, different site or organ system, separate incision/excision, separate lesion, or separate injury (or area of injury in extensive injuries).

Subsection Information

Several of the subheadings or subsections have special needs or instructions unique to that section. Where these are indicated (eg, "Radiation Oncology") special **"Notes"** will be presented preceding those procedural terminology listings, referring to that subsection specifically. If there is an "Unlisted Procedure" code number (see section below) for the individual subsection, it will be shown. Those subsections with **"Notes"** are as follows:

Aorta and Arteries	75600-75790
▶**Veins and Lymphatics**	75801-75893◀
▶**Transcatheter Procedures**	75894-75989◀
Diagnostic Ultrasound	76506-76999
▶**Abdomen and Retroperitoneum**	76700-76778◀
▶**Obstetrical**	76801-76828◀
▶**Non-Obstetrical**	76830-76857◀
Radiation Oncology	77261-77799
Clinical Treatment Planning	77261-77299
Radiation Treatment Management	77427-77499
Proton Beam Treatment Delivery	77520-77525
Hyperthermia	77600-77620
Clinical Brachytherapy	77750-77799
Nuclear Medicine	78000-78299
Musculoskeletal System	78300-78399
Cardiovascular System	78414-78499
▶**Therapeutic**	79005-79999◀

Unlisted Service or Procedure

A service or procedure may be provided that is not listed in this edition of *CPT.* When reporting such a service, the appropriate "Unlisted Procedure" code may be used to indicate the service, identifying it by "Special Report" as discussed below. The "Unlisted Procedures" and accompanying codes for **Radiology (Including Nuclear Medicine and Diagnostic Ultrasound)** are as follows:

76496 Unlisted fluoroscopic procedure (eg, diagnostic, interventional)

76497 Unlisted computed tomography procedure (eg, diagnostic, interventional)

76498 Unlisted magnetic resonance procedure (eg, diagnostic, interventional)

76499 Unlisted diagnostic radiographic procedure

76999	Unlisted ultrasound procedure (eg, diagnostic, interventional)
77299	Unlisted procedure, therapeutic radiology clinical treatment planning
77399	Unlisted procedure, medical radiation physics, dosimetry and treatment devices, and special services
77499	Unlisted procedure, therapeutic radiology treatment management
77799	Unlisted procedure, clinical brachytherapy
78099	Unlisted endocrine procedure, diagnostic nuclear medicine
78199	Unlisted hematopoietic, reticuloendothelial and lymphatic procedure, diagnostic nuclear medicine
78299	Unlisted gastrointestinal procedure, diagnostic nuclear medicine
78399	Unlisted musculoskeletal procedure, diagnostic nuclear medicine
78499	Unlisted cardiovascular procedure, diagnostic nuclear medicine
78599	Unlisted respiratory procedure, diagnostic nuclear medicine
78699	Unlisted nervous system procedure, diagnostic nuclear medicine
78799	Unlisted genitourinary procedure, diagnostic nuclear medicine
78999	Unlisted miscellaneous procedure, diagnostic nuclear medicine
▲ 79999	Radiopharmaceutical therapy, unlisted procedure

Special Report

A service that is rarely provided, unusual, variable, or new may require a special report in determining medical appropriateness of the service. Pertinent information should include an adequate definition or description of the nature, extent, and need for the procedure; and the time, effort, and equipment necessary to provide the service. Additional items which may be included are:

- complexity of symptoms;
- final diagnosis;
- pertinent physical findings;
- diagnostic and therapeutic procedures;
- concurrent problems;
- follow-up care.

Supervision and Interpretation

When a procedure is performed by two physicians, the radiologic portion of the procedure is designated as "radiological supervision and interpretation." When a

physician performs both the procedure and provides imaging supervision and interpretation, a combination of procedure codes outside the 70000 series and imaging supervision and interpretation codes are to be used.

(The Radiological Supervision and Interpretation codes are not applicable to the Radiation Oncology subsection.)

Administration of Contrast Material(s)

The phrase "with contrast" used in the codes for procedures performed using contrast for imaging enhancement represents contrast material administered intravascularly, intra-articularly or intrathecally.

For intra-articular injection, use the appropriate joint injection code. If radiographic arthrography is performed, also use the arthrography supervision and interpretation code for the appropriate joint (which includes fluoroscopy). If CT or MR arthrography are performed without radiographic arthrography, use the appropriate joint injection code, the appropriate CT or MR code ("with contrast" or "without followed by contrast"), and the appropriate imaging guidance code for needle placement for contrast injection.

For spine examinations using computed tomography, magnetic resonance imaging, magnetic resonance angiography, "with contrast" includes intrathecal or intravascular injection. For intrathecal injection, use also 61055 or 62284.

Injection of intravascular contrast material is part of the "with contrast" CT, CTA, MRI, MRA procedure.

Oral and/or rectal contrast administration alone does not qualify as a study "with contrast."

Written Report(s)

A written report, signed by the interpreting physician, should be considered an integral part of a radiologic procedure or interpretation.

Radiology

Diagnostic Radiology (Diagnostic Imaging)

Head and Neck

70010 Myelography, posterior fossa, radiological supervision and interpretation

70015 Cisternography, positive contrast, radiological supervision and interpretation

70030 Radiologic examination, eye, for detection of foreign body

70100 Radiologic examination, mandible; partial, less than four views

70110 complete, minimum of four views

70120 Radiologic examination, mastoids; less than three views per side

70130 complete, minimum of three views per side

70134 Radiologic examination, internal auditory meati, complete

70140 Radiologic examination, facial bones; less than three views

70150 complete, minimum of three views

70160 Radiologic examination, nasal bones, complete, minimum of three views

70170 Dacryocystography, nasolacrimal duct, radiological supervision and interpretation

70190 Radiologic examination; optic foramina

70200 orbits, complete, minimum of four views

70210 Radiologic examination, sinuses, paranasal, less than three views

70220 Radiologic examination, sinuses, paranasal, complete, minimum of three views

70240 Radiologic examination, sella turcica

70250 Radiologic examination, skull; less than four views

70260 complete, minimum of four views

70300 Radiologic examination, teeth; single view

70310 partial examination, less than full mouth

70320 complete, full mouth

70328 Radiologic examination, temporomandibular joint, open and closed mouth; unilateral

70330 bilateral

70332 Temporomandibular joint arthrography, radiological supervision and interpretation

(Do not report 76003 in addition to 70332)

70336 Magnetic resonance (eg, proton) imaging, temporomandibular joint(s)

70350 Cephalogram, orthodontic

70355 Orthopantogram

70360 Radiologic examination; neck, soft tissue

70370 pharynx or larynx, including fluoroscopy and/or magnification technique

70371 Complex dynamic pharyngeal and speech evaluation by cine or video recording

70373 Laryngography, contrast, radiological supervision and interpretation

70380 Radiologic examination, salivary gland for calculus

70390 Sialography, radiological supervision and interpretation

70450 Computed tomography, head or brain; without contrast material

70460 with contrast material(s)

70470 without contrast material, followed by contrast material(s) and further sections

(For coronal, sagittal, and/or oblique sections, use 76375)

70480 Computed tomography, orbit, sella, or posterior fossa or outer, middle, or inner ear; without contrast material

70481 with contrast material(s)

70482 without contrast material, followed by contrast material(s) and further sections

(For coronal, sagittal, and/or oblique sections, use 76375)

70486 Computed tomography, maxillofacial area; without contrast material

70487 with contrast material(s)

70488 without contrast material, followed by contrast material(s) and further sections

(For coronal, sagittal, and/or oblique sections, use 76375)

70490 Computed tomography, soft tissue neck; without contrast material

70491 with contrast material(s)

70492 without contrast material followed by contrast material(s) and further sections

(For coronal, sagittal, and/or oblique sections, use 76375)

(For cervical spine, see 72125, 72126)

70496 Computed tomographic angiography, head, without contrast material(s), followed by contrast material(s) and further sections, including image post-processing

70498 Computed tomographic angiography, neck, without contrast material(s), followed by contrast material(s) and further sections, including image post-processing

70540 Magnetic resonance (eg, proton) imaging, orbit, face, and neck; without contrast material(s)

(For head or neck magnetic resonance angiography studies, see 70544-70546, 70547-70549)

70542 with contrast material(s)

70543 without contrast material(s), followed by contrast material(s) and further sequences

70544 Magnetic resonance angiography, head; without contrast material(s)

70545 with contrast material(s)

70546 without contrast material(s), followed by contrast material(s) and further sequences

70547 Magnetic resonance angiography, neck; without contrast material(s)

70548 with contrast material(s)

70549 without contrast material(s), followed by contrast material(s) and further sequences

70551 Magnetic resonance (eg, proton) imaging, brain (including brain stem); without contrast material

70552 with contrast material(s)

70553 without contrast material, followed by contrast material(s) and further sequences

(For magnetic spectroscopy, use 76390)

70557 Magnetic resonance (eg, proton) imaging, brain (including brain stem and skull base), during open intracranial procedure (eg, to assess for residual tumor or residual vascular malformation); without contrast material

70558 with contrast material(s)

70559 without contrast material(s), followed by contrast material(s) and further sequences

(For stereotactic biopsy of intracranial lesion with magnetic resonance guidance, use 61751. 70557, 70558 or 70559 may be reported only if a separate report is generated. Report only one of the above codes once per operative session. Do not use these codes in conjunction with 61751, 76393, 76394)

Chest

(For fluoroscopic or ultrasonic guidance for needle placement procedures (eg, biopsy, aspiration, injection, localization device) of the thorax, see 76003, 76942)

71010 Radiologic examination, chest; single view, frontal

71015 stereo, frontal

71020 Radiologic examination, chest, two views, frontal and lateral;

71021 with apical lordotic procedure

71022 with oblique projections

71023 with fluoroscopy

71030 Radiologic examination, chest, complete, minimum of four views;

71034 with fluoroscopy

(For separate chest fluoroscopy, use 76000)

71035 Radiologic examination, chest, special views (eg, lateral decubitus, Bucky studies)

71040 Bronchography, unilateral, radiological supervision and interpretation

71060 Bronchography, bilateral, radiological supervision and interpretation

71090 Insertion pacemaker, fluoroscopy and radiography, radiological supervision and interpretation

(For procedure, see appropriate organ or site)

71100 Radiologic examination, ribs, unilateral; two views

71101 including posteroanterior chest, minimum of three views

71110 Radiologic examination, ribs, bilateral; three views

71111 including posteroanterior chest, minimum of four views

71120 Radiologic examination; sternum, minimum of two views

71130 sternoclavicular joint or joints, minimum of three views

71250 Computed tomography, thorax; without contrast material

71260 with contrast material(s)

71270 without contrast material, followed by contrast material(s) and further sections

(For coronal, sagittal, and/or oblique sections, use 76375)

71275 Computed tomographic angiography, chest, without contrast material(s), followed by contrast material(s) and further sections, including image post-processing

71550 Magnetic resonance (eg, proton) imaging, chest (eg, for evaluation of hilar and mediastinal lymphadenopathy); without contrast material(s)

71551 with contrast material(s)

71552 without contrast material(s), followed by contrast material(s) and further sequences

(For breast MRI, see 76093 and 76094)

71555 Magnetic resonance angiography, chest (excluding myocardium), with or without contrast material(s)

Spine and Pelvis

72010   Radiologic examination, spine, entire, survey study, anteroposterior and lateral

72020   Radiologic examination, spine, single view, specify level

72040   Radiologic examination, spine, cervical; two or three views

72050   minimum of four views

72052   complete, including oblique and flexion and/or extension studies

72069   Radiologic examination, spine, thoracolumbar, standing (scoliosis)

72070   Radiologic examination, spine; thoracic, two views

72072   thoracic, three views

72074   thoracic, minimum of four views

72080   thoracolumbar, two views

72090   scoliosis study, including supine and erect studies

72100   Radiologic examination, spine, lumbosacral; two or three views

72110   minimum of four views

72114   complete, including bending views

72120   Radiologic examination, spine, lumbosacral, bending views only, minimum of four views

(Contrast material in CT of spine is either by intrathecal or intravenous injection. For intrathecal injection, use also 61055 or 62284. IV injection of contrast material is part of the CT procedure)

72125   Computed tomography, cervical spine; without contrast material

72126   with contrast material

72127   without contrast material, followed by contrast material(s) and further sections

(For intrathecal injection procedure, see 61055, 62284)

72128   Computed tomography, thoracic spine; without contrast material

72129   with contrast material

(For intrathecal injection procedure, see 61055, 62284)

72130   without contrast material, followed by contrast material(s) and further sections

(For intrathecal injection procedure, see 61055, 62284)

72131   Computed tomography, lumbar spine; without contrast material

72132   with contrast material

72133   without contrast material, followed by contrast material(s) and further sections

(For intrathecal injection procedure, see 61055, 62284)

(For coronal, sagittal, and/or oblique sections, use 76375)

72141   Magnetic resonance (eg, proton) imaging, spinal canal and contents, cervical; without contrast material

72142   with contrast material(s)

(For cervical spinal canal imaging without contrast material followed by contrast material, use 72156)

72146   Magnetic resonance (eg, proton) imaging, spinal canal and contents, thoracic; without contrast material

72147   with contrast material(s)

(For thoracic spinal canal imaging without contrast material followed by contrast material, use 72157)

72148   Magnetic resonance (eg, proton) imaging, spinal canal and contents, lumbar; without contrast material

72149   with contrast material(s)

(For lumbar spinal canal imaging without contrast material followed by contrast material, use 72158)

72156   Magnetic resonance (eg, proton) imaging, spinal canal and contents, without contrast material, followed by contrast material(s) and further sequences; cervical

72157   thoracic

72158   lumbar

72159   Magnetic resonance angiography, spinal canal and contents, with or without contrast material(s)

72170   Radiologic examination, pelvis; one or two views

72190   complete, minimum of three views

(For pelvimetry, use 74710)

72191   Computed tomographic angiography, pelvis, without contrast material(s), followed by contrast material(s) and further sections, including image post-processing

(For CTA aorto-iliofemoral runoff, use 75635)

72192   Computed tomography, pelvis; without contrast material

72193   with contrast material(s)

72194   without contrast material, followed by contrast material(s) and further sections

(For coronal, sagittal, and/or oblique sections, use 76375)

►(For computed tomographic colonography, see Category III codes 0066T, 0067T. Do not report 72192-72194 in conjunction with 0066T, 0067T)◄

72195   Magnetic resonance (eg, proton) imaging, pelvis; without contrast material(s)

72196   with contrast material(s)

72197   without contrast material(s), followed by contrast material(s) and further sequences

72198   Magnetic resonance angiography, pelvis, with or without contrast material(s)

72200   Radiologic examination, sacroiliac joints; less than three views

72202   three or more views

Radiology

72220 Radiologic examination, sacrum and coccyx, minimum of two views

72240 Myelography, cervical, radiological supervision and interpretation

(For complete cervical myelography, see 61055, 62284, 72240)

72255 Myelography, thoracic, radiological supervision and interpretation

(For complete thoracic myelography, see 61055, 62284, 72255)

72265 Myelography, lumbosacral, radiological supervision and interpretation

(For complete lumbosacral myelography, see 61055, 62284, 72265)

72270 Myelography, two or more regions (eg, lumbar/thoracic, cervical/thoracic, lumbar/cervical, lumbar/thoracic/cervical), radiological supervision and interpretation

(For complete myelography of entire spinal canal, see 61055, 62284, 72270)

72275 Epidurography, radiological supervision and interpretation

(72275 includes 76005)

(For injection procedure, see 62280-62282, 62310-62319, 64479-64484, 0027T)

(Use 72275 only when an epidurogram is performed, images documented, and a formal radiologic report is issued)

72285 Diskography, cervical or thoracic, radiological supervision and interpretation

72295 Diskography, lumbar, radiological supervision and interpretation

Upper Extremities

(For stress views, any joint, use 76006)

73000 Radiologic examination; clavicle, complete

73010 scapula, complete

73020 Radiologic examination, shoulder; one view

73030 complete, minimum of two views

73040 Radiologic examination, shoulder, arthrography, radiological supervision and interpretation

(Do not report 76003 in addition to 73040)

73050 Radiologic examination; acromioclavicular joints, bilateral, with or without weighted distraction

73060 humerus, minimum of two views

73070 Radiologic examination, elbow; two views

73080 complete, minimum of three views

73085 Radiologic examination, elbow, arthrography, radiological supervision and interpretation

(Do not report 76003 in addition to 73085)

73090 Radiologic examination; forearm, two views

73092 upper extremity, infant, minimum of two views

73100 Radiologic examination, wrist; two views

73110 complete, minimum of three views

73115 Radiologic examination, wrist, arthrography, radiological supervision and interpretation

(Do not report 76003 in addition to 73115)

73120 Radiologic examination, hand; two views

73130 minimum of three views

73140 Radiologic examination, finger(s), minimum of two views

73200 Computed tomography, upper extremity; without contrast material

73201 with contrast material(s)

73202 without contrast material, followed by contrast material(s) and further sections

(For coronal, sagittal, and/or oblique sections, use 76375)

73206 Computed tomographic angiography, upper extremity, without contrast material(s), followed by contrast material(s) and further sections, including image post-processing

73218 Magnetic resonance (eg, proton) imaging, upper extremity, other than joint; without contrast material(s)

73219 with contrast material(s)

73220 without contrast material(s), followed by contrast material(s) and further sequences

73221 Magnetic resonance (eg, proton) imaging, any joint of upper extremity; without contrast material(s)

73222 with contrast material(s)

73223 without contrast material(s), followed by contrast material(s) and further sequences

73225 Magnetic resonance angiography, upper extremity, with or without contrast material(s)

Lower Extremities

(For stress views, any joint, use 76006)

73500 Radiologic examination, hip, unilateral; one view

73510 complete, minimum of two views

73520 Radiologic examination, hips, bilateral, minimum of two views of each hip, including anteroposterior view of pelvis

73525 Radiologic examination, hip, arthrography, radiological supervision and interpretation

(Do not report 76003 in addition to 73525)

Radiology

73530	Radiologic examination, hip, during operative procedure
73540	Radiologic examination, pelvis and hips, infant or child, minimum of two views
73542	Radiological examination, sacroiliac joint arthrography, radiological supervision and interpretation

(Do not report 76003 in addition to 73542)

(For procedure, use 27096. If formal arthrography is not performed, recorded, and a formal radiologic report is not issued, use 76005 for fluoroscopic guidance for sacroiliac joint injections)

73550	Radiologic examination, femur, two views
73560	Radiologic examination, knee; one or two views
73562	three views
73564	complete, four or more views
73565	both knees, standing, anteroposterior
73580	Radiologic examination, knee, arthrography, radiological supervision and interpretation

(Do not report 76003 in addition to 73580)

73590	Radiologic examination; tibia and fibula, two views
73592	lower extremity, infant, minimum of two views
73600	Radiologic examination, ankle; two views
73610	complete, minimum of three views
73615	Radiologic examination, ankle, arthrography, radiological supervision and interpretation

(Do not report 76003 in addition to 73615)

73620	Radiologic examination, foot; two views
73630	complete, minimum of three views
73650	Radiologic examination; calcaneus, minimum of two views
73660	toe(s), minimum of two views
73700	Computed tomography, lower extremity; without contrast material
73701	with contrast material(s)
73702	without contrast material, followed by contrast material(s) and further sections

(For coronal, sagittal, and/or oblique sections, use 76375)

73706	Computed tomographic angiography, lower extremity, without contrast material(s), followed by contrast material(s) and further sections, including image post-processing

(For CTA aorto-iliofemoral runoff, use 75635)

73718	Magnetic resonance (eg, proton) imaging, lower extremity other than joint; without contrast material(s)
73719	with contrast material(s)
73720	without contrast material(s), followed by contrast material(s) and further sequences
73721	Magnetic resonance (eg, proton) imaging, any joint of lower extremity; without contrast material
73722	with contrast material(s)
73723	without contrast material(s), followed by contrast material(s) and further sequences
73725	Magnetic resonance angiography, lower extremity, with or without contrast material(s)

Abdomen

74000	Radiologic examination, abdomen; single anteroposterior view
74010	anteroposterior and additional oblique and cone views
74020	complete, including decubitus and/or erect views
74022	complete acute abdomen series, including supine, erect, and/or decubitus views, single view chest
74150	Computed tomography, abdomen; without contrast material
74160	with contrast material(s)
74170	without contrast material, followed by contrast material(s) and further sections

(For coronal, sagittal, and/or oblique sections, use 76375)

▶(For computed tomographic colonography, see Category III codes 0066T, 0067T. Do not report 74150-74170 in conjunction with 0066T, 0067T)◀

74175	Computed tomographic angiography, abdomen, without contrast material(s), followed by contrast material(s) and further sections, including image post-processing

(For CTA aorto-iliofemoral runoff, use 75635)

74181	Magnetic resonance (eg, proton) imaging, abdomen; without contrast material(s)
74182	with contrast material(s)
74183	without contrast material(s), followed by with contrast material(s) and further sequences
74185	Magnetic resonance angiography, abdomen, with or without contrast material(s)
74190	Peritoneogram (eg, after injection of air or contrast), radiological supervision and interpretation

(For procedure, use 49400)

(For computed tomography, see 72192 or 74150)

Gastrointestinal Tract

(For percutaneous placement of gastrostomy tube, use 43750)

74210	Radiologic examination; pharynx and/or cervical esophagus
74220	esophagus
74230	Swallowing function, with cineradiography/videoradiography

Radiology

74235 Removal of foreign body(s), esophageal, with use of balloon catheter, radiological supervision and interpretation

(For procedure, see 43215, 43247)

74240 Radiologic examination, gastrointestinal tract, upper; with or without delayed films, without KUB

74241 with or without delayed films, with KUB

74245 with small intestine, includes multiple serial films

74246 Radiological examination, gastrointestinal tract, upper, air contrast, with specific high density barium, effervescent agent, with or without glucagon; with or without delayed films, without KUB

74247 with or without delayed films, with KUB

74249 with small intestine follow-through

74250 Radiologic examination, small intestine, includes multiple serial films;

74251 via enteroclysis tube

74260 Duodenography, hypotonic

74270 Radiologic examination, colon; barium enema, with or without KUB

74280 air contrast with specific high density barium, with or without glucagon

74283 Therapeutic enema, contrast or air, for reduction of intussusception or other intraluminal obstruction (eg, meconium ileus)

74290 Cholecystography, oral contrast;

74291 additional or repeat examination or multiple day examination

74300 Cholangiography and/or pancreatography; intraoperative, radiological supervision and interpretation

+ 74301 additional set intraoperative, radiological supervision and interpretation (List separately in addition to code for primary procedure)

(Use 74301 in conjunction with 74300)

74305 through existing catheter, radiological supervision and interpretation

(For procedure, see 47505, 48400, 47560-47561, 47563)

(For biliary duct stone extraction, percutaneous, see 47630, 74327)

74320 Cholangiography, percutaneous, transhepatic, radiological supervision and interpretation

74327 Postoperative biliary duct calculus removal, percutaneous via T-tube tract, basket, or snare (eg, Burhenne technique), radiological supervision and interpretation

(For procedure, use 47630)

74328 Endoscopic catheterization of the biliary ductal system, radiological supervision and interpretation

(For procedure, see 43260-43272 as appropriate)

74329 Endoscopic catheterization of the pancreatic ductal system, radiological supervision and interpretation

(For procedure, see 43260-43272 as appropriate)

74330 Combined endoscopic catheterization of the biliary and pancreatic ductal systems, radiological supervision and interpretation

(For procedure, see 43260-43272 as appropriate)

74340 Introduction of long gastrointestinal tube (eg, Miller-Abbott), including multiple fluoroscopies and films, radiological supervision and interpretation

(For tube placement, use 44500)

74350 Percutaneous placement of gastrostomy tube, radiological supervision and interpretation

74355 Percutaneous placement of enteroclysis tube, radiological supervision and interpretation

74360 Intraluminal dilation of strictures and/or obstructions (eg, esophagus), radiological supervision and interpretation

74363 Percutaneous transhepatic dilation of biliary duct stricture with or without placement of stent, radiological supervision and interpretation

(For procedure, see 47510, 47511, 47555, 47556)

Urinary Tract

74400 Urography (pyelography), intravenous, with or without KUB, with or without tomography

74410 Urography, infusion, drip technique and/or bolus technique;

74415 with nephrotomography

74420 Urography, retrograde, with or without KUB

74425 Urography, antegrade, (pyelostogram, nephrostogram, loopogram), radiological supervision and interpretation

74430 Cystography, minimum of three views, radiological supervision and interpretation

74440 Vasography, vesiculography, or epididymography, radiological supervision and interpretation

74445 Corpora cavernosography, radiological supervision and interpretation

74450 Urethrocystography, retrograde, radiological supervision and interpretation

74455 Urethrocystography, voiding, radiological supervision and interpretation

74470 Radiologic examination, renal cyst study, translumbar, contrast visualization, radiological supervision and interpretation

74475 Introduction of intracatheter or catheter into renal pelvis for drainage and/or injection, percutaneous, radiological supervision and interpretation

Radiology

74480 Introduction of ureteral catheter or stent into ureter through renal pelvis for drainage and/or injection, percutaneous, radiological supervision and interpretation

(For transurethral surgery (ureter and pelvis), see 52320-52355)

74485 Dilation of nephrostomy, ureters, or urethra, radiological supervision and interpretation

(For dilation of ureter without radiologic guidance, use 52341, 52344)

(For change of nephrostomy or pyelostomy tube, use 50398)

Gynecological and Obstetrical

(For abdomen and pelvis, see 72170-72190, 74000-74170)

74710 Pelvimetry, with or without placental localization

74740 Hysterosalpingography, radiological supervision and interpretation

(For introduction of saline or contrast for hysterosalpingography, see 58340)

74742 Transcervical catheterization of fallopian tube, radiological supervision and interpretation

(For procedure, use 58345)

74775 Perineogram (eg, vaginogram, for sex determination or extent of anomalies)

Heart

(For separate injection procedures for vascular radiology, see **Surgery** section, 36000-36299)

(For cardiac catheterization procedures, see 93501-93556)

75552 Cardiac magnetic resonance imaging for morphology; without contrast material

75553   with contrast material

75554 Cardiac magnetic resonance imaging for function, with or without morphology; complete study

75555   limited study

75556 Cardiac magnetic resonance imaging for velocity flow mapping

▶Vascular Procedures◀

Aorta and Arteries

Selective vascular catheterizations should be coded to include introduction and all lesser order selective catheterizations used in the approach (eg, the description for a selective right middle cerebral artery catheterization includes the introduction and placement catheterization of the right common and internal carotid arteries).

Additional second and/or third order arterial catheterizations within the same family of arteries supplied by a single first order artery should be expressed by 36218 or 36248. Additional first order or higher catheterizations in vascular families supplied by a first order vessel different from a previously selected and coded family should be separately coded using the conventions described above.

▶For angiography performed in conjunction with therapeutic transcatheter radiological supervision and interpretation services, see the Radiology Transcatheter Procedures guidelines.◀

▶Diagnostic angiography (radiological supervision and interpretation) codes should NOT be used with interventional procedures for:◀

▶1) Contrast injections, angiography, roadmapping, and/or fluoroscopic guidance for the intervention,◀

▶2) Vessel measurement, and◀

▶3) Post-angioplasty/stent angiography◀

▶as this work is captured in the interventional procedure code(s).◀

▶Diagnostic angiography performed at the time of an interventional procedure is separately reportable if:◀

▶1) No prior catheter-based angiographic study is available and a full diagnostic study is performed, and the decision to intervene is based on the diagnostic study, OR◀

▶2) A prior study is available, but as documented in the medical record:◀

▶a) The patient's condition with respect to the clinical indication has changed since the prior study, OR◀

▶b) There is inadequate visualization of the anatomy and/or pathology, OR◀

▶c) There is a clinical change during the procedure that requires new evaluation outside the target area of intervention◀

▶Diagnostic angiography performed at a separate setting from an interventional procedure is separately reported.◀

▶Diagnostic angiography performed at the time of an interventional procedure is NOT separately reportable if it is specifically included in the interventional code descriptor.◀

(For intravenous procedure, see 36000-36013, 36400-36425 and 36100-36248 for intra-arterial procedure)

(For radiological supervision and interpretation, see 75600-75978)

75600 Aortography, thoracic, without serialography, radiological supervision and interpretation

(For injection procedure, use 93544)

75605 Aortography, thoracic, by serialography, radiological supervision and interpretation

(For injection procedure, use 93544)

75625 Aortography, abdominal, by serialography, radiological supervision and interpretation

(For injection procedure, use 93544)

75630 Aortography, abdominal plus bilateral iliofemoral lower extremity, catheter, by serialography, radiological supervision and interpretation

75635 Computed tomographic angiography, abdominal aorta and bilateral iliofemoral lower extremity runoff, radiological supervision and interpretation, without contrast material(s), followed by contrast material(s) and further sections, including image post-processing

75650 Angiography, cervicocerebral, catheter, including vessel origin, radiological supervision and interpretation

75658 Angiography, brachial, retrograde, radiological supervision and interpretation

75660 Angiography, external carotid, unilateral, selective, radiological supervision and interpretation

75662 Angiography, external carotid, bilateral, selective, radiological supervision and interpretation

75665 Angiography, carotid, cerebral, unilateral, radiological supervision and interpretation

75671 Angiography, carotid, cerebral, bilateral, radiological supervision and interpretation

75676 Angiography, carotid, cervical, unilateral, radiological supervision and interpretation

75680 Angiography, carotid, cervical, bilateral, radiological supervision and interpretation

75685 Angiography, vertebral, cervical, and/or intracranial, radiological supervision and interpretation

75705 Angiography, spinal, selective, radiological supervision and interpretation

75710 Angiography, extremity, unilateral, radiological supervision and interpretation

75716 Angiography, extremity, bilateral, radiological supervision and interpretation

75722 Angiography, renal, unilateral, selective (including flush aortogram), radiological supervision and interpretation

75724 Angiography, renal, bilateral, selective (including flush aortogram), radiological supervision and interpretation

75726 Angiography, visceral, selective or supraselective, (with or without flush aortogram), radiological supervision and interpretation

(For selective angiography, each additional visceral vessel studied after basic examination, use 75774)

75731 Angiography, adrenal, unilateral, selective, radiological supervision and interpretation

75733 Angiography, adrenal, bilateral, selective, radiological supervision and interpretation

75736 Angiography, pelvic, selective or supraselective, radiological supervision and interpretation

75741 Angiography, pulmonary, unilateral, selective, radiological supervision and interpretation

(For injection procedure, use 93541)

75743 Angiography, pulmonary, bilateral, selective, radiological supervision and interpretation

(For injection procedure, use 93541)

75746 Angiography, pulmonary, by nonselective catheter or venous injection, radiological supervision and interpretation

(For injection procedure, use 93541)

(For introduction of catheter, injection procedure, see 93501-93533, 93539, 93540, 93545, 93556)

(For introduction of catheter, injection procedure, see 93501-93533, 93545, 93556)

(For introduction of catheter, injection procedure, see 93501-93533, 93539, 93540, 93545, 93556)

75756 Angiography, internal mammary, radiological supervision and interpretation

(For introduction of catheter, injection procedure, see 93501-93533, 93545, 93556)

+ 75774 Angiography, selective, each additional vessel studied after basic examination, radiological supervision and interpretation (List separately in addition to code for primary procedure)

(Use 75774 in addition to code for specific initial vessel studied)

(For angiography, see codes 75600-75790)

(For catheterizations, see codes 36215-36248)

(For introduction of catheter, injection procedure, see 93501-93533, 93545, 93555, 93556)

75790 Angiography, arteriovenous shunt (eg, dialysis patient), radiological supervision and interpretation

(For introduction of catheter, use 36140, 36145, 36215-36217, 36245-36247)

Veins and Lymphatics

▶For venography performed in conjunction with therapeutic transcatheter radiological supervision and interpretation services, see the Radiology Transcatheter Procedures guidelines.◀

▶Diagnostic venography (radiological supervision and interpretation) codes should NOT be used with interventional procedures for:◀

▶1) Contrast injections, venography, roadmapping, and/or fluoroscopic guidance for the intervention,◀

▶2) Vessel measurement, and◀

▶3) Post-angioplasty/stent venography◀

▶as this work is captured in the interventional procedure code(s).◀

▶Diagnostic venography performed at the time of an interventional procedure is separately reportable if:◀

▶1) No prior catheter-based venographic study is available and a full diagnostic study is performed, and decision to intervene is based on the diagnostic study, OR◀

▶2) A prior study is available, but as documented in the medical record:◀

▶a) The patient's condition with respect to the clinical indication has changed since the prior study, OR◀

▶b) There is inadequate visualization of the anatomy and/or pathology, OR◀

▶c) There is a clinical change during the procedure that requires new evaluation outside the target area of intervention◀

▶Diagnostic venography performed at a separate setting from an interventional procedure is separately reported.◀

▶Diagnostic venography performed at the time of an interventional procedure is NOT separately reportable if it is specifically included in the interventional code descriptor.◀

(For injection procedure for venous system, see 36000-36015, 36400-36510)

(For injection procedure for lymphatic system, use 38790)

75801 Lymphangiography, extremity only, unilateral, radiological supervision and interpretation

75803 Lymphangiography, extremity only, bilateral, radiological supervision and interpretation

75805 Lymphangiography, pelvic/abdominal, unilateral, radiological supervision and interpretation

75807 Lymphangiography, pelvic/abdominal, bilateral, radiological supervision and interpretation

75809 Shuntogram for investigation of previously placed indwelling nonvascular shunt (eg, LeVeen shunt, ventriculoperitoneal shunt, indwelling infusion pump), radiological supervision and interpretation

(For procedure, see 49427 or 61070)

75810 Splenoportography, radiological supervision and interpretation

75820 Venography, extremity, unilateral, radiological supervision and interpretation

75822 Venography, extremity, bilateral, radiological supervision and interpretation

75825 Venography, caval, inferior, with serialography, radiological supervision and interpretation

75827 Venography, caval, superior, with serialography, radiological supervision and interpretation

75831 Venography, renal, unilateral, selective, radiological supervision and interpretation

75833 Venography, renal, bilateral, selective, radiological supervision and interpretation

75840 Venography, adrenal, unilateral, selective, radiological supervision and interpretation

75842 Venography, adrenal, bilateral, selective, radiological supervision and interpretation

75860 Venography, venous sinus (eg, petrosal and inferior sagittal) or jugular, catheter, radiological supervision and interpretation

75870 Venography, superior sagittal sinus, radiological supervision and interpretation

75872 Venography, epidural, radiological supervision and interpretation

75880 Venography, orbital, radiological supervision and interpretation

75885 Percutaneous transhepatic portography with hemodynamic evaluation, radiological supervision and interpretation

75887 Percutaneous transhepatic portography without hemodynamic evaluation, radiological supervision and interpretation

75889 Hepatic venography, wedged or free, with hemodynamic evaluation, radiological supervision and interpretation

75891 Hepatic venography, wedged or free, without hemodynamic evaluation, radiological supervision and interpretation

75893 Venous sampling through catheter, with or without angiography (eg, for parathyroid hormone, renin), radiological supervision and interpretation

(For procedure, use 36500)

Transcatheter Procedures

▶Therapeutic transcatheter radiological supervision and interpretation code(s) include the following services associated with that intervention:◀

▶1) Contrast injections, angiography/venography, roadmapping, and fluoroscopic guidance for the intervention,◀

▶2) Vessel measurement, and◀

▶3) Completion angiography/venography (except for those uses permitted by 75898).◀

▶Unless specifically included in the code descriptor, diagnostic angiography/venography performed at the time of transcatheter therapeutic radiological and interpretation service(s) is separately reportable (eg, no prior catheter-based diagnostic angiography/venography study of the target vessel is available, prior diagnostic study is inadequate, patient's condition with respect to the clinical indication has changed since the prior study or during the intervention). See 75600-75893.◄

75894   Transcatheter therapy, embolization, any method, radiological supervision and interpretation

75896   Transcatheter therapy, infusion, any method (eg, thrombolysis other than coronary), radiological supervision and interpretation

(For infusion for coronary disease, see 92975, 92977)

75898   Angiography through existing catheter for follow-up study for transcatheter therapy, embolization or infusion

75900   Exchange of a previously placed arterial catheter during thrombolytic therapy with contrast monitoring, radiological supervision and interpretation

(For procedure, use 37209)

75901   Mechanical removal of pericatheter obstructive material (eg, fibrin sheath) from central venous device via separate venous access, radiologic supervision and interpretation

(For procedure, use 36595)

(For venous catheterization, see 36010-36012)

75902   Mechanical removal of intraluminal (intracatheter) obstructive material from central venous device through device lumen, radiologic supervision and interpretation

(For procedure, use 36596)

(For venous catheterization, see 36010-36012)

75940   Percutaneous placement of IVC filter, radiological supervision and interpretation

75945   Intravascular ultrasound (non-coronary vessel), radiological supervision and interpretation; initial vessel

+ 75946   each additional non-coronary vessel (List separately in addition to code for primary procedure)

(Use 75946 in conjunction with 75945)

(For catheterizations, see codes 36215-36248)

(For transcatheter therapies, see codes 37200-37208, 61624, 61626)

(For procedure, see 37250, 37251)

75952   Endovascular repair of infrarenal abdominal aortic aneurysm or dissection, radiological supervision and interpretation

(For implantation of endovascular grafts, see 34800-34808)

►(For radiologic supervision and interpretation of endovascular repair of abdominal aortic aneurysm involving visceral vessels, see Category III codes 0078T-0081T)◄

75953   Placement of proximal or distal extension prosthesis for endovascular repair of infrarenal aortic or iliac artery aneurysm, pseudoaneurysm, or dissection, radiological supervision and interpretation

(For implantation of endovascular extension prostheses, see 34825, 34826)

75954   Endovascular repair of iliac artery aneurysm, pseudoaneurysm, arteriovenous malformation, or trauma, radiological supervision and interpretation

(For implantation of endovascular graft, see 34900)

▲ **75960**   Transcatheter introduction of intravascular stent(s), (except coronary, carotid, and vertebral vessel), percutaneous and/or open, radiological supervision and interpretation, each vessel

(For procedure, see 37205-37208)

(For radiologic supervision and interpretation for transcatheter placement of extracranial ►vertebral or intrathoracic carotid◄ artery stent(s), ►see◄ Category III codes ►0075T, 0076T◄)

75961   Transcatheter retrieval, percutaneous, of intravascular foreign body (eg, fractured venous or arterial catheter), radiological supervision and interpretation

(For procedure, use 37203)

75962   Transluminal balloon angioplasty, peripheral artery, radiological supervision and interpretation

+ 75964   Transluminal balloon angioplasty, each additional peripheral artery, radiological supervision and interpretation (List separately in addition to code for primary procedure)

(Use 75964 in conjunction with 75962)

75966   Transluminal balloon angioplasty, renal or other visceral artery, radiological supervision and interpretation

+ 75968   Transluminal balloon angioplasty, each additional visceral artery, radiological supervision and interpretation (List separately in addition to code for primary procedure)

(Use 75968 in conjunction with 75966)

(For percutaneous transluminal coronary angioplasty, see 92982-92984)

75970   Transcatheter biopsy, radiological supervision and interpretation

(For injection procedure only for transcatheter therapy or biopsy, see 36100-36299)

(For transcatheter renal and ureteral biopsy, use 52007)

(For percutaneous needle biopsy of pancreas, use 48102; of retroperitoneal lymph node or mass, use 49180)

75978   Transluminal balloon angioplasty, venous (eg, subclavian stenosis), radiological supervision and interpretation

75980   Percutaneous transhepatic biliary drainage with contrast monitoring, radiological supervision and interpretation

Radiology

75982 Percutaneous placement of drainage catheter for combined internal and external biliary drainage or of a drainage stent for internal biliary drainage in patients with an inoperable mechanical biliary obstruction, radiological supervision and interpretation

75984 Change of percutaneous tube or drainage catheter with contrast monitoring (eg, gastrointestinal system, genitourinary system, abscess), radiological supervision and interpretation

(For change of nephrostomy or pyelostomy tube only, use 50398)

(For introduction procedure only for percutaneous biliary drainage, see 47510, 47511)

(For percutaneous cholecystostomy, use 47490)

(For change of percutaneous biliary drainage catheter only, use 47525)

(For percutaneous nephrostolithotomy or pyelostolithotomy, see 50080, 50081)

75989 Radiological guidance (ie, fluoroscopy, ultrasound, or computed tomography), for percutaneous drainage (eg, abscess, specimen collection), with placement of catheter, radiological supervision and interpretation

Transluminal Atherectomy

75992 Transluminal atherectomy, peripheral artery, radiological supervision and interpretation

(For procedure, see 35481-35485, 35491-35495)

+ 75993 Transluminal atherectomy, each additional peripheral artery, radiological supervision and interpretation (List separately in addition to code for primary procedure)

(Use 75993 in conjunction with 75992)

(For procedure, see 35481-35485, 35491-35495)

75994 Transluminal atherectomy, renal, radiological supervision and interpretation

(For procedure, see 35480, 35490)

75995 Transluminal atherectomy, visceral, radiological supervision and interpretation

(For procedure, see 35480, 35490)

+ 75996 Transluminal atherectomy, each additional visceral artery, radiological supervision and interpretation (List separately in addition to code for primary procedure)

(Use 75996 in conjunction with 75995)

(For procedure, see 35480, 35490)

Other Procedures

(For computed tomography cerebral perfusion analysis, see Category III code 0042T)

(For arthrography of shoulder, use 73040; elbow, use 73085; wrist, use 73115; hip, use 73525; knee, use 73580; ankle, use 73615)

+ 75998 Fluoroscopic guidance for central venous access device placement, replacement (catheter only or complete), or removal (includes fluoroscopic guidance for vascular access and catheter manipulation, any necessary contrast injections through access site or catheter with related venography radiologic supervision and interpretation, and radiographic documentation of final catheter position) (List separately in addition to code for primary procedure)

(Do not use 76003 in conjunction with 75998)

(If formal extremity venography is performed from separate venous access and separately interpreted, use 36005 and 75820, 75822, 75825 or 75827)

76000 Fluoroscopy (separate procedure), up to one hour physician time, other than 71023 or 71034 (eg, cardiac fluoroscopy)

76001 Fluoroscopy, physician time more than one hour, assisting a non-radiologic physician (eg, nephrostolithotomy, ERCP, bronchoscopy, transbronchial biopsy)

76003 Fluoroscopic guidance for needle placement (eg, biopsy, aspiration, injection, localization device)

(See appropriate surgical code for procedure and anatomic location)

(Fluoroscopy 76003 is considered inclusive of all radiographic arthrography with the exception of supervision and interpretation for CT and MR arthrography)

(Do not report 76003 in addition to 70332, 73040, 73085, 73115, 73525, 73580, 73615)

(Fluoroscopy 76003 is considered inclusive of organ/anatomic specific radiological supervision and interpretation procedures 74320, 74350, 74355, 74445, 74470, 74475, 75809, 75810, 75885, 75887, 75980, 75982, 75989)

76005 Fluoroscopic guidance and localization of needle or catheter tip for spine or paraspinous diagnostic or therapeutic injection procedures (epidural, transforaminal epidural, subarachnoid, paravertebral facet joint, paravertebral facet joint nerve or sacroiliac joint), including neurolytic agent destruction

(Injection of contrast during fluoroscopic guidance and localization is an inclusive component of codes 62263, 62264, 62270-62273, 62280-62282, 62310-62319, 0027T)

(Fluoroscopic guidance for subarachnoid puncture for diagnostic radiographic myelography is included in supervision and interpretation codes 72240, 72255, 72265, 72270)

(For epidural or subarachnoid needle or catheter placement and injection, see codes 62270-62273, 62280-62282, 62310-62319)

(For sacroiliac joint arthrography, see 27096, 73542. If formal arthrography is not performed, recorded, and a formal radiographic report is not issued, use 76005 for fluoroscopic guidance for sacroiliac joint injections)

Radiology

(For paravertebral facet joint injection, see 64470-64476. For transforaminal epidural needle placement and injection, see 64479-64484)

(For destruction by neurolytic agent, see 64600-64680)

(For percutaneous or endoscopic lysis of epidural adhesions, codes 62263, 62264, 0027T include fluoroscopic guidance and localization)

76006 Manual application of stress performed by physician for joint radiography, including contralateral joint if indicated

(For radiographic interpretation of stressed images, see appropriate anatomic site and number of views)

76010 Radiologic examination from nose to rectum for foreign body, single view, child

76012 Radiological supervision and interpretation, percutaneous vertebroplasty, per vertebral body; under fluoroscopic guidance

76013 under CT guidance

(For procedure, see 22520-22522)

76020 Bone age studies

76040 Bone length studies (orthoroentgenogram, scanogram)

76061 Radiologic examination, osseous survey; limited (eg, for metastases)

76062 complete (axial and appendicular skeleton)

76065 Radiologic examination, osseous survey, infant

76066 Joint survey, single view, two or more joints (specify)

76070 Computed tomography, bone mineral density study, one or more sites; axial skeleton (eg, hips, pelvis, spine)

76071 appendicular skeleton (peripheral) (eg, radius, wrist, heel)

▲ **76075** Dual energy x-ray absorptiometry (DXA), bone density study, one or more sites; axial skeleton (eg, hips, pelvis, spine)

76076 appendicular skeleton (peripheral) (eg, radius, wrist, heel)

● **76077** vertebral fracture assessment

(To report dual energy x-ray absorptiometry (►DXA◄) body composition study, one or more sites, use Category III code 0028T)

76078 Radiographic absorptiometry (eg, photodensitometry, radiogrammetry), one or more sites

76080 Radiologic examination, abscess, fistula or sinus tract study, radiological supervision and interpretation

+ **76082** Computer aided detection (computer algorithm analysis of digital image data for lesion detection) with further physician review for interpretation, with or without digitization of film radiographic images; diagnostic mammography (List separately in addition to code for primary procedure)

(Use 76082 in conjunction with 76090 or 76091)

+ **76083** screening mammography (List separately in addition to code for primary procedure)

(Use 76083 in conjunction with 76092)

(76085 has been deleted. To report, see 76082, 76083)

76086 Mammary ductogram or galactogram, single duct, radiological supervision and interpretation

(For mammary ductogram or galactogram injection, use 19030)

76088 Mammary ductogram or galactogram, multiple ducts, radiological supervision and interpretation

76090 Mammography; unilateral

76091 bilateral

(Use 76082 in conjunction with 76090 or 76091 for computer aided detection applied to a diagnostic mammogram)

76092 Screening mammography, bilateral (two view film study of each breast)

(Use 76083 in conjunction with 76092 for computer aided detection applied to a screening mammogram)

(To report electrical impedance scan of the breast, bilateral, use Category III code 0060T)

76093 Magnetic resonance imaging, breast, without and/or with contrast material(s); unilateral

76094 bilateral

76095 Stereotactic localization guidance for breast biopsy or needle placement (eg, for wire localization or for injection), each lesion, radiological supervision and interpretation

(For procedure, see 10022, 19000, 19001, 19102, 19103, 19290, 19291)

(For injection for sentinel node localization without lymphoscintigraphy, use 38792)

76096 Mammographic guidance for needle placement, breast (eg, for wire localization or for injection), each lesion, radiological supervision and interpretation

(For procedure, see 10022, 19000, 19102, 19103, 19290, 19291)

(For injection for sentinel node localization without lymphoscintigraphy, use 38792)

76098 Radiological examination, surgical specimen

76100 Radiologic examination, single plane body section (eg, tomography), other than with urography

76101 Radiologic examination, complex motion (ie, hypercycloidal) body section (eg, mastoid polytomography), other than with urography; unilateral

76102 bilateral

(For nephrotomography, use 74415)

76120 Cineradiography/videoradiography, except where specifically included

+ 76125   Cineradiography/videoradiography to complement routine examination (List separately in addition to code for primary procedure)

76140   Consultation on x-ray examination made elsewhere, written report

76150   Xeroradiography

(76150 is to be used for non-mammographic studies only)

76350   Subtraction in conjunction with contrast studies

76355   Computed tomography guidance for stereotactic localization

76360   Computed tomography guidance for needle placement (eg, biopsy, aspiration, injection, localization device), radiological supervision and interpretation

76362   Computed tomography guidance for, and monitoring of, visceral tissue ablation

(For percutaneous radiofrequency ablation, use 47382)

76370   Computed tomography guidance for placement of radiation therapy fields

76375   Coronal, sagittal, multiplanar, oblique, 3-dimensional and/or holographic reconstruction of computed tomography, magnetic resonance imaging, or other tomographic modality

(Use 76375 in addition to code for imaging procedure)

►(For computed tomographic colonography, see Category III codes 0066T, 0067T. Do not report 76375 in conjunction with 0066T, 0067T)◄

76380   Computed tomography, limited or localized follow-up study

76390   Magnetic resonance spectroscopy

(For magnetic resonance imaging, use appropriate MRI body site code)

76393   Magnetic resonance guidance for needle placement (eg, for biopsy, needle aspiration, injection, or placement of localization device) radiological supervision and interpretation

(For procedure see appropriate organ or site)

76394   Magnetic resonance guidance for, and monitoring of, visceral tissue ablation

(For percutaneous radiofrequency ablation, use 47382)

►(For focused ultrasound ablation treatment of uterine leiomyomata, see Category III codes 0071T, 0072T)◄

76400   Magnetic resonance (eg, proton) imaging, bone marrow blood supply

(76490 has been deleted. To report, use 76940)

76496   Unlisted fluoroscopic procedure (eg, diagnostic, interventional)

76497   Unlisted computed tomography procedure (eg, diagnostic, interventional)

76498   Unlisted magnetic resonance procedure (eg, diagnostic, interventional)

76499   Unlisted diagnostic radiographic procedure

Diagnostic Ultrasound

►All diagnostic ultrasound examinations require permanently recorded images with measurements, when such measurements are clinically indicated. For those codes whose sole diagnostic goal is a biometric measure (ie, 76514, 76516, and 76519), permanently recorded images are not required. A final, written report should be issued for inclusion in the patient's medical record. The prescription form for the intraocular lens satisfies the written report requirement for 76519. For those anatomic regions that have "complete" and "limited" ultrasound codes, note the elements that comprise a "complete" exam. The report should contain a description of these elements or the reason that an element could not be visualized (eg, obscured by bowel gas, surgically absent etc.).◄

►If less than the required elements for a "complete" exam are reported (eg, limited number of organs or limited portion of region evaluated), the "limited" code for that anatomic region should be used once per patient exam session. A "limited" exam of an anatomic region should not be reported for the same exam session as a "complete" exam of that same region.◄

►Doppler evaluation of vascular structures (other than color flow used only for anatomic structure identification) is separately reportable. To report, see Non-Invasive Vascular Diagnostic Studies (93875-93990).◄

►Ultrasound guidance procedures also require permanently recorded images of the site to be localized, as well as a documented description of the localization process, either separately or within the report of the procedure for which the guidance is utilized.◄

►Use of ultrasound, without thorough evaluation of organ(s) or anatomic region, image documentation, and final, written report, is not separately reportable.◄

Definitions

A-mode implies a one-dimensional ultrasonic measurement procedure.

M-mode implies a one-dimensional ultrasonic measurement procedure with movement of the trace to record amplitude and velocity of moving echo-producing structures.

B-scan implies a two-dimensional ultrasonic scanning procedure with a two-dimensional display.

Real-time scan implies a two-dimensional ultrasonic scanning procedure with display of both two-dimensional structure and motion with time.

Radiology

(To report diagnostic vascular ultrasound studies, see 93875-93990)

▶(For focused ultrasound ablation treatment of uterine leiomyomata, see Category III codes 0071T, 0072T)◀

Head and Neck

76506 Echoencephalography, B-scan and/or real time with image documentation (gray scale) (for determination of ventricular size, delineation of cerebral contents and detection of fluid masses or other intracranial abnormalities), including A-mode encephalography as secondary component where indicated

● **76510** Ophthalmic ultrasound, diagnostic; B-scan and quantitative A-scan performed during the same patient encounter

▲ **76511**   quantitative A-scan only

▲ **76512**   B-scan (with or without superimposed non-quantitative A-scan)

76513   anterior segment ultrasound, immersion (water bath) B-scan or high resolution biomicroscopy

76514   corneal pachymetry, unilateral or bilateral (determination of corneal thickness)

76516 Ophthalmic biometry by ultrasound echography, A-scan;

76519   with intraocular lens power calculation

(For partial coherence interferometry, use 92136)

76529 Ophthalmic ultrasonic foreign body localization

76536 Ultrasound, soft tissues of head and neck (eg, thyroid, parathyroid, parotid), B-scan and/or real time with image documentation

Chest

76604 Ultrasound, chest, B-scan (includes mediastinum) and/or real time with image documentation

76645 Ultrasound, breast(s) (unilateral or bilateral), B-scan and/or real time with image documentation

Abdomen and Retroperitoneum

▶A complete ultrasound examination of the abdomen (76700) consists of B mode scans of: liver, gall bladder, common bile duct, pancreas, spleen, kidneys, and the upper abdominal aorta and inferior vena cava including any demonstrated abdominal abnormality.◀

▶A complete ultrasound examination of the retroperitoneum (76770) consists of B mode scans of: kidneys, abdominal aorta, common iliac artery origins, and inferior vena cava, including any demonstrated retroperitoneal abnormality. Alternatively, if clinical history suggests urinary tract pathology, complete evaluation of the kidneys and urinary bladder also comprises a complete retroperitoneal ultrasound.◀

▶Use of ultrasound, without thorough evaluation of organ(s) or anatomic region, image documentation and final, written report, is not separately reportable.◀

76700 Ultrasound, abdominal, B-scan and/or real time with image documentation; complete

76705   limited (eg, single organ, quadrant, follow-up)

76770 Ultrasound, retroperitoneal (eg, renal, aorta, nodes), B-scan and/or real time with image documentation; complete

76775   limited

76778 Ultrasound, transplanted kidney, B-scan and/or real time with image documentation, with or without duplex Doppler study

Spinal Canal

76800 Ultrasound, spinal canal and contents

Pelvis

Obstetrical

Codes 76801 and 76802 include determination of the number of gestational sacs and fetuses, gestational sac/fetal measurements appropriate for gestation (<14 weeks 0 days), survey of visible fetal and placental anatomic structure, qualitative assessment of amniotic fluid volume/gestational sac shape and examination of the maternal uterus and adnexa.

Codes 76805 and 76810 include determination of number of fetuses and amniotic/chorionic sacs, measurements appropriate for gestational age (> or = 14 weeks 0 days), survey of intracranial/spinal/abdominal anatomy, 4 chambered heart, umbilical cord insertion site, placenta location and amniotic fluid assessment and, when visible, examination of maternal adnexa.

Codes 76811 and 76812 include all elements of codes 76805 and 76810 plus detailed anatomic evaluation of the fetal brain/ventricles, face, heart/outflow tracts and chest anatomy, abdominal organ specific anatomy, number/length/architecture of limbs and detailed evaluation of the umbilical cord and placenta and other fetal anatomy as clinically indicated.

Report should document the results of the evaluation of each element described above or the reason for non-visualization.

Code 76815 represents a focused "quick look" exam limited to the assessment of one or more of the elements listed in code 76815.

Code 76816 describes an examination designed to reassess fetal size and interval growth or reevaluate one or more anatomic abnormalities of a fetus previously demonstrated on ultrasound, and should be coded once for each fetus requiring reevaluation using modifier 59 for each fetus after the first.

Code 76817 describes a transvaginal obstetric ultrasound performed separately or in addition to one of the transabdominal examinations described above. For transvaginal examinations performed for non-obstetrical purposes, use code 76830.

76801 Ultrasound, pregnant uterus, real time with image documentation, fetal and maternal evaluation, first trimester (<14 weeks 0 days), transabdominal approach; single or first gestation

+ 76802   each additional gestation (List separately in addition to code for primary procedure)

(Use 76802 in conjunction with 76801)

76805 Ultrasound, pregnant uterus, real time with image documentation, fetal and maternal evaluation, after first trimester (> or = 14 weeks 0 days), transabdominal approach; single or first gestation

+ 76810   each additional gestation (List separately in addition to code for primary procedure)

(Use 76810 in conjunction with 76805)

76811 Ultrasound, pregnant uterus, real time with image documentation, fetal and maternal evaluation plus detailed fetal anatomic examination, transabdominal approach; single or first gestation

+ 76812   each additional gestation (List separately in addition to code for primary procedure)

(Use 76812 in conjunction with 76811)

76815 Ultrasound, pregnant uterus, real time with image documentation, limited (eg, fetal heart beat, placental location, fetal position and/or qualitative amniotic fluid volume), one or more fetuses

(Use 76815 only once per exam and not per element)

76816 Ultrasound, pregnant uterus, real time with image documentation, follow-up (eg, re-evaluation of fetal size by measuring standard growth parameters and amniotic fluid volume, re-evaluation of organ system(s) suspected or confirmed to be abnormal on a previous scan), transabdominal approach, per fetus

(Report 76816 with modifier 59 for each additional fetus examined in a multiple pregnancy)

76817 Ultrasound, pregnant uterus, real time with image documentation, transvaginal

(For non-obstetrical transvaginal ultrasound, use 76830)

(If transvaginal examination is done in addition to transabdominal obstetrical ultrasound exam, use 76817 in addition to appropriate transabdominal exam code)

76818 Fetal biophysical profile; with non-stress testing

76819   without non-stress testing

(Fetal biophysical profile assessments for the second and any additional fetuses, should be reported separately by code 76818 or 76819 with the modifier 59 appended)

(For amniotic fluid index without non-stress test, use 76815)

● **76820** Doppler velocimetry, fetal; umbilical artery

● **76821**   middle cerebral artery

76825 Echocardiography, fetal, cardiovascular system, real time with image documentation (2D), with or without M-mode recording;

76826   follow-up or repeat study

▲ **76827** Doppler echocardiography, fetal, pulsed wave and/or continuous wave with spectral display; complete

76828   follow-up or repeat study

(To report the use of color mapping, use 93325)

Non-Obstetrical

►Code 76856 includes the complete evaluation of the female pelvic anatomy. Elements of this examination include a description and measurements of the uterus and adnexal structures, measurement of the endometrium, measurement of the bladder (when applicable), and a description of any pelvic pathology (eg, ovarian cysts, uterine leiomyomata, free pelvic fluid).◄

►Code 76856 is also applicable to a complete evaluation of the male pelvis. Elements of the examination include evaluation and measurement (when applicable) of the urinary bladder, evaluation of the prostate and seminal vesicles to the extent that they are visualized transabdominally, and any pelvic pathology (eg, bladder tumor, enlarged prostate, free pelvic fluid, pelvic abscess).◄

►Code 76857 represents a focused examination limited to the assessment of one or more elements listed in code 76856 and/or the reevaluation of one or more pelvic abnormalities previously demonstrated on ultrasound. Code 76857, rather than 76770, should be utilized if the urinary bladder alone (ie, not including the kidneys) is imaged, whereas code 51798 should be utilized if a bladder volume or post-void residual measurement is obtained without imaging the bladder.◄

►Use of ultrasound, without thorough evaluation of organ(s) or anatomic region, image documentation, and final, written report, is not separately reportable.◄

76830 Ultrasound, transvaginal

(For obstetrical transvaginal ultrasound, use 76817)

(If transvaginal examination is done in addition to transabdominal non-obstetrical ultrasound exam, use 76830 in addition to appropriate transabdominal exam code)

76831 Saline infusion sonohysterography (SIS), including color flow Doppler, when performed

(For introduction of saline for saline infusion sonohysterography, use 58340)

Radiology

76856   Ultrasound, pelvic (nonobstetric), B-scan and/or real time with image documentation; complete

76857   limited or follow-up (eg, for follicles)

Genitalia

76870   Ultrasound, scrotum and contents

76872   Ultrasound, transrectal;

76873   prostate volume study for brachytherapy treatment planning (separate procedure)

Extremities

76880   Ultrasound, extremity, non-vascular, B-scan and/or real time with image documentation

76885   Ultrasound, infant hips, real time with imaging documentation; dynamic (requiring physician manipulation)

76886   limited, static (not requiring physician manipulation)

Ultrasonic Guidance Procedures

76930   Ultrasonic guidance for pericardiocentesis, imaging supervision and interpretation

76932   Ultrasonic guidance for endomyocardial biopsy, imaging supervision and interpretation

76936   Ultrasound guided compression repair of arterial pseudoaneurysm or arteriovenous fistulae (includes diagnostic ultrasound evaluation, compression of lesion and imaging)

+ 76937 Ultrasound guidance for vascular access requiring ultrasound evaluation of potential access sites, documentation of selected vessel patency, concurrent realtime ultrasound visualization of vascular needle entry, with permanent recording and reporting (List separately in addition to code for primary procedure)

(Do not use 76937 in conjunction with 76942)

(If extremity venous non-invasive vascular diagnostic study is performed separate from venous access guidance, use 93965, 93970 or 93971)

76940   Ultrasound guidance for, and monitoring of, visceral tissue ablation

(Do not report 76940 in conjunction with 76986)

(For ablation, see 47370-47382)

76941   Ultrasonic guidance for intrauterine fetal transfusion or cordocentesis, imaging supervision and interpretation

(For procedure, see 36460, 59012)

76942   Ultrasonic guidance for needle placement (eg, biopsy, aspiration, injection, localization device), imaging supervision and interpretation

(Do not report 76942 in conjunction with 43232, 43237, 43242, 45341, 45342, or 76975)

(For microwave thermotherapy of the breast, use Category III code 0061T)

76945   Ultrasonic guidance for chorionic villus sampling, imaging supervision and interpretation

(For procedure, use 59015)

76946   Ultrasonic guidance for amniocentesis, imaging supervision and interpretation

76948   Ultrasonic guidance for aspiration of ova, imaging supervision and interpretation

76950   Ultrasonic guidance for placement of radiation therapy fields

76965   Ultrasonic guidance for interstitial radioelement application

Other Procedures

76970   Ultrasound study follow-up (specify)

76975   Gastrointestinal endoscopic ultrasound, supervision and interpretation

(Do not report 76975 in conjunction with 43231, 43232, 43237, 43238, 43242, 43259, 45341, 45342, or 76942)

76977   Ultrasound bone density measurement and interpretation, peripheral site(s), any method

76986   Ultrasonic guidance, intraoperative

(Do not report 76986 in addition to 47370-47382)

(For ultrasound guidance for open and laparoscopic radiofrequency tissue ablation, use 76940)

76999   Unlisted ultrasound procedure (eg, diagnostic, interventional)

Radiation Oncology

Listings for Radiation Oncology provide for teletherapy and brachytherapy to include initial consultation, clinical treatment planning, simulation, medical radiation physics, dosimetry, treatment devices, special services, and clinical treatment management procedures. They include normal follow-up care during course of treatment and for three months following its completion.

When a service or procedure is provided that is not listed in this edition of *CPT* it should be identified by a Special Report (see page 218) and one of the unlisted procedure codes listed below:

77299 Unlisted procedure, therapeutic radiology clinical treatment planning

77399 Unlisted procedure, medical radiation physics, dosimetry and treatment devices, and special services

77499 Unlisted procedure, therapeutic radiology treatment management

77799 Unlisted procedure, clinical brachytherapy

For treatment by injectable or ingestible isotopes, see subsection **Nuclear Medicine.**

Radiology

Consultation: Clinical Management

Preliminary consultation, evaluation of patient prior to decision to treat, or full medical care (in addition to treatment management) when provided by the therapeutic radiologist may be identified by the appropriate procedure codes from **Evaluation and Management, Medicine,** or **Surgery** sections.

Clinical Treatment Planning (External and Internal Sources)

The clinical treatment planning process is a complex service including interpretation of special testing, tumor localization, treatment volume determination, treatment time/dosage determination, choice of treatment modality, determination of number and size of treatment ports, selection of appropriate treatment devices, and other procedures.

Definitions

Simple planning requires a single treatment area of interest encompassed in a single port or simple parallel opposed ports with simple or no blocking.

Intermediate planning requires three or more converging ports, two separate treatment areas, multiple blocks, or special time dose constraints.

Complex planning requires highly complex blocking, custom shielding blocks, tangential ports, special wedges or compensators, three or more separate treatment areas, rotational or special beam considerations, combination of therapeutic modalities.

77261   Therapeutic radiology treatment planning; simple

77262   intermediate

77263   complex

Definitions

Simple simulation of a single treatment area with either a single port or parallel opposed ports. Simple or no blocking.

Intermediate simulation of three or more converging ports, two separate treatment areas, multiple blocks.

Complex simulation of tangential portals, three or more treatment areas, rotation or arc therapy, complex blocking, custom shielding blocks, brachytherapy source verification, hyperthermia probe verification, any use of contrast materials.

Three-dimensional computer-generated three dimensional reconstruction of tumor volume and surrounding critical normal tissue structures from direct CT scans and/or MRI data in preparation for non-coplanar or coplanar therapy. The simulation utilizes documented three-dimensional beam's eye view volume-dose displays of multiple or moving beams. Documentation with three-dimensional volume reconstruction and dose distribution is required.

Simulation may be carried out on a dedicated simulator, a radiation therapy treatment unit, or diagnostic x-ray machine.

77280   Therapeutic radiology simulation-aided field setting; simple

77285   intermediate

77290   complex

77295   three-dimensional

77299   Unlisted procedure, therapeutic radiology clinical treatment planning

Medical Radiation Physics, Dosimetry, Treatment Devices, and Special Services

77300   Basic radiation dosimetry calculation, central axis depth dose calculation, TDF, NSD, gap calculation, off axis factor, tissue inhomogeneity factors, calculation of non-ionizing radiation surface and depth dose, as required during course of treatment, only when prescribed by the treating physician

77301   Intensity modulated radiotherapy plan, including dose-volume histograms for target and critical structure partial tolerance specifications

(Dose plan is optimized using inverse or forward planning technique for modulated beam delivery (eg, binary, dynamic MLC) to create highly conformal dose distribution. Computer plan distribution must be verified for positional accuracy based on dosimetric verification of the intensity map with verification of treatment set-up and interpretation of verification methodology)

77305   Teletherapy, isodose plan (whether hand or computer calculated); simple (one or two parallel opposed unmodified ports directed to a single area of interest)

77310   intermediate (three or more treatment ports directed to a single area of interest)

77315   complex (mantle or inverted Y, tangential ports, the use of wedges, compensators, complex blocking, rotational beam, or special beam considerations)

(Only one teletherapy isodose plan may be reported for a given course of therapy to a specific treatment area)

77321   Special teletherapy port plan, particles, hemibody, total body

77326   Brachytherapy isodose plan; simple (calculation made from single plane, one to four sources/ribbon application, remote afterloading brachytherapy, 1 to 8 sources)

(For definition of source/ribbon, see page 237)

77327   intermediate (multiplane dosage calculations, application involving 5 to 10 sources/ribbons, remote afterloading brachytherapy, 9 to 12 sources)

77328   complex (multiplane isodose plan, volume implant calculations, over 10 sources/ribbons used, special spatial reconstruction, remote afterloading brachytherapy, over 12 sources)

77331   Special dosimetry (eg, TLD, microdosimetry) (specify), only when prescribed by the treating physician

77332   Treatment devices, design and construction; simple (simple block, simple bolus)

77333   intermediate (multiple blocks, stents, bite blocks, special bolus)

77334   complex (irregular blocks, special shields, compensators, wedges, molds or casts)

77336   Continuing medical physics consultation, including assessment of treatment parameters, quality assurance of dose delivery, and review of patient treatment documentation in support of the radiation oncologist, reported per week of therapy

77370   Special medical radiation physics consultation

77399   Unlisted procedure, medical radiation physics, dosimetry and treatment devices, and special services

Radiation Treatment Delivery

(Radiation treatment delivery (77401-77416) recognizes the technical component and the various energy levels.)

▶(For stereotactic body radiation therapy treatment delivery, use Category III code 0082T)◀

77401   Radiation treatment delivery, superficial and/or ortho voltage

77402   Radiation treatment delivery, single treatment area, single port or parallel opposed ports, simple blocks or no blocks; up to 5 MeV

77403   6-10 MeV

77404   11-19 MeV

77406   20 MeV or greater

77407   Radiation treatment delivery, two separate treatment areas, three or more ports on a single treatment area, use of multiple blocks; up to 5 MeV

77408   6-10 MeV

77409   11-19 MeV

77411   20 MeV or greater

77412   Radiation treatment delivery, three or more separate treatment areas, custom blocking, tangential ports, wedges, rotational beam, compensators, special particle beam (eg, electron or neutrons); up to 5 MeV

77413   6-10 MeV

77414   11-19 MeV

77416   20 MeV or greater

77417   Therapeutic radiology port film(s)

▲ **77418**   Intensity modulated treatment delivery, single or multiple fields/arcs, via narrow spatially and temporally modulated beams, binary, dynamic MLC, per treatment session

(For intensity modulated treatment planning, use 77301)

▶(For compensator-based beam modulation treatment delivery, use Category III code 0073T)◀

Radiation Treatment Management

Radiation treatment management is reported in units of five fractions or treatment sessions, regardless of the actual time period in which the services are furnished. The services need not be furnished on consecutive days. Multiple fractions representing two or more treatment sessions furnished on the same day may be counted separately as long as there has been a distinct break in therapy sessions, and the fractions are of the character usually furnished on different days. Code 77427 is also reported if there are three or four fractions beyond a multiple of five at the end of a course of treatment; one or two fractions beyond a multiple of five at the end of a course of treatment are not reported separately. The professional services furnished during treatment management typically consist of:

- Review of port films;

- Review of dosimetry, dose delivery, and treatment parameters;

- Review of patient treatment set-up;

- Examination of patient for medical evaluation and management (eg, assessment of the patient's response to treatment, coordination of care and treatment, review of imaging and/or lab test results).

77427   Radiation treatment management, five treatments

77431   Radiation therapy management with complete course of therapy consisting of one or two fractions only

(77431 is not to be used to fill in the last week of a long course of therapy)

77432   Stereotactic radiation treatment management of cerebral lesion(s) (complete course of treatment consisting of one session)

▶(For stereotactic body radiation therapy treatment management, use Category III code 0083T)◀

77470   Special treatment procedure (eg, total body irradiation, hemibody radiation, per oral, endocavitary or intraoperative cone irradiation)

(77470 assumes that the procedure is performed one or more times during the course of therapy, in addition to daily or weekly patient management)

77499   Unlisted procedure, therapeutic radiology treatment management

Radiology

Proton Beam Treatment Delivery

Definitions

Simple proton treatment delivery to a single treatment area utilizing a single non-tangential/oblique port, custom block with compensation (77522) and without compensation (77520).

Intermediate proton treatment delivery to one or more treatment areas utilizing two or more ports or one or more tangential/oblique ports, with custom blocks and compensators.

Complex proton treatment delivery to one or more treatment areas utilizing two or more ports per treatment area with matching or patching fields and/or multiple isocenters, with custom blocks and compensators.

77520   Proton treatment delivery; simple, without compensation

77522   simple, with compensation

77523   intermediate

77525   complex

Hyperthermia

Hyperthermia treatments as listed in this section include external (superficial and deep), interstitial, and intracavitary.

Radiation therapy when given concurrently is listed separately.

Hyperthermia is used only as an adjunct to radiation therapy or chemotherapy. It may be induced by a variety of sources (eg, microwave, ultrasound, low energy radio-frequency conduction, or by probes).

The listed treatments include management during the course of therapy and follow-up care for three months after completion.

Preliminary consultation is not included (see **Medicine** 99241-99263).

Physics planning and interstitial insertion of temperature sensors, and use of external or interstitial heat generating sources are included.

The following descriptors are included in the treatment schedule:

⊙ **77600**   Hyperthermia, externally generated; superficial (ie, heating to a depth of 4 cm or less)

⊙ **77605**   deep (ie, heating to depths greater than 4 cm)

⊙ **77610**   Hyperthermia generated by interstitial probe(s); 5 or fewer interstitial applicators

⊙ **77615**   more than 5 interstitial applicators

Clinical Intracavitary Hyperthermia

77620   Hyperthermia generated by intracavitary probe(s)

Clinical Brachytherapy

Clinical brachytherapy requires the use of either natural or man-made radioelements applied into or around a treatment field of interest. The supervision of radioelements and dose interpretation are performed solely by the therapeutic radiologist.

Services 77750-77799 include admission to the hospital and daily visits.

For insertion of ovoids and tandems, use 57155.

For insertion of Heyman capsules, use 58346.

Definitions

(Sources refer to intracavitary placement or permanent interstitial placement; ribbons refer to temporary interstitial placement)

A simple application has one to four sources/ribbons.

An intermediate application has five to ten sources/ribbons.

A complex application has greater than ten sources/ribbons.

▲ **77750**   Infusion or instillation of radioelement solution (includes three months follow-up care)

(For administration of radiolabeled monoclonal antibodies, ►use◄ 79403)

►(For non-antibody radiopharmaceutical therapy by intravenous administration only, not including three month follow-up care, use 79101)◄

77761   Intracavitary radiation source application; simple

77762   intermediate

77763   complex

77776   Interstitial radiation source application; simple

77777   intermediate

77778   complex

77781   Remote afterloading high intensity brachytherapy; 1-4 source positions or catheters

77782   5-8 source positions or catheters

77783   9-12 source positions or catheters

77784   over 12 source positions or catheters

77789   Surface application of radiation source

77790   Supervision, handling, loading of radiation source

77799   Unlisted procedure, clinical brachytherapy

Radiology

Nuclear Medicine

Listed procedures may be performed independently or in the course of overall medical care. If the physician providing these services is also responsible for diagnostic work-up and/or follow-up care of patient, see appropriate sections also.

Radioimmunoassay tests are found in the **Clinical Pathology** section (codes 82000-84999). These codes can be appropriately used by any specialist performing such tests in a laboratory licensed and/or certified for radioimmunoassays. The reporting of these tests is not confined to clinical pathology laboratories alone.

The services listed do not include the provision of radium or other radioelements. ▶Diagnostic and therapeutic radiopharmaceuticals supplied by the physician should be reported separately.◀

Diagnostic

Endocrine System

78000	Thyroid uptake; single determination
78001	multiple determinations
78003	stimulation, suppression or discharge (not including initial uptake studies)
78006	Thyroid imaging, with uptake; single determination
78007	multiple determinations
78010	Thyroid imaging; only
78011	with vascular flow
78015	Thyroid carcinoma metastases imaging; limited area (eg, neck and chest only)
78016	with additional studies (eg, urinary recovery)
78018	whole body
✚ **78020**	Thyroid carcinoma metastases uptake (List separately in addition to code for primary procedure)
	(Use 78020 in conjunction with 78018 only)
78070	Parathyroid imaging
78075	Adrenal imaging, cortex and/or medulla
78099	Unlisted endocrine procedure, diagnostic nuclear medicine
	(For chemical analysis, see **Chemistry** section)

Hematopoietic, Reticuloendothelial and Lymphatic System

78102	Bone marrow imaging; limited area
78103	multiple areas
78104	whole body

78110	Plasma volume, radiopharmaceutical volume-dilution technique (separate procedure); single sampling
78111	multiple samplings
78120	Red cell volume determination (separate procedure); single sampling
78121	multiple samplings
78122	Whole blood volume determination, including separate measurement of plasma volume and red cell volume (radiopharmaceutical volume-dilution technique)
78130	Red cell survival study;
78135	differential organ/tissue kinetics, (eg, splenic and/or hepatic sequestration)
78140	Labeled red cell sequestration, differential organ/tissue, (eg, splenic and/or hepatic)
78160	Plasma radioiron disappearance (turnover) rate
78162	Radioiron oral absorption
78170	Radioiron red cell utilization
78172	Chelatable iron for estimation of total body iron
78185	Spleen imaging only, with or without vascular flow
	(If combined with liver study, use procedures 78215 and 78216)
78190	Kinetics, study of platelet survival, with or without differential organ/tissue localization
78191	Platelet survival study
78195	Lymphatics and lymph nodes imaging
	(For sentinel node identification without scintigraphy imaging, use 38792)
	(For sentinal node excision, see 38500-38542)
78199	Unlisted hematopoietic, reticuloendothelial and lymphatic procedure, diagnostic nuclear medicine
	(For chemical analysis, see **Chemistry** section)

Gastrointestinal System

78201	Liver imaging; static only
78202	with vascular flow
	(For spleen imaging only, use 78185)
78205	Liver imaging (SPECT);
78206	with vascular flow
78215	Liver and spleen imaging; static only
78216	with vascular flow
78220	Liver function study with hepatobiliary agents, with serial images

Radiology

78223 Hepatobiliary ductal system imaging, including gallbladder, with or without pharmacologic intervention, with or without quantitative measurement of gallbladder function

78230 Salivary gland imaging;

78231 with serial images

78232 Salivary gland function study

78258 Esophageal motility

78261 Gastric mucosa imaging

78262 Gastroesophageal reflux study

78264 Gastric emptying study

▲ **78267** Urea breath test, C-14 (isotopic); acquisition for analysis

78268 analysis

78270 Vitamin B-12 absorption study (eg, Schilling test); without intrinsic factor

78271 with intrinsic factor

78272 Vitamin B-12 absorption studies combined, with and without intrinsic factor

78278 Acute gastrointestinal blood loss imaging

78282 Gastrointestinal protein loss

78290 Intestine imaging (eg, ectopic gastric mucosa, Meckel's localization, volvulus)

78291 Peritoneal-venous shunt patency test (eg, for LeVeen, Denver shunt)

(For injection procedure, use 49427)

78299 Unlisted gastrointestinal procedure, diagnostic nuclear medicine

Musculoskeletal System

Bone and joint imaging can be used in the diagnosis of a variety of inflammatory processes (eg, osteomyelitis), as well as for localization of primary and/or metastatic neoplasms.

78300 Bone and/or joint imaging; limited area

78305 multiple areas

78306 whole body

78315 three phase study

78320 tomographic (SPECT)

78350 Bone density (bone mineral content) study, one or more sites; single photon absorptiometry

78351 dual photon absorptiometry, one or more sites

(For radiographic bone density (photodensitometry), use 76078)

78399 Unlisted musculoskeletal procedure, diagnostic nuclear medicine

Cardiovascular System

Myocardial perfusion and cardiac blood pool imaging studies may be performed at rest and/or during stress. When performed during exercise and/or pharmacologic stress, the appropriate stress testing code from the 93015-93018 series should be reported in addition to 78460-78465, 78472-78492.

78414 Determination of central c-v hemodynamics (non-imaging) (eg, ejection fraction with probe technique) with or without pharmacologic intervention or exercise, single or multiple determinations

78428 Cardiac shunt detection

78445 Non-cardiac vascular flow imaging (ie, angiography, venography)

78455 Venous thrombosis study (eg, radioactive fibrinogen)

78456 Acute venous thrombosis imaging, peptide

78457 Venous thrombosis imaging, venogram; unilateral

78458 bilateral

78459 Myocardial imaging, positron emission tomography (PET), metabolic evaluation

(For myocardial perfusion study, see 78491-78492)

78460 Myocardial perfusion imaging; (planar) single study, at rest or stress (exercise and/or pharmacologic), with or without quantification

78461 multiple studies, (planar) at rest and/or stress (exercise and/or pharmacologic), and redistribution and/or rest injection, with or without quantification

▲ **78464** tomographic (SPECT), single study (including attenuation correction when performed), at rest or stress (exercise and/or pharmacologic), with or without quantification

▲ **78465** tomographic (SPECT), multiple studies (including attenuation correction when performed), at rest and/or stress (exercise and/or pharmacologic) and redistribution and/or rest injection, with or without quantification

78466 Myocardial imaging, infarct avid, planar; qualitative or quantitative

78468 with ejection fraction by first pass technique

78469 tomographic SPECT with or without quantification

78472 Cardiac blood pool imaging, gated equilibrium; planar, single study at rest or stress (exercise and/or pharmacologic), wall motion study plus ejection fraction, with or without additional quantitative processing

(For assessment of cardiac function by first pass technique, use 78496)

78473 multiple studies, wall motion study plus ejection fraction, at rest and stress (exercise and/or pharmacologic), with or without additional quantification

Radiology

+ **78478** Myocardial perfusion study with wall motion, qualitative or quantitative study (List separately in addition to code for primary procedure)

(Use 78478 in conjunction with 78460, 78461, 78464, 78465)

+ **78480** Myocardial perfusion study with ejection fraction (List separately in addition to code for primary procedure)

(Use 78480 in conjunction with 78460, 78461, 78464, 78465)

78481 Cardiac blood pool imaging, (planar), first pass technique; single study, at rest or with stress (exercise and/or pharmacologic), wall motion study plus ejection fraction, with or without quantification

78483 multiple studies, at rest and with stress (exercise and/ or pharmacologic), wall motion study plus ejection fraction, with or without quantification

(For cerebral blood flow study, use 78615)

78491 Myocardial imaging, positron emission tomography (PET), perfusion; single study at rest or stress

78492 multiple studies at rest and/or stress

78494 Cardiac blood pool imaging, gated equilibrium, SPECT, at rest, wall motion study plus ejection fraction, with or without quantitative processing

+ **78496** Cardiac blood pool imaging, gated equilibrium, single study, at rest, with right ventricular ejection fraction by first pass technique (List separately in addition to code for primary procedure)

(Use 78496 in conjunction with 78472)

78499 Unlisted cardiovascular procedure, diagnostic nuclear medicine

Respiratory System

78580 Pulmonary perfusion imaging, particulate

78584 Pulmonary perfusion imaging, particulate, with ventilation; single breath

78585 rebreathing and washout, with or without single breath

78586 Pulmonary ventilation imaging, aerosol; single projection

78587 multiple projections (eg, anterior, posterior, lateral views)

78588 Pulmonary perfusion imaging, particulate, with ventilation imaging, aerosol, one or multiple projections

78591 Pulmonary ventilation imaging, gaseous, single breath, single projection

78593 Pulmonary ventilation imaging, gaseous, with rebreathing and washout with or without single breath; single projection

78594 multiple projections (eg, anterior, posterior, lateral views)

78596 Pulmonary quantitative differential function (ventilation/perfusion) study

78599 Unlisted respiratory procedure, diagnostic nuclear medicine

Nervous System

78600 Brain imaging, limited procedure; static

78601 with vascular flow

78605 Brain imaging, complete study; static

78606 with vascular flow

78607 tomographic (SPECT)

78608 Brain imaging, positron emission tomography (PET); metabolic evaluation

78609 perfusion evaluation

78610 Brain imaging, vascular flow only

78615 Cerebral vascular flow

78630 Cerebrospinal fluid flow, imaging (not including introduction of material); cisternography

(For injection procedure, see 61000-61070, 62270-62319)

78635 ventriculography

(For injection procedure, see 61000-61070, 62270-62294)

78645 shunt evaluation

(For injection procedure, see 61000-61070, 62270-62294)

78647 tomographic (SPECT)

78650 Cerebrospinal fluid leakage detection and localization

(For injection procedure, see 61000-61070, 62270-62294)

78660 Radiopharmaceutical dacryocystography

78699 Unlisted nervous system procedure, diagnostic nuclear medicine

Genitourinary System

78700 Kidney imaging; static only

78701 with vascular flow

78704 with function study (ie, imaging renogram)

78707 Kidney imaging with vascular flow and function; single study without pharmacological intervention

78708 single study, with pharmacological intervention (eg, angiotensin converting enzyme inhibitor and/or diuretic)

78709 multiple studies, with and without pharmacological intervention (eg, angiotensin converting enzyme inhibitor and/or diuretic)

Radiology

78710	Kidney imaging, tomographic (SPECT)
78715	Kidney vascular flow only
78725	Kidney function study, non-imaging radioisotopic study
78730	Urinary bladder residual study

(For introduction of radioactive substance in association with cystotomy or cystostomy, use 51020; in association with cystourethroscopy, use 52250)

| 78740 | Ureteral reflux study (radiopharmaceutical voiding cystogram) |

(For catheterization, see 51701, 51702, 51703)

78760	Testicular imaging;
78761	with vascular flow
78799	Unlisted genitourinary procedure, diagnostic nuclear medicine

(For chemical analysis, see **Chemistry** section)

Other Procedures

(For specific organ, see appropriate heading)

(For radiophosphorus tumor identification, ocular, see 78800)

| 78800 | Radiopharmaceutical localization of tumor or distribution of radiopharmaceutical agent(s); limited area |

(For specific organ, see appropriate heading)

78801	multiple areas
78802	whole body, single day imaging
78803	tomographic (SPECT)
78804	whole body, requiring two or more days imaging
78805	Radiopharmaceutical localization of inflammatory process; limited area
78806	whole body
78807	tomographic (SPECT)

(For imaging bone infectious or inflammatory disease with a bone imaging radiopharmaceutical, see 78300, 78305, 78306)

►(78810 has been deleted. To report, see 78811-78813)◄

►(For PET of brain, see 78608, 78609)◄

►(For PET myocardial imaging, see 78491, 78492)◄

● 78811	Tumor imaging, positron emission tomography (PET); limited area (eg, chest, head/neck)
● 78812	skull base to mid-thigh
● 78813	whole body

● 78814	Tumor imaging, positron emission tomography (PET) with concurrently acquired computed tomography (CT) for attenuation correction and anatomical localization; limited area (eg, chest, head/neck)
● 78815	skull base to mid-thigh
● 78816	whole body

►(Report 78811-78816 only once per imaging session)◄

►(Computed tomography (CT) performed for other than attenuation correction and anatomical localization is reported using the appropriate site specific CT code with modifier 59)◄

| 78890 | Generation of automated data: interactive process involving nuclear physician and/or allied health professional personnel; simple manipulations and interpretation, not to exceed 30 minutes |
| 78891 | complex manipulations and interpretation, exceeding 30 minutes |

(Use 78890 or 78891 in addition to primary procedure)

►(78990 has been deleted)◄

| 78999 | Unlisted miscellaneous procedure, diagnostic nuclear medicine |

Therapeutic

►The oral and intravenous administration codes in this section are inclusive of the mode of administration. For intra-arterial, intra-cavitary, and intra-articular administration, also use the appropriate injection and/or procedure codes, as well as imaging guidance and radiological supervision and interpretation codes, when appropriate.◄

►(79000, 79001 have been deleted. To report, use 79005)◄

| ● 79005 | Radiopharmaceutical therapy, by oral administration |

►(79020, 79030, 79035 have been deleted. To report, use 79005)◄

►(79100 has been deleted. To report, use 79101)◄

(For monoclonal antibody therapy, use 79403)

| ● 79101 | Radiopharmaceutical therapy, by intravenous administration |

►(Do not report 79101 in conjunction with 36400, 36410, 79403, 90780, 90784, 96408)◄

►(For radiolabeled monoclonal antibody by intravenous infusion, use 79403)◄

►(For infusion or instillation of non-antibody radioelement solution that includes three months follow-up care, use 77750)◄

Radiology

▲ **79200**   Radiopharmaceutical therapy, by intracavitary
              administration

▲ **79300**   Radiopharmaceutical therapy, by interstitial radioactive
              colloid administration

              ►(79400 has been deleted. To report, use 79101)◄

79403   Radiopharmaceutical therapy, radiolabeled monoclonal
            antibody by intravenous infusion

            (For pre-treatment imaging, see 78802, 78804)

            (Do not report 79403 in conjunction with ►79101◄)

            ►(79420 has been deleted. To report use 79445)◄

▲ **79440**   Radiopharmaceutical therapy, by intra-articular
              administration

● **79445**   Radiopharmaceutical therapy, by intra-arterial particulate
              administration

              ►(Do not report 79445 in conjunction with 90783,
              96420)◄

              ►(Use appropriate procedural and radiological
              supervision and interpretation codes for the angiographic
              and interventional procedures provided pre-requisite to
              intra-arterial radiopharmaceutical therapy)◄

              ►(79900 has been deleted)◄

▲ **79999**   Radiopharmaceutical therapy, unlisted procedure

Pathology and Laboratory Guidelines

Items used by all physicians in reporting their services are presented in the **Introduction.** Some of the commonalities are repeated here for the convenience of those physicians referring to this section on **Pathology and Laboratory.** Other definitions and items unique to Pathology and Laboratory are also listed.

Services in Pathology and Laboratory

Services in Pathology and Laboratory are provided by a physician or by technologists under responsible supervision of a physician.

Separate or Multiple Procedures

It is appropriate to designate multiple procedures that are rendered on the same date by separate entries.

Subsection Information

Several of the subheadings or subsections have special needs or instructions unique to that section. Where these are indicated, (eg, "Panel Tests"), special **"Notes"** will be presented preceding those procedural terminology listings referring to that subsection specifically. If there is an "Unlisted Procedure" code number (see section below) for the individual subsection, it will be shown. Those subsections with **"Notes"** are as follows:

Organ or Disease Panels 80048-80076
Drug Testing 80100-80103
Therapeutic Drug Assays 80150-80299
Evocative/Suppression Testing 80400-80440
Consultations
   (Clinical Pathology) 80500-80502
Urinalysis 81000-81099
Chemistry 82000-84999
Molecular Diagnostics 83890-83912
Infectious Agent: Detection
   of Antibodies 86602-86804
Microbiology 87001-87255
   Infectious Agent Detection 87260-87999
Anatomic Pathology 88000-88099
Cytopathology 88104-88199
▶Cytogenetic Studies . . . . 88230-88299◀
Surgical Pathology 88300-88399

Unlisted Service or Procedure

A service or procedure may be provided that is not listed in this edition of *CPT.* When reporting such a service, the appropriate "Unlisted Procedure" code may be used to indicate the service, identifying it by "Special Report" as discussed below. The "Unlisted Procedures" and accompanying codes for **Pathology and Laboratory** are as follows:

81099	Unlisted urinalysis procedure
84999	Unlisted chemistry procedure
85999	Unlisted hematology and coagulation procedure
86586	Unlisted antigen, each
86849	Unlisted immunology procedure
86999	Unlisted transfusion medicine procedure
87999	Unlisted microbiology procedure
88099	Unlisted necropsy (autopsy) procedure
88199	Unlisted cytopathology procedure
88299	Unlisted cytogenetic study
88399	Unlisted surgical pathology procedure
89240	Unlisted miscellaneous pathology test

Special Report

A service that is rarely provided, unusual, variable, or new may require a special report in determining medical appropriateness of the service. Pertinent information should include an adequate definition or description of the nature, extent, and need for the procedure; and the time, effort, and equipment necessary to provide the service. Additional items which may be included are:

- complexity of symptoms;
- final diagnosis;
- pertinent physical findings;
- diagnostic and therapeutic procedures;
- concurrent problems;
- follow-up care.

Notes

○=Modifier 51 Exempt   ⊙=Conscious Sedation   ✚=Add-on Code

Pathology and Laboratory

Organ or Disease Oriented Panels

These panels were developed for coding purposes only and should not be interpreted as clinical parameters. The tests listed with each panel identify the defined components of that panel.

These panel components are not intended to limit the performance of other tests. If one performs tests in addition to those specifically indicated for a particular panel, those tests should be reported separately in addition to the panel code.

80048 Basic metabolic panel ·

This panel must include the following:

Calcium (82310)

Carbon dioxide (82374)

Chloride (82435)

Creatinine (82565)

Glucose (82947)

Potassium (84132)

Sodium (84295)

Urea nitrogen (BUN) (84520)

(Do not use 80048 in addition to 80053)

80050 General health panel

This panel must include the following:

Comprehensive metabolic panel (80053)

Blood count, complete (CBC), automated and automated differential WBC count (85025 or 85027 and 85004)

OR

Blood count, complete (CBC), automated (85027) and appropriate manual differential WBC count (85007 or 85009)

Thyroid stimulating hormone (TSH) (84443)

80051 Electrolyte panel

This panel must include the following:

Carbon dioxide (82374)

Chloride (82435)

Potassium (84132)

Sodium (84295)

80053 Comprehensive metabolic panel

This panel must include the following:

Albumin (82040)

Bilirubin, total (82247)

Calcium (82310)

Carbon dioxide (bicarbonate) (82374)

Chloride (82435)

Creatinine (82565)

Glucose (82947)

Phosphatase, alkaline (84075)

Potassium (84132)

Protein, total (84155)

Sodium (84295)

Transferase, alanine amino (ALT) (SGPT) (84460)

Transferase, aspartate amino (AST) (SGOT) (84450)

Urea nitrogen (BUN) (84520)

(Do not use 80053 in addition to 80048, 80076)

80055 Obstetric panel

This panel must include the following:

Blood count, complete (CBC), automated and automated differential WBC count (85025 or 85027 and 85004)

OR

Blood count, complete (CBC), automated (85027) and appropriate manual differential WBC count (85007 or 85009)

Hepatitis B surface antigen (HBsAg) (87340)

Antibody, rubella (86762)

Syphilis test, qualitative (eg, VDRL, RPR, ART) (86592)

Antibody screen, RBC, each serum technique (86850)

Blood typing, ABO (86900) AND

Blood typing, Rh (D) (86901)

80061 Lipid panel

This panel must include the following:

Cholesterol, serum, total (82465)

Lipoprotein, direct measurement, high density cholesterol (HDL cholesterol) (83718)

Triglycerides (84478)

80069 Renal function panel

This panel must include the following:

Albumin (82040)

Calcium (82310)

Carbon dioxide (bicarbonate) (82374)

Chloride (82435)

Creatinine (82565)

Glucose (82947)

Phosphorus inorganic (phosphate) (84100)

Potassium (84132)

Sodium (84295)

Urea nitrogen (BUN) (84520)

80074 Acute hepatitis panel

This panel must include the following:

Hepatitis A antibody (HAAb), IgM antibody (86709)

Hepatitis B core antibody (HBcAb), IgM antibody (86705)

Hepatitis B surface antigen (HBsAg) (87340)

Hepatitis C antibody (86803)

80076 Hepatic function panel

This panel must include the following:

Albumin (82040)

Bilirubin, total (82247)

Bilirubin, direct (82248)

Phosphatase, alkaline (84075)

Protein, total (84155)

Transferase, alanine amino (ALT) (SGPT) (84460)

Transferase, aspartate amino (AST) (SGOT) (84450)

(Do not use 80076 in addition to 80053)

(80090 has been deleted. To report, see codes for specific tests)

Drug Testing

The following list contains examples of drugs or classes of drugs that are commonly assayed by qualitative screen, followed by confirmation with a second method.

Alcohols

Amphetamines

Barbiturates

Benzodiazepines

Cocaine and Metabolites

Methadones

Methaqualones

Opiates

Phencyclidines

Phenothiazines

Propoxyphenes

Tetrahydrocannabinoids

Tricyclic Antidepressants

Confirmed drugs may also be quantitated.

Use 80100 for each multiple drug class chromatographic procedure. Use 80102 for each procedure necessary for confirmation. For chromatography, each combination of stationary and mobile phase is to be counted as one procedure. For example, if detection of three drugs by chromatography requires one stationary phase with three mobile phases, use 80100 three (3) times. However, if multiple drugs can be detected using a single analysis (eg, one stationary phase with one mobile phase), use 80100 only once.

For quantitation of drugs screened, use appropriate code in **Chemistry** section (82000-84999) or **Therapeutic Drug Assay** section (80150-80299).

80100 Drug screen, qualitative; multiple drug classes chromatographic method, each procedure

80101   single drug class method (eg, immunoassay, enzyme assay), each drug class

80102 Drug confirmation, each procedure

80103 Tissue preparation for drug analysis

Therapeutic Drug Assays

The material for examination may be from any source. Examination is quantitative. For nonquantitative testing, see Drug Testing (80100-80103).

80150 Amikacin

80152 Amitriptyline

80154 Benzodiazepines

80156 Carbamazepine; total

80157   free

80158 Cyclosporine

80160 Desipramine

80162 Digoxin

80164 Dipropylacetic acid (valproic acid)

80166 Doxepin

80168 Ethosuximide

80170 Gentamicin

80172 Gold

80173 Haloperidol

80174 Imipramine

80176 Lidocaine

80178 Lithium

80182 Nortriptyline

80184 Phenobarbital

80185 Phenytoin; total

80186   free

80188 Primidone

80190   Procainamide;

80192   with metabolites (eg, n-acetyl procainamide)

80194   Quinidine

80196   Salicylate

80197   Tacrolimus

80198   Theophylline

80200   Tobramycin

80201   Topiramate

80202   Vancomycin

80299   Quantitation of drug, not elsewhere specified

Evocative/Suppression Testing

The following test panels involve the administration of evocative or suppressive agents, and the baseline and subsequent measurement of their effects on chemical constituents. These codes are to be used for the reporting of the laboratory component of the overall testing protocol. For the physician's administration of the evocative or suppressive agents, see 90780-90784; for the supplies and drugs, see 99070. To report physician attendance and monitoring during the testing, use the appropriate evaluation and management code, including the prolonged physician care codes if required. Prolonged physician care codes are not separately reported when evocative/suppression testing involves prolonged infusions reported with 90780 and 90781. In the code descriptors where reference is made to a particular analyte (eg, Cortisol (82533 x 2)) the "x 2" refers to the number of times the test for that particular analyte is performed.

80400   ACTH stimulation panel; for adrenal insufficiency

This panel must include the following:

Cortisol (82533 x 2)

80402   for 21 hydroxylase deficiency

This panel must include the following:

Cortisol (82533 x 2)

17 hydroxyprogesterone (83498 x 2)

80406   for 3 beta-hydroxydehydrogenase deficiency

This panel must include the following:

Cortisol (82533 x 2)

17 hydroxypregnenolone (84143 x 2)

80408   Aldosterone suppression evaluation panel (eg, saline infusion)

This panel must include the following:

Aldosterone (82088 x 2)

Renin (84244 x 2)

80410   Calcitonin stimulation panel (eg, calcium, pentagastrin)

This panel must include the following:

Calcitonin (82308 x 3)

80412   Corticotropic releasing hormone (CRH) stimulation panel

This panel must include the following:

Cortisol (82533 x 6)

Adrenocorticotropic hormone (ACTH) (82024 x 6)

80414   Chorionic gonadotropin stimulation panel; testosterone response

This panel must include the following:

Testosterone (84403 x 2 on three pooled blood samples)

80415   estradiol response

This panel must include the following:

Estradiol (82670 x 2 on three pooled blood samples)

80416   Renal vein renin stimulation panel (eg, captopril)

This panel must include the following:

Renin (84244 x 6)

80417   Peripheral vein renin stimulation panel (eg, captopril)

This panel must include the following:

Renin (84244 x 2)

80418   Combined rapid anterior pituitary evaluation panel

This panel must include the following:

Adrenocorticotropic hormone (ACTH) (82024 x 4)

Luteinizing hormone (LH) (83002 x 4)

Follicle stimulating hormone (FSH) (83001 x 4)

Prolactin (84146 x 4)

Human growth hormone (HGH) (83003 x 4)

Cortisol (82533 x 4)

Thyroid stimulating hormone (TSH) (84443 x 4)

80420   Dexamethasone suppression panel, 48 hour

This panel must include the following:

Free cortisol, urine (82530 x 2)

Cortisol (82533 x 2)

Volume measurement for timed collection (81050 x 2)

(For single dose dexamethasone, use 82533)

80422   Glucagon tolerance panel; for insulinoma

This panel must include the following:

Glucose (82947 x 3)

Insulin (83525 x 3)

80424   for pheochromocytoma

This panel must include the following:

Catecholamines, fractionated (82384 x 2)

Pathology and Laboratory

Pathology and Laboratory

80426 Gonadotropin releasing hormone stimulation panel

This panel must include the following:

Follicle stimulating hormone (FSH) (83001 x 4)

Luteinizing hormone (LH) (83002 x 4)

80428 Growth hormone stimulation panel (eg, arginine infusion, l-dopa administration)

This panel must include the following:

Human growth hormone (HGH) (83003 x 4)

80430 Growth hormone suppression panel (glucose administration)

This panel must include the following:

Glucose (82947 x 3)

Human growth hormone (HGH) (83003 x 4)

80432 Insulin-induced C-peptide suppression panel

This panel must include the following:

Insulin (83525)

C-peptide (84681 x 5)

Glucose (82947 x 5)

80434 Insulin tolerance panel; for ACTH insufficiency

This panel must include the following:

Cortisol (82533 x 5)

Glucose (82947 x 5)

80435 for growth hormone deficiency

This panel must include the following:

Glucose (82947 x 5)

Human growth hormone (HGH) (83003 x 5)

80436 Metyrapone panel

This panel must include the following:

Cortisol (82533 x 2)

11 deoxycortisol (82634 x 2)

80438 Thyrotropin releasing hormone (TRH) stimulation panel; one hour

This panel must include the following:

Thyroid stimulating hormone (TSH) (84443 x 3)

80439 two hour

This panel must include the following:

Thyroid stimulating hormone (TSH) (84443 x 4)

80440 for hyperprolactinemia

This panel must include the following:

Prolactin (84146 x 3)

Consultations (Clinical Pathology)

A clinical pathology consultation is a service, including a written report, rendered by the pathologist in response to a request from an attending physician in relation to a test result(s) requiring additional medical interpretive judgment.

Reporting of a test result(s) without medical interpretive judgment is not considered a clinical pathology consultation.

80500 Clinical pathology consultation; limited, without review of patient's history and medical records

80502 comprehensive, for a complex diagnostic problem, with review of patient's history and medical records

(These codes may also be used for pharmacokinetic consultations)

(For consultations involving the examination and evaluation of the patient, see 99241-99275)

Urinalysis

For specific analyses, see appropriate section.

(For urinalysis, infectious agent detection, semi-quantitative analysis of volatile compounds, use Category III code 0041T)

81000 Urinalysis, by dip stick or tablet reagent for bilirubin, glucose, hemoglobin, ketones, leukocytes, nitrite, pH, protein, specific gravity, urobilinogen, any number of these constituents; non-automated, with microscopy

81001 automated, with microscopy

81002 non-automated, without microscopy

81003 automated, without microscopy

81005 Urinalysis; qualitative or semiquantitative, except immunoassays

(For non-immunoassay reagent strip urinalysis, see 81000, 81002)

(For immunoassay, qualitative or semiquantitative, use 83518)

(For microalbumin, see 82043, 82044)

81007 bacteriuria screen, except by culture or dipstick

(For culture, see 87086-87088)

(For dipstick, use 81000 or 81002)

81015 microscopic only

81020 two or three glass test

81025 Urine pregnancy test, by visual color comparison methods

81050 Volume measurement for timed collection, each

81099 Unlisted urinalysis procedure

Chemistry

The material for examination may be from any source unless otherwise specified in the code descriptor. When an analyte is measured in multiple specimens from different sources, or in specimens that are obtained at different times, the analyte is reported separately for each source and for each specimen. The examination is quantitative unless specified. To report an organ or disease oriented panel, see codes 80048-80076.

When a code describes a method where measurement of multiple analytes may require one or several procedures, each procedure is coded separately (eg, 82491-82492, 82541-82544). For example, if two (2) analytes are measured using column chromatography using a single stationary or mobile phase, use 82492. If the same two analytes are measured using different stationary or mobile phase conditions, 82491 would be used twice. If a total of four (4) analytes are measured where two (2) analytes are measured with a single stationary and mobile phase, and the other two (2) analytes are measured using a different stationary and mobile phase, use 82492 twice. If a total of three (3) analytes are measured where two (2) analytes are measured using a single stationary or mobile phase condition, and the third analyte is measured separately using a different stationary or mobile phase procedure, use 82492 once for the (2) analytes measured under the same condition, and use 82491 once for the third analyte measured separately.

Clinical information derived from the results of laboratory data that is mathematically calculated (eg, free thyroxine index (T7)) is considered part of the test procedure and therefore is not a separately reportable service.

82000	Acetaldehyde, blood
82003	Acetaminophen
82009	Acetone or other ketone bodies, serum; qualitative
82010	quantitative
82013	Acetylcholinesterase
	(Acid, gastric, see gastric acid, 82926, 82928)
	(Acid phosphatase, see 84060-84066)
82016	Acylcarnitines; qualitative, each specimen
82017	quantitative, each specimen
	(For carnitine, use 82379)
82024	Adrenocorticotropic hormone (ACTH)
82030	Adenosine, 5-monophosphate, cyclic (cyclic AMP)
82040	Albumin; serum
82042	urine or other source, quantitative, each specimen

82043	urine, microalbumin, quantitative
82044	urine, microalbumin, semiquantitative (eg, reagent strip assay)
	(For prealbumin, use 84134)
● 82045	ischemia modified
82055	Alcohol (ethanol); any specimen except breath
	(For other volatiles, alcohol, use 84600)
82075	breath
82085	Aldolase
82088	Aldosterone
	(Alkaline phosphatase, see 84075, 84080)
82101	Alkaloids, urine, quantitative
	(Alphaketoglutarate, see 82009, 82010)
	(Alpha tocopherol (Vitamin E), use 84446)
82103	Alpha-1-antitrypsin; total
82104	phenotype
82105	Alpha-fetoprotein; serum
82106	amniotic fluid
82108	Aluminum
82120	Amines, vaginal fluid, qualitative
	(For combined pH and amines test for vaginitis, use 82120 and 83986)
82127	Amino acids; single, qualitative, each specimen
82128	multiple, qualitative, each specimen
82131	single, quantitative, each specimen
82135	Aminolevulinic acid, delta (ALA)
82136	Amino acids, 2 to 5 amino acids, quantitative, each specimen
82139	Amino acids, 6 or more amino acids, quantitative, each specimen
82140	Ammonia
82143	Amniotic fluid scan (spectrophotometric)
	(For L/S ratio, use 83661)
	(Amobarbital, see 80100-80103 for qualitative analysis, 82205 for quantitative analysis)
82145	Amphetamine or methamphetamine
	(For qualitative analysis, see 80100-80103)
82150	Amylase
82154	Androstanediol glucuronide
82157	Androstenedione
82160	Androsterone
82163	Angiotensin II

Pathology and Laboratory

82164	Angiotensin I - converting enzyme (ACE)
	(Antidiuretic hormone (ADH), use 84588)
	(Antimony, use 83015)
	(Antitrypsin, alpha-1-, see 82103, 82104)
82172	Apolipoprotein, each
82175	Arsenic
	(For heavy metal screening, use 83015)
82180	Ascorbic acid (Vitamin C), blood
	(Aspirin, see acetylsalicylic acid, 80196)
	(Atherogenic index, blood, ultracentrifugation, quantitative, use 83716)
82190	Atomic absorption spectroscopy, each analyte
82205	Barbiturates, not elsewhere specified
	(For qualitative analysis, see 80100-80103)
	(For B-Natriuretic peptide, use 83880)
82232	Beta-2 microglobulin
	(Bicarbonate, use 82374)
82239	Bile acids; total
82240	cholylglycine
	(For bile pigments, urine, see 81000-81005)
82247	Bilirubin; total
82248	direct
82252	feces, qualitative
82261	Biotinidase, each specimen
82270	Blood, occult, by peroxidase activity (eg, guaiac), qualitative; feces, 1-3 simultaneous determinations
82273	other sources
	(Blood urea nitrogen (BUN), see 84520, 84525)
82274	Blood, occult, by fecal hemoglobin determination by immunoassay, qualitative, feces, 1-3 simultaneous determinations
82286	Bradykinin
82300	Cadmium
82306	Calcifediol (25-OH Vitamin D-3)
82307	Calciferol (Vitamin D)
	(For 1,25-Dihydroxyvitamin D, use 82652)
82308	Calcitonin
82310	Calcium; total
82330	ionized
82331	after calcium infusion test
82340	urine quantitative, timed specimen
82355	Calculus; qualitative analysis
82360	quantitative analysis, chemical

82365	infrared spectroscopy
82370	x-ray diffraction
	(Carbamates, see individual listings)
82373	Carbohydrate deficient transferrin
82374	Carbon dioxide (bicarbonate)
	(See also 82803)
82375	Carbon monoxide, (carboxyhemoglobin); quantitative
82376	qualitative
	(To report end-tidal carbon monoxide, use Category III code 0043T)
82378	Carcinoembryonic antigen (CEA)
82379	Carnitine (total and free), quantitative, each specimen
	(For acylcarnitine, see 82016, 82017)
82380	Carotene
82382	Catecholamines; total urine
82383	blood
82384	fractionated
	(For urine metabolites, see 83835, 84585)
82387	Cathepsin-D
82390	Ceruloplasmin
82397	Chemiluminescent assay
82415	Chloramphenicol
82435	Chloride; blood
82436	urine
82438	other source
	(For sweat collection by iontophoresis, use 89230)
82441	Chlorinated hydrocarbons, screen
	(Chlorpromazine, use 84022)
	(Cholecalciferol (Vitamin D), use 82307)
82465	Cholesterol, serum or whole blood, total
	(For high density lipoprotein (HDL), use 83718)
82480	Cholinesterase; serum
82482	RBC
82485	Chondroitin B sulfate, quantitative
	(Chorionic gonadotropin, see gonadotropin, 84702, 84703)
82486	Chromatography, qualitative; column (eg, gas liquid or HPLC), analyte not elsewhere specified
82487	paper, 1-dimensional, analyte not elsewhere specified
82488	paper, 2-dimensional, analyte not elsewhere specified
82489	thin layer, analyte not elsewhere specified

82491	Chromatography, quantitative, column (eg, gas liquid or HPLC); single analyte not elsewhere specified, single stationary and mobile phase	
82492	multiple analytes, single stationary and mobile phase	
82495	Chromium	
82507	Citrate	
82520	Cocaine or metabolite	

(Cocaine, qualitative analysis, see 80100-80103)

(Codeine, qualitative analysis, see 80100-80103)

(Codeine, quantitative analysis, see 82101)

(Complement, see 86160-86162)

82523 Collagen cross links, any method

82525 Copper

(Coproporphyrin, see 84119, 84120)

(Corticosteroids, use 83491)

82528 Corticosterone

82530 Cortisol; free

82533 total

(C-peptide, use 84681)

82540 Creatine

82541 Column chromatography/mass spectrometry (eg, GC/MS, or HPLC/MS), analyte not elsewhere specified; qualitative, single stationary and mobile phase

82542 quantitative, single stationary and mobile phase

82543 stable isotope dilution, single analyte, quantitative, single stationary and mobile phase

82544 stable isotope dilution, multiple analytes, quantitative, single stationary and mobile phase

82550 Creatine kinase (CK), (CPK); total

82552 isoenzymes

82553 MB fraction only

82554 isoforms

82565 Creatinine; blood

82570 other source

82575 clearance

82585 Cryofibrinogen

82595 Cryoglobulin, qualitative or semi-quantitative (eg, cryocrit)

(For quantitative, cryoglobulin, see 82784, 82785)

(Crystals, pyrophosphate vs. urate, use 89060)

82600 Cyanide

82607 Cyanocobalamin (Vitamin B-12);

82608 unsaturated binding capacity

(Cyclic AMP, use 82030)

(Cyclic GMP, use 83008)

(Cyclosporine, use 80158)

82615 Cystine and homocystine, urine, qualitative

82626 Dehydroepiandrosterone (DHEA)

82627 Dehydroepiandrosterone-sulfate (DHEA-S)

(Delta-aminolevulinic acid (ALA), use 82135)

82633 Desoxycorticosterone, 11-

82634 Deoxycortisol, 11-

(Dexamethasone suppression test, use 80420)

(Diastase, urine, use 82150)

82638 Dibucaine number

(Dichloroethane, use 84600)

(Dichloromethane, use 84600)

(Diethylether, use 84600)

82646 Dihydrocodeinone

(For qualitative analysis, see 80100-80103)

82649 Dihydromorphinone

(For qualitative analysis, see 80100-80103)

82651 Dihydrotestosterone (DHT)

82652 Dihydroxyvitamin D, 1,25-

82654 Dimethadione

(For qualitative analysis, see 80100-80103)

(Diphenylhydantoin, use 80185)

(Dipropylacetic acid, use 80164)

(Dopamine, see 82382-82384)

(Duodenal contents, see individual enzymes; for intubation and collection, use 89100)

● **82656** Elastase, pancreatic (EL-1), fecal, qualitative or semi-quantitative

82657 Enzyme activity in blood cells, cultured cells, or tissue, not elsewhere specified; nonradioactive substrate, each specimen

82658 radioactive substrate, each specimen

82664 Electrophoretic technique, not elsewhere specified

(Endocrine receptor assays, see 84233-84235)

82666 Epiandrosterone

(Epinephrine, see 82382-82384)

82668 Erythropoietin

82670 Estradiol

82671 Estrogens; fractionated

82672 total

(Estrogen receptor assay, use 84233)

82677 Estriol

Pathology and Laboratory

Pathology and Laboratory

82679	Estrone
	(Ethanol, see 82055 and 82075)
82690	Ethchlorvynol
	(Ethyl alcohol, see 82055 and 82075)
82693	Ethylene glycol
82696	Etiocholanolone
	(For fractionation of ketosteroids, use 83593)
82705	Fat or lipids, feces; qualitative
82710	quantitative
82715	Fat differential, feces, quantitative
82725	Fatty acids, nonesterified
82726	Very long chain fatty acids
82728	Ferritin
	(Fetal hemoglobin, see hemoglobin 83030, 83033, and 85460)
	(Fetoprotein, alpha-1, see 82105, 82106)
82731	Fetal fibronectin, cervicovaginal secretions, semi-quantitative
82735	Fluoride
82742	Flurazepam
	(For qualitative analysis, see 80100-80103)
	(Foam stability test, use 83662)
82746	Folic acid; serum
82747	RBC
	(Follicle stimulating hormone (FSH), use 83001)
82757	Fructose, semen
	(Fructosamine, use 82985)
	(Fructose, TLC screen, use 84375)
82759	Galactokinase, RBC
82760	Galactose
82775	Galactose-1-phosphate uridyl transferase; quantitative
82776	screen
82784	Gammaglobulin; IgA, IgD, IgG, IgM, each
82785	IgE
	(For allergen specific IgE, see 86003, 86005)
82787	immunoglobulin subclasses, (IgG1, 2, 3, or 4), each
	(Gamma-glutamyltransferase (GGT), use 82977)
82800	Gases, blood, pH only
82803	Gases, blood, any combination of pH, pCO_2, pO_2, CO_2, HCO_3 (including calculated O_2 saturation);
	(Use 82803 for two or more of the above listed analytes)
82805	with O_2 saturation, by direct measurement, except pulse oximetry

82810	Gases, blood, O_2 saturation only, by direct measurement, except pulse oximetry
	(For pulse oximetry, use 94760)
82820	Hemoglobin-oxygen affinity (pO_2 for 50% hemoglobin saturation with oxygen)
82926	Gastric acid, free and total, each specimen
82928	Gastric acid, free or total, each specimen
82938	Gastrin after secretin stimulation
82941	Gastrin
	(Gentamicin, use 80170)
	(GGT, use 82977)
	(GLC, gas liquid chromatography, use 82486)
82943	Glucagon
82945	Glucose, body fluid, other than blood
82946	Glucagon tolerance test
82947	Glucose; quantitative, blood (except reagent strip)
82948	blood, reagent strip
82950	post glucose dose (includes glucose)
82951	tolerance test (GTT), three specimens (includes glucose)
82952	tolerance test, each additional beyond three specimens
82953	tolbutamide tolerance test
	(For insulin tolerance test, see 80434, 80435)
	(For leucine tolerance test, use 80428)
	(For semiquantitative urine glucose, see 81000, 81002, 81005, 81099)
82955	Glucose-6-phosphate dehydrogenase (G6PD); quantitative
82960	screen
	(For glucose tolerance test with medication, use 90784 in addition)
82962	Glucose, blood by glucose monitoring device(s) cleared by the FDA specifically for home use
82963	Glucosidase, beta
82965	Glutamate dehydrogenase
82975	Glutamine (glutamic acid amide)
82977	Glutamyltransferase, gamma (GGT)
82978	Glutathione
82979	Glutathione reductase, RBC
82980	Glutethimide
	(Glycohemoglobin, use 83036)
82985	Glycated protein
	(Gonadotropin, chorionic, see 84702, 84703)

83001	Gonadotropin; follicle stimulating hormone (FSH)
83002	luteinizing hormone (LH)

(For luteinizing releasing factor (LRH), use 83727)

83003 Growth hormone, human (HGH) (somatotropin)

(For antibody to human growth hormone, use 86277)

83008 Guanosine monophosphate (GMP), cyclic

● **83009** Helicobacter pylori, blood test analysis for urease activity, non-radioactive isotope (eg, C-13)

►(For H. pylori, breath test analysis for urease activity, see 83013, 83014)◄

83010 Haptoglobin; quantitative

83012 phenotypes

▲ **83013** Helicobacter pylori; breath test analysis for urease activity, non-radioactive isotope (eg, C-13)

▲ **83014** drug administration

(For H. pylori, stool, use 87338. For H. pylori, liquid scintillation counter, see 78267, 78268. For H. pylori, enzyme immunoassay, use 87339)

►(For H. pylori, blood test analysis for urease activity, use 83009)◄

83015 Heavy metal (eg, arsenic, barium, beryllium, bismuth, antimony, mercury); screen

83018 quantitative, each

83020 Hemoglobin fractionation and quantitation; electrophoresis (eg, A2, S, C, and/or F)

83021 chromatography (eg, A2, S, C, and/or F)

83026 Hemoglobin; by copper sulfate method, non-automated

83030 F (fetal), chemical

83033 F (fetal), qualitative

83036 glycated

(For fecal hemoglobin detection by immunoassay, use 82274)

83045 methemoglobin, qualitative

83050 methemoglobin, quantitative

83051 plasma

83055 sulfhemoglobin, qualitative

83060 sulfhemoglobin, quantitative

83065 thermolabile

83068 unstable, screen

83069 urine

83070 Hemosiderin; qualitative

83071 quantitative

(Heroin, see 80100-80103)

(HIAA, use 83497)

(High performance liquid chromatography (HPLC), use 82486)

83080 b-Hexosaminidase, each assay

83088 Histamine

(Hollander test, use 91052)

83090 Homocystine

83150 Homovanillic acid (HVA)

(Hormones, see individual alphabetic listings in **Chemistry** section)

(Hydrogen breath test, use 91065)

83491 Hydroxycorticosteroids, 17- (17-OHCS)

(For cortisol, see 82530, 82533. For deoxycortisol, use 82634)

83497 Hydroxyindolacetic acid, 5-(HIAA)

(For urine qualitative test, use 81005)

(5-Hydroxytryptamine, use 84260)

83498 Hydroxyprogesterone, 17-d

83499 Hydroxyprogesterone, 20-

83500 Hydroxyproline; free

83505 total

83516 Immunoassay for analyte other than infectious agent antibody or infectious agent antigen, qualitative or semiquantitative; multiple step method

83518 single step method (eg, reagent strip)

83519 Immunoassay, analyte, quantitative; by radiopharmaceutical technique (eg, RIA)

83520 not otherwise specified

(For immunoassays for antibodies to infectious agent antigens, see analyte and method specific codes in the **Immunology** section)

(For immunoassay of tumor antigen not elsewhere specified, use 86316)

(Immunoglobulins, see 82784, 82785)

83525 Insulin; total

(For proinsulin, use 84206)

83527 free

83528 Intrinsic factor

(For intrinsic factor antibodies, use 86340)

83540 Iron

83550 Iron binding capacity

83570 Isocitric dehydrogenase (IDH)

(Isonicotinic acid hydrazide, INH, see code for specific method)

(Isopropyl alcohol, use 84600)

Pathology and Laboratory

▲=Revised Code   ●=New Code   ► ◄=New or Revised Text

83582   Ketogenic steroids, fractionation

(Ketone bodies, for serum, see 82009, 82010; for urine, see 81000-81003)

83586   Ketosteroids, 17- (17-KS); total

83593   fractionation

83605   Lactate (lactic acid)

83615   Lactate dehydrogenase (LD), (LDH);

83625   isoenzymes, separation and quantitation

● **83630**   Lactoferrin, fecal, qualitative

83632   Lactogen, human placental (HPL) human chorionic somatomammotropin

83633   Lactose, urine; qualitative

83634   quantitative

(For tolerance, see 82951, 82952)

(For breath hydrogen test for lactase deficiency, use 91065)

83655   Lead

83661   Fetal lung maturity assessment; lecithin sphingomyelin (L/S) ratio

83662   foam stability test

83663   fluorescence polarization

83664   lamellar body density

(For phosphatidylglycerol, use 84081)

83670   Leucine aminopeptidase (LAP)

83690   Lipase

83715   Lipoprotein, blood; electrophoretic separation and quantitation

83716   high resolution fractionation and quantitation of lipoproteins including lipoprotein subclasses when performed (eg, electrophoresis, nuclear magnetic resonance, ultracentrifugation)

83718   Lipoprotein, direct measurement; high density cholesterol (HDL cholesterol)

83719   direct measurement, VLDL cholesterol

83721   direct measurement, LDL cholesterol

(For fractionation by nuclear magnetic resonance or high resolution electrophoresis, use 83716)

(To report direct measurement, intermediate density lipoproteins (remnant lipoproteins), use Category III code 0026T)

(Luteinizing hormone (LH), use 83002)

83727   Luteinizing releasing factor (LRH)

(For qualitative analysis, see 80100-80103)

(Macroglobulins, alpha-2, use 86329)

83735   Magnesium

83775   Malate dehydrogenase

(Maltose tolerance, see 82951, 82952)

(Mammotropin, use 84146)

83785   Manganese

(Marijuana, see 80100-80103)

83788   Mass spectrometry and tandem mass spectrometry (MS, MS/MS), analyte not elsewhere specified; qualitative, each specimen

83789   quantitative, each specimen

83805   Meprobamate

(For qualitative analysis, see 80100-80103)

83825   Mercury, quantitative

(Mercury screen, use 83015)

83835   Metanephrines

(For catecholamines, see 82382-82384)

83840   Methadone

(For methadone qualitative analysis, see 80100-80103)

(Methamphetamine, see 80100-80103, 82145)

(Methanol, use 84600)

83857   Methemalbumin

(Methemoglobin, see hemoglobin 83045, 83050)

83858   Methsuximide

(Methyl alcohol, use 84600)

(Microalbumin, see 82043 for quantitative, see 82044 for semiquantitative)

(Microglobulin, beta-2, use 82232)

83864   Mucopolysaccharides, acid; quantitative

83866   screen

83872   Mucin, synovial fluid (Ropes test)

83873   Myelin basic protein, cerebrospinal fluid

(For oligoclonal bands, use 83916)

83874   Myoglobin

(Nalorphine, use 83925)

83880   Natriuretic peptide

83883   Nephelometry, each analyte not elsewhere specified

83885   Nickel

83887   Nicotine

Codes 83890-83912 are intended for use with molecular diagnostic techniques for analysis of nucleic acids.

Codes 83890-83912 are coded by procedure rather than analyte.

Code separately for each procedure used in an analysis. For example, a procedure requiring isolation of DNA, restriction endonuclease digestion, electrophoresis, and nucleic acid probe amplification would be coded 83890, 83892, 83894, and 83898.

►When molecular diagnostic procedures are performed to test for infectious disease, oncology, hematology, neurology or inherited disorder, use the appropriate modifier to specify probe type or condition tested. (See **Appendix I**).◄

(For microbial identification, see 87797, 87798)

83890	Molecular diagnostics; molecular isolation or extraction
83891	isolation or extraction of highly purified nucleic acid
83892	enzymatic digestion
83893	dot/slot blot production
83894	separation by gel electrophoresis (eg, agarose, polyacrylamide)
83896	nucleic acid probe, each
83897	nucleic acid transfer (eg, Southern, Northern)
83898	amplification of patient nucleic acid (eg, PCR, LCR), single primer pair, each primer pair
83901	amplification of patient nucleic acid, multiplex, each multiplex reaction
83902	reverse transcription
83903	mutation scanning, by physical properties (eg, single strand conformational polymorphisms (SSCP), heteroduplex, denaturing gradient gel electrophoresis (DGGE), RNA'ase A), single segment, each
83904	mutation identification by sequencing, single segment, each segment
83905	mutation identification by allele specific transcription, single segment, each segment
83906	mutation identification by allele specific translation, single segment, each segment
83912	interpretation and report
83915	Nucleotidase 5-
83916	Oligoclonal immune (oligoclonal bands)
83918	Organic acids; total, quantitative, each specimen
83919	qualitative, each specimen
83921	Organic acid, single, quantitative
83925	Opiates, (eg, morphine, meperidine)
83930	Osmolality; blood
83935	urine
83937	Osteocalcin (bone g1a protein)
83945	Oxalate
83950	Oncoprotein, HER-2/neu

(For tissue, see 88342, 88365)

83970	Parathormone (parathyroid hormone)

(Pesticide, quantitative, see code for specific method. For screen for chlorinated hydrocarbons, use 82441)

83986	pH, body fluid, except blood

(For blood pH, see 82800, 82803)

83992	Phencyclidine (PCP)

(For qualitative analysis, see 80100-80103)

(Phenobarbital, use 80184)

84022	Phenothiazine

(For qualitative analysis, see 80100, 80101)

84030	Phenylalanine (PKU), blood

(Phenylalanine-tyrosine ratio, see 84030, 84510)

84035	Phenylketones, qualitative
84060	Phosphatase, acid; total
84061	forensic examination
84066	prostatic
84075	Phosphatase, alkaline;
84078	heat stable (total not included)
84080	isoenzymes
84081	Phosphatidylglycerol

(Phosphates inorganic, use 84100)

(Phosphates, organic, see code for specific method. For cholinesterase, see 82480, 82482)

84085	Phosphogluconate, 6-, dehydrogenase, RBC
84087	Phosphohexose isomerase
84100	Phosphorus inorganic (phosphate);
84105	urine

(Pituitary gonadotropins, see 83001-83002)

(PKU, see 84030, 84035)

84106	Porphobilinogen, urine; qualitative
84110	quantitative
84119	Porphyrins, urine; qualitative
84120	quantitation and fractionation
84126	Porphyrins, feces; quantitative
84127	qualitative

(Porphyrin precursors, see 82135, 84106, 84110)

(For protoporphyrin, RBC, see 84202, 84203)

84132	Potassium; serum
84133	urine
84134	Prealbumin

(For microalbumin, see 82043, 82044)

84135	Pregnanediol

Pathology and Laboratory

84138	Pregnanetriol	
84140	Pregnenolone	
84143	17-hydroxypregnenolone	
84144	Progesterone	
	(Progesterone receptor assay, use 84234)	
	(For proinsulin, use 84206)	
84146	Prolactin	
84150	Prostaglandin, each	
84152	Prostate specific antigen (PSA); complexed (direct measurement)	
84153	total	
84154	free	
84155	Protein, total, except by refractometry; serum	
84156	urine	
84157	other source (eg, synovial fluid, cerebrospinal fluid)	
84160	Protein, total, by refractometry, any source	
	(For urine total protein by dipstick method, use 81000-81003)	
● 84163	Pregnancy-associated plasma protein-A (PAPP-A)	
▲ 84165	Protein; electrophoretic fractionation and quantitation, serum	
● 84166	electrophoretic fractionation and quantitation, other fluids with concentration (eg, urine, CSF)	
84181	Western Blot, with interpretation and report, blood or other body fluid	
84182	Western Blot, with interpretation and report, blood or other body fluid, immunological probe for band identification, each	
	(For Western Blot tissue analysis, use 88371)	
84202	Protoporphyrin, RBC; quantitative	
84203	screen	
84206	Proinsulin	
	(Pseudocholinesterase, use 82480)	
84207	Pyridoxal phosphate (Vitamin B-6)	
84210	Pyruvate	
84220	Pyruvate kinase	
84228	Quinine	
84233	Receptor assay; estrogen	
84234	progesterone	
84235	endocrine, other than estrogen or progesterone (specify hormone)	
84238	non-endocrine (eg, acetylcholine) (specify receptor)	
84244	Renin	

84252	Riboflavin (Vitamin B-2)
	(Salicylates, use 80196)
	(Secretin test, see 99070, 89100 and appropriate analyses)
84255	Selenium
84260	Serotonin
	(For urine metabolites (HIAA), use 83497)
84270	Sex hormone binding globulin (SHBG)
84275	Sialic acid
	(Sickle hemoglobin, use 85660)
84285	Silica
84295	Sodium; serum
84300	urine
84302	other source
	(Somatomammotropin, use 83632)
	(Somatotropin, use 83003)
84305	Somatomedin
84307	Somatostatin
84311	Spectrophotometry, analyte not elsewhere specified
84315	Specific gravity (except urine)
	(For specific gravity, urine, see 81000-81003)
	(Stone analysis, see 82355-82370)
84375	Sugars, chromatographic, TLC or paper chromatography
84376	Sugars (mono-, di-, and oligosaccharides); single qualitative, each specimen
84377	multiple qualitative, each specimen
84378	single quantitative, each specimen
84379	multiple quantitative, each specimen
84392	Sulfate, urine
	(Sulfhemoglobin, see hemoglobin, 83055, 83060)
	(T-3, see 84479-84481)
	(T-4, see 84436-84439)
84402	Testosterone; free
84403	total
84425	Thiamine (Vitamin B-1)
84430	Thiocyanate
84432	Thyroglobulin
	(Thyroglobulin, antibody, use 86800)
	(Thyrotropin releasing hormone (TRH) test, see 80438, 80439)
84436	Thyroxine; total
84437	requiring elution (eg, neonatal)
84439	free

Pathology and Laboratory

84442	Thyroxine binding globulin (TBG)
84443	Thyroid stimulating hormone (TSH)
84445	Thyroid stimulating immune globulins (TSI)
	(Tobramycin, use 80200)
84446	Tocopherol alpha (Vitamin E)
	(Tolbutamide tolerance, use 82953)
84449	Transcortin (cortisol binding globulin)
84450	Transferase; aspartate amino (AST) (SGOT)
84460	alanine amino (ALT) (SGPT)
84466	Transferrin
	(Iron binding capacity, use 83550)
84478	Triglycerides
84479	Thyroid hormone (T3 or T4) uptake or thyroid hormone binding ratio (THBR)
84480	Triiodothyronine T3; total (TT-3)
84481	free
84482	reverse
84484	Troponin, quantitative
	(For troponin, qualitative assay, use 84512)
84485	Trypsin; duodenal fluid
84488	feces, qualitative
84490	feces, quantitative, 24-hour collection
84510	Tyrosine
	(Urate crystal identification, use 89060)
84512	Troponin, qualitative
	(For troponin, quantitative assay, use 84484)
84520	Urea nitrogen; quantitative
84525	semiquantitative (eg, reagent strip test)
84540	Urea nitrogen, urine
84545	Urea nitrogen, clearance
84550	Uric acid; blood
84560	other source
84577	Urobilinogen, feces, quantitative
84578	Urobilinogen, urine; qualitative
84580	quantitative, timed specimen
84583	semiquantitative
	(Uroporphyrins, use 84120)
	(Valproic acid (dipropylacetic acid), use 80164)
84585	Vanillylmandelic acid (VMA), urine
84586	Vasoactive intestinal peptide (VIP)
84588	Vasopressin (antidiuretic hormone, ADH)

84590	Vitamin A
	(Vitamin B-1, use 84425)
	(Vitamin B-2, use 84252)
	(Vitamin B-6, use 84207)
	(Vitamin B-12, use 82607)
	(Vitamin B-12, absorption (Schilling), see 78270, 78271)
	(Vitamin C, use 82180)
	(Vitamin D, see 82306, 82307, 82652)
	(Vitamin E, use 84446)
84591	Vitamin, not otherwise specified
84597	Vitamin K
	(VMA, use 84585)
84600	Volatiles (eg, acetic anhydride, carbon tetrachloride, dichloroethane, dichloromethane, diethylether, isopropyl alcohol, methanol)
	(For acetaldehyde, use 82000)
	(Volume, blood, RISA or Cr-51, see 78110, 78111)
84620	Xylose absorption test, blood and/or urine
	(For administration, use 99070)
84630	Zinc
84681	C-peptide
84702	Gonadotropin, chorionic (hCG); quantitative
84703	qualitative
	(For urine pregnancy test by visual color comparison, use 81025)
84830	Ovulation tests, by visual color comparison methods for human luteinizing hormone
84999	Unlisted chemistry procedure

Hematology and Coagulation

(For blood banking procedures, see **Transfusion Medicine**)

(Agglutinins, see **Immunology**)

(Antiplasmin, use 85410)

(Antithrombin III, see 85300, 85301)

85002	Bleeding time
85004	Blood count; automated differential WBC count
85007	blood smear, microscopic examination with manual differential WBC count
85008	blood smear, microscopic examination without manual differential WBC count

(For other fluids (eg, CSF), see 89050, 89051)

85009	manual differential WBC count, buffy coat

(Eosinophils, nasal smear, use 89190)

85013	spun microhematocrit
85014	hematocrit (Hct)
85018	hemoglobin (Hgb)

(For other hemoglobin determination, see 83020-83069)

(For immunoassay, hemoglobin, fecal, use 82274)

(85021 has been deleted)

(85022 has been deleted)

(85023 has been deleted. To report, use 85007 and 85027)

(85024 has been deleted. To report, use 85025)

85025	complete (CBC), automated (Hgb, Hct, RBC, WBC and platelet count) and automated differential WBC count
85027	complete (CBC), automated (Hgb, Hct, RBC, WBC and platelet count)

(85031 has been deleted. To report, use 85014, 85018 and 85032)

85032	manual cell count (erythrocyte, leukocyte, or platelet) each
85041	red blood cell (RBC), automated

(Do not report code 85041 in conjunction with 85025 or 85027)

85044	reticulocyte, manual
85045	reticulocyte, automated
▲ 85046	reticulocytes, automated, including one or more cellular parameters (eg, reticulocyte hemoglobin content (CHr), immature reticulocyte fraction (IRF), reticulocyte volume (MRV), RNA content), direct measurement
85048	leukocyte (WBC), automated
85049	platelet, automated
85055	Reticulated platelet assay
85060	Blood smear, peripheral, interpretation by physician with written report
85097	Bone marrow, smear interpretation

(For special stains, see 85540, 88312, 88313)

(For bone biopsy, see 20220, 20225, 20240, 20245, 20250, 20251)

85130	Chromogenic substrate assay

(Circulating anti-coagulant screen (mixing studies), see 85611, 85732)

85170	Clot retraction
85175	Clot lysis time, whole blood dilution

(Clotting factor I (fibrinogen), see 85384, 85385)

85210	Clotting; factor II, prothrombin, specific

(See also 85610-85613)

85220	factor V (AcG or proaccelerin), labile factor
85230	factor VII (proconvertin, stable factor)
85240	factor VIII (AHG), one stage
85244	factor VIII related antigen
85245	factor VIII, VW factor, ristocetin cofactor
85246	factor VIII, VW factor antigen
85247	factor VIII, von Willebrand factor, multimetric analysis
85250	factor IX (PTC or Christmas)
85260	factor X (Stuart-Prower)
85270	factor XI (PTA)
85280	factor XII (Hageman)
85290	factor XIII (fibrin stabilizing)
85291	factor XIII (fibrin stabilizing), screen solubility
85292	prekallikrein assay (Fletcher factor assay)
85293	high molecular weight kininogen assay (Fitzgerald factor assay)
85300	Clotting inhibitors or anticoagulants; antithrombin III, activity
85301	antithrombin III, antigen assay
85302	protein C, antigen
85303	protein C, activity
85305	protein S, total
85306	protein S, free
85307	Activated Protein C (APC) resistance assay
85335	Factor inhibitor test
85337	Thrombomodulin

(For mixing studies for inhibitors, use 85732)

85345	Coagulation time; Lee and White
85347	activated
85348	other methods

(Differential count, see 85007 et seq)

(Duke bleeding time, use 85002)

(Eosinophils, nasal smear, use 89190)

85360	Euglobulin lysis

(Fetal hemoglobin, see 83030, 83033, 85460)

85362	Fibrin(ogen) degradation (split) products (FDP)(FSP); agglutination slide, semiquantitative

(Immunoelectrophoresis, use 86320)

85366	paracoagulation
85370	quantitative

Pathology and Laboratory

85378   Fibrin degradation products, D-dimer; qualitative or semiquantitative

85379   quantitative

(For ultrasensitive and standard sensitivity quantitative D-dimer, use 85379)

85380   ultrasensitive (eg, for evaluation for venous thromboembolism), qualitative or semiquantitative

85384   Fibrinogen; activity

85385   antigen

85390   Fibrinolysins or coagulopathy screen, interpretation and report

85396   Coagulation/fibrinolysis assay, whole blood (eg, viscoelastic clot assessment), including use of any pharmacologic additive(s), as indicated, including interpretation and written report, per day

85400   Fibrinolytic factors and inhibitors; plasmin

85410   alpha-2 antiplasmin

85415   plasminogen activator

85420   plasminogen, except antigenic assay

85421   plasminogen, antigenic assay

(Fragility, red blood cell, see 85547, 85555-85557)

85441   Heinz bodies; direct

85445   induced, acetyl phenylhydrazine

(Hematocrit (PCV), see 85014, 85025, 85027)

(Hemoglobin, see 83020-83068, 85018, 85025, 85027)

85460   Hemoglobin or RBCs, fetal, for fetomaternal hemorrhage; differential lysis (Kleihauer-Betke)

(See also 83030, 83033)

(Hemolysins, see 86940, 86941)

85461   rosette

85475   Hemolysin, acid

(See also 86940, 86941)

85520   Heparin assay

85525   Heparin neutralization

85530   Heparin-protamine tolerance test

85536   Iron stain, peripheral blood

(For iron stains on bone marrow or other tissues with physician evaluation, use 88313)

85540   Leukocyte alkaline phosphatase with count

85547   Mechanical fragility, RBC

85549   Muramidase

(Nitroblue tetrazolium dye test, use 86384)

85555   Osmotic fragility, RBC; unincubated

85557   incubated

(Packed cell volume, use 85013)

(Partial thromboplastin time, see 85730, 85732)

(Parasites, blood (eg, malaria smears), use 87207)

(Plasmin, use 85400)

(Plasminogen, use 85420)

(Plasminogen activator, use 85415)

85576   Platelet, aggregation (in vitro), each agent

(85585 has been deleted. To report, use 85008)

(85590 has been deleted. To report, use 85032)

(85595 has been deleted. To report, use 85049)

85597   Platelet neutralization

85610   Prothrombin time;

85611   substitution, plasma fractions, each

85612   Russell viper venom time (includes venom); undiluted

85613   diluted

(Red blood cell count, see 85025, 85027, 85041)

85635   Reptilase test

(Reticulocyte count, see 85044, 85045)

85651   Sedimentation rate, erythrocyte; non-automated

85652   automated

85660   Sickling of RBC, reduction

(Hemoglobin electrophoresis, use 83020)

(Smears (eg, for parasites, malaria), use 87207)

85670   Thrombin time; plasma

85675   titer

85705   Thromboplastin inhibition, tissue

(For individual clotting factors, see 85245-85247)

85730   Thromboplastin time, partial (PTT); plasma or whole blood

85732   substitution, plasma fractions, each

85810   Viscosity

(von Willebrand factor assay, see 85245-85247)

(WBC count, see 85025, 85027, 85048, 89050)

85999   Unlisted hematology and coagulation procedure

Immunology

(Acetylcholine receptor antibody, see 86255, 86256)

(Actinomyces, antibodies to, use 86602)

(Adrenal cortex antibodies, see 86255, 86256)

(For tuberculosis test, cell mediated immunity measurement of gamma interferon antigen response, use Category III code 0010T)

Pathology and Laboratory

Pathology and Laboratory

86000 Agglutinins, febrile (eg, Brucella, Francisella, Murine typhus, Q fever, Rocky Mountain spotted fever, scrub typhus), each antigen

(For antibodies to infectious agents, see 86602-86804)

86001 Allergen specific IgG quantitative or semiquantitative, each allergen

(Agglutinins and autohemolysins, see 86940, 86941)

86003 Allergen specific IgE; quantitative or semiquantitative, each allergen

(For total quantitative IgE, use 82785)

86005 qualitative, multiallergen screen (dipstick, paddle or disk)

(For total qualitative IgE, use 83518)

(Alpha-1 antitrypsin, see 82103, 82104)

(Alpha-1 feto-protein, see 82105, 82106)

(Anti-AChR (acetylcholine receptor) antibody titer, see 86255, 86256)

(Anticardiolipin antibody, use 86147)

(Anti-DNA, use 86225)

(Anti-deoxyribonuclease titer, use 86215)

86021 Antibody identification; leukocyte antibodies

86022 platelet antibodies

86023 platelet associated immunoglobulin assay

86038 Antinuclear antibodies (ANA);

86039 titer

(Antistreptococcal antibody, ie, anti-DNAse, use 86215)

(Antistreptokinase titer, use 86590)

86060 Antistreptolysin O; titer

(For antibodies to infectious agents, see 86602-86804)

86063 screen

(For antibodies to infectious agents, see 86602-86804)

(Blastomyces, antibodies to, use 86612)

● **86064** B cells, total count

►(For flow cytometric immunophenotyping for the assessment of potential hematolymphoid neoplasia, see 88182, 88184-88189)◄

86077 Blood bank physician services; difficult cross match and/or evaluation of irregular antibody(s), interpretation and written report

86078 investigation of transfusion reaction including suspicion of transmissible disease, interpretation and written report

86079 authorization for deviation from standard blood banking procedures (eg, use of outdated blood, transfusion of Rh incompatible units), with written report

(Brucella, antibodies to, use 86622)

(Candida, antibodies to, use 86628. For skin testing, use 86485)

86140 C-reactive protein;

(Candidiasis, use 86628)

86141 high sensitivity (hsCRP)

86146 Beta 2 Glycoprotein I antibody, each

86147 Cardiolipin (phospholipid) antibody, each Ig class

86148 Anti-phosphatidylserine (phospholipid) antibody

(To report antiprothrombin (phospholipid cofactor) antibody, use Category III code 0030T)

86155 Chemotaxis assay, specify method

(Clostridium difficile toxin, use 87230)

(Coccidioides, antibodies to, see 86635. For skin testing, use 86490)

86156 Cold agglutinin; screen

86157 titer

86160 Complement; antigen, each component

86161 functional activity, each component

86162 total hemolytic (CH50)

86171 Complement fixation tests, each antigen

(Coombs test, see 86880-86886)

86185 Counterimmunoelectrophoresis, each antigen

(Cryptococcus, antibodies to, use 86641)

86215 Deoxyribonuclease, antibody

86225 Deoxyribonucleic acid (DNA) antibody; native or double stranded

(Echinococcus, antibodies to, see code for specific method)

(For HIV antibody tests, see 86701-86703)

86226 single stranded

(Anti D.S., DNA, IFA, eg, using C.Lucilae, see 86255 and 86256)

86235 Extractable nuclear antigen, antibody to, any method (eg, nRNP, SS-A, SS-B, Sm, RNP, Sc170, J01), each antibody

86243 Fc receptor

(Filaria, antibodies to, see code for specific method)

86255 Fluorescent noninfectious agent antibody; screen, each antibody

86256 titer, each antibody

(Fluorescent technique for antigen identification in tissue, use 88346; for indirect fluorescence, use 88347)

(FTA, see 86781)

(Gel (agar) diffusion tests, use 86331)

86277	Growth hormone, human (HGH), antibody
86280	Hemagglutination inhibition test (HAI)
	(For rubella, use 86762)
	(For antibodies to infectious agents, see 86602-86804)
86294	Immunoassay for tumor antigen, qualitative or semiquantitative (eg, bladder tumor antigen)
86300	Immunoassay for tumor antigen, quantitative; CA 15-3 (27.29)
86301	CA 19-9
86304	CA 125
	(For measurement of serum HER-2/neu oncoprotein, see 83950)
	(For hepatitis delta agent, antibody, use 86692)
86308	Heterophile antibodies; screening
	(For antibodies to infectious agents, see 86602-86804)
86309	titer
	(For antibodies to infectious agents, see 86602-86804)
86310	titers after absorption with beef cells and guinea pig kidney
	(Histoplasma, antibodies to, use 86698. For skin testing, use 86510)
	(For antibodies to infectious agents, see 86602-86804)
	(Human growth hormone antibody, use 86277)
86316	Immunoassay for tumor antigen, other antigen, quantitative (eg, CA 50, 72-4, 549), each
86317	Immunoassay for infectious agent antibody, quantitative, not otherwise specified
	(For immunoassay techniques for antigens, see 83516, 83518, 83519, 83520, 87301-87450, 87810-87899)
	(For particle agglutination procedures, use 86403)
86318	Immunoassay for infectious agent antibody, qualitative or semiquantitative, single step method (eg, reagent strip)
86320	Immunoelectrophoresis; serum
86325	other fluids (eg, urine, cerebrospinal fluid) with concentration
86327	crossed (2-dimensional assay)
86329	Immunodiffusion; not elsewhere specified
86331	gel diffusion, qualitative (Ouchterlony), each antigen or antibody
86332	Immune complex assay
▲ 86334	Immunofixation electrophoresis; serum
● 86335	other fluids with concentration (eg, urine, CSF)
86336	Inhibin A
86337	Insulin antibodies

86340	Intrinsic factor antibodies
	(Leptospira, antibodies to, use 86720)
	(Leukoagglutinins, use 86021)
86341	Islet cell antibody
86343	Leukocyte histamine release test (LHR)
86344	Leukocyte phagocytosis
86353	Lymphocyte transformation, mitogen (phytomitogen) or antigen induced blastogenesis
	(Lymphocytes immunophenotyping, ►see 88182, 88189◄ for cytometry; see 88342, 88346 for microscopic techniques)
	(Malaria antibodies, use 86750)
86359	T cells; total count
86360	absolute CD4 and CD8 count, including ratio
86361	absolute CD4 count
86376	Microsomal antibodies (eg, thyroid or liver-kidney), each
86378	Migration inhibitory factor test (MIF)
	(Mitochondrial antibody, liver, see 86255, 86256)
	(Mononucleosis, see 86308-86310)
● 86379	Natural killer (NK) cells, total count
	►(For flow cytometric immunophenotyping for the assessment of potential hematolymphoid neoplasia, see 88182, 88184-88189)◄
86382	Neutralization test, viral
86384	Nitroblue tetrazolium dye test (NTD)
	(Ouchterlony diffusion, use 86331)
	(Platelet antibodies, see 86022, 86023)
86403	Particle agglutination; screen, each antibody
86406	titer, each antibody
	(Pregnancy test, see 84702, 84703)
	(Rapid plasma reagin test (RPR), see 86592, 86593)
86430	Rheumatoid factor; qualitative
86431	quantitative
	(Serologic test for syphilis, see 86592, 86593)
86485	Skin test; candida
	(For antibody, candida, use 86628)
86490	coccidioidomycosis
86510	histoplasmosis
	(For histoplasma, antibody, use 86698)
86580	tuberculosis, intradermal
86585	tuberculosis, tine test
	(For tuberculosis test, cell mediated immunity measurement of gamma interferon antigen response, use Category III code 0010T)

Pathology and Laboratory

(For skin tests for allergy, see 95010-95199)

(Smooth muscle antibody, see 86255, 86256)

(Sporothrix, antibodies to, see code for specific method)

86586 Unlisted antigen, each

● **86587** Stem cells (ie, CD34), total count

▶(For flow cytometric immunophenotyping for the assessment of potential hematolymphoid neoplasia, see 88182, 88189)◀

86590 Streptokinase, antibody

(For antibodies to infectious agents, see 86602-86804)

(Streptolysin O antibody, see antistreptolysin O, 86060, 86063)

86592 Syphilis test; qualitative (eg, VDRL, RPR, ART)

(For antibodies to infectious agents, see 86602-86804)

86593 quantitative

(For antibodies to infectious agents, see 86602-86804)

(Tetanus antibody, use 86774)

(Thyroglobulin antibody, use 86800)

(Thyroglobulin, use 84432)

(Thyroid microsomal antibody, use 86376)

(For toxoplasma antibody, see 86777-86778)

The following codes (86602-86804) are qualitative or semiquantitative immunoassays performed by multiple step methods for the detection of antibodies to infectious agents. For immunoassays by single step method (eg, reagent strips), use code 86318. Procedures for the identification of antibodies should be coded as precisely as possible. For example, an antibody to a virus could be coded with increasing specificity for virus, family, genus, species, or type. In some cases, further precision may be added to codes by specifying the class of immunoglobulin being detected. When multiple tests are done to detect antibodies to organisms classified more precisely than the specificity allowed by available codes, it is appropriate to code each as a separate service. For example, a test for antibody to an enterovirus is coded as 86658. Coxsackie viruses are enteroviruses, but there are no codes for the individual species of enterovirus. If assays are performed for antibodies to coxsackie A and B species, each assay should be separately coded. Similarly, if multiple assays are performed for antibodies of different immunoglobulin classes, each assay should be coded separately.

(For the detection of antibodies other than those to infectious agents, see specific antibody (eg, 86021, 86022, 86023, 86376, 86800, 86850-86870) or specific method (eg, 83516, 86255, 86256)).

(For infectious agent/antigen detection, see 87260-87899)

86602 Antibody; actinomyces

86603 adenovirus

86606 Aspergillus

86609 bacterium, not elsewhere specified

86611 Bartonella

86612 Blastomyces

86615 Bordetella

86617 Borrelia burgdorferi (Lyme disease) confirmatory test (eg, Western Blot or immunoblot)

86618 Borrelia burgdorferi (Lyme disease)

86619 Borrelia (relapsing fever)

86622 Brucella

86625 Campylobacter

86628 Candida

(For skin test, candida, use 86485)

86631 Chlamydia

86632 Chlamydia, IgM

(For chlamydia antigen, see 87270, 87320. For fluorescent antibody technique, see 86255, 86256)

86635 Coccidioides

86638 Coxiella burnetii (Q fever)

86641 Cryptococcus

86644 cytomegalovirus (CMV)

86645 cytomegalovirus (CMV), IgM

86648 Diphtheria

86651 encephalitis, California (La Crosse)

86652 encephalitis, Eastern equine

86653 encephalitis, St. Louis

86654 encephalitis, Western equine

86658 enterovirus (eg, coxsackie, echo, polio)

(Trichinella, antibodies to, use 86784)

(Trypanosoma, antibodies to, see code for specific method)

(Tuberculosis, use 86580 for skin testing)

(Viral antibodies, see code for specific method)

86663 Epstein-Barr (EB) virus, early antigen (EA)

86664 Epstein-Barr (EB) virus, nuclear antigen (EBNA)

86665 Epstein-Barr (EB) virus, viral capsid (VCA)

86666 Ehrlichia

86668 Francisella tularensis

86671 fungus, not elsewhere specified

86674 Giardia lamblia

86677 Helicobacter pylori

86682	helminth, not elsewhere specified
86684	Haemophilus influenza
86687	HTLV-I
86688	HTLV-II
86689	HTLV or HIV antibody, confirmatory test (eg, Western Blot)
86692	hepatitis, delta agent
	(For hepatitis delta agent, antigen, use 87380)
86694	herpes simplex, non-specific type test
86695	herpes simplex, type 1
86696	herpes simplex, type 2
86698	histoplasma
86701	HIV-1
86702	HIV-2
86703	HIV-1 and HIV-2, single assay
	(For HIV-1 antigen, use 87390)
	(For HIV-2 antigen, use 87391)
	(For confirmatory test for HIV antibody (eg, Western Blot), use 86689)
86704	Hepatitis B core antibody (HBcAb); total
86705	IgM antibody
86706	Hepatitis B surface antibody (HBsAb)
86707	Hepatitis Be antibody (HBeAb)
86708	Hepatitis A antibody (HAAb); total
86709	IgM antibody
86710	Antibody; influenza virus
86713	Legionella
86717	Leishmania
86720	Leptospira
86723	Listeria monocytogenes
86727	lymphocytic choriomeningitis
86729	lymphogranuloma venereum
86732	mucormycosis
86735	mumps
86738	mycoplasma
86741	Neisseria meningitidis
86744	Nocardia
86747	parvovirus
86750	Plasmodium (malaria)
86753	protozoa, not elsewhere specified
86756	respiratory syncytial virus
86757	Rickettsia

86759	rotavirus
86762	rubella
86765	rubeola
86768	Salmonella
86771	Shigella
86774	tetanus
86777	Toxoplasma
86778	Toxoplasma, IgM
86781	Treponema pallidum, confirmatory test (eg, FTA-abs)
86784	Trichinella
86787	varicella-zoster
86790	virus, not elsewhere specified
86793	Yersinia
86800	Thyroglobulin antibody
	(For thyroglobulin, use 84432)
86803	Hepatitis C antibody;
86804	confirmatory test (eg, immunoblot)

Tissue Typing

	(For pretransplant cross-match, see appropriate code or codes)
86805	Lymphocytotoxicity assay, visual crossmatch; with titration
86806	without titration
86807	Serum screening for cytotoxic percent reactive antibody (PRA); standard method
86808	quick method
86812	HLA typing; A, B, or C (eg, A10, B7, B27), single antigen
86813	A, B, or C, multiple antigens
86816	DR/DQ, single antigen
86817	DR/DQ, multiple antigens
86821	lymphocyte culture, mixed (MLC)
86822	lymphocyte culture, primed (PLC)
86849	Unlisted immunology procedure

Transfusion Medicine

	(For apheresis, use 36511, 36512)
	(For therapeutic phlebotomy, use 99195)
86850	Antibody screen, RBC, each serum technique
86860	Antibody elution (RBC), each elution
86870	Antibody identification, RBC antibodies, each panel for each serum technique

86880 Antihuman globulin test (Coombs test); direct, each antiserum

86885   indirect, qualitative, each antiserum

86886   indirect, titer, each antiserum

86890 Autologous blood or component, collection processing and storage; predeposited

86891   intra- or postoperative salvage

(For physician services to autologous donors, see 99201-99204)

86900 Blood typing; ABO

86901   Rh (D)

86903   antigen screening for compatible blood unit using reagent serum, per unit screened

86904   antigen screening for compatible unit using patient serum, per unit screened

86905   RBC antigens, other than ABO or Rh (D), each

86906   Rh phenotyping, complete

86910 Blood typing, for paternity testing, per individual; ABO, Rh and MN

86911   each additional antigen system

(86915 has been deleted. To report, see 38210-38213)

86920 Compatibility test each unit; immediate spin technique

86921   incubation technique

86922   antiglobulin technique

86927 Fresh frozen plasma, thawing, each unit

86930 Frozen blood, each unit; freezing (includes preparation)

86931   thawing

86932   freezing (includes preparation) and thawing

86940 Hemolysins and agglutinins; auto, screen, each

86941   incubated

86945 Irradiation of blood product, each unit

86950 Leukocyte transfusion

(For leukapheresis, use 36511)

86965 Pooling of platelets or other blood products

86970 Pretreatment of RBCs for use in RBC antibody detection, identification, and/or compatibility testing; incubation with chemical agents or drugs, each

86971   incubation with enzymes, each

86972   by density gradient separation

86975 Pretreatment of serum for use in RBC antibody identification; incubation with drugs, each

86976   by dilution

86977   incubation with inhibitors, each

86978   by differential red cell absorption using patient RBCs or RBCs of known phenotype, each absorption

86985 Splitting of blood or blood products, each unit

86999 Unlisted transfusion medicine procedure

Microbiology

Includes bacteriology, mycology, parasitology, and virology.

Presumptive identification of microorganisms is defined as identification by colony morphology, growth on selective media, Gram stains, or up to three tests (eg, catalase, oxidase, indole, urease). Definitive identification of microorganisms is defined as an identification to the genus or species level that requires additional tests (eg, biochemical panels, slide cultures). If additional studies involve molecular probes, chromatography, or immunologic techniques, these should be separately coded in addition to definitive identification codes (87140-87158). For multiple specimens/sites use modifier 59. For repeat laboratory tests performed on the same day, use modifier 91.

87001 Animal inoculation, small animal; with observation

87003   with observation and dissection

87015 Concentration (any type), for infectious agents

(Do not report 87015 in conjunction with 87177)

87040 Culture, bacterial; blood, aerobic, with isolation and presumptive identification of isolates (includes anaerobic culture, if appropriate)

87045   stool, aerobic, with isolation and preliminary examination (eg, KIA, LIA), Salmonella and Shigella species

▲ **87046**   stool, aerobic, additional pathogens, isolation and presumptive identification of isolates, each plate

87070   any other source except urine, blood or stool, aerobic, with isolation and presumptive identification of isolates

(For urine, use 87088)

87071   quantitative, aerobic with isolation and presumptive identification of isolates, any source except urine, blood or stool

(For urine, use 87088)

87073   quantitative, anaerobic with isolation and presumptive identification of isolates, any source except urine, blood or stool

(For definitive identification of isolates, use 87076 or 87077. For typing of isolates see 87140-87158)

87075   any source, except blood, anaerobic with isolation and presumptive identification of isolates

87076   anaerobic isolate, additional methods required for definitive identification, each isolate

(For gas liquid chromatography (GLC) or high pressure liquid chromatography (HPLC), use 87143)

87077   aerobic isolate, additional methods required for definitive identification, each isolate

(For gas liquid chromatography (GLC) or high pressure liquid chromatography (HPLC), use 87143)

87081   Culture, presumptive, pathogenic organisms, screening only;

87084   with colony estimation from density chart

87086   Culture, bacterial; quantitative colony count, urine

87088   with isolation and presumptive identification of isolates, urine

87101   Culture, fungi (mold or yeast) isolation, with presumptive identification of isolates; skin, hair, or nail

87102   other source (except blood)

87103   blood

87106   Culture, fungi, definitive identification, each organism; yeast

(Use 87106 in addition to codes 87101, 87102, or 87103 when appropriate)

87107   mold

87109   Culture, mycoplasma, any source

87110   Culture, chlamydia, any source

(For immunofluorescence staining of shell vials, use 87140)

87116   Culture, tubercle or other acid-fast bacilli (eg, TB, AFB, mycobacteria) any source, with isolation and presumptive identification of isolates

(For concentration, use 87015)

87118   Culture, mycobacterial, definitive identification, each isolate

(For nucleic acid probe identification, use 87149)

(For GLC or HPLC identification, use 87143)

87140   Culture, typing; immunofluorescent method, each antiserum

87143   gas liquid chromatography (GLC) or high pressure liquid chromatography (HPLC) method

87147   immunologic method, other than immunofluoresence (eg, agglutination grouping), per antiserum

87149   identification by nucleic acid probe

87152   identification by pulse field gel typing

87158   other methods

87164   Dark field examination, any source (eg, penile, vaginal, oral, skin); includes specimen collection

87166   without collection

87168   Macroscopic examination; arthropod

87169   parasite

87172   Pinworm exam (eg, cellophane tape prep)

87176   Homogenization, tissue, for culture

87177   Ova and parasites, direct smears, concentration and identification

(Do not report 87177 in conjunction with 87015)

(For direct smears from a primary source, use 87207)

(For coccidia or microsporidia exam, use 87207)

(For trichrome, iron hemotoxylin and other special stains, use 88313)

(For nucleic acid probes in cytologic material, use 88365)

(For molecular diagnostics, see 83890-83898, 87470-87799)

87181   Susceptibility studies, antimicrobial agent; agar dilution method, per agent (eg, antibiotic gradient strip)

87184   disk method, per plate (12 or fewer agents)

87185   enzyme detection (eg, beta lactamase), per enzyme

87186   microdilution or agar dilution (minimum inhibitory concentration (MIC) or breakpoint), each multi-antimicrobial, per plate

+ 87187   microdilution or agar dilution, minimum lethal concentration (MLC), each plate (List separately in addition to code for primary procedure)

(Use 87187 in conjunction with 87186 or 87188)

87188   macrobroth dilution method, each agent

87190   mycobacteria, proportion method, each agent

(For other mycobacterial susceptibility studies, see 87181, 87184, 87186, or 87188)

87197   Serum bactericidal titer (Schlicter test)

87205   Smear, primary source with interpretation; Gram or Giemsa stain for bacteria, fungi, or cell types

87206   fluorescent and/or acid fast stain for bacteria, fungi, parasites, viruses or cell types

87207   special stain for inclusion bodies or parasites (eg, malaria, coccidia, microsporidia, trypanosomes, herpes viruses)

(For direct smears with concentration and identification, use 87177)

(For thick smear preparation, use 87015)

(For complex special stains, see 88312, 88313)

(For fat, meat, fibers, nasal eosinophils, and starch, see miscellaneous section)

87210   wet mount for infectious agents (eg, saline, India ink, KOH preps)

(For KOH examination of skin, hair or nails, see 87220)

Pathology and Laboratory

87220   Tissue examination by KOH slide of samples from skin, hair, or nails for fungi or ectoparasite ova or mites (eg, scabies)

87230   Toxin or antitoxin assay, tissue culture (eg, Clostridium difficile toxin)

87250   Virus isolation; inoculation of embryonated eggs, or small animal, includes observation and dissection

87252   tissue culture inoculation, observation, and presumptive identification by cytopathic effect

87253   tissue culture, additional studies or definitive identification (eg, hemabsorption, neutralization, immunofluoresence stain), each isolate

(Electron microscopy, use 88348)

(Inclusion bodies in tissue sections, see 88304-88309; in smears, see 87207-87210; in fluids, use 88106)

87254   centrifuge enhanced (shell vial) technique, includes identification with immunofluorescence stain, each virus

(Report 87254 in addition to 87252 as appropriate)

87255   including identification by non-immunologic method, other than by cytopathic effect (eg, virus specific enzymatic activity)

These codes are intended for primary source only. For similar studies on culture material, refer to codes 87140-87158. Infectious agents by antigen detection, immunofluorescence microscopy, or nucleic acid probe techniques should be reported as precisely as possible. The most specific code possible should be reported. If there is no specific agent code, the general methodology code (eg, 87299, 87449, 87450, 87797, 87798, 87799, 87899) should be used. For identification of antibodies to many of the listed infectious agents, see 86602-86804. When separate assays are performed for different species or strain(s) of organisms, each assay should be reported separately.

87260   Infectious agent antigen detection by immunofluorescent technique; adenovirus

87265   Bordetella pertussis/parapertussis

87267   Enterovirus, direct fluorescent antibody (DFA)

87269   giardia

87270   Chlamydia trachomatis

87271   Cytomegalovirus, direct fluorescent antibody (DFA)

87272   cryptosporidium

87273   Herpes simplex virus type 2

87274   Herpes simplex virus type 1

87275   influenza B virus

87276   influenza A virus

87277   Legionella micdadei

87278   Legionella pneumophila

87279   Parainfluenza virus, each type

87280   respiratory syncytial virus

87281   Pneumocystis carinii

87283   Rubeola

87285   Treponema pallidum

87290   Varicella zoster virus

87299   not otherwise specified, each organism

87300   Infectious agent antigen detection by immunofluorescent technique, polyvalent for multiple organisms, each polyvalent antiserum

(For physician evaluation of infectious disease agents by immunofluorescence, use 88346)

87301   Infectious agent antigen detection by enzyme immunoassay technique, qualitative or semiquantitative, multiple step method; adenovirus enteric types 40/41

87320   Chlamydia trachomatis

87324   Clostridium difficile toxin(s)

87327   Cryptococcus neoformans

(For Cryptococcus latex agglutination, use 86403)

87328   cryptosporidium

87329   giardia

87332   cytomegalovirus

87335   Escherichia coli 0157

(For giardia antigen, use ►87329◄)

87336   Entamoeba histolytica dispar group

87337   Entamoeba histolytica group

87338   Helicobacter pylori, stool

87339   Helicobacter pylori

(For H. pylori, stool, use 87338. For H. pylori, breath and blood by mass spectrometry, see 83013, 83014. For H. pylori, liquid scintillation counter, see 78267, 78268)

87340   hepatitis B surface antigen (HBsAg)

87341   hepatitis B surface antigen (HBsAg) neutralization

87350   hepatitis Be antigen (HBeAg)

87380   hepatitis, delta agent

87385   Histoplasma capsulatum

87390   HIV-1

87391   HIV-2

87400   Influenza, A or B, each

87420   respiratory syncytial virus

87425   rotavirus

87427   Shiga-like toxin

87430   Streptococcus, group A

87449	Infectious agent antigen detection by enzyme immunoassay technique qualitative or semiquantitative; multiple step method, not otherwise specified, each organism
87450	single step method, not otherwise specified, each organism
87451	multiple step method, polyvalent for multiple organisms, each polyvalent antiserum
87470	Infectious agent detection by nucleic acid (DNA or RNA); Bartonella henselae and Bartonella quintana, direct probe technique
87471	Bartonella henselae and Bartonella quintana, amplified probe technique
87472	Bartonella henselae and Bartonella quintana, quantification
87475	Borrelia burgdorferi, direct probe technique
87476	Borrelia burgdorferi, amplified probe technique
87477	Borrelia burgdorferi, quantification
87480	Candida species, direct probe technique
87481	Candida species, amplified probe technique
87482	Candida species, quantification
87485	Chlamydia pneumoniae, direct probe technique
87486	Chlamydia pneumoniae, amplified probe technique
87487	Chlamydia pneumoniae, quantification
87490	Chlamydia trachomatis, direct probe technique
87491	Chlamydia trachomatis, amplified probe technique
87492	Chlamydia trachomatis, quantification
87495	cytomegalovirus, direct probe technique
87496	cytomegalovirus, amplified probe technique
87497	cytomegalovirus, quantification
87510	Gardnerella vaginalis, direct probe technique
87511	Gardnerella vaginalis, amplified probe technique
87512	Gardnerella vaginalis, quantification
87515	hepatitis B virus, direct probe technique
87516	hepatitis B virus, amplified probe technique
87517	hepatitis B virus, quantification
87520	hepatitis C, direct probe technique
87521	hepatitis C, amplified probe technique
87522	hepatitis C, quantification
87525	hepatitis G, direct probe technique
87526	hepatitis G, amplified probe technique
87527	hepatitis G, quantification
87528	Herpes simplex virus, direct probe technique
87529	Herpes simplex virus, amplified probe technique

87530	Herpes simplex virus, quantification
87531	Herpes virus-6, direct probe technique
87532	Herpes virus-6, amplified probe technique
87533	Herpes virus-6, quantification
87534	HIV-1, direct probe technique
87535	HIV-1, amplified probe technique
87536	HIV-1, quantification
87537	HIV-2, direct probe technique
87538	HIV-2, amplified probe technique
87539	HIV-2, quantification
87540	Legionella pneumophila, direct probe technique
87541	Legionella pneumophila, amplified probe technique
87542	Legionella pneumophila, quantification
87550	Mycobacteria species, direct probe technique
87551	Mycobacteria species, amplified probe technique
87552	Mycobacteria species, quantification
87555	Mycobacteria tuberculosis, direct probe technique
87556	Mycobacteria tuberculosis, amplified probe technique
87557	Mycobacteria tuberculosis, quantification
87560	Mycobacteria avium-intracellulare, direct probe technique
87561	Mycobacteria avium-intracellulare, amplified probe technique
87562	Mycobacteria avium-intracellulare, quantification
87580	Mycoplasma pneumoniae, direct probe technique
87581	Mycoplasma pneumoniae, amplified probe technique
87582	Mycoplasma pneumoniae, quantification
87590	Neisseria gonorrhoeae, direct probe technique
87591	Neisseria gonorrhoeae, amplified probe technique
87592	Neisseria gonorrhoeae, quantification
87620	papillomavirus, human, direct probe technique
87621	papillomavirus, human, amplified probe technique
87622	papillomavirus, human, quantification
87650	Streptococcus, group A, direct probe technique
87651	Streptococcus, group A, amplified probe technique
87652	Streptococcus, group A, quantification
87660	Trichomonas vaginalis, direct probe technique
87797	Infectious agent detection by nucleic acid (DNA or RNA), not otherwise specified; direct probe technique, each organism
87798	amplified probe technique, each organism
87799	quantification, each organism

Pathology and Laboratory

87800 Infectious agent detection by nucleic acid (DNA or RNA), multiple organisms; direct probe(s) technique

87801   amplified probe(s) technique

87802 Infectious agent antigen detection by immunoassay with direct optical observation; Streptococcus, group B

87803   Clostridium difficile toxin A

87804   Influenza

● **87807**   respiratory syncytial virus

87810 Infectious agent detection by immunoassay with direct optical observation; Chlamydia trachomatis

87850   Neisseria gonorrhoeae

87880   Streptococcus, group A

87899   not otherwise specified

87901 Infectious agent genotype analysis by nucleic acid (DNA or RNA); HIV 1, reverse transcriptase and protease

(For infectious agent drug susceptibility phenotype prediction for HIV-1, use Category III code 0023T)

87902   Hepatitis C virus

87903 Infectious agent phenotype analysis by nucleic acid (DNA or RNA) with drug resistance tissue culture analysis, HIV 1; first through 10 drugs tested

+ **87904**   each additional 1 through 5 drugs tested (List separately in addition to code for primary procedure)

(Use 87904 in conjunction with 87903)

87999 Unlisted microbiology procedure

Anatomic Pathology

Postmortem Examination

Procedures 88000 through 88099 represent physician services only. Use modifier 90 for outside laboratory services.

88000 Necropsy (autopsy), gross examination only; without CNS

88005   with brain

88007   with brain and spinal cord

88012   infant with brain

88014   stillborn or newborn with brain

88016   macerated stillborn

88020 Necropsy (autopsy), gross and microscopic; without CNS

88025   with brain

88027   with brain and spinal cord

88028   infant with brain

88029   stillborn or newborn with brain

88036 Necropsy (autopsy), limited, gross and/or microscopic; regional

88037   single organ

88040 Necropsy (autopsy); forensic examination

88045   coroner's call

88099 Unlisted necropsy (autopsy) procedure

Cytopathology

(For cervicography, see Category III code 0003T)

(For collection of cytology specimens via mammary duct catheter lavage, report 0045T-0046T)

88104 Cytopathology, fluids, washings or brushings, except cervical or vaginal; smears with interpretation

88106   filter method only with interpretation

88107   smears and filter preparation with interpretation

88108 Cytopathology, concentration technique, smears and interpretation (eg, Saccomanno technique)

(For cervical or vaginal smears, see 88150-88155)

(For gastric intubation with lavage, see 89130-89141, 91055)

(For x-ray localization, use 74340)

88112 Cytopathology, selective cellular enhancement technique with interpretation (eg, liquid based slide preparation method), except cervical or vaginal

(Do not report 88112 with 88108)

88125 Cytopathology, forensic (eg, sperm)

88130 Sex chromatin identification; Barr bodies

88140   peripheral blood smear, polymorphonuclear drumsticks

(For Guard stain, use 88313)

Codes 88141-88155, 88164-88167, 88174-88175 are used to report cervical or vaginal screening by various methods and to report physician interpretation services. Use codes 88150-88154 to report Pap smears that are examined using non-Bethesda reporting. Use codes 88164-88167 to report Pap smears that are examined using the Bethesda System of reporting. Use codes 88142-88143 to report specimens collected in fluid medium with automated thin layer preparation that are examined using any system of reporting (Bethesda or non-Bethesda). Use codes 88174-88175 to report automated screening of specimens collected in fluid medium with automated thin layer preparation that are examined using any system of reporting (Bethesda or non-Bethesda). Within each of these three code families choose the one code that describes the screening method(s) used. Codes 88141 and 88155 should be reported in addition to the screening code chosen when the additional services are provided.

+ 88141   Cytopathology, cervical or vaginal (any reporting system), requiring interpretation by physician (List separately in addition to code for technical service)

(Use 88141 in conjunction with 88142-88154, 88164-88167, 88174-88175)

88142   Cytopathology, cervical or vaginal (any reporting system), collected in preservative fluid, automated thin layer preparation; manual screening under physician supervision

88143   with manual screening and rescreening under physician supervision

(88144 has been deleted)

(88145 has been deleted)

(For automated screening of automated thin layer preparation, see 88174, 88175)

88147   Cytopathology smears, cervical or vaginal; screening by automated system under physician supervision

88148   screening by automated system with manual rescreening under physician supervision

88150   Cytopathology, slides, cervical or vaginal; manual screening under physician supervision

88152   with manual screening and computer-assisted rescreening under physician supervision

88153   with manual screening and rescreening under physician supervision

88154   with manual screening and computer-assisted rescreening using cell selection and review under physician supervision

+ 88155   Cytopathology, slides, cervical or vaginal, definitive hormonal evaluation (eg, maturation index, karyopyknotic index, estrogenic index) (List separately in addition to code(s) for other technical and interpretation services)

(Use 88155 in conjunction with 88142-88154, 88164-88167, 88174-88175)

88160   Cytopathology, smears, any other source; screening and interpretation

88161   preparation, screening and interpretation

88162   extended study involving over 5 slides and/or multiple stains

(For obtaining specimen, see percutaneous needle biopsy under individual organ in **Surgery**)

(For aerosol collection of sputum, use 89220)

(For special stains, see 88312-88314)

88164   Cytopathology, slides, cervical or vaginal (the Bethesda System); manual screening under physician supervision

88165   with manual screening and rescreening under physician supervision

88166   with manual screening and computer-assisted rescreening under physician supervision

88167   with manual screening and computer-assisted rescreening using cell selection and review under physician supervision

(88170 has been deleted. To report, see 10021, 10022)

(88171 has been deleted. To report, see 10021, 10022)

88172   Cytopathology, evaluation of fine needle aspirate; immediate cytohistologic study to determine adequacy of specimen(s)

88173   interpretation and report

88174   Cytopathology, cervical or vaginal (any reporting system), collected in preservative fluid, automated thin layer preparation; screening by automated system, under physician supervision

88175   with screening by automated system and manual rescreening, under physician supervision

(For manual screening, see 88142, 88143)

▶(88180 has been deleted. To report, see 88182, 88189)◀

88182   Flow cytometry; cell cycle or DNA analysis

(For tumor morphometry and DNA and ploidy analysis by imaging techniques, use 88358)

● **88184**   Flow cytometry, cell surface, cytoplasmic, or nuclear marker, technical component only; first marker

+● **88185**   each additional marker (List separately in addition to code for first marker)

▶(Report 88185 in conjunction with 88184)◀

● **88187**   Flow cytometry, interpretation; 2 to 8 markers

● **88188**   9 to 15 markers

● **88189**   16 or more markers

88199   Unlisted cytopathology procedure

(For electron microscopy, see 88348, 88349)

Cytogenetic Studies

▶When molecular diagnostic procedures are performed to test for oncologic or inherited disorder, use the appropriate modifier to specify probe type or condition tested. (See **Appendix I**).◀

(For acetylcholinesterase, use 82013)

(For alpha-fetoprotein, serum or amniotic fluid, see 82105, 82106)

(For laser microdissection of cells from tissue sample, see 88380)

88230   Tissue culture for non-neoplastic disorders; lymphocyte

88233   skin or other solid tissue biopsy

88235   amniotic fluid or chorionic villus cells

Pathology and Laboratory

Pathology and Laboratory

88237 Tissue culture for neoplastic disorders; bone marrow, blood cells

88239   solid tumor

88240 Cryopreservation, freezing and storage of cells, each cell line

(For therapeutic cryopreservation and storage, use 38207)

88241 Thawing and expansion of frozen cells, each aliquot

(For therapeutic thawing of previous harvest, use 38208)

88245 Chromosome analysis for breakage syndromes; baseline Sister Chromatid Exchange (SCE), 20-25 cells

88248   baseline breakage, score 50-100 cells, count 20 cells, 2 karyotypes (eg, for ataxia telangiectasia, Fanconi anemia, fragile X)

88249   score 100 cells, clastogen stress (eg, diepoxybutane, mitomycin C, ionizing radiation, UV radiation)

88261 Chromosome analysis; count 5 cells, 1 karyotype, with banding

88262   count 15-20 cells, 2 karyotypes, with banding

88263   count 45 cells for mosaicism, 2 karyotypes, with banding

88264   analyze 20-25 cells

88267 Chromosome analysis, amniotic fluid or chorionic villus, count 15 cells, 1 karyotype, with banding

88269 Chromosome analysis, in situ for amniotic fluid cells, count cells from 6-12 colonies, 1 karyotype, with banding

88271 Molecular cytogenetics; DNA probe, each (eg, FISH)

88272   chromosomal in situ hybridization, analyze 3-5 cells (eg, for derivatives and markers)

88273   chromosomal in situ hybridization, analyze 10-30 cells (eg, for microdeletions)

88274   interphase in situ hybridization, analyze 25-99 cells

88275   interphase in situ hybridization, analyze 100-300 cells

88280 Chromosome analysis; additional karyotypes, each study

88283   additional specialized banding technique (eg, NOR, C-banding)

88285   additional cells counted, each study

88289   additional high resolution study

88291 Cytogenetics and molecular cytogenetics, interpretation and report

88299 Unlisted cytogenetic study

Surgical Pathology

Services 88300 through 88309 include accession, examination, and reporting. They do not include the services designated in codes 88311 through 88365 and 88399, which are coded in addition when provided.

The unit of service for codes 88300 through 88309 is the specimen.

A specimen is defined as tissue or tissues that is (are) submitted for individual and separate attention, requiring individual examination and pathologic diagnosis. Two or more such specimens from the same patient (eg, separately identified endoscopic biopsies, skin lesions, etc.) are each appropriately assigned an individual code reflective of its proper level of service.

Service code 88300 is used for any specimen that in the opinion of the examining pathologist can be accurately diagnosed without microscopic examination. Service code 88302 is used when gross and microscopic examination is performed on a specimen to confirm identification and the absence of disease. Service codes 88304 through 88309 describe all other specimens requiring gross and microscopic examination, and represent additional ascending levels of physician work. Levels 88302 through 88309 are specifically defined by the assigned specimens.

Any unlisted specimen should be assigned to the code which most closely reflects the physician work involved when compared to other specimens assigned to that code.

88300   **Level I** - Surgical pathology, gross examination only

88302   **Level II** - Surgical pathology, gross and microscopic examination

    Appendix, Incidental

    Fallopian Tube, Sterilization

    Fingers/Toes, Amputation, Traumatic

    Foreskin, Newborn

    Hernia Sac, Any Location

    Hydrocele Sac

    Nerve

    Skin, Plastic Repair

    Sympathetic Ganglion

    Testis, Castration

    Vaginal Mucosa, Incidental

    Vas Deferens, Sterilization

88304   **Level III** - Surgical pathology, gross and microscopic examination

    Abortion, Induced

    Abscess

    Aneurysm - Arterial/Ventricular

    Anus, Tag

    Appendix, Other than Incidental

    Artery, Atheromatous Plaque

    Bartholin's Gland Cyst

    Bone Fragment(s), Other than Pathologic Fracture

    Bursa/Synovial Cyst

Carpal Tunnel Tissue

Cartilage, Shavings

Cholesteatoma

Colon, Colostomy Stoma

Conjunctiva - Biopsy/Pterygium

Cornea

Diverticulum - Esophagus/Small Intestine

Dupuytren's Contracture Tissue

Femoral Head, Other than Fracture

Fissure/Fistula

Foreskin, Other than Newborn

Gallbladder

Ganglion Cyst

Hematoma

Hemorrhoids

Hydatid of Morgagni

Intervertebral Disc

Joint, Loose Body

Meniscus

Mucocele, Salivary

Neuroma - Morton's/Traumatic

Pilonidal Cyst/Sinus

Polyps, Inflammatory - Nasal/Sinusoidal

Skin - Cyst/Tag/Debridement

Soft Tissue, Debridement

Soft Tissue, Lipoma

Spermatocele

Tendon/Tendon Sheath

Testicular Appendage

Thrombus or Embolus

Tonsil and/or Adenoids

Varicocele

Vas Deferens, Other than Sterilization

Vein, Varicosity

88305   **Level IV** - Surgical pathology, gross and microscopic examination

Abortion - Spontaneous/Missed

Artery, Biopsy

Bone Marrow, Biopsy

Bone Exostosis

Brain/Meninges, Other than for Tumor Resection

Breast, Biopsy, Not Requiring Microscopic Evaluation of Surgical Margins

Breast, Reduction Mammoplasty

Bronchus, Biopsy

Cell Block, Any Source

Cervix, Biopsy

Colon, Biopsy

Duodenum, Biopsy

Endocervix, Curettings/Biopsy

Endometrium, Curettings/Biopsy

Esophagus, Biopsy

Extremity, Amputation, Traumatic

Fallopian Tube, Biopsy

Fallopian Tube, Ectopic Pregnancy

Femoral Head, Fracture

Fingers/Toes, Amputation, Non-traumatic

Gingiva/Oral Mucosa, Biopsy

Heart Valve

Joint, Resection

Kidney, Biopsy

Larynx, Biopsy

Leiomyoma(s), Uterine Myomectomy - without Uterus

Lip, Biopsy/Wedge Resection

Lung, Transbronchial Biopsy

Lymph Node, Biopsy

Muscle, Biopsy

Nasal Mucosa, Biopsy

Nasopharynx/Oropharynx, Biopsy

Nerve, Biopsy

Odontogenic/Dental Cyst

Omentum, Biopsy

Ovary with or without Tube, Non-neoplastic

Ovary, Biopsy/Wedge Resection

Parathyroid Gland

Peritoneum, Biopsy

Pituitary Tumor

Placenta, Other than Third Trimester

Pleura/Pericardium - Biopsy/Tissue

Polyp, Cervical/Endometrial

Polyp, Colorectal

Polyp, Stomach/Small Intestine

Prostate, Needle Biopsy

Prostate, TUR

Salivary Gland, Biopsy

Sinus, Paranasal Biopsy

Skin, Other than Cyst/Tag/Debridement/Plastic Repair

Small Intestine, Biopsy

Soft Tissue, Other than Tumor/Mass/Lipoma/Debridement

Spleen

Stomach, Biopsy

Synovium

Testis, Other than Tumor/Biopsy/Castration

Thyroglossal Duct/Brachial Cleft Cyst

Tongue, Biopsy

Tonsil, Biopsy

Trachea, Biopsy

Ureter, Biopsy

Urethra, Biopsy

Urinary Bladder, Biopsy

Uterus, with or without Tubes and Ovaries, for Prolapse

Vagina, Biopsy

Vulva/Labia, Biopsy

88307   **Level V** - Surgical pathology, gross and microscopic examination

Adrenal, Resection

Bone - Biopsy/Curettings

Bone Fragment(s), Pathologic Fracture

Brain, Biopsy

Brain/Meninges, Tumor Resection

Breast, Excision of Lesion, Requiring Microscopic Evaluation of Surgical Margins

Breast, Mastectomy - Partial/Simple

Cervix, Conization

Colon, Segmental Resection, Other than for Tumor

Extremity, Amputation, Non-traumatic

Eye, Enucleation

Kidney, Partial/Total Nephrectomy

Larynx, Partial/Total Resection

Liver, Biopsy - Needle/Wedge

Liver, Partial Resection

Lung, Wedge Biopsy

Lymph Nodes, Regional Resection

Mediastinum, Mass

Myocardium, Biopsy

Odontogenic Tumor

Ovary with or without Tube, Neoplastic

Pancreas, Biopsy

Placenta, Third Trimester

Prostate, Except Radical Resection

Salivary Gland

Sentinel Lymph Node

Small Intestine, Resection, Other than for Tumor

Soft Tissue Mass (except Lipoma) - Biopsy/Simple Excision

Stomach - Subtotal/Total Resection, Other than for Tumor

Testis, Biopsy

Thymus, Tumor

Thyroid, Total/Lobe

Ureter, Resection

Urinary Bladder, TUR

Uterus, with or without Tubes and Ovaries, Other than Neoplastic/Prolapse

88309   **Level VI** - Surgical pathology, gross and microscopic examination

Bone Resection

Breast, Mastectomy - with Regional Lymph Nodes

Colon, Segmental Resection for Tumor

Colon, Total Resection

Esophagus, Partial/Total Resection

Extremity, Disarticulation

Fetus, with Dissection

Larynx, Partial/Total Resection - with Regional Lymph Nodes

Lung - Total/Lobe/Segment Resection

Pancreas, Total/Subtotal Resection

Prostate, Radical Resection

Small Intestine, Resection for Tumor

Soft Tissue Tumor, Extensive Resection

Stomach - Subtotal/Total Resection for Tumor

Testis, Tumor

Tongue/Tonsil - Resection for Tumor

Urinary Bladder, Partial/Total Resection

Uterus, with or without Tubes and Ovaries, Neoplastic

Vulva, Total/Subtotal Resection

(For fine needle aspiration, see 10021, 10022)

(For evaluation of fine needle aspirate, see 88172-88173)

+ 88311   Decalcification procedure (List separately in addition to code for surgical pathology examination)

+ 88312   Special stains (List separately in addition to code for primary service); Group I for microorganisms (eg, Gridley, acid fast, methenamine silver), each

+ 88313   Group II, all other, (eg, iron, trichrome), except immunocytochemistry and immunoperoxidase stains, each

(For immunocytochemistry and immunoperoxidase tissue studies, use 88342)

+ 88314   histochemical staining with frozen section(s)

88318   Determinative histochemistry to identify chemical components (eg, copper, zinc)

88319   Determinative histochemistry or cytochemistry to identify enzyme constituents, each

88321   Consultation and report on referred slides prepared elsewhere

88323   Consultation and report on referred material requiring preparation of slides

88325   Consultation, comprehensive, with review of records and specimens, with report on referred material

88329   Pathology consultation during surgery;

88331   first tissue block, with frozen section(s), single specimen

88332   each additional tissue block with frozen section(s)

88342   Immunohistochemistry (including tissue immunoperoxidase), each antibody

▶(Do not report 88342 in conjunction with 88360 or 88361 for the same antibody)◀

(For quantitative or semiquantitative immunohistochemistry, ▶see 88360,◀ 88361)

88346   Immunofluorescent study, each antibody; direct method

88347   indirect method

88348   Electron microscopy; diagnostic

88349   scanning

88355   Morphometric analysis; skeletal muscle

88356   nerve

88358   tumor (eg, DNA ploidy)

(Do not report 88358 with 88313 unless each procedure is for a different special stain)

● **88360**   Morphometric analysis, tumor immunohistochemistry (eg, Her-2/neu, estrogen receptor/progesterone receptor), quantitative or semiquantitative, each antibody; manual

▲ **88361**   using computer-assisted technology

(Do not report ▶88360,◀ 88361 with 88342 unless each procedure is for a different antibody)

▶(For morphometric analysis, in situ hybridization, see 88367, 88368)◀

(When semi-thin plastic-embedded sections are performed in conjunction with morphometric analysis, only the morphometric analysis should be reported; if performed as an independent procedure, see codes 88300-88309 for surgical pathology.)

88362   Nerve teasing preparations

▲ **88365**   In situ hybridization (eg, FISH), each probe

▶(Do not report 88365 in conjunction with 88367, 88368 for the same probe)◀

● **88367**   Morphometric analysis, in situ hybridization, (quantitative or semi-quantitative) each probe; using computer-assisted technology

● **88368**   manual

88371   Protein analysis of tissue by Western Blot, with interpretation and report;

88372   immunological probe for band identification, each

88380   Microdissection (eg, mechanical, laser capture)

88399   Unlisted surgical pathology procedure

Transcutaneous Procedures

88400   Bilirubin, total, transcutaneous

Other Procedures

89050   Cell count, miscellaneous body fluids (eg, cerebrospinal fluid, joint fluid), except blood;

89051   with differential count

89055   Leukocyte assessment, fecal, qualitative or semiquantitative

89060   Crystal identification by light microscopy with or without polarizing lens analysis, any body fluid (except urine)

89100   Duodenal intubation and aspiration; single specimen (eg, simple bile study or afferent loop culture) plus appropriate test procedure

89105   collection of multiple fractional specimens with pancreatic or gallbladder stimulation, single or double lumen tube

(For radiological localization, use 74340)

(For chemical analyses, see **Chemistry,** this section)

(Electrocardiogram, see 93000-93268)

(Esophagus acid perfusion test (Bernstein), see 91030)

89125   Fat stain, feces, urine, or respiratory secretions

89130   Gastric intubation and aspiration, diagnostic, each specimen, for chemical analyses or cytopathology;

89132   after stimulation

Pathology and Laboratory

89135 Gastric intubation, aspiration, and fractional collections (eg, gastric secretory study); one hour

89136 two hours

89140 two hours including gastric stimulation (eg, histalog, pentagastrin)

89141 three hours, including gastric stimulation

(For gastric lavage, therapeutic, use 91105)

(For radiologic localization of gastric tube, use 74340)

(For chemical analyses, see 82926, 82928)

(Joint fluid chemistry, see **Chemistry,** this section)

89160 Meat fibers, feces

89190 Nasal smear for eosinophils

(Occult blood, feces, use 82270)

(Paternity tests, use 86910)

89220 Sputum, obtaining specimen, aerosol induced technique (separate procedure)

89225 Starch granules, feces

89230 Sweat collection by iontophoresis

89235 Water load test

89240 Unlisted miscellaneous pathology test

Reproductive Medicine Procedures

89250 Culture of oocyte(s)/embryo(s), less than 4 days;

89251 with co-culture of oocyte(s)/embryos

(For extended culture of oocyte(s)/embryo(s), see 89272)

(89252 has been deleted. To report, use 89280-89281)

89253 Assisted embryo hatching, microtechniques (any method)

89254 Oocyte identification from follicular fluid

89255 Preparation of embryo for transfer (any method)

(89256 has been deleted. To report, use 89352)

89257 Sperm identification from aspiration (other than seminal fluid)

(For semen analysis, see 89300-89320)

(For sperm identification from testis tissue, use 89264)

89258 Cryopreservation; embryo(s)

89259 sperm

(For cryopreservation of reproductive tissue, testicular, use 89335)

(For cryopreservation of reproductive tissue, ovarian, use Category III code 0058T)

(For cryopreservation of oocyte(s), use Category III code 0059T)

89260 Sperm isolation; simple prep (eg, sperm wash and swim-up) for insemination or diagnosis with semen analysis

89261 complex prep (eg, Percoll gradient, albumin gradient) for insemination or diagnosis with semen analysis

(For semen analysis without sperm wash or swim-up, use 89320)

89264 Sperm identification from testis tissue, fresh or cryopreserved

(For biopsy of testis, see 54500, 54505)

(For sperm identification from aspiration, use 89257)

(For semen analysis, see 89300-89320)

89268 Insemination of oocytes

89272 Extended culture of oocyte(s)/embryo(s), 4-7 days

89280 Assisted oocyte fertilization, microtechnique; less than or equal to 10 oocytes

89281 greater than 10 oocytes

89290 Biopsy, oocyte polar body or embryo blastomere, microtechnique (for pre-implantation genetic diagnosis); less than or equal to 5 embryos

89291 greater than 5 embryos

89300 Semen analysis; presence and/or motility of sperm including Huhner test (post coital)

89310 motility and count (not including Huhner test)

89320 complete (volume, count, motility, and differential)

(Skin tests, see 86485-86585 and 95010-95199)

89321 Semen analysis, presence and/or motility of sperm

►(To report Hyaluronan binding assay (HBA), use Category III code 0087T)◄

89325 Sperm antibodies

(For medicolegal identification of sperm, use 88125)

89329 Sperm evaluation; hamster penetration test

89330 cervical mucus penetration test, with or without spinnbarkeit test

89335 Cryopreservation, reproductive tissue, testicular

(For cryopreservation of embryo(s), use 89258. For cryopreservation of sperm, use 89259)

(For cryopreservation of reproductive tissue, ovarian, use Category III code 0058T)

(For cryopreservation of oocyte, use Category III code 0059T)

89342 Storage, (per year); embryo(s)

89343 sperm/semen

89344 reproductive tissue, testicular/ovarian

▲ **89346** oocyte(s)

(89350 has been deleted. To report, use 89220)

89352   Thawing of cryopreserved; embryo(s)

89353   sperm/semen, each aliquot

89354   reproductive tissue, testicular/ovarian

            (89355 has been deleted. To report, use 89225)

89356   oocytes, each aliquot

            (89360 has been deleted. To report, use 89230)

            (89365 has been deleted. To report, use 89235)

            (89399 has been deleted. To report, use 89240)

Pathology and Laboratory

Notes

⊘=Modifier 51 Exempt   ⊙=Conscious Sedation   ✛=Add-on Code

Medicine Guidelines

In addition to the definitions and commonly used terms presented in the **Introduction**, several other items unique to this section on **Medicine** are defined or identified here.

Multiple Procedures

It is appropriate to designate multiple procedures that are rendered on the same date by separate entries. For example: If individual medical psychotherapy (90829) is rendered in addition to subsequent hospital care (eg, 99231), the psychotherapy would be reported separately from the hospital visit. In this instance, both 99231 and 90829 would be reported.

Add-on Codes

Some of the listed procedures are commonly carried out in addition to the primary procedure performed. All add-on codes found in *CPT* are exempt from the multiple procedure concept. They are exempt from the use of modifier 51, as these procedures are not reported as stand-alone codes. These additional or supplemental procedures are designated as "add-on" codes. Add-on codes in *CPT* can be readily identified by specific descriptor nomenclature which includes phrases such as "each additional" or "(List separately in addition to primary procedure)."

Separate Procedures

Some of the procedures or services listed in *CPT* that are commonly carried out as an integral component of a total service or procedure have been identified by the inclusion of the term "separate procedure." The codes designated as "separate procedure" should not be reported in addition to the code for the total procedure or service of which it is considered an integral component.

However, when a procedure or service that is designated as a "separate procedure" is carried out independently or considered to be unrelated or distinct from other procedures/services provided at that time, it may be reported by itself, or in addition to other procedures/services by appending modifier 59 to the specific "separate procedure" code to indicate that the procedure is not considered to be a component of another procedure, but is a distinct, independent procedure. This may represent a different session or patient encounter, different procedure or surgery, different site or organ system, separate incision/excision, separate lesion, or separate injury (or area of injury in extensive injuries).

Subsection Information

Several of the subheadings or subsections have special instructions unique to that section. These special instructions will be presented preceding those procedural terminology listings, referring to that subsection specifically. If there is an "Unlisted Procedure" code number (see section below) for the individual subsection, it will also be shown. Those subsections within the **Medicine** section that have special instructions are as follows:

Immune Globulins	90281-90399
Immunization Administration for Vaccines/Toxoids	90465-90474
Vaccines, Toxoids	90476-90749
Therapeutic or Diagnostic Infusions	90780-90781
Psychiatry	90801-90899
Dialysis	90918-90999
Ophthalmology	92002-92499
Contact Lens Services	92310-92326
Spectacle Services	92340-92396
Otorhinolaryngology	92502-92700
Audiologic Function Tests	92551-92597
Evaluative and Therapeutic Services	92601-92625
Echocardiography	93303-93350
Cardiac Catheterization	93501-93581
Intracardiac Electrophysiological Procedures/Studies	93600-93662
Peripheral Arterial Disease Rehabilitation	93668
Non-Invasive Vascular Diagnostic Studies	93875-93990
Pulmonary	94010-94799
Allergy and Clinical Immunology	95004-95199
Neurology and Neuromuscular	95805-95999
Neurostimulators, Analysis-Programming	95970-95979
Motion Analysis	96000-96004
Central Nervous System Assessments/Tests	96100-96117
Health and Behavior Assessment/Intervention	96150-96155
Chemotherapy Administration	96400-96549
Dermatological Procedures	96900-96999
Physical Medicine and Rehabilitation	97001-97755
Modalities	97010-97039
Constant Attendance	97032-97039

Unlisted Service or Procedure

A service or procedure may be provided that is not listed in this edition of *CPT*. When reporting such a service, the appropriate "Unlisted Procedure" code may be used to indicate the service, identifying it by "Special Report" as discussed on this page. The "Unlisted Procedures" and accompanying codes for **Medicine** are as follows:

⊘ **90399**   Unlisted immune globulin

⊘ **90749**   Unlisted vaccine/toxoid

90799   Unlisted therapeutic, prophylactic or diagnostic injection

90899   Unlisted psychiatric service or procedure

90999   Unlisted dialysis procedure, inpatient or outpatient

91299   Unlisted diagnostic gastroenterology procedure

92499   Unlisted ophthalmological service or procedure

92700   Unlisted otorhinolaryngological service or procedure

93799   Unlisted cardiovascular service or procedure

94799   Unlisted pulmonary service or procedure

95199   Unlisted allergy/clinical immunologic service or procedure

95999   Unlisted neurological or neuromuscular diagnostic procedure

96549   Unlisted chemotherapy procedure

96999   Unlisted special dermatological service or procedure

97039   Unlisted modality (specify type and time if constant attendance)

97139   Unlisted therapeutic procedure (specify)

97799   Unlisted physical medicine/rehabilitation service or procedure

99199   Unlisted special service, procedure or report

99600   Unlisted home visit service or procedure

Special Report

A service that is rarely provided, unusual, variable, or new may require a special report in determining medical appropriateness of the service. Pertinent information should include an adequate definition or description of the nature, extent, and need for the procedure; and the time, effort, and equipment necessary to provide the service. Additional items which may be included are:

- complexity of symptoms;
- final diagnosis;
- pertinent physical findings;
- diagnostic and therapeutic procedures;
- concurrent problems;
- follow-up care.

Materials Supplied by Physician

Supplies and materials provided by the physician (eg, sterile trays/drugs), over and above those usually included with the procedure(s) rendered are reported separately. List drugs, trays, supplies, and materials provided. Identify as 99070 or specific supply code.

Medicine

Immune Globulins

Codes 90281-90399 identify the immune globulin product only and must be reported in addition to the administration codes 90780-90784 as appropriate. Immune globulin products listed here include broad-spectrum and anti-infective immune globulins, antitoxins, and various isoantibodies.

⊘ **90281**   Immune globulin (Ig), human, for intramuscular use

⊘ **90283**   Immune globulin (IgIV), human, for intravenous use

⊘ **90287**   Botulinum antitoxin, equine, any route

⊘ **90288**   Botulism immune globulin, human, for intravenous use

⊘ **90291**   Cytomegalovirus immune globulin (CMV-IgIV), human, for intravenous use

⊘ **90296**   Diphtheria antitoxin, equine, any route

⊘ **90371**   Hepatitis B immune globulin (HBIg), human, for intramuscular use

⊘ **90375**   Rabies immune globulin (RIg), human, for intramuscular and/or subcutaneous use

⊘ **90376**   Rabies immune globulin, heat-treated (RIg-HT), human, for intramuscular and/or subcutaneous use

⊘ **90378**   Respiratory syncytial virus immune globulin (RSV-IgIM), for intramuscular use, 50 mg, each

⊘ **90379**   Respiratory syncytial virus immune globulin (RSV-IgIV), human, for intravenous use

⊘ **90384**   Rho(D) immune globulin (RhIg), human, full-dose, for intramuscular use

⊘ **90385**   Rho(D) immune globulin (RhIg), human, mini-dose, for intramuscular use

⊘ **90386**   Rho(D) immune globulin (RhIgIV), human, for intravenous use

⊘ **90389**   Tetanus immune globulin (TIg), human, for intramuscular use

⊘ **90393**   Vaccinia immune globulin, human, for intramuscular use

⊘ **90396**   Varicella-zoster immune globulin, human, for intramuscular use

⊘ **90399**   Unlisted immune globulin

Immunization Administration for Vaccines/Toxoids

Codes ▶90465◀-90474 must be reported in addition to the vaccine and toxoid code(s) 90476-90749.

▶Report codes 90465-90468 only when the physician provides face-to-face counseling of the patient and family during the administration of a vaccine. For immunization administration of any vaccine that is not accompanied by face-to-face physician counseling to the patient/family, report codes 90471-90474.◀

If a significant separately identifiable Evaluation and Management service (eg, office or other outpatient services, preventive medicine services) is performed, the appropriate E/M service code should be reported in addition to the vaccine and toxoid administration codes.

(For allergy testing, see 95004 et seq)

(For skin testing of bacterial, viral, fungal extracts, see 86485-86586)

(For therapeutic or diagnostic injections, see 90782-90799)

● **90465**   Immunization administration under 8 years of age (includes percutaneous, intradermal, subcutaneous, or intramuscular injections) when the physician counsels the patient/family; first injection (single or combination vaccine/toxoid), per day

▶(Do not report 90465 in conjunction with 90467)◀

+● **90466**   each additional injection (single or combination vaccine/toxoid), per day (List separately in addition to code for primary procedure)

▶(Use 90466 in conjunction with 90465 or 90467)◀

● **90467**   Immunization administration under age 8 years (includes intranasal or oral routes of administration) when the physician counsels the patient/family; first administration (single or combination vaccine/toxoid), per day

▶(Do not report 90467 in conjunction with 90465)◀

+● **90468**   each additional administration (single or combination vaccine/toxoid), per day (List separately in addition to code for primary procedure)

▶(Use 90468 in conjunction with 90465 or 90467)◀

Medicine

Medicine

▲ **90471** Immunization administration (includes percutaneous, intradermal, subcutaneous, or intramuscular injections); one vaccine (single or combination vaccine/toxoid)

▶(Do not report 90471 in conjunction with 90473)◀

+ **90472** each additional vaccine (single or combination vaccine/toxoid) (List separately in addition to code for primary procedure)

(Use 90472 in conjunction with 90471 ▶or 90473◀)

(For administration of immune globulins, use 90780-90784, and see 90281-90399)

(For intravesical administration of BCG vaccine, use 51720, and see 90586)

90473 Immunization administration by intranasal or oral route; one vaccine (single or combination vaccine/toxoid)

▶(Do not report 90473 in conjunction with 90471)◀

+ **90474** each additional vaccine (single or combination vaccine/toxoid) (List separately in addition to code for primary procedure)

(Use 90474 in conjunction with ▶90471 or◀ 90473)

Vaccines, Toxoids

Codes 90476-90748 identify the vaccine product **only.** To report the administration of a vaccine/toxoid, the vaccine/toxoid product codes 90476-90749 must be used in addition to an immunization administration code(s) ▶90465-90474◀. Do not append modifier 51 to the vaccine/toxoid product codes 90476-90749.

If a significantly separately identifiable Evaluation and Management service (eg, office or other outpatient services, preventive medicine services) is performed, the appropriate E/M service code should be reported in addition to the vaccine and toxoid administration codes.

To meet the reporting requirements of immunization registries, vaccine distribution programs, and reporting systems (eg, Vaccine Adverse Event Reporting System) the exact vaccine product administered needs to be reported. Multiple codes for a particular vaccine are provided in *CPT* when the schedule (number of doses or timing) differs for two or more products of the same vaccine type (eg, hepatitis A, Hib) or the vaccine product is available in more than one chemical formulation, dosage, or route of administration.

Separate codes are available for combination vaccines (eg, DTP-Hib, DtaP-Hib, HepB-Hib). It is inappropriate to code each component of a combination vaccine separately. If a specific vaccine code is not available, the unlisted procedure code should be reported, until a new code becomes available.

(For immune globulins, see codes 90281-90399, and 90780-90784 for administration of immune globulins)

⊘ **90476** Adenovirus vaccine, type 4, live, for oral use

⊘ **90477** Adenovirus vaccine, type 7, live, for oral use

⊘ **90581** Anthrax vaccine, for subcutaneous use

⊘ **90585** Bacillus Calmette-Guerin vaccine (BCG) for tuberculosis, live, for percutaneous use

⊘ **90586** Bacillus Calmette-Guerin vaccine (BCG) for bladder cancer, live, for intravesical use

⊘ **90632** Hepatitis A vaccine, adult dosage, for intramuscular use

⊘ **90633** Hepatitis A vaccine, pediatric/adolescent dosage-2 dose schedule, for intramuscular use

⊘ **90634** Hepatitis A vaccine, pediatric/adolescent dosage-3 dose schedule, for intramuscular use

⊘ **90636** Hepatitis A and hepatitis B vaccine (HepA-HepB), adult dosage, for intramuscular use

⊘ **90645** Hemophilus influenza b vaccine (Hib), HbOC conjugate (4 dose schedule), for intramuscular use

⊘ **90646** Hemophilus influenza b vaccine (Hib), PRP-D conjugate, for booster use only, intramuscular use

⊘ **90647** Hemophilus influenza b vaccine (Hib), PRP-OMP conjugate (3 dose schedule), for intramuscular use

⊘ **90648** Hemophilus influenza b vaccine (Hib), PRP-T conjugate (4 dose schedule), for intramuscular use

⊘ **90655** Influenza virus vaccine, split virus, preservative free, for children 6-35 months of age, for intramuscular use

⊘● **90656** Influenza virus vaccine, split virus, preservative free, for use in individuals 3 years and above, for intramuscular use

⊘ **90657** Influenza virus vaccine, split virus, for children 6-35 months of age, for intramuscular use

⊘ **90658** Influenza virus vaccine, split virus, for use in individuals 3 years of age and above, for intramuscular use

(90659 has been deleted. To report influenza virus vaccine, split virus, see 90657 or 90658)

⊘ **90660** Influenza virus vaccine, live, for intranasal use

⊘ **90665** Lyme disease vaccine, adult dosage, for intramuscular use

⊘ **90669** Pneumococcal conjugate vaccine, polyvalent, for children under 5 years, for intramuscular use

⊘ **90675** Rabies vaccine, for intramuscular use

⊘ **90676** Rabies vaccine, for intradermal use

⊘ **90680** Rotavirus vaccine, tetravalent, live, for oral use

⊘ **90690** Typhoid vaccine, live, oral

⊘ **90691** Typhoid vaccine, Vi capsular polysaccharide (ViCPs), for intramuscular use

⊘ **90692** Typhoid vaccine, heat- and phenol-inactivated (H-P), for subcutaneous or intradermal use

⊘ **90693** Typhoid vaccine, acetone-killed, dried (AKD), for subcutaneous use (U.S. military)

⊘ **90698**   Diphtheria, tetanus toxoids, acellular pertussis vaccine, haemophilus influenza Type B, and poliovirus vaccine, inactivated (DTaP - Hib - IPV), for intramuscular use

⊘▲ **90700**   Diphtheria, tetanus toxoids, and acellular pertussis vaccine (DTaP), for use in individuals younger than 7 years, for intramuscular use

⊘ **90701**   Diphtheria, tetanus toxoids, and whole cell pertussis vaccine (DTP), for intramuscular use

⊘ **90702**   Diphtheria and tetanus toxoids (DT) adsorbed for use in individuals younger than 7 years, for intramuscular use

⊘ **90703**   Tetanus toxoid adsorbed, for intramuscular use

⊘ **90704**   Mumps virus vaccine, live, for subcutaneous use

⊘ **90705**   Measles virus vaccine, live, for subcutaneous use

⊘ **90706**   Rubella virus vaccine, live, for subcutaneous use

⊘ **90707**   Measles, mumps and rubella virus vaccine (MMR), live, for subcutaneous use

⊘ **90708**   Measles and rubella virus vaccine, live, for subcutaneous use

(90709 has been deleted)

⊘ **90710**   Measles, mumps, rubella, and varicella vaccine (MMRV), live, for subcutaneous use

⊘ **90712**   Poliovirus vaccine, (any type(s)) (OPV), live, for oral use

⊘ **90713**   Poliovirus vaccine, inactivated, (IPV), for subcutaneous use

⊘ **90715**   Tetanus, diphtheria toxoids and acellular pertussis vaccine (TdaP), for use in individuals 7 years or older, for intramuscular use

⊘ **90716**   Varicella virus vaccine, live, for subcutaneous use

⊘ **90717**   Yellow fever vaccine, live, for subcutaneous use

⊘ **90718**   Tetanus and diphtheria toxoids (Td) adsorbed for use in individuals 7 years or older, for intramuscular use

⊘ **90719**   Diphtheria toxoid, for intramuscular use

⊘ **90720**   Diphtheria, tetanus toxoids, and whole cell pertussis vaccine and Hemophilus influenza B vaccine (DTP-Hib), for intramuscular use

⊘ **90721**   Diphtheria, tetanus toxoids, and acellular pertussis vaccine and Hemophilus influenza B vaccine (DtaP-Hib), for intramuscular use

⊘ **90723**   Diphtheria, tetanus toxoids, acellular pertussis vaccine, Hepatitis B, and poliovirus vaccine, inactivated (DtaP-HepB-IPV), for intramuscular use

⊘ **90725**   Cholera vaccine for injectable use

⊘ **90727**   Plague vaccine, for intramuscular use

⊘ **90732**   Pneumococcal polysaccharide vaccine, 23-valent, adult or immunosuppressed patient dosage, for use in individuals 2 years or older, for subcutaneous or intramuscular use

⊘ **90733**   Meningococcal polysaccharide vaccine (any group(s)), for subcutaneous use

⊘ **90734**   Meningococcal conjugate vaccine, serogroups A, C, Y and W-135 (tetravalent), for intramuscular use

⊘ **90735**   Japanese encephalitis virus vaccine, for subcutaneous use

⊘ **90740**   Hepatitis B vaccine, dialysis or immunosuppressed patient dosage (3 dose schedule), for intramuscular use

⊘ **90743**   Hepatitis B vaccine, adolescent (2 dose schedule), for intramuscular use

⊘ **90744**   Hepatitis B vaccine, pediatric/adolescent dosage (3 dose schedule), for intramuscular use

⊘ **90746**   Hepatitis B vaccine, adult dosage, for intramuscular use

⊘ **90747**   Hepatitis B vaccine, dialysis or immunosuppressed patient dosage (4 dose schedule), for intramuscular use

⊘ **90748**   Hepatitis B and Hemophilus influenza b vaccine (HepB-Hib), for intramuscular use

⊘ **90749**   Unlisted vaccine/toxoid

Therapeutic or Diagnostic Infusions (Excludes Chemotherapy)

These procedures encompass prolonged intravenous injections.

These codes require the presence of the physician during the infusion. These codes are not to be used for intradermal, subcutaneous or intramuscular or routine IV drug injections. For these services, see 90782-90788.

These codes may not be used in addition to prolonged services codes.

90780   Intravenous infusion for therapy/diagnosis, administered by physician or under direct supervision of physician; up to one hour

+ **90781**   each additional hour, up to eight (8) hours (List separately in addition to code for primary procedure)

(Use 90781 in conjunction with 90780)

Therapeutic, Prophylactic or Diagnostic Injections

90782   Therapeutic, prophylactic or diagnostic injection (specify material injected); subcutaneous or intramuscular

(For administration of vaccines/toxoids, see ▶90465◀-90472)

90783   intra-arterial

90784   intravenous

(90782-90784 do not include injections for allergen immunotherapy. For allergen immunotherapy injections, see 95115-95117)

Medicine

90788   Intramuscular injection of antibiotic (specify)

(For chemotherapy administration and infusion services, see 95990, 96408-96414, 96420-96425, 96440, 96450, 96530, 96545, 96549)

90799   Unlisted therapeutic, prophylactic or diagnostic injection

(For allergy immunizations, see 95004 et seq)

Psychiatry

(For repetitive transcranial magnetic stimulation for treatment of clinical depression, use Category III code 0018T)

Hospital care by the attending physician in treating a psychiatric inpatient or partial hospitalization may be initial or subsequent in nature (see 99221-99233) and may include exchanges with nursing and ancillary personnel. Hospital care services involve a variety of responsibilities unique to the medical management of inpatients, such as physician hospital orders, interpretation of laboratory or other medical diagnostic studies and observations.

Some patients receive hospital evaluation and management services only and others receive evaluation and management services and other procedures. If other procedures such as electroconvulsive therapy or psychotherapy are rendered in addition to hospital evaluation and management services, these should be listed separately (ie, hospital care service plus electroconvulsive therapy or when psychotherapy is done, an appropriate code defining psychotherapy with medical evaluation and management services). Modifier 22 may be used to indicate a more extensive service. Modifier 52 may be used to signify a service that is reduced or less extensive than the usual procedure.

Other evaluation and management services, such as office medical service or other patient encounters, may be described as listed in the section on **Evaluation and Management,** if appropriate.

The evaluation and management services should not be reported separately, when reporting codes 90805, 90807, 90809, 90811, 90813, 90815, 90817, 90819, 90822, 90824, 90827, 90829.

Consultation for psychiatric evaluation of a patient includes examination of a patient and exchange of information with the primary physician and other informants such as nurses or family members, and preparation of a report. These consultation services (99241-99263) are limited to initial or follow-up evaluation and do not involve psychiatric treatment.

Psychiatric Diagnostic or Evaluative Interview Procedures

Psychiatric diagnostic interview examination includes a history, mental status, and a disposition, and may include communication with family or other sources, ordering and medical interpretation of laboratory or other medical diagnostic studies. In certain circumstances other informants will be seen in lieu of the patient.

Interactive psychiatric diagnostic interview examination is typically furnished to children. It involves the use of physical aids and non-verbal communication to overcome barriers to therapeutic interaction between the clinician and a patient who has not yet developed, or has lost, either the expressive language communication skills to explain his/her symptoms and response to treatment, or the receptive communication skills to understand the clinician if he/she were to use ordinary adult language for communication.

90801   Psychiatric diagnostic interview examination

90802   Interactive psychiatric diagnostic interview examination using play equipment, physical devices, language interpreter, or other mechanisms of communication

Psychiatric Therapeutic Procedures

Psychotherapy is the treatment for mental illness and behavioral disturbances in which the clinician establishes a professional contract with the patient and, through definitive therapeutic communication, attempts to alleviate the emotional disturbances, reverse or change maladaptive patterns of behavior, and encourage personality growth and development. The codes for reporting psychotherapy are divided into two broad categories: Interactive Psychotherapy; and Insight Oriented, Behavior Modifying and/or Supportive Psychotherapy.

Interactive psychotherapy is typically furnished to children. It involves the use of physical aids and non-verbal communication to overcome barriers to therapeutic interaction between the clinician and a patient who has not yet developed, or has lost, either the expressive language communication skills to explain his/her symptoms and response to treatment, or the receptive communication skills to understand the clinician if he/she were to use ordinary adult language for communication.

Insight oriented, behavior modifying and/or supportive psychotherapy refers to the development of insight or affective understanding, the use of behavior modification techniques, the use of supportive interactions, the use of cognitive discussion of reality, or any combination of the above to provide therapeutic change.

Medicine

Some patients receive psychotherapy only and others receive psychotherapy and medical evaluation and management services. These evaluation and management services involve a variety of responsibilities unique to the medical management of psychiatric patients, such as medical diagnostic evaluation (eg, evaluation of comorbid medical conditions, drug interactions, and physical examinations), drug management when indicated, physician orders, interpretation of laboratory or other medical diagnostic studies and observations.

In reporting psychotherapy, the appropriate code is chosen on the basis of the type of psychotherapy (interactive using non-verbal techniques versus insight oriented, behavior modifying and/or supportive using verbal techniques), the place of service (office versus inpatient), the face-to-face time spent with the patient during psychotherapy, and whether evaluation and management services are furnished on the same date of service as psychotherapy.

To report medical evaluation and management services furnished on a day when psychotherapy is not provided, select the appropriate code from the **Evaluation and Management Services Guidelines.**

Office or Other Outpatient Facility

Insight Oriented, Behavior Modifying and/or Supportive Psychotherapy

90804   Individual psychotherapy, insight oriented, behavior modifying and/or supportive, in an office or outpatient facility, approximately 20 to 30 minutes face-to-face with the patient;

90805   with medical evaluation and management services

90806   Individual psychotherapy, insight oriented, behavior modifying and/or supportive, in an office or outpatient facility, approximately 45 to 50 minutes face-to-face with the patient;

90807   with medical evaluation and management services

90808   Individual psychotherapy, insight oriented, behavior modifying and/or supportive, in an office or outpatient facility, approximately 75 to 80 minutes face-to-face with the patient;

90809   with medical evaluation and management services

Interactive Psychotherapy

90810   Individual psychotherapy, interactive, using play equipment, physical devices, language interpreter, or other mechanisms of non-verbal communication, in an office or outpatient facility, approximately 20 to 30 minutes face-to-face with the patient;

90811   with medical evaluation and management services

90812   Individual psychotherapy, interactive, using play equipment, physical devices, language interpreter, or other mechanisms of non-verbal communication, in an office or outpatient facility, approximately 45 to 50 minutes face-to-face with the patient;

90813   with medical evaluation and management services

90814   Individual psychotherapy, interactive, using play equipment, physical devices, language interpreter, or other mechanisms of non-verbal communication, in an office or outpatient facility, approximately 75 to 80 minutes face-to-face with the patient;

90815   with medical evaluation and management services

Inpatient Hospital, Partial Hospital or Residential Care Facility

Insight Oriented, Behavior Modifying and/or Supportive Psychotherapy

90816   Individual psychotherapy, insight oriented, behavior modifying and/or supportive, in an inpatient hospital, partial hospital or residential care setting, approximately 20 to 30 minutes face-to-face with the patient;

90817   with medical evaluation and management services

90818   Individual psychotherapy, insight oriented, behavior modifying and/or supportive, in an inpatient hospital, partial hospital or residential care setting, approximately 45 to 50 minutes face-to-face with the patient;

90819   with medical evaluation and management services

90821   Individual psychotherapy, insight oriented, behavior modifying and/or supportive, in an inpatient hospital, partial hospital or residential care setting, approximately 75 to 80 minutes face-to-face with the patient;

90822   with medical evaluation and management services

Interactive Psychotherapy

90823   Individual psychotherapy, interactive, using play equipment, physical devices, language interpreter, or other mechanisms of non-verbal communication, in an inpatient hospital, partial hospital or residential care setting, approximately 20 to 30 minutes face-to-face with the patient;

90824   with medical evaluation and management services

90826   Individual psychotherapy, interactive, using play equipment, physical devices, language interpreter, or other mechanisms of non-verbal communication, in an inpatient hospital, partial hospital or residential care setting, approximately 45 to 50 minutes face-to-face with the patient;

90827   with medical evaluation and management services

Medicine

90828   Individual psychotherapy, interactive, using play equipment, physical devices, language interpreter, or other mechanisms of non-verbal communication, in an inpatient hospital, partial hospital or residential care setting, approximately 75 to 80 minutes face-to-face with the patient;

90829   with medical evaluation and management services

Other Psychotherapy

90845   Psychoanalysis

90846   Family psychotherapy (without the patient present)

90847   Family psychotherapy (conjoint psychotherapy) (with patient present)

90849   Multiple-family group psychotherapy

90853   Group psychotherapy (other than of a multiple-family group)

90857   Interactive group psychotherapy

Other Psychiatric Services or Procedures

90862   Pharmacologic management, including prescription, use, and review of medication with no more than minimal medical psychotherapy

90865   Narcosynthesis for psychiatric diagnostic and therapeutic purposes (eg, sodium amobarbital (Amytal) interview)

90870   Electroconvulsive therapy (includes necessary monitoring); single seizure

90871   multiple seizures, per day

90875   Individual psychophysiological therapy incorporating biofeedback training by any modality (face-to-face with the patient), with psychotherapy (eg, insight oriented, behavior modifying or supportive psychotherapy); approximately 20-30 minutes

90876   approximately 45-50 minutes

90880   Hypnotherapy

90882   Environmental intervention for medical management purposes on a psychiatric patient's behalf with agencies, employers, or institutions

90885   Psychiatric evaluation of hospital records, other psychiatric reports, psychometric and/or projective tests, and other accumulated data for medical diagnostic purposes

90887   Interpretation or explanation of results of psychiatric, other medical examinations and procedures, or other accumulated data to family or other responsible persons, or advising them how to assist patient

90889   Preparation of report of patient's psychiatric status, history, treatment, or progress (other than for legal or consultative purposes) for other physicians, agencies, or insurance carriers

90899   Unlisted psychiatric service or procedure

Biofeedback

(For psychophysiological therapy incorporating biofeedback training, see 90875, 90876)

90901   Biofeedback training by any modality

90911   Biofeedback training, perineal muscles, anorectal or urethral sphincter, including EMG and/or manometry

(For incontinence treatment by pulsed magnetic neuromodulation, use Category III code 0029T)

►(For testing of rectal sensation, tone and compliance, use 91120)◄

Dialysis

Codes 90918-90921 are reported ONCE per month to distinguish age-specific services related to the patient's end-stage renal disease (ESRD) performed in an outpatient setting. ESRD-related physician services include establishment of a dialyzing cycle, outpatient evaluation and management of the dialysis visits, telephone calls, and patient management during the dialysis, provided during a full month. These codes are not used if the physician also submits hospitalization codes during the month.

Codes 90918-90921 describe a full month of ESRD-related services provided in an outpatient setting. For ESRD and non-ESRD dialysis services performed in an inpatient setting, and for non-ESRD dialysis services performed in an outpatient setting, see 90935-90937 and 90945-90947.

Evaluation and management services unrelated to ESRD services that cannot be performed during the dialysis session may be reported separately.

Codes 90922-90925 are reported when outpatient ESRD-related services are not performed consecutively during an entire full month (eg, when the patient spends part of the month as a hospital inpatient, or when the outpatient ESRD-related services are initiated after the first of the month). The appropriate age-related code from this series (90922-90925) is reported daily less the days of hospitalization. For reporting purposes, each month is considered 30 days.

Example:

Outpatient ESRD-related services are initiated on July 1 for a 57-year-old male. On July 11, he is admitted to the hospital as an inpatient and is discharged on July 27.

In this example, code 90925 should be reported for each day outside of the inpatient hospitalization (30 days/month less 17 days/hospitalization = 13 days). Report inpatient E/M services as appropriate. Dialysis procedures rendered during the hospitalization (July 11-27) should be reported as appropriate (90935-90937, 90945-90947).

Medicine

End Stage Renal Disease Services

90918 End stage renal disease (ESRD) related services per full month; for patients under two years of age to include monitoring for the adequacy of nutrition, assessment of growth and development, and counseling of parents

90919 for patients between two and eleven years of age to include monitoring for the adequacy of nutrition, assessment of growth and development, and counseling of parents

90920 for patients between twelve and nineteen years of age to include monitoring for the adequacy of nutrition, assessment of growth and development, and counseling of parents

90921 for patients twenty years of age and over

90922 End stage renal disease (ESRD) related services (less than full month), per day; for patients under two years of age

90923 for patients between two and eleven years of age

90924 for patients between twelve and nineteen years of age

90925 for patients twenty years of age and over

Hemodialysis

Codes 90935, 90937 are reported to describe the hemodialysis procedure with all evaluation and management services related to the patient's renal disease on the day of the hemodialysis procedure. These codes are used for inpatient ESRD and non-ESRD procedures or for outpatient non-ESRD dialysis services. Code 90935 is reported if only one evaluation of the patient is required related to that hemodialysis procedure. Code 90937 is reported when patient re-evaluation(s) is required during a hemodialysis procedure. Utilize modifier 25 with Evaluation and Management codes for separately identifiable services unrelated to the dialysis procedure or renal failure which cannot be rendered during the dialysis session.

(For home visit hemodialysis services performed by a non-physician health care professional, use 99512)

(For cannula declotting, see 36831, 36833, 36860, 36861)

(For declotting of implanted vascular access device or catheter by thrombolytic agent, use 36550)

(For collection of blood specimen from a partially or completely implantable venous access device, use 36540)

(For prolonged physician attendance, see 99354-99360)

90935 Hemodialysis procedure with single physician evaluation

90937 Hemodialysis procedure requiring repeated evaluation(s) with or without substantial revision of dialysis prescription

90939 Hemodialysis access flow study to determine blood flow in grafts and arteriovenous fistulae by an indicator dilution method, hook-up; transcutaneous measurement and disconnection

90940 measurement and disconnection

(For duplex scan of hemodialysis access, use 93990)

Miscellaneous Dialysis Procedures

Codes 90945, 90947 describe dialysis procedures other than hemodialysis (eg, peritoneal dialysis, hemofiltration or continuous renal replacement therapies), and all evaluation and management services related to the patient's renal disease on the day of the procedure. Code 90945 is reported if only one evaluation of the patient is required related to that procedure. Code 90947 is reported when patient re-evaluation(s) is required during a procedure. Utilize modifier 25 with Evaluation and Management codes for separately identifiable services unrelated to the procedure or the renal failure which cannot be rendered during the dialysis session.

(For insertion of intraperitoneal cannula or catheter, see 49420, 49421)

(For prolonged physician attendance, see 99354-99360)

90945 Dialysis procedure other than hemodialysis (eg, peritoneal dialysis, hemofiltration, or other continuous renal replacement therapies), with single physician evaluation

(For home infusion of peritoneal dialysis, use 99601, 99602)

90947 Dialysis procedure other than hemodialysis (eg, peritoneal dialysis, hemofiltration, or other continuous renal replacement therapies) requiring repeated physician evaluations, with or without substantial revision of dialysis prescription

90989 Dialysis training, patient, including helper where applicable, any mode, completed course

90993 Dialysis training, patient, including helper where applicable, any mode, course not completed, per training session

90997 Hemoperfusion (eg, with activated charcoal or resin)

90999 Unlisted dialysis procedure, inpatient or outpatient

Gastroenterology

(For duodenal intubation and aspiration, see 89100-89105)

(For gastrointestinal radiologic procedures, see 74210-74363)

(For esophagoscopy procedures, see 43200-43228; upper GI endoscopy 43234-43259; endoscopy, small intestine and stomal 44360-44393; proctosigmoidoscopy 45300-45321; sigmoidoscopy 45330-45339; colonoscopy 45355-45385; anoscopy 46600-46615)

Medicine

91000   Esophageal intubation and collection of washings for cytology, including preparation of specimens (separate procedure)

91010   Esophageal motility (manometric study of the esophagus and/or gastroesophageal junction) study;

91011   with mecholyl or similar stimulant

91012   with acid perfusion studies

91020   Gastric motility (manometric) studies

91030   Esophagus, acid perfusion (Bernstein) test for esophagitis

►(91032 and 91033 have been deleted. To report, see 91034, 91035)◄

● **91034**   Esophagus, gastroesophageal reflux test; with nasal catheter pH electrode(s) placement, recording, analysis and interpretation

● **91035**   with mucosal attached telemetry pH electrode placement, recording, analysis and interpretation

● **91037**   Esophageal function test, gastroesophageal reflux test with nasal catheter intraluminal impedance electrode(s) placement, recording, analysis and interpretation;

● **91038**   prolonged (greater than 1 hour, up to 24 hours)

● **91040**   Esophageal balloon distension provocation study

►(For balloon dilatation with endoscopy, see 43220, 43249, 43456, or 43458)◄

91052   Gastric analysis test with injection of stimulant of gastric secretion (eg, histamine, insulin, pentagastrin, calcium and secretin)

(For gastric biopsy by capsule, peroral, via tube, one or more specimens, use 43600)

(For gastric laboratory procedures, see also 89130-89141)

91055   Gastric intubation, washings, and preparing slides for cytology (separate procedure)

(For gastric lavage, therapeutic, use 91105)

91060   Gastric saline load test

(For biopsy by capsule, small intestine, per oral, via tube (one or more specimens), use 44100)

▲ **91065**   Breath hydrogen test (eg, for detection of lactase deficiency), fructose intolerance, bacterial overgrowth, or oro-cecal gastrointestinal transit)

►(For H. pylori breath test analysis, use 83013 for non-radioactive (C-13) isotope or 78268 for radioactive (C-14) isotope)◄

91100   Intestinal bleeding tube, passage, positioning and monitoring

91105   Gastric intubation, and aspiration or lavage for treatment (eg, for ingested poisons)

(For cholangiography, see 47500, 74320)

(For abdominal paracentesis, see 49080, 49081; with instillation of medication, see 96440, 96445)

(For peritoneoscopy, use 49320; with biopsy, use 49321)

(For peritoneoscopy and guided transhepatic cholangiography, use 47560; with biopsy, use 47561)

(For splenoportography, see 38200, 75810)

91110   Gastrointestinal tract imaging, intraluminal (eg, capsule endoscopy), esophagus through ileum, with physician interpretation and report

(Visualization of the colon is not reported separately)

(Append modifier 52 if the ileum is not visualized)

● **91120**   Rectal sensation, tone, and compliance test (ie, response to graded balloon distention)

►(For biofeedback training, use 90911)◄

►(For anorectal manometry, use 91122)◄

91122   Anorectal manometry

91123   Pulsed irrigation of fecal impaction

Gastric Physiology

91132   Electrogastrography, diagnostic, transcutaneous;

91133   with provocative testing

Other Procedures

91299   Unlisted diagnostic gastroenterology procedure

Ophthalmology

(For surgical procedures, see **Surgery,** Eye and Ocular Adnexa, 65091 et seq)

Definitions

Intermediate ophthalmological services describes an evaluation of a new or existing condition complicated with a new diagnostic or management problem not necessarily relating to the primary diagnosis, including history, general medical observation, external ocular and adnexal examination and other diagnostic procedures as indicated; may include the use of mydriasis for ophthalmoscopy.

For example:

a. Review of history, external examination, ophthalmoscopy, biomicroscopy for an acute complicated condition (eg, iritis) not requiring comprehensive ophthalmological services.

b. Review of interval history, external examination, ophthalmoscopy, biomicroscopy and tonometry in established patient with known cataract not requiring comprehensive ophthalmological services.

Medicine

Comprehensive ophthalmological services describes a general evaluation of the complete visual system. The comprehensive services constitute a single service entity but need not be performed at one session. The service includes history, general medical observation, external and ophthalmoscopic examinations, gross visual fields and basic sensorimotor examination. It often includes, as indicated: biomicroscopy, examination with cycloplegia or mydriasis and tonometry. It always includes initiation of diagnostic and treatment programs.

Intermediate and comprehensive ophthalmological services constitute integrated services in which medical decision making cannot be separated from the examining techniques used. Itemization of service components, such as slit lamp examination, keratometry, routine ophthalmoscopy, retinoscopy, tonometry, or motor evaluation is not applicable.

For example:

The comprehensive services required for diagnosis and treatment of a patient with symptoms indicating possible disease of the visual system, such as glaucoma, cataract or retinal disease, or to rule out disease of the visual system, new or established patient.

Initiation of diagnostic and treatment program includes the prescription of medication, and arranging for special ophthalmological diagnostic or treatment services, consultations, laboratory procedures and radiological services.

Special ophthalmological services describes services in which a special evaluation of part of the visual system is made, which goes beyond the services included under general ophthalmological services, or in which special treatment is given. Special ophthalmological services may be reported in addition to the general ophthalmological services or evaluation and management services.

For example:

Fluorescein angioscopy, quantitative visual field examination, refraction or extended color vision examination (such as Nagel's anomaloscope) should be separately reported.

Prescription of lenses, when required, is included in 92015. It includes specification of lens type (monofocal, bifocal, other), lens power, axis, prism, absorptive factor, impact resistance, and other factors.

Interpretation and report by the physician is an integral part of special ophthalmological services where indicated. Technical procedures (which may or may not be performed by the physician personally) are often part of the service, but should not be mistaken to constitute the service itself.

General Ophthalmological Services

New Patient

Solely for the purposes of distinguishing between new and established patients, **professional services** are those face-to-face services rendered by a physician and reported by a specific code(s). A new patient is one who has not received any professional services from the physician or another physician of the same specialty who belongs to the same group practice within the past three years.

92002   Ophthalmological services: medical examination and evaluation with initiation of diagnostic and treatment program; intermediate, new patient

92004   comprehensive, new patient, one or more visits

Established Patient

Solely for the purposes of distinguishing between new and established patients, **professional services** are those face-to-face services rendered by a physician and reported by a specific code(s). An established patient is one who has received professional services from the physician or another physician of the same specialty who belongs to the same group practice within the past three years.

92012   Ophthalmological services: medical examination and evaluation, with initiation or continuation of diagnostic and treatment program; intermediate, established patient

92014   comprehensive, established patient, one or more visits

(For surgical procedures, see **Surgery,** Eye and Ocular Adnexa, 65091 et seq)

Special Ophthalmological Services

92015   Determination of refractive state

92018   Ophthalmological examination and evaluation, under general anesthesia, with or without manipulation of globe for passive range of motion or other manipulation to facilitate diagnostic examination; complete

92019   limited

92020   Gonioscopy (separate procedure)

(For gonioscopy under general anesthesia, use 92018)

92060   Sensorimotor examination with multiple measurements of ocular deviation (eg, restrictive or paretic muscle with diplopia) with interpretation and report (separate procedure)

92065   Orthoptic and/or pleoptic training, with continuing medical direction and evaluation

92070   Fitting of contact lens for treatment of disease, including supply of lens

Medicine

92081   Visual field examination, unilateral or bilateral, with interpretation and report; limited examination (eg, tangent screen, Autoplot, arc perimeter, or single stimulus level automated test, such as Octopus 3 or 7 equivalent)

92082   intermediate examination (eg, at least 2 isopters on Goldmann perimeter, or semiquantitative, automated suprathreshold screening program, Humphrey suprathreshold automatic diagnostic test, Octopus program 33)

92083   extended examination (eg, Goldmann visual fields with at least 3 isopters plotted and static determination within the central 30°, or quantitative, automated threshold perimetry, Octopus program G-1, 32 or 42, Humphrey visual field analyzer full threshold programs 30-2, 24-2, or 30/60-2)

(Gross visual field testing (eg, confrontation testing) is a part of general ophthalmological services and is not reported separately)

92100   Serial tonometry (separate procedure) with multiple measurements of intraocular pressure over an extended time period with interpretation and report, same day (eg, diurnal curve or medical treatment of acute elevation of intraocular pressure)

92120   Tonography with interpretation and report, recording indentation tonometer method or perilimbal suction method

92130   Tonography with water provocation

92135   Scanning computerized ophthalmic diagnostic imaging (eg, scanning laser) with interpretation and report, unilateral

92136   Ophthalmic biometry by partial coherence interferometry with intraocular lens power calculation

92140   Provocative tests for glaucoma, with interpretation and report, without tonography

Ophthalmoscopy

Routine ophthalmoscopy is part of general and special ophthalmologic services whenever indicated. It is a non-itemized service and is not reported separately.

92225   Ophthalmoscopy, extended, with retinal drawing (eg, for retinal detachment, melanoma), with interpretation and report; initial

92226   subsequent

92230   Fluorescein angioscopy with interpretation and report

92235   Fluorescein angiography (includes multiframe imaging) with interpretation and report

92240   Indocyanine-green angiography (includes multiframe imaging) with interpretation and report

92250   Fundus photography with interpretation and report

92260   Ophthalmodynamometry

(For ophthalmoscopy under general anesthesia, use 92018)

Other Specialized Services

92265   Needle oculoelectromyography, one or more extraocular muscles, one or both eyes, with interpretation and report

92270   Electro-oculography with interpretation and report

92275   Electroretinography with interpretation and report

(For electronystagmography for vestibular function studies, see 92541 et seq)

(For ophthalmic echography (diagnostic ultrasound), see 76511-76529)

92283   Color vision examination, extended, eg, anomaloscope or equivalent

(Color vision testing with pseudoisochromatic plates (such as HRR or Ishihara) is not reported separately. It is included in the appropriate general or ophthalmological service, or 99172)

92284   Dark adaptation examination with interpretation and report

92285   External ocular photography with interpretation and report for documentation of medical progress (eg, close-up photography, slit lamp photography, goniophotography, stereo-photography)

92286   Special anterior segment photography with interpretation and report; with specular endothelial microscopy and cell count

92287   with fluorescein angiography

Contact Lens Services

The prescription of contact lens includes specification of optical and physical characteristics (such as power, size, curvature, flexibility, gas-permeability). It is NOT a part of the general ophthalmological services.

The fitting of contact lens includes instruction and training of the wearer and incidental revision of the lens during the training period.

Follow-up of successfully fitted extended wear lenses is reported as part of a general ophthalmological service (92012 et seq).

The supply of contact lenses may be reported as part of the service of fitting. It may also be reported separately by using 92391 or 92396 and modifier 26 for the service of fitting without supply.

(For therapeutic or surgical use of contact lens, see 68340, 92070)

92310   Prescription of optical and physical characteristics of and fitting of contact lens, with medical supervision of adaptation; corneal lens, both eyes, except for aphakia

(For prescription and fitting of one eye, add modifier 52)

92311   corneal lens for aphakia, one eye

92312   corneal lens for aphakia, both eyes

92313   corneoscleral lens

92314 Prescription of optical and physical characteristics of contact lens, with medical supervision of adaptation and direction of fitting by independent technician; corneal lens, both eyes except for aphakia

(For prescription and fitting of one eye, add modifier 52)

92315 corneal lens for aphakia, one eye

92316 corneal lens for aphakia, both eyes

92317 corneoscleral lens

92325 Modification of contact lens (separate procedure), with medical supervision of adaptation

92326 Replacement of contact lens

Ocular Prosthetics, Artificial Eye

92330 Prescription, fitting, and supply of ocular prosthesis (artificial eye), with medical supervision of adaptation

(If supply is not included, use modifier 26; to report supply separately, use 92393)

92335 Prescription of ocular prosthesis (artificial eye) and direction of fitting and supply by independent technician, with medical supervision of adaptation

Spectacle Services (Including Prosthesis for Aphakia)

Prescription of lenses, when required, is included in 92015 Determination of refractive state. It includes specification of lens type (monofocal, bifocal, other), lens power, axis, prism, absorptive factor, impact resistance, and other factors.

Fitting of spectacles is a separate service; when provided by the physician, it is reported as indicated by 92340-92371.

Fitting includes measurement of anatomical facial characteristics, the writing of laboratory specifications, and the final adjustment of the spectacles to the visual axes and anatomical topography. Presence of physician is not required.

Supply of materials is a separate service component; it is not part of the service of fitting spectacles.

92340 Fitting of spectacles, except for aphakia; monofocal

92341 bifocal

92342 multifocal, other than bifocal

92352 Fitting of spectacle prosthesis for aphakia; monofocal

92353 multifocal

92354 Fitting of spectacle mounted low vision aid; single element system

92355 telescopic or other compound lens system

92358 Prosthesis service for aphakia, temporary (disposable or loan, including materials)

92370 Repair and refitting spectacles; except for aphakia

92371 spectacle prosthesis for aphakia

Supply of Materials

92390 Supply of spectacles, except prosthesis for aphakia and low vision aids

92391 Supply of contact lenses, except prosthesis for aphakia

(For supply of contact lenses reported as part of the service of fitting, see 92310-92313)

(For replacement of contact lens, use 92326)

92392 Supply of low vision aids (A low vision aid is any lens or device used to aid or improve visual function in a person whose vision cannot be normalized by conventional spectacle correction. Includes reading additions up to 4D.)

92393 Supply of ocular prosthesis (artificial eye)

(For supply reported as part of the service of fitting, use 92330)

92395 Supply of permanent prosthesis for aphakia; spectacles

(For temporary spectacle correction, use 92358)

92396 contact lenses

(For supply reported as part of the service of fitting, see 92311, 92312)

(Use 99070 for the supply of other materials, drugs, trays, etc.)

Other Procedures

92499 Unlisted ophthalmological service or procedure

Special Otorhinolaryngologic Services

Diagnostic or treatment procedures usually included in a comprehensive otorhinolaryngologic evaluation or office visit, are reported as an integrated medical service, using appropriate descriptors from the 99201 series.
Itemization of component procedures (eg, otoscopy, rhinoscopy, tuning fork test) does not apply.

Special otorhinolaryngologic services are those diagnostic and treatment services not usually included in a comprehensive otorhinolaryngologic evaluation or office visit. These services are reported separately, using codes 92502-92700.

Medicine

All services include medical diagnostic evaluation. Technical procedures (which may or may not be performed by the physician personally) are often part of the service, but should not be mistaken to constitute the service itself.

(For laryngoscopy with stroboscopy, use 31579)

92502   Otolaryngologic examination under general anesthesia

92504   Binocular microscopy (separate diagnostic procedure)

92506   Evaluation of speech, language, voice, communication, auditory processing, and/or aural rehabilitation status

92507   Treatment of speech, language, voice, communication, and/or auditory processing disorder (includes aural rehabilitation); individual

92508   group, two or more individuals

92510   Aural rehabilitation following cochlear implant (includes evaluation of aural rehabilitation status and hearing, therapeutic services) with or without speech processor programming

92511   Nasopharyngoscopy with endoscope (separate procedure)

92512   Nasal function studies (eg, rhinomanometry)

92516   Facial nerve function studies (eg, electroneuronography)

92520   Laryngeal function studies

(92525 has been deleted. To report, see 92610-92611 for specific evaluation)

92526   Treatment of swallowing dysfunction and/or oral function for feeding

Vestibular Function Tests, With Observation and Evaluation by Physician, Without Electrical Recording

92531   Spontaneous nystagmus, including gaze

92532   Positional nystagmus test

92533   Caloric vestibular test, each irrigation (binaural, bithermal stimulation constitutes four tests)

92534   Optokinetic nystagmus test

Vestibular Function Tests, With Recording (eg, ENG, PENG), and Medical Diagnostic Evaluation

92541   Spontaneous nystagmus test, including gaze and fixation nystagmus, with recording

92542   Positional nystagmus test, minimum of 4 positions, with recording

92543   Caloric vestibular test, each irrigation (binaural, bithermal stimulation constitutes four tests), with recording

92544   Optokinetic nystagmus test, bidirectional, foveal or peripheral stimulation, with recording

92545   Oscillating tracking test, with recording

92546   Sinusoidal vertical axis rotational testing

+ 92547   Use of vertical electrodes (List separately in addition to code for primary procedure)

(Use 92547 in conjunction with 92541-92546)

(For unlisted vestibular tests, use 92700)

92548   Computerized dynamic posturography

Audiologic Function Tests With Medical Diagnostic Evaluation

The audiometric tests listed below imply the use of calibrated electronic equipment. Other hearing tests (such as whispered voice, tuning fork) are considered part of the general otorhinolaryngologic services and are not reported separately. All services include testing of both ears. Use modifier 52 if a test is applied to one ear instead of to two ears. All codes (except 92559) apply to testing of individuals; for testing of groups, use 92559 and specify test(s) used.

(For evaluation of speech, language and/or hearing problems through observation and assessment of performance, use 92506)

92551   Screening test, pure tone, air only

92552   Pure tone audiometry (threshold); air only

92553   air and bone

92555   Speech audiometry threshold;

92556   with speech recognition

92557   Comprehensive audiometry threshold evaluation and speech recognition (92553 and 92556 combined)

(For hearing aid evaluation and selection, see 92590-92595)

92559   Audiometric testing of groups

92560   Bekesy audiometry; screening

92561   diagnostic

92562   Loudness balance test, alternate binaural or monaural

92563   Tone decay test

92564   Short increment sensitivity index (SISI)

92565   Stenger test, pure tone

92567   Tympanometry (impedance testing)

92568   Acoustic reflex testing

92569   Acoustic reflex decay test

92571   Filtered speech test

92572   Staggered spondaic word test

92573   Lombard test

92575   Sensorineural acuity level test

92576   Synthetic sentence identification test

92577   Stenger test, speech

92579   Visual reinforcement audiometry (VRA)

92582   Conditioning play audiometry

92583   Select picture audiometry

92584   Electrocochleography

92585   Auditory evoked potentials for evoked response audiometry and/or testing of the central nervous system; comprehensive

92586   limited

92587   Evoked otoacoustic emissions; limited (single stimulus level, either transient or distortion products)

92588   comprehensive or diagnostic evaluation (comparison of transient and/or distortion product otoacoustic emissions at multiple levels and frequencies)

          ►(92589 has been deleted)◄

          ►(For central auditory function evaluation, see 92620, 92621)◄

92590   Hearing aid examination and selection; monaural

92591   binaural

92592   Hearing aid check; monaural

92593   binaural

92594   Electroacoustic evaluation for hearing aid; monaural

92595   binaural

92596   Ear protector attenuation measurements

92597   Evaluation for use and/or fitting of voice prosthetic device to supplement oral speech

          (To report augmentative and alternative communication device services, see 92605, 92607, 92608)

          (92598 has been deleted)

          (92599 has been deleted. To report use 92700)

Evaluative and Therapeutic Services

Codes 92601 and 92603 describe post-operative analysis and fitting of previously placed external devices, connection to the cochlear implant, and programming of the stimulator. Codes 92602 and 92604 describe subsequent sessions for measurements and adjustment of the external transmitter and re-programming of the internal stimulator.

          (For placement of cochlear implant, use 69930)

92601   Diagnostic analysis of cochlear implant, patient under 7 years of age; with programming

92602   subsequent reprogramming

          (Do not report 92602 in addition to 92601)

          (For aural rehabilitation services following cochlear implant, including evaluation of rehabilitation status, use 92510)

92603   Diagnostic analysis of cochlear implant, age 7 years or older; with programming

92604   subsequent reprogramming

          (Do not report 92604 in addition to 92603)

92605   Evaluation for prescription of non-speech-generating augmentative and alternative communication device

92606   Therapeutic service(s) for the use of non-speech-generating device, including programming and modification

92607   Evaluation for prescription for speech-generating augmentative and alternative communication device, face-to-face with the patient; first hour

          (For evaluation for prescription of a non-speech-generating device, use 92605)

+ 92608   each additional 30 minutes (List separately in addition to code for primary procedure)

          (Use 92608 in conjunction with 92607)

92609   Therapeutic services for the use of speech-generating device, including programming and modification

          (For therapeutic service(s) for the use of a non-speech-generating device, use 92606)

92610   Evaluation of oral and pharyngeal swallowing function

          (For motion fluoroscopic evaluation of swallowing function, use 92611)

          (For flexible endoscopic examination, use 92612-92617)

92611   Motion fluoroscopic evaluation of swallowing function by cine or video recording

          (For radiological supervision and interpretation, use 74230)

          (For evaluation of oral and pharyngeal swallowing function, use 92610)

          (For flexible fiberoptic diagnostic laryngoscopy, use 31575. Do not report 31575 in conjunction with 92612-92617)

92612   Flexible fiberoptic endoscopic evaluation of swallowing by cine or video recording;

          (If flexible fiberoptic or endoscopic evaluation of swallowing is performed without cine or video recording, use 92700)

92613   physician interpretation and report only

          (To report an evaluation of oral and pharyngeal swallowing function, use 92610)

          (To report motion fluoroscopic evaluation of swallowing function, use 92611)

Medicine

92614 Flexible fiberoptic endoscopic evaluation, laryngeal sensory testing by cine or video recording;

(If flexible fiberoptic or endoscopic evaluation of swallowing is performed without cine or video recording, use 92700)

92615 physician interpretation and report only

92616 Flexible fiberoptic endoscopic evaluation of swallowing and laryngeal sensory testing by cine or video recording;

(If flexible fiberoptic or endoscopic evaluation of swallowing is performed without cine or video recording, use 92700)

92617 physician interpretation and report only

● 92620 Evaluation of central auditory function, with report; initial 60 minutes

● 92621 each additional 15 minutes

▶(Do not report 92620, 92621 in conjunction with 92506)◀

● 92625 Assessment of tinnitus (includes pitch, loudness matching, and masking)

▶(Do not report 92625 in conjunction with 92562)◀

▶(For unilateral assessment, use modifier 52)◀

Other Procedures

92700 Unlisted otorhinolaryngological service or procedure

Cardiovascular

Therapeutic Services

(For non-surgical septal reduction therapy (eg, alcohol ablation), use Category III code 0024T)

92950 Cardiopulmonary resuscitation (eg, in cardiac arrest)

(See also critical care services, 99291, 99292)

⊙ 92953 Temporary transcutaneous pacing

(For physician direction of ambulance or rescue personnel outside the hospital, use 99288)

⊙ 92960 Cardioversion, elective, electrical conversion of arrhythmia; external

⊙ 92961 internal (separate procedure)

(Do not report 92961 in addition to codes 93662, 93618-93624, 93631, 93640-93642, 93650-93652, 93741-93744)

92970 Cardioassist-method of circulatory assist; internal

92971 external

(For balloon atrial-septostomy, use 92992)

(For placement of catheters for use in circulatory assist devices such as intra-aortic balloon pump, use 33970)

⊙+ 92973 Percutaneous transluminal coronary thrombectomy (List separately in addition to code for primary procedure)

(Use 92973 in conjunction with 92980, 92982)

⊙+ 92974 Transcatheter placement of radiation delivery device for subsequent coronary intravascular brachytherapy (List separately in addition to code for primary procedure)

(Use 92974 in conjunction with 92980, 92982, 92995, 93508)

(For intravascular radioelement application, see 77781-77784)

⊙ 92975 Thrombolysis, coronary; by intracoronary infusion, including selective coronary angiography

92977 by intravenous infusion

(For thrombolysis of vessels other than coronary, see 37201, 75896)

(For cerebral thrombolysis, use 37195)

⊙+ 92978 Intravascular ultrasound (coronary vessel or graft) during diagnostic evaluation and/or therapeutic intervention including imaging supervision, interpretation and report; initial vessel (List separately in addition to code for primary procedure)

⊙+ 92979 each additional vessel (List separately in addition to code for primary procedure)

(Use 92979 in conjunction with 92978)

(Intravascular ultrasound services include all transducer manipulations and repositioning within the specific vessel being examined, both before and after therapeutic intervention (eg, stent placement))

⊙ 92980 Transcatheter placement of an intracoronary stent(s), percutaneous, with or without other therapeutic intervention, any method; single vessel

⊙+ 92981 each additional vessel (List separately in addition to code for primary procedure)

(Use 92981 in conjunction with 92980)

▶(Codes 92980, 92981 are used to report coronary artery stenting. Coronary angioplasty (92982, 92984) or atherectomy (92995, 92996), in the same artery, is considered part of the stenting procedure and is not reported separately. Codes 92973 (percutaneous transluminal coronary thombectomy), 92974 (coronary brachytherapy) and 92978, 92979 (intravascular ultrasound) are add-on codes for reporting procedures performed in addition to coronary stenting, atherectomy, and angioplasty and are not included in the "therapeutic interventions" in 92980)◀

(To report additional vessels treated by angioplasty or atherectomy only during the same session, see 92984, 92996)

(To report transcatheter placement of radiation delivery device for coronary intravascular brachytherapy, use 92974)

(For intravascular radioelement application, see 77781-77784)

⊙ **92982**   Percutaneous transluminal coronary balloon angioplasty; single vessel

⊙+ **92984**   each additional vessel (List separately in addition to code for primary procedure)

(Use 92984 in conjunction with 92980, 92982, 92995)

(For stent placement following completion of angioplasty or atherectomy, see 92980, 92981)

(To report transcatheter placement of radiation delivery device for coronary intravascular brachytherapy, use 92974)

(For intravascular radioelement application, see 77781-77784)

⊙ **92986**   Percutaneous balloon valvuloplasty; aortic valve

⊙ **92987**   mitral valve

92990   pulmonary valve

92992   Atrial septectomy or septostomy; transvenous method, balloon (eg, Rashkind type) (includes cardiac catheterization)

92993   blade method (Park septostomy) (includes cardiac catheterization)

⊙ **92995**   Percutaneous transluminal coronary atherectomy, by mechanical or other method, with or without balloon angioplasty; single vessel

⊙+ **92996**   each additional vessel (List separately in addition to code for primary procedure)

(Use 92996 in conjunction with 92980, 92982, 92995)

(For stent placement following completion of angioplasty or atherectomy, see 92980, 92981)

(To report additional vessels treated by angioplasty only during the same session, use 92984)

92997   Percutaneous transluminal pulmonary artery balloon angioplasty; single vessel

+ **92998**   each additional vessel (List separately in addition to code for primary procedure)

(Use 92998 in conjunction with 92997)

Cardiography

(For echocardiography, see 93303-93350)

93000   Electrocardiogram, routine ECG with at least 12 leads; with interpretation and report

93005   tracing only, without interpretation and report

93010   interpretation and report only

(For ECG monitoring, see 99354-99360)

93012   Telephonic transmission of post-symptom electrocardiogram rhythm strip(s), 24-hour attended monitoring, per 30 day period of time; tracing only

93014   physician review with interpretation and report only

93015   Cardiovascular stress test using maximal or submaximal treadmill or bicycle exercise, continuous electrocardiographic monitoring, and/or pharmacological stress; with physician supervision, with interpretation and report

93016   physician supervision only, without interpretation and report

93017   tracing only, without interpretation and report

93018   interpretation and report only

93024   Ergonovine provocation test

93025   Microvolt T-wave alternans for assessment of ventricular arrhythmias

93040   Rhythm ECG, one to three leads; with interpretation and report

93041   tracing only without interpretation and report

93042   interpretation and report only

93224   Electrocardiographic monitoring for 24 hours by continuous original ECG waveform recording and storage, with visual superimposition scanning; includes recording, scanning analysis with report, physician review and interpretation

93225   recording (includes hook-up, recording, and disconnection)

93226   scanning analysis with report

93227   physician review and interpretation

93230   Electrocardiographic monitoring for 24 hours by continuous original ECG waveform recording and storage without superimposition scanning utilizing a device capable of producing a full miniaturized printout; includes recording, microprocessor-based analysis with report, physician review and interpretation

93231   recording (includes hook-up, recording, and disconnection)

93232   microprocessor-based analysis with report

93233   physician review and interpretation

93235   Electrocardiographic monitoring for 24 hours by continuous computerized monitoring and non-continuous recording, and real-time data analysis utilizing a device capable of producing intermittent full-sized waveform tracings, possibly patient activated; includes monitoring and real-time data analysis with report, physician review and interpretation

93236   monitoring and real-time data analysis with report

93237   physician review and interpretation

93268   Patient demand single or multiple event recording with presymptom memory loop, 24-hour attended monitoring, per 30 day period of time; includes transmission, physician review and interpretation

93270   recording (includes hook-up, recording, and disconnection)

Medicine

93271	monitoring, receipt of transmissions, and analysis
93272	physician review and interpretation only

(For postsymptom recording, see 93012, 93014)

(For implanted patient activated cardiac event recording, see 33282, 93727)

93278   Signal-averaged electrocardiography (SAECG), with or without ECG

(For interpretation and report only, use 93278 with modifier 26)

(For unlisted cardiographic procedure, use 93799)

Echocardiography

Echocardiography includes obtaining ultrasonic signals from the heart and great arteries, with two-dimensional image and/or Doppler ultrasonic signal documentation, and interpretation and report. When interpretation is performed separately use modifier 26.

►Echocardiography is an ultrasound examination of the cardiac chambers and valves, the adjacent great vessels, and the pericardium. A complete transthoracic echocardiogram (93307) is a comprehensive procedure that includes 2-dimensional and selected M-mode examination of the left and right atria, left and right ventricles, the aortic, mitral, and tricuspid valves, the pericardium, and adjacent portions of the aorta. These structures are assessed using multiple views as required to obtain a complete functional and anatomic evaluation, and appropriate measurements are obtained and recorded. Despite significant effort, identification and measurement of some structures may not always be possible. In such instances, the reason that an element could not be visualized must be documented. Additional structures that may be visualized (eg, pulmonary veins, pulmonary artery, pulmonic valve, inferior vena cava) would be included as part of the service.◄

►A follow-up or limited echocardiographic study (93308) is an examination that does not evaluate or document the attempt to evaluate all the structures that comprise the complete echocardiographic exam. This is typically performed in follow-up of a complete echocardiographic examination when a repeat complete exam is unnecessary due to the more focused clinical concern. In some emergent clinical situations, a limited echocardiographic study may be performed primarily.◄

►Report of an echocardiographic study, whether complete or limited, includes an interpretation of all obtained information, documentation of all clinically relevant findings including quantitative measurements obtained, plus a description of any recognized abnormalities. Pertinent images, videotape, and/or digital data are archived for permanent storage and are available for subsequent review. Use of echocardiography not meeting these criteria is not separately reportable.◄

►Use of ultrasound, without thorough evaluation of organ(s) or anatomic region, image documentation and final, written report, is not separately reportable.◄

(For fetal echocardiography, see 76825-76828)

93303   Transthoracic echocardiography for congenital cardiac anomalies; complete

93304   follow-up or limited study

93307   Echocardiography, transthoracic, real-time with image documentation (2D) with or without M-mode recording; complete

93308   follow-up or limited study

⊙ **93312**   Echocardiography, transesophageal, real time with image documentation (2D) (with or without M-mode recording); including probe placement, image acquisition, interpretation and report

⊙ **93313**   placement of transesophageal probe only

⊙ **93314**   image acquisition, interpretation and report only

⊙ **93315**   Transesophageal echocardiography for congenital cardiac anomalies; including probe placement, image acquisition, interpretation and report

⊙ **93316**   placement of transesophageal probe only

⊙ **93317**   image acquisition, interpretation and report only

⊙ **93318**   Echocardiography, transesophageal (TEE) for monitoring purposes, including probe placement, real time 2-dimensional image acquisition and interpretation leading to ongoing (continuous) assessment of (dynamically changing) cardiac pumping function and to therapeutic measures on an immediate time basis

+ **93320**   Doppler echocardiography, pulsed wave and/or continuous wave with spectral display (List separately in addition to codes for echocardiographic imaging); complete

(Use 93320 in conjunction with 93303, 93304, 93307, 93308, 93312, 93314, 93315, 93317, 93350)

+ **93321**   follow-up or limited study (List separately in addition to codes for echocardiographic imaging)

(Use 93321 in conjunction with 93303, 93304, 93307, 93308, 93312, 93314, 93315, 93317, 93350)

+ **93325**   Doppler echocardiography color flow velocity mapping (List separately in addition to codes for echocardiography)

(Use 93325 in conjunction with 76825, 76826, 76827, 76828, 93303, 93304, 93307, 93308, 93312, 93314, 93315, 93317, 93320, 93321, 93350)

93350   Echocardiography, transthoracic, real-time with image documentation (2D), with or without M-mode recording, during rest and cardiovascular stress test using treadmill, bicycle exercise and/or pharmacologically induced stress, with interpretation and report

(The appropriate stress testing code from the 93015-93018 series should be reported in addition to 93350 to capture the exercise stress portion of the study)

Cardiac Catheterization

Cardiac catheterization is a diagnostic medical procedure which includes introduction, positioning and repositioning of catheter(s), when necessary, recording of intracardiac and intravascular pressure, obtaining blood samples for measurement of blood gases or dilution curves and cardiac output measurements (Fick or other method, with or without rest and exercise and/or studies) with or without electrode catheter placement, final evaluation and report of procedure. When selective injection procedures are performed without a preceding cardiac catheterization, these services should be reported using codes in the Vascular Injection Procedures section, 36011-36015 and 36215-36218.

When coronary artery, arterial coronary conduit or venous bypass graft angiography is performed without concomitant left heart cardiac catheterization, use 93508. Injection procedures 93539, 93540, 93544, and 93545 represent separate identifiable services and may be reported in conjunction with one another in addition to 93508, as appropriate. To report imaging supervision, interpretation and report in conjunction with 93508, use 93556.

Modifier 51 should not be appended to 93501-93533, 93539-93556.

⊙⊘ **93501**   Right heart catheterization

(For bundle of His recording, use 93600)

⊘ **93503**   Insertion and placement of flow directed catheter (eg, Swan-Ganz) for monitoring purposes

(For subsequent monitoring, see 99356-99357)

⊙⊘ **93505**   Endomyocardial biopsy

⊙⊘ **93508**   Catheter placement in coronary artery(s), arterial coronary conduit(s), and/or venous coronary bypass graft(s) for coronary angiography without concomitant left heart catheterization

(93508 is to be used only when left heart catheterization 93510, 93511, 93524, 93526 is not performed)

(93508 is to be used only once per procedure)

(To report transcatheter placement of radiation delivery device for coronary intravascular brachytherapy, use 92974)

(For intravascular radioelement application, see 77781-77784)

⊙⊘ **93510**   Left heart catheterization, retrograde, from the brachial artery, axillary artery or femoral artery; percutaneous

⊙⊘ **93511**   by cutdown

⊙⊘ **93514**   Left heart catheterization by left ventricular puncture

⊙⊘ **93524**   Combined transseptal and retrograde left heart catheterization

⊙⊘ **93526**   Combined right heart catheterization and retrograde left heart catheterization

⊙⊘ **93527**   Combined right heart catheterization and transseptal left heart catheterization through intact septum (with or without retrograde left heart catheterization)

⊙⊘ **93528**   Combined right heart catheterization with left ventricular puncture (with or without retrograde left heart catheterization)

⊙⊘ **93529**   Combined right heart catheterization and left heart catheterization through existing septal opening (with or without retrograde left heart catheterization)

⊙⊘ **93530**   Right heart catheterization, for congenital cardiac anomalies

⊘ **93531**   Combined right heart catheterization and retrograde left heart catheterization, for congenital cardiac anomalies

⊘ **93532**   Combined right heart catheterization and transseptal left heart catheterization through intact septum with or without retrograde left heart catheterization, for congenital cardiac anomalies

⊘ **93533**   Combined right heart catheterization and transseptal left heart catheterization through existing septal opening, with or without retrograde left heart catheterization, for congenital cardiac anomalies

(When injection procedures are performed in conjunction with cardiac catheterization, these services do not include introduction of catheters but do include repositioning of catheters when necessary and use of automatic power injectors. Injection procedures 93539-93545 represent separate identifiable services and may be coded in conjunction with one another when appropriate. The technical details of angiography, supervision of filming and processing, interpretation and report are not included. To report imaging supervision, interpretation and report, use 93555 and/or 93556. Modifier 51 should not be appended to 93539-93556.)

⊙⊘ **93539**   Injection procedure during cardiac catheterization; for selective opacification of arterial conduits (eg, internal mammary), whether native or used for bypass

⊙⊘ **93540**   for selective opacification of aortocoronary venous bypass grafts, one or more coronary arteries

⊙⊘ **93541**   for pulmonary angiography

⊙⊘ **93542**   for selective right ventricular or right atrial angiography

⊙⊘ **93543**   for selective left ventricular or left atrial angiography

⊙⊘ **93544**   for aortography

⊙⊘ **93545**   for selective coronary angiography (injection of radiopaque material may be by hand)

(To report imaging supervision and interpretation, use 93555)

Medicine

⊙⊘ **93555** Imaging supervision, interpretation and report for injection procedure(s) during cardiac catheterization; ventricular and/or atrial angiography

⊙⊘ **93556** pulmonary angiography, aortography, and/or selective coronary angiography including venous bypass grafts and arterial conduits (whether native or used in bypass)

(Codes 93561 and 93562 are not to be used with cardiac catheterization codes)

⊙ **93561** Indicator dilution studies such as dye or thermal dilution, including arterial and/or venous catheterization; with cardiac output measurement (separate procedure)

⊙ **93562** subsequent measurement of cardiac output

(For radioisotope method of cardiac output, see 78472, 78473, or 78481)

⊙✚ **93571** Intravascular Doppler velocity and/or pressure derived coronary flow reserve measurement (coronary vessel or graft) during coronary angiography including pharmacologically induced stress; initial vessel (List separately in addition to code for primary procedure)

⊙✚ **93572** each additional vessel (List separately in addition to code for primary procedure)

(Intravascular distal coronary blood flow velocity measurements include all Doppler transducer manipulations and repositioning within the specific vessel being examined, during coronary angiography or therapeutic intervention (eg, angioplasty))

(For unlisted cardiac catheterization procedure, use 93799)

Repair of Septal Defect

93580 Percutaneous transcatheter closure of congenital interatrial communication (ie, Fontan fenestration, atrial septal defect) with implant

(Percutaneous transcatheter closure of atrial septal defect includes a right heart catheterization procedure. Code 93580 includes injection of contrast for atrial and ventricular angiograms. Codes 93501, 93529-93533, 93539, 93543, 93555 should not be reported separately in addition to code 93580)

93581 Percutaneous transcatheter closure of a congenital ventricular septal defect with implant

(Percutaneous transcatheter closure of ventricular septal defect includes a right heart catheterization procedure. Code 93581 includes injection of contrast for atrial and ventricular angiograms. Codes 93501, 93529-93533, 93539, 93543, 93555 should not be reported separately in addition to code 93581)

(For echocardiographic services performed in addition to 93580, 93581, see 93303-93317, 93662 as appropriate)

Intracardiac Electrophysiological Procedures/Studies

Intracardiac electrophysiologic studies (EPS) are an invasive diagnostic medical procedure which include the insertion and repositioning of electrode catheters, recording of electrograms before and during pacing or programmed stimulation of multiple locations in the heart, analysis of recorded information, and report of the procedure. Electrophysiologic studies are most often performed with two or more electrode catheters. In many circumstances, patients with arrhythmias are evaluated and treated at the same encounter. In this situation, a diagnostic *electrophysiologic study* is performed, induced tachycardia(s) are *mapped*, and on the basis of the diagnostic and mapping information, the tissue is *ablated*. Electrophysiologic study(ies), mapping, and ablation represent distinctly different procedures, requiring individual reporting whether performed on the same or subsequent dates.

Definitions

Arrhythmia Induction: In most electrophysiologic studies, an attempt is made to induce arrhythmia(s) from single or multiple sites within the heart. Arrhythmia induction is achieved by performing pacing at different rates, programmed stimulation (introduction of critically timed electrical impulses), and other techniques. Because arrhythmia induction occurs via the same catheter(s) inserted for the electrophysiologic study(ies), catheter insertion and temporary pacemaker codes are not additionally reported. Codes 93600-93603, 93610-93612 and 93618 are used to describe unusual situations where there may be recording, pacing or an attempt at arrhythmia induction from only one site in the heart. Code 93619 describes only evaluation of the sinus node, atrioventricular node and His-Purkinje conduction system, without arrhythmia induction. Codes 93620-93624 and 93640-93642 all include recording, pacing and attempted arrhythmia induction from one or more site(s) in the heart.

Mapping: Mapping is a distinct procedure performed in addition to a diagnostic electrophysiologic procedure and should be separately reported using 93609 or 93613. Do not report standard mapping (93609) in addition to 3-D mapping (93613). When a tachycardia is induced, the site of tachycardia origination or its electrical path through the heart is often defined by mapping. Mapping creates a multidimensional depiction of a tachycardia by recording multiple electrograms obtained sequentially or simultaneously from multiple catheter sites in the heart. Depending upon the technique, certain types of mapping catheters may be repositioned from point-to-point within the heart, allowing sequential recording from the various sites to construct maps. Other types of mapping catheters allow mapping without a point-to-point technique by allowing simultaneous recording from many electrodes on the same catheter and computer-assisted three dimensional reconstruction of the tachycardia activation sequence.

Ablation: Once the part of the heart involved in the tachycardia is localized, the tachycardia may be treated by ablation (the delivery of a radiofrequency energy to the area to selectively destroy cardiac tissue). Ablation procedures (93651-93652) may be performed: independently on a date subsequent to a diagnostic electrophysiologic study and mapping; or, at the time a diagnostic electrophysiologic study, tachycardia(s) induction and mapping is performed. When an electrophysiologic study, mapping, and ablation are performed on the same date, each procedure should be separately reported. In reporting catheter ablation, 93651 and/or 93652 should be reported once to describe ablation of cardiac arrhythmias, regardless of the number of arrhythmias ablated.

Modifier 51 should not be appended to 93600-93660.

⊘ **93600** Bundle of His recording

⊘ **93602** Intra-atrial recording

⊘ **93603** Right ventricular recording

⊙+ **93609** Intraventricular and/or intra-atrial mapping of tachycardia site(s) with catheter manipulation to record from multiple sites to identify origin of tachycardia (List separately in addition to code for primary procedure)

(Use 93609 in conjunction with 93620, 93651, 93652)

(Do not report 93609 in addition to 93613)

⊘ **93610** Intra-atrial pacing

⊘ **93612** Intraventricular pacing

(Do not report 93612 in conjunction with 93620-93622)

⊙+ **93613** Intracardiac electrophysiologic 3-dimensional mapping (List separately in addition to code for primary procedure)

(Use 93613 in conjunction with 93620, 93651, 93652)

(Do not report 93613 in addition to 93609)

⊙⊘ **93615** Esophageal recording of atrial electrogram with or without ventricular electrogram(s);

⊙⊘ **93616**   with pacing

⊙⊘ **93618** Induction of arrhythmia by electrical pacing

(For intracardiac phonocardiogram, use 93799)

⊙⊘ **93619** Comprehensive electrophysiologic evaluation with right atrial pacing and recording, right ventricular pacing and recording, His bundle recording, including insertion and repositioning of multiple electrode catheters, without induction or attempted induction of arrhythmia

(Do not report 93619 in conjunction with 93600, 93602, 93610, 93612, 93618, or 93620-93622)

⊙⊘ **93620** Comprehensive electrophysiologic evaluation including insertion and repositioning of multiple electrode catheters with induction or attempted induction of arrhythmia; with right atrial pacing and recording, right ventricular pacing and recording, His bundle recording

(Do not report 93620 in conjunction with 93600, 93602, 93610, 93612, 93618 or 93619)

⊙+ **93621**   with left atrial pacing and recording from coronary sinus or left atrium (List separately in addition to code for primary procedure)

(Use 93621 in conjunction with 93620)

⊙+ **93622**   with left ventricular pacing and recording (List separately in addition to code for primary procedure)

(Use 93622 in conjunction with 93620)

+ **93623** Programmed stimulation and pacing after intravenous drug infusion (List separately in addition to code for primary procedure)

(Use 93623 in conjunction with 93619, 93620)

⊙⊘ **93624** Electrophysiologic follow-up study with pacing and recording to test effectiveness of therapy, including induction or attempted induction of arrhythmia

⊘ **93631** Intra-operative epicardial and endocardial pacing and mapping to localize the site of tachycardia or zone of slow conduction for surgical correction

⊙⊘ **93640** Electrophysiologic evaluation of single or dual chamber pacing cardioverter-defibrillator leads including defibrillation threshold evaluation (induction of arrhythmia, evaluation of sensing and pacing for arrhythmia termination) at time of initial implantation or replacement;

⊙⊘ **93641**   with testing of single or dual chamber pacing cardioverter-defibrillator pulse generator

(For subsequent or periodic electronic analysis and/or reprogramming of single or dual chamber pacing cardioverter-defibrillators, see 93642, 93741-93744)

⊙⊘ **93642** Electrophysiologic evaluation of single or dual chamber pacing cardioverter-defibrillator (includes defibrillation threshold evaluation, induction of arrhythmia, evaluation of sensing and pacing for arrhythmia termination, and programming or reprogramming of sensing or therapeutic parameters)

⊙⊘ **93650** Intracardiac catheter ablation of atrioventricular node function, atrioventricular conduction for creation of complete heart block, with or without temporary pacemaker placement

⊙⊘ **93651** Intracardiac catheter ablation of arrhythmogenic focus; for treatment of supraventricular tachycardia by ablation of fast or slow atrioventricular pathways, accessory atrioventricular connections or other atrial foci, singly or in combination

⊙⊘ **93652**   for treatment of ventricular tachycardia

Medicine

⊘ **93660** Evaluation of cardiovascular function with tilt table evaluation, with continuous ECG monitoring and intermittent blood pressure monitoring, with or without pharmacological intervention

(For testing of autonomic nervous system function, see 95921-95923)

✛ **93662** Intracardiac echocardiography during therapeutic/diagnostic intervention, including imaging supervision and interpretation (List separately in addition to code for primary procedure)

(Use 93662 in conjunction with 93580, 93581, 93621, 93622, 93651, or 93652, as appropriate)

(Do not report 92961 in addition to 93662)

Peripheral Arterial Disease Rehabilitation

Peripheral arterial disease (PAD) rehabilitative physical exercise consists of a series of sessions, lasting 45-60 minutes per session, involving use of either a motorized treadmill or a track to permit each patient to achieve symptom-limited claudication. Each session is supervised by an exercise physiologist or nurse. The supervising provider monitors the individual patient's claudication threshold and other cardiovascular limitations for adjustment of workload. During this supervised rehabilitation program, the development of new arrhythmias, symptoms that might suggest angina or the continued inability of the patient to progress to an adequate level of exercise may require physician review and examination of the patient. These physician services would be separately reported with an appropriate level E/M service code.

93668 Peripheral arterial disease (PAD) rehabilitation, per session

Other Vascular Studies

(For arterial cannulization and recording of direct arterial pressure, use 36620)

(For radiographic injection procedures, see 36000-36299)

(For vascular cannulization for hemodialysis, see 36800-36821)

(For chemotherapy for malignant disease, see 96408-96549)

(For penile plethysmography, use 54240)

93701 Bioimpedance, thoracic, electrical

93720 Plethysmography, total body; with interpretation and report

93721 tracing only, without interpretation and report

93722 interpretation and report only

(For regional plethysmography, see 93875-93931)

93724 Electronic analysis of antitachycardia pacemaker system (includes electrocardiographic recording, programming of device, induction and termination of tachycardia via implanted pacemaker, and interpretation of recordings)

93727 Electronic analysis of implantable loop recorder (ILR) system (includes retrieval of recorded and stored ECG data, physician review and interpretation of retrieved ECG data and reprogramming)

93731 Electronic analysis of dual-chamber pacemaker system (includes evaluation of programmable parameters at rest and during activity where applicable, using electrocardiographic recording and interpretation of recordings at rest and during exercise, analysis of event markers and device response); without reprogramming

93732 with reprogramming

93733 Electronic analysis of dual chamber internal pacemaker system (may include rate, pulse amplitude and duration, configuration of wave form, and/or testing of sensory function of pacemaker), telephonic analysis

93734 Electronic analysis of single chamber pacemaker system (includes evaluation of programmable parameters at rest and during activity where applicable, using electrocardiographic recording and interpretation of recordings at rest and during exercise, analysis of event markers and device response); without reprogramming

93735 with reprogramming

93736 Electronic analysis of single chamber internal pacemaker system (may include rate, pulse amplitude and duration, configuration of wave form, and/or testing of sensory function of pacemaker), telephonic analysis

93740 Temperature gradient studies

▲ **93741** Electronic analysis of pacing cardioverter-defibrillator (includes interrogation, evaluation of pulse generator status, evaluation of programmable parameters at rest and during activity where applicable, using electrocardiographic recording and interpretation of recordings at rest and during exercise, analysis of event markers and device response); single chamber or wearable cardioverter-defibrillator system, without reprogramming

►(Do not report 93741 in conjunction with 93745)◄

▲ **93742** single chamber or wearable cardioverter-defibrillator system, with reprogramming

►(Do not report 93742 in conjunction with 93745)◄

93743 dual chamber, without reprogramming

93744 dual chamber, with reprogramming

● **93745** Initial set-up and programming by a physician of wearable cardioverter-defibrillator includes initial programming of system, establishing baseline electronic ECG, transmission of data to data repository, patient instruction in wearing system and patient reporting of problems or events

►(Do not report 93745 in conjunction with 93741, 93742)◄

93760 Thermogram; cephalic

93762 peripheral

93770 Determination of venous pressure

(For central venous cannulization see 36555-36556, 36500)

93784 Ambulatory blood pressure monitoring, utilizing a system such as magnetic tape and/or computer disk, for 24 hours or longer; including recording, scanning analysis, interpretation and report

93786 recording only

93788 scanning analysis with report

93790 physician review with interpretation and report

Other Procedures

93797 Physician services for outpatient cardiac rehabilitation; without continuous ECG monitoring (per session)

93798 with continuous ECG monitoring (per session)

93799 Unlisted cardiovascular service or procedure

Non-Invasive Vascular Diagnostic Studies

Vascular studies include patient care required to perform the studies, supervision of the studies and interpretation of study results with copies for patient records of hard copy output with analysis of all data, including bidirectional vascular flow or imaging when provided.

The use of a simple hand-held or other Doppler device that does not produce hard copy output, or that produces a record that does not permit analysis of bidirectional vascular flow, is considered to be part of the physical examination of the vascular system and is not separately reported.

Duplex scan (eg, 93880, 93882) describes an ultrasonic scanning procedure for characterizing the pattern and direction of blood flow in arteries or veins with the production of real time images integrating B-mode two-dimensional vascular structure with spectral and/or color flow Doppler mapping or imaging.

Non-invasive physiologic studies are performed using equipment separate and distinct from the duplex scanner. Codes 93875, 93965, 93922, 93923, and 93924 describe the evaluation of non-imaging physiologic recordings of pressures, Doppler analysis of bi-directional blood flow, plethysmography, and/or oxygen tension measurements appropriate for the anatomic area studied.

Cerebrovascular Arterial Studies

►A complete transcranial Doppler (TCD) study (93886) includes ultrasound evaluation of the right and left anterior circulation territories and the posterior circulation territory (to include vertebral arteries and basilar artery). In a limited TCD study (93888) there is ultrasound evaluation of two or fewer of these territories. For TCD, ultrasound evaluation is a reasonable and concerted attempt to identify arterial signals through an acoustic window.◄

93875 Non-invasive physiologic studies of extracranial arteries, complete bilateral study (eg, periorbital flow direction with arterial compression, ocular pneumoplethysmography, Doppler ultrasound spectral analysis)

93880 Duplex scan of extracranial arteries; complete bilateral study

93882 unilateral or limited study

93886 Transcranial Doppler study of the intracranial arteries; complete study

93888 limited study

● **93890** vasoreactivity study

● **93892** emboli detection without intravenous microbubble injection

● **93893** emboli detection with intravenous microbubble injection

►(Do not report 93890-93893 in conjunction with 93888)◄

Extremity Arterial Studies (Including Digits)

93922 Non-invasive physiologic studies of upper or lower extremity arteries, single level, bilateral (eg, ankle/brachial indices, Doppler waveform analysis, volume plethysmography, transcutaneous oxygen tension measurement)

93923 Non-invasive physiologic studies of upper or lower extremity arteries, multiple levels or with provocative functional maneuvers, complete bilateral study (eg, segmental blood pressure measurements, segmental Doppler waveform analysis, segmental volume plethysmography, segmental transcutaneous oxygen tension measurements, measurements with postural provocative tests, measurements with reactive hyperemia)

93924 Non-invasive physiologic studies of lower extremity arteries, at rest and following treadmill stress testing, complete bilateral study

93925 Duplex scan of lower extremity arteries or arterial bypass grafts; complete bilateral study

93926 unilateral or limited study

Medicine

93930 Duplex scan of upper extremity arteries or arterial bypass grafts; complete bilateral study

93931 unilateral or limited study

Extremity Venous Studies (Including Digits)

93965 Non-invasive physiologic studies of extremity veins, complete bilateral study (eg, Doppler waveform analysis with responses to compression and other maneuvers, phleborheography, impedance plethysmography)

93970 Duplex scan of extremity veins including responses to compression and other maneuvers; complete bilateral study

93971 unilateral or limited study

Visceral and Penile Vascular Studies

93975 Duplex scan of arterial inflow and venous outflow of abdominal, pelvic, scrotal contents and/or retroperitoneal organs; complete study

93976 limited study

93978 Duplex scan of aorta, inferior vena cava, iliac vasculature, or bypass grafts; complete study

93979 unilateral or limited study

93980 Duplex scan of arterial inflow and venous outflow of penile vessels; complete study

93981 follow-up or limited study

Extremity Arterial-Venous Studies

93990 Duplex scan of hemodialysis access (including arterial inflow, body of access and venous outflow)

(For measurement of hemodialysis access flow using indicator dilution methods, use 90940)

Pulmonary

Codes 94010-94799 include laboratory procedure(s) and interpretation of test results. If a separate identifiable Evaluation and Management service is performed, the appropriate E/M service code should be reported in addition to 94010-94799.

94010 Spirometry, including graphic record, total and timed vital capacity, expiratory flow rate measurement(s), with or without maximal voluntary ventilation

94014 Patient-initiated spirometric recording per 30-day period of time; includes reinforced education, transmission of spirometric tracing, data capture, analysis of transmitted data, periodic recalibration and physician review and interpretation

94015 recording (includes hook-up, reinforced education, data transmission, data capture, trend analysis, and periodic recalibration)

94016 physician review and interpretation only

▲ **94060** Bronchodilation responsiveness, spirometry as in 94010, pre- and post-bronchodilator administration

►(Report bronchodilator supply separately with 99070 or appropriate supply code)◄

(For prolonged exercise test for bronchospasm with pre- and post-spirometry, use 94620)

▲ **94070** Bronchospasm provocation evaluation, multiple spirometric determinations as in 94010, with administered agents (eg, antigen(s), cold air, methacholine)

►(Report antigen(s) administration separately with 99070 or appropriate supply code)◄

94150 Vital capacity, total (separate procedure)

94200 Maximum breathing capacity, maximal voluntary ventilation

94240 Functional residual capacity or residual volume: helium method, nitrogen open circuit method, or other method

94250 Expired gas collection, quantitative, single procedure (separate procedure)

94260 Thoracic gas volume

(For plethysmography, see 93720-93722)

94350 Determination of maldistribution of inspired gas: multiple breath nitrogen washout curve including alveolar nitrogen or helium equilibration time

94360 Determination of resistance to airflow, oscillatory or plethysmographic methods

94370 Determination of airway closing volume, single breath tests

94375 Respiratory flow volume loop

94400 Breathing response to CO_2 (CO_2 response curve)

94450 Breathing response to hypoxia (hypoxia response curve)

►(For high altitude simulation test (HAST), see 94452, 94453)◄

● **94452** High altitude simulation test (HAST), with physician interpretation and report;

►(For obtaining arterial blood gases, use 36600)◄

►(Do not report 94452 in conjunction with 94453, 94760, 94761)◄

● **94453** with supplemental oxygen titration

►(For obtaining arterial blood gases, use 36600)◄

►(Do not report 94453 in conjunction with 94452, 94760, 94761)◄

Medicine

94620   Pulmonary stress testing; simple (eg, prolonged exercise test for bronchospasm with pre- and post-spirometry)

94621   complex (including measurements of CO_2 production, O_2 uptake, and electrocardiographic recordings)

94640   Pressurized or nonpressurized inhalation treatment for acute airway obstruction or for sputum induction for diagnostic purposes (eg, with an aerosol generator, nebulizer, metered dose inhaler or intermittent positive pressure breathing (IPPB) device)

(For more than one inhalation treatment performed on the same date, append modifier 76)

94642   Aerosol inhalation of pentamidine for pneumocystis carinii pneumonia treatment or prophylaxis

(94650, 94651, 94652 have been deleted)

94656   Ventilation assist and management, initiation of pressure or volume preset ventilators for assisted or controlled breathing; first day

94657   subsequent days

94660   Continuous positive airway pressure ventilation (CPAP), initiation and management

94662   Continuous negative pressure ventilation (CNP), initiation and management

94664   Demonstration and/or evaluation of patient utilization of an aerosol generator, nebulizer, metered dose inhaler or IPPB device

(94664 can be reported one time only per day of service)

(94665 has been deleted)

94667   Manipulation chest wall, such as cupping, percussing, and vibration to facilitate lung function; initial demonstration and/or evaluation

94668   subsequent

94680   Oxygen uptake, expired gas analysis; rest and exercise, direct, simple

94681   including CO_2 output, percentage oxygen extracted

94690   rest, indirect (separate procedure)

(For single arterial puncture, use 36600)

94720   Carbon monoxide diffusing capacity (eg, single breath, steady state)

94725   Membrane diffusion capacity

94750   Pulmonary compliance study (eg, plethysmography, volume and pressure measurements)

94760   Noninvasive ear or pulse oximetry for oxygen saturation; single determination

(For blood gases, see 82803-82810)

94761   multiple determinations (eg, during exercise)

94762   by continuous overnight monitoring (separate procedure)

94770   Carbon dioxide, expired gas determination by infrared analyzer

(For bronchoscopy, see 31622-31656)

(For placement of flow directed catheter, use 93503)

(For venipuncture, use 36410)

(For central venous catheter placement, see 36555-36556)

(For arterial puncture, use 36600)

(For arterial catheterization, use 36620)

(For thoracentesis, use 32000)

(For phlebotomy, therapeutic, use 99195)

(For lung biopsy, needle, use 32405)

(For intubation, orotracheal or nasotracheal, use 31500)

94772   Circadian respiratory pattern recording (pediatric pneumogram), 12 to 24 hour continuous recording, infant

(Separate procedure codes for electromyograms, EEG, ECG, and recordings of respiration are excluded when 94772 is reported)

94799   Unlisted pulmonary service or procedure

Allergy and Clinical Immunology

Definitions

Allergy sensitivity tests describe the performance and evaluation of selective cutaneous and mucous membrane tests in correlation with the history, physical examination, and other observations of the patient. The number of tests performed should be judicious and dependent upon the history, physical findings, and clinical judgment. All patients should not necessarily receive the same tests nor the same number of sensitivity tests.

Immunotherapy (desensitization, hyposensitization) is the parenteral administration of allergenic extracts as antigens at periodic intervals, usually on an increasing dosage scale to a dosage which is maintained as maintenance therapy. Indications for immunotherapy are determined by appropriate diagnostic procedures coordinated with clinical judgment and knowledge of the natural history of allergic diseases.

Other therapy: for medical conferences on the use of mechanical and electronic devices (precipitators, air conditioners, air filters, humidifiers, dehumidifiers), climatotherapy, physical therapy, occupational and recreational therapy, see **Evaluation and Management** section.

Medicine

Allergy Testing

95004   Percutaneous tests (scratch, puncture, prick) with allergenic extracts, immediate type reaction, specify number of tests

95010   Percutaneous tests (scratch, puncture, prick) sequential and incremental, with drugs, biologicals or venoms, immediate type reaction, specify number of tests

95015   Intracutaneous (intradermal) tests, sequential and incremental, with drugs, biologicals, or venoms, immediate type reaction, specify number of tests

95024   Intracutaneous (intradermal) tests with allergenic extracts, immediate type reaction, specify number of tests

95027   Intracutaneous (intradermal) tests, sequential and incremental, with allergenic extracts for airborne allergens, immediate type reaction, specify number of tests

95028   Intracutaneous (intradermal) tests with allergenic extracts, delayed type reaction, including reading, specify number of tests

95044   Patch or application test(s) (specify number of tests)

95052   Photo patch test(s) (specify number of tests)

95056   Photo tests

95060   Ophthalmic mucous membrane tests

95065   Direct nasal mucous membrane test

95070   Inhalation bronchial challenge testing (not including necessary pulmonary function tests); with histamine, methacholine, or similar compounds

95071   with antigens or gases, specify

(For pulmonary function tests, see 94060, 94070)

95075   Ingestion challenge test (sequential and incremental ingestion of test items, eg, food, drug or other substance such as metabisulfite)

95078   Provocative testing (eg, Rinkel test)

(For allergy laboratory tests, see 86000-86999)

(For intravenous therapy for severe or intractable allergic disease, see 90780, 90781, 90784)

Allergen Immunotherapy

Codes 95115-95199 include the professional services necessary for allergen immunotherapy. Office visit codes may be used in addition to allergen immunotherapy if other identifiable services are provided at that time.

95115   Professional services for allergen immunotherapy not including provision of allergenic extracts; single injection

95117   two or more injections

95120   Professional services for allergen immunotherapy in prescribing physicians office or institution, including provision of allergenic extract; single injection

95125   two or more injections

95130   single stinging insect venom

95131   two stinging insect venoms

95132   three stinging insect venoms

95133   four stinging insect venoms

95134   five stinging insect venoms

95144   Professional services for the supervision of preparation and provision of antigens for allergen immunotherapy, single dose vial(s) (specify number of vials)

(A single dose vial contains a single dose of antigen administered in one injection)

95145   Professional services for the supervision of preparation and provision of antigens for allergen immunotherapy (specify number of doses); single stinging insect venom

95146   two single stinging insect venoms

95147   three single stinging insect venoms

95148   four single stinging insect venoms

95149   five single stinging insect venoms

95165   Professional services for the supervision of preparation and provision of antigens for allergen immunotherapy; single or multiple antigens (specify number of doses)

95170   whole body extract of biting insect or other arthropod (specify number of doses)

(For allergy immunotherapy reporting, a dose is the amount of antigen(s) administered in a single injection from a multiple dose vial)

95180   Rapid desensitization procedure, each hour (eg, insulin, penicillin, equine serum)

95199   Unlisted allergy/clinical immunologic service or procedure

(For skin testing of bacterial, viral, fungal extracts, see 95028, 86485-86586)

(For special reports on allergy patients, use 99080)

(For testing procedures such as radioallergosorbent testing (RAST), rat mast cell technique (RMCT), mast cell degranulation test (MCDT), lymphocytic transformation test (LTT), leukocyte histamine release (LHR), migration inhibitory factor test (MIF), transfer factor test (TFT), nitroblue tetrazolium dye test (NTD), see Immunology section in **Pathology** or use 95199)

Endocrinology

95250   Glucose monitoring for up to 72 hours by continuous recording and storage of glucose values from interstitial tissue fluid via a subcutaneous sensor (includes hook-up, calibration, patient initiation and training, recording, disconnection, downloading with printout of data)

(Do not report 95250 in conjunction with 99091)

(To report physician review, interpretation and written report associated with code 95250, see **Evaluation and Management** services codes)

Neurology and Neuromuscular Procedures

Neurologic services are typically consultative, and any of the levels of consultation (99241-99263) may be appropriate.

In addition, services and skills outlined under **Evaluation and Management** levels of service appropriate to neurologic illnesses should be reported similarly.

The EEG, autonomic function, evoked potential, ▶reflex tests, EMG, NCV, and MEG◀ services (95812-95829 and ▶95860-95967◀) include recording, interpretation by a physician, and report. For interpretation only, use modifier 26.

(For repetitive transcranial magnetic stimulation for treatment of clinical depression, use Category III code 0018T)

(Do not report codes 95860-95875 in addition to 96000-96004)

Sleep Testing

Sleep studies and polysomnography refer to the continuous and simultaneous monitoring and recording of various physiological and pathophysiological parameters of sleep for 6 or more hours with physician review, interpretation and report. The studies are performed to diagnose a variety of sleep disorders and to evaluate a patient's response to therapies such as nasal continuous positive airway pressure (NCPAP). Polysomnography is distinguished from sleep studies by the inclusion of sleep staging which is defined to include a 1-4 lead electroencephalogram (EEG), an electro-oculogram (EOG), and a submental electromyogram (EMG). Additional parameters of sleep include: 1) ECG; 2) airflow; 3) ventilation and respiratory effort; 4) gas exchange by oximetry, transcutaneous monitoring, or end tidal gas analysis; 5) extremity muscle activity, motor activity-movement; 6) extended EEG monitoring; 7) penile tumescence; 8) gastroesophageal reflux; 9) continuous blood pressure monitoring; 10) snoring; 11) body positions; etc.

The sleep services (95805-95811) include recording, interpretation and report. For interpretation only, use modifier 26.

For a study to be reported as polysomnography, sleep must be recorded and staged.

(Report with modifier 52 if less than 6 hours of recording or in other cases of reduced services as appropriate)

(For unattended sleep study, use 95806)

95805   Multiple sleep latency or maintenance of wakefulness testing, recording, analysis and interpretation of physiological measurements of sleep during multiple trials to assess sleepiness

95806   Sleep study, simultaneous recording of ventilation, respiratory effort, ECG or heart rate, and oxygen saturation, unattended by a technologist

95807   Sleep study, simultaneous recording of ventilation, respiratory effort, ECG or heart rate, and oxygen saturation, attended by a technologist

95808   Polysomnography; sleep staging with 1-3 additional parameters of sleep, attended by a technologist

95810   sleep staging with 4 or more additional parameters of sleep, attended by a technologist

95811   sleep staging with 4 or more additional parameters of sleep, with initiation of continuous positive airway pressure therapy or bilevel ventilation, attended by a technologist

Routine Electroencephalography (EEG)

EEG codes 95812-95822 include hyperventilation and/or photic stimulation when appropriate. Routine EEG codes 95816-95822 include 20 to 40 minutes of recording. Extended EEG codes 95812-95813 include reporting times longer than 40 minutes.

95812   Electroencephalogram (EEG) extended monitoring; 41-60 minutes

95813   greater than one hour

95816   Electroencephalogram (EEG); including recording awake and drowsy

95819   including recording awake and asleep

95822   recording in coma or sleep only

95824   cerebral death evaluation only

95827   all night recording

(For 24-hour EEG monitoring, see 95950-95953 or 95956)

(For EEG during nonintracranial surgery, use 95955)

(For Wada test, use 95958)

(For digital analysis of EEG, use 95957)

Medicine

95829   Electrocorticogram at surgery (separate procedure)

95830   Insertion by physician of sphenoidal electrodes for electroencephalographic (EEG) recording

Muscle and Range of Motion Testing

95831   Muscle testing, manual (separate procedure) with report; extremity (excluding hand) or trunk

95832   hand, with or without comparison with normal side

95833   total evaluation of body, excluding hands

95834   total evaluation of body, including hands

95851   Range of motion measurements and report (separate procedure); each extremity (excluding hand) or each trunk section (spine)

95852   hand, with or without comparison with normal side

95857   Tensilon test for myasthenia gravis;

95858   with electromyographic recording

Electromyography and Nerve Conduction Tests

95860   Needle electromyography; one extremity with or without related paraspinal areas

95861   two extremities with or without related paraspinal areas

(For dynamic electromyography performed during motion analysis studies, see 96002-96003)

95863   three extremities with or without related paraspinal areas

95864   four extremities with or without related paraspinal areas

95867   cranial nerve supplied muscle(s), unilateral

95868   cranial nerve supplied muscles, bilateral

95869   thoracic paraspinal muscles (excluding T1 or T12)

95870   limited study of muscles in one extremity or non-limb (axial) muscles (unilateral or bilateral), other than thoracic paraspinal, cranial nerve supplied muscles, or sphincters

(To report a complete study of the extremities, see 95860-95864)

(For anal or urethral sphincter, detrusor, urethra, perineum musculature, see 51785-51792)

(For eye muscles, use 92265)

95872   Needle electromyography using single fiber electrode, with quantitative measurement of jitter, blocking and/or fiber density, any/all sites of each muscle studied

95875   Ischemic limb exercise test with serial specimen(s) acquisition for muscle(s) metabolite(s)

⊘ **95900**   Nerve conduction, amplitude and latency/velocity study, each nerve; motor, without F-wave study

⊘ **95903**   motor, with F-wave study

⊘ **95904**   sensory

(Report 95900, 95903, and/or 95904 only once when multiple sites on the same nerve are stimulated or recorded)

Intraoperative Neurophysiology

+ **95920**   Intraoperative neurophysiology testing, per hour (List separately in addition to code for primary procedure)

(Use 95920 in conjunction with the study performed, 92585, 95822, 95860, 95861, 95867, 95868, ▶95870,◀ 95900, 95904, 95925▶-◀95937.)

(Code 95920 describes ongoing electrophysiologic testing and monitoring performed during surgical procedures. Code 95920 is reported per hour of service, and includes only the ongoing electrophysiologic monitoring time distinct from performance of specific type(s) of baseline electrophysiologic study(s) (95860, 95861, 95867, 95868, ▶95870,◀ 95900, 95904, ▶95928, 95929,◀ 95933▶-◀95937) or interpretation of specific type(s) of baseline electrophysiologic study(s) (92585, 95822, ▶95870, 95925-95928, 95929, 95930◀). The time spent performing or interpreting the baseline electrophysiologic study(s) should not be counted as intraoperative monitoring, but represents separately reportable procedures. Code 95920 should be used once per hour even if multiple electrophysiologic studies are performed. The baseline electrophysiologic study(s) should be used once per operative session.)

(For electrocorticography, use 95829)

(For intraoperative EEG during nonintracranial surgery, use 95955)

(For intraoperative functional cortical or subcortical mapping, see 95961-95962)

(For intraoperative neurostimulator programming and analysis, see 95970-95975)

Autonomic Function Tests

95921   Testing of autonomic nervous system function; cardiovagal innervation (parasympathetic function), including two or more of the following: heart rate response to deep breathing with recorded R-R interval, Valsalva ratio, and 30:15 ratio

95922   vasomotor adrenergic innervation (sympathetic adrenergic function), including beat-to-beat blood pressure and R-R interval changes during Valsalva maneuver and at least five minutes of passive tilt

95923   sudomotor, including one or more of the following: quantitative sudomotor axon reflex test (QSART), silastic sweat imprint, thermoregulatory sweat test, and changes in sympathetic skin potential

Medicine

Evoked Potentials and Reflex Tests

95925   Short-latency somatosensory evoked potential study, stimulation of any/all peripheral nerves or skin sites, recording from the central nervous system; in upper limbs

95926   in lower limbs

95927   in the trunk or head

(To report a unilateral study, use modifier 52)

(For auditory evoked potentials, use 92585)

● **95928**   Central motor evoked potential study (transcranial motor stimulation); upper limbs

● **95929**   lower limbs

95930   Visual evoked potential (VEP) testing central nervous system, checkerboard or flash

95933   Orbicularis oculi (blink) reflex, by electrodiagnostic testing

95934   H-reflex, amplitude and latency study; record gastrocnemius/soleus muscle

95936   record muscle other than gastrocnemius/soleus muscle

(To report a bilateral study, use modifier 50)

95937   Neuromuscular junction testing (repetitive stimulation, paired stimuli), each nerve, any one method

Special EEG Tests

95950   Monitoring for identification and lateralization of cerebral seizure focus, electroencephalographic (eg, 8 channel EEG) recording and interpretation, each 24 hours

95951   Monitoring for localization of cerebral seizure focus by cable or radio, 16 or more channel telemetry, combined electroencephalographic (EEG) and video recording and interpretation (eg, for presurgical localization), each 24 hours

95953   Monitoring for localization of cerebral seizure focus by computerized portable 16 or more channel EEG, electroencephalographic (EEG) recording and interpretation, each 24 hours

95954   Pharmacological or physical activation requiring physician attendance during EEG recording of activation phase (eg, thiopental activation test)

95955   Electroencephalogram (EEG) during nonintracranial surgery (eg, carotid surgery)

95956   Monitoring for localization of cerebral seizure focus by cable or radio, 16 or more channel telemetry, electroencephalographic (EEG) recording and interpretation, each 24 hours

95957   Digital analysis of electroencephalogram (EEG) (eg, for epileptic spike analysis)

95958   Wada activation test for hemispheric function, including electroencephalographic (EEG) monitoring

95961   Functional cortical and subcortical mapping by stimulation and/or recording of electrodes on brain surface, or of depth electrodes, to provoke seizures or identify vital brain structures; initial hour of physician attendance

+ **95962**   each additional hour of physician attendance (List separately in addition to code for primary procedure)

(Use 95962 in conjunction with 95961)

95965   Magnetoencephalography (MEG), recording and analysis; for spontaneous brain magnetic activity (eg, epileptic cerebral cortex localization)

95966   for evoked magnetic fields, single modality (eg, sensory, motor, language, or visual cortex localization)

+ **95967**   for evoked magnetic fields, each additional modality (eg, sensory, motor, language, or visual cortex localization) (List separately in addition to code for primary procedure)

(Use 95967 in conjunction with 95966)

(For electroencephalography performed in addition to magnetoencephalography, see 95812-95827)

(For somatosensory evoked potentials, auditory evoked potentials, and visual evoked potentials performed in addition to magnetic evoked field responses, see 92585, 95925, 95926, and/or 95930)

(For computerized tomography performed in addition to magnetoencephalography, see 70450-70470, 70496)

(For magnetic resonance imaging performed in addition to magnetoencephalography, see 70551-70553)

Neurostimulators, Analysis-Programming

A simple neurostimulator pulse generator/transmitter (95970, 95971) is one capable of affecting 3 or fewer of the following: pulse amplitude, pulse duration, pulse frequency, 8 or more electrode contacts, cycling, stimulation train duration, train spacing, number of programs, number of channels, alternating electrode polarities, dose time (stimulation parameters changing in time periods of minutes including dose lockout times), more than 1 clinical feature (eg, rigidity, dyskinesia, tremor). A complex neurostimulator pulse generator/transmitter (95970-95975) is one capable of affecting more than 3 of the above.

Code 95970 describes subsequent electronic analysis of a previously-implanted simple or complex brain, spinal cord, or peripheral neurostimulator pulse generator system, without reprogramming. Code 95971 describes intraoperative or subsequent electronic analysis of an implanted simple spinal cord or peripheral (ie, peripheral nerve, autonomic nerve, neuromuscular) neurostimulator pulse generator system, with programming. Codes 95972

Medicine

and 95973 describe intraoperative (at initial insertion/revision) or subsequent electronic analysis of an implanted complex spinal cord or peripheral (except cranial nerve) neurostimulator pulse generator system, with programming. Codes 95974 and 95975 describe intraoperative (at initial insertion/revision) or subsequent electronic analysis of an implanted complex cranial nerve neurostimulator pulse generator system, with programming. ►Codes 95978 and 95979 describe initial or subsequent electronic analysis of an implanted brain neurostimulator pulse generator system, with programming.◄

(For insertion of neurostimulator pulse generator, see 61885, 63685, 63688, 64590)

(For revision or removal of neurostimulator pulse generator or receiver, see 61888, 63688, 64595)

(For implantation of neurostimulator electrodes, see 61850-61875, 63650-63655, 64553-64580. For revision or removal of neurostimulator electrodes, see 61880, 63660, 64585)

95970 Electronic analysis of implanted neurostimulator pulse generator system (eg, rate, pulse amplitude and duration, configuration of wave form, battery status, electrode selectability, output modulation, cycling, impedance and patient compliance measurements); simple or complex brain, spinal cord, or peripheral (ie, cranial nerve, peripheral nerve, autonomic nerve, neuromuscular) neurostimulator pulse generator/transmitter, without reprogramming

▲ **95971** simple spinal cord, or peripheral (ie, peripheral nerve, autonomic nerve, neuromuscular) neurostimulator pulse generator/transmitter, with intraoperative or subsequent programming

▲ **95972** complex spinal cord, or peripheral (except cranial nerve) neurostimulator pulse generator/transmitter, with intraoperative or subsequent programming, first hour

+▲ **95973** complex spinal cord, or peripheral (except cranial nerve) neurostimulator pulse generator/transmitter, with intraoperative or subsequent programming, each additional 30 minutes after first hour (List separately in addition to code for primary procedure)

(Use 95973 in conjunction with 95972)

95974 complex cranial nerve neurostimulator pulse generator/transmitter, with intraoperative or subsequent programming, with or without nerve interface testing, first hour

+ **95975** complex cranial nerve neurostimulator pulse generator/transmitter, with intraoperative or subsequent programming, each additional 30 minutes after first hour (List separately in addition to code for primary procedure)

(Use 95975 in conjunction with 95974)

● **95978** Electronic analysis of implanted neurostimulator pulse generator system (eg, rate, pulse amplitude and duration, battery status, electrode selectability and polarity, impedance and patient compliance measurements), complex deep brain neurostimulator pulse generator/transmitter, with initial or subsequent programming; first hour

+● **95979** each additional 30 minutes after first hour (List separately in addition to code for primary procedure)

►(Use 95979 in conjunction with 95978)◄

Other Procedures

95990 Refilling and maintenance of implantable pump or reservoir for drug delivery, spinal (intrathecal, epidural) or brain (intraventricular);

(For analysis and/or reprogramming of implantable infusion pump, see 62367-62368)

(For refill and maintenance of implanted infusion pump or reservoir for systemic drug therapy (eg, chemotherapy or insulin, use 96530)

95991 administered by physician

95999 Unlisted neurological or neuromuscular diagnostic procedure

Motion Analysis

Codes 96000-96004 describe services performed as part of a major therapeutic or diagnostic decision making process. Motion analysis is performed in a dedicated motion analysis laboratory (ie, a facility capable of performing videotaping from the front, back and both sides, computerized 3-D kinematics, 3-D kinetics, and dynamic electromyography). Code 96000 may include 3-D kinetics and stride characteristics. Codes 96002-96003 describe dynamic electromyography.

Code 96004 should only be reported once regardless of the number of study(ies) reviewed/interpreted.

(For performance of needle electromyography procedures, see 95860-95875)

(For gait training, use 97116)

96000 Comprehensive computer-based motion analysis by video-taping and 3-D kinematics;

96001 with dynamic plantar pressure measurements during walking

96002 Dynamic surface electromyography, during walking or other functional activities, 1-12 muscles

96003 Dynamic fine wire electromyography, during walking or other functional activities, 1 muscle

(Do not report 96002, 96003 in conjunction with 95860-►95864, 95869-95872◄)

Medicine

96004   Physician review and interpretation of comprehensive computer based motion analysis, dynamic plantar pressure measurements, dynamic surface electromyography during walking or other functional activities, and dynamic fine wire electromyography, with written report

Central Nervous System Assessments/Tests (eg, Neuro-Cognitive, Mental Status, Speech Testing)

The following codes are used to report the services provided during testing of the cognitive function of the central nervous system. The testing of cognitive processes, visual motor responses, and abstractive abilities is accomplished by the combination of several types of testing procedures. It is expected that the administration of these tests will generate material that will be formulated into a report.

(For development of cognitive skills, see 97532, 97533)

96100   Psychological testing (includes psychodiagnostic assessment of personality, psychopathology, emotionality, intellectual abilities, eg, WAIS-R, Rorschach, MMPI) with interpretation and report, per hour

96105   Assessment of aphasia (includes assessment of expressive and receptive speech and language function, language comprehension, speech production ability, reading, spelling, writing, eg, by Boston Diagnostic Aphasia Examination) with interpretation and report, per hour

96110   Developmental testing; limited (eg, Developmental Screening Test II, Early Language Milestone Screen), with interpretation and report

▲ 96111   extended (includes assessment of motor, language, social, adaptive and/or cognitive functioning by standardized developmental instruments) with interpretation and report

96115   Neurobehavioral status exam (clinical assessment of thinking, reasoning and judgment, eg, acquired knowledge, attention, memory, visual spatial abilities, language functions, planning) with interpretation and report, per hour

(For mini-mental status examination performed by a physician, see **Evaluation and Management** services codes)

96117   Neuropsychological testing battery (eg, Halstead-Reitan, Luria, WAIS-R) with interpretation and report, per hour

Health and Behavior Assessment/Intervention

Health and behavior assessment procedures are used to identify the psychological, behavioral, emotional, cognitive, and social factors important to the prevention, treatment, or management of physical health problems.

The focus of the assessment is not on mental health but on the biopsychosocial factors important to physical health problems and treatments. The focus of the intervention is to improve the patient's health and well-being utilizing cognitive, behavioral, social, and/or psychophysiological procedures designed to ameliorate specific disease-related problems.

Codes 96150-96155 describe services offered to patients who present with established illnesses or symptoms, who are not diagnosed with mental illness, and may benefit from evaluations that focus on the biopsychosocial factors related to the patient's physical health status. These services do not represent preventive medicine counseling and risk factor reduction interventions.

For patients that require psychiatric services (90801-90899) as well as health and behavior assessment/intervention (96150-96155), report the predominant service performed. Do not report 96150-96155 in conjunction with 90801-90899 on the same date.

Evaluation and Management services codes (including **Preventive Medicine, Individual Counseling** codes 99401-99404, and **Preventive Medicine, Group Counseling** codes 99411-99412), should not be reported on the same day.

(For health and behavior assessment and/or intervention performed by a physician, see **Evaluation and Management** or **Preventive Medicine** services codes)

96150   Health and behavior assessment (eg, health-focused clinical interview, behavioral observations, psychophysiological monitoring, health-oriented questionnaires), each 15 minutes face-to-face with the patient; initial assessment

96151   re-assessment

96152   Health and behavior intervention, each 15 minutes, face-to-face; individual

96153   group (2 or more patients)

96154   family (with the patient present)

96155   family (without the patient present)

Medicine

Chemotherapy Administration

Codes 96400-96549 are independent of the patient's visit.

If a significant separately identifiable Evaluation and Management service is performed, the appropriate E/M service code should be reported in addition to 96400-96549.

Either may occur independently on any date of service, or they may occur sequentially on the same day.

Preparation of chemotherapy agent(s) is included in the service for administration of the agent.

Regional (isolation) chemotherapy perfusion should be reported using the codes for arterial infusion (96420-96425). Placement of the intra-arterial catheter should be reported using the appropriate code from the **Cardiovascular Surgery** section. Placement of arterial and venous cannula(s) for extracorporeal circulation via a membrane oxygenator perfusion pump should be reported using 36823. Code 36823 includes dose calculation and administration of the chemotherapy agent by injection into the perfusate. Do not report 96408-96425 in conjunction with 36823.

Report separate codes for each parenteral method of administration employed when chemotherapy is administered by different techniques. Medications (eg, antibiotics, steroidal agents, antiemetics, narcotics, analgesics, biological agents) administered independently or sequentially as supportive management of chemotherapy administration, should be separately reported using 90780-90788, as appropriate.

96400   Chemotherapy administration, subcutaneous or intramuscular, with or without local anesthesia

96405   Chemotherapy administration, intralesional; up to and including 7 lesions

96406   more than 7 lesions

96408   Chemotherapy administration, intravenous; push technique

96410   infusion technique, up to one hour

+ 96412   infusion technique, one to 8 hours, each additional hour (List separately in addition to code for primary procedure)

(Use 96412 in conjunction with 96410)

96414   infusion technique, initiation of prolonged infusion (more than 8 hours), requiring the use of a portable or implantable pump

(For refilling and maintenance of a portable pump or an implantable infusion pump or reservoir for drug delivery, see 96520, 96530)

96420   Chemotherapy administration, intra-arterial; push technique

96422   infusion technique, up to one hour

+ 96423   infusion technique, one to 8 hours, each additional hour (List separately in addition to code for primary procedure)

(Use 96423 in conjunction with 96422)

(For regional chemotherapy perfusion via membrane oxygenator perfusion pump to an extremity, use 36823)

96425   infusion technique, initiation of prolonged infusion (more than 8 hours), requiring the use of a portable or implantable pump

(For refilling and maintenance of a portable pump or an implantable infusion pump or reservoir for drug delivery, see 96520, 96530)

96440   Chemotherapy administration into pleural cavity, requiring and including thoracentesis

96445   Chemotherapy administration into peritoneal cavity, requiring and including peritoneocentesis

96450   Chemotherapy administration, into CNS (eg, intrathecal), requiring and including spinal puncture

(For intravesical (bladder) chemotherapy administration, use 51720)

(For insertion of subarachnoid catheter and reservoir for infusion of drug, see 62350, 62351, 62360-62362; for insertion of intraventricular catheter and reservoir, see 61210, 61215)

96520   Refilling and maintenance of portable pump

96530   Refilling and maintenance of implantable pump or reservoir for drug delivery, systemic (eg, intravenous, intra-arterial)

(For refilling and maintenance of an implantable infusion pump for spinal or brain drug infusion, use 95990)

(For collection of blood specimen from a completely implantable venous access device, use 36540)

96542   Chemotherapy injection, subarachnoid or intraventricular via subcutaneous reservoir, single or multiple agents

96545   Provision of chemotherapy agent

(For radioactive isotope therapy, ►use 79005◄)

96549   Unlisted chemotherapy procedure

Medicine

Photodynamic Therapy

(To report ocular photodynamic therapy, use 67221)

96567   Photodynamic therapy by external application of light to destroy premalignant and/or malignant lesions of the skin and adjacent mucosa (eg, lip) by activation of photosensitive drug(s), each phototherapy exposure session

+ 96570   Photodynamic therapy by endoscopic application of light to ablate abnormal tissue via activation of photosensitive drug(s); first 30 minutes (List separately in addition to code for endoscopy or bronchoscopy procedures of lung and esophagus)

+ 96571   each additional 15 minutes (List separately in addition to code for endoscopy or bronchoscopy procedures of lung and esophagus)

(96570, 96571 are to be used in addition to bronchoscopy, endoscopy codes)

(Use 96570, 96571 in conjunction with 31641, 43228 as appropriate)

Special Dermatological Procedures

Dermatologic services are typically consultative, and any of the five levels of consultation (99241-99263) may be appropriate.

In addition, services and skills outlined under **Evaluation and Management** levels of service appropriate to dermatologic illnesses should be coded similarly.

(For whole body photography, see Category III code 0044T, 0045T)

(For intralesional injections, see 11900, 11901)

(For Tzanck smear, use 87207)

96900   Actinotherapy (ultraviolet light)

96902   Microscopic examination of hairs plucked or clipped by the examiner (excluding hair collected by the patient) to determine telogen and anagen counts, or structural hair shaft abnormality

96910   Photochemotherapy; tar and ultraviolet B (Goeckerman treatment) or petrolatum and ultraviolet B

96912   psoralens and ultraviolet A (PUVA)

96913   Photochemotherapy (Goeckerman and/or PUVA) for severe photoresponsive dermatoses requiring at least four to eight hours of care under direct supervision of the physician (includes application of medication and dressings)

96920   Laser treatment for inflammatory skin disease (psoriasis); total area less than 250 sq cm

96921   250 sq cm to 500 sq cm

96922   over 500 sq cm

96999   Unlisted special dermatological service or procedure

Physical Medicine and Rehabilitation

►Codes 97001-97755 should be used to report each distinct procedure performed. Do not append modifier 51 to 97001-97755.◄

(For muscle testing, range of joint motion, electromyography, see 95831 et seq)

(For biofeedback training by EMG, use 90901)

(For transcutaneous nerve stimulation (TNS), use 64550)

97001   Physical therapy evaluation

97002   Physical therapy re-evaluation

97003   Occupational therapy evaluation

97004   Occupational therapy re-evaluation

97005   Athletic training evaluation

97006   Athletic training re-evaluation

Modalities

Any physical agent applied to produce therapeutic changes to biologic tissue; includes but not limited to thermal, acoustic, light, mechanical, or electric energy.

Supervised

The application of a modality that does not require direct (one-on-one) patient contact by the provider.

97010   Application of a modality to one or more areas; hot or cold packs

97012   traction, mechanical

97014   electrical stimulation (unattended)

(For acupuncture with electrical stimulation, ►see 97813, 97814◄)

97016   vasopneumatic devices

97018   paraffin bath

97020   microwave

97022   whirlpool

97024   diathermy

97026   infrared

97028   ultraviolet

Medicine

▲=Revised Code   ●=New Code   ► ◄=New or Revised Text

Constant Attendance

The application of a modality that requires direct (one-on-one) patient contact by the provider.

97032 Application of a modality to one or more areas; electrical stimulation (manual), each 15 minutes

97033 iontophoresis, each 15 minutes

97034 contrast baths, each 15 minutes

97035 ultrasound, each 15 minutes

97036 Hubbard tank, each 15 minutes

97039 Unlisted modality (specify type and time if constant attendance)

Therapeutic Procedures

A manner of effecting change through the application of clinical skills and/or services that attempt to improve function.

Physician or therapist required to have direct (one-on-one) patient contact.

97110 Therapeutic procedure, one or more areas, each 15 minutes; therapeutic exercises to develop strength and endurance, range of motion and flexibility

97112 neuromuscular reeducation of movement, balance, coordination, kinesthetic sense, posture, and/or proprioception for sitting and/or standing activities

97113 aquatic therapy with therapeutic exercises

97116 gait training (includes stair climbing)

(Use 96000-96003 to report comprehensive gait and motion analysis procedures)

97124 massage, including effleurage, petrissage and/or tapotement (stroking, compression, percussion)

(For myofascial release, use 97140)

97139 Unlisted therapeutic procedure (specify)

97140 Manual therapy techniques (eg, mobilization/manipulation, manual lymphatic drainage, manual traction), one or more regions, each 15 minutes

97150 Therapeutic procedure(s), group (2 or more individuals)

(Report 97150 for each member of group)

(Group therapy procedures involve constant attendance of the physician or therapist, but by definition do not require one-on-one patient contact by the physician or therapist)

(For manipulation under general anesthesia, see appropriate anatomic section in **Musculoskeletal System**)

(For osteopathic manipulative treatment (OMT), see 98925-98929)

97504 Orthotic(s) fitting and training, upper extremity(ies), lower extremity(ies), and/or trunk, each 15 minutes

(Code 97504 should not be reported with 97116)

(For casting and strapping of fracture, injury or dislocation, see 29000, 29590)

97520 Prosthetic training, upper and/or lower extremities, each 15 minutes

97530 Therapeutic activities, direct (one-on-one) patient contact by the provider (use of dynamic activities to improve functional performance), each 15 minutes

97532 Development of cognitive skills to improve attention, memory, problem solving, (includes compensatory training), direct (one-on-one) patient contact by the provider, each 15 minutes

97533 Sensory integrative techniques to enhance sensory processing and promote adaptive responses to environmental demands, direct (one-on-one) patient contact by the provider, each 15 minutes

97535 Self-care/home management training (eg, activities of daily living (ADL) and compensatory training, meal preparation, safety procedures, and instructions in use of assistive technology devices/adaptive equipment) direct one-on-one contact by provider, each 15 minutes

97537 Community/work reintegration training (eg, shopping, transportation, money management, avocational activities and/or work environment/modification analysis, work task analysis, use of assistive technology device/adaptive equipment), direct one-on-one contact by provider, each 15 minutes

(For wheelchair management/propulsion training, use 97542)

97542 Wheelchair management/propulsion training, each 15 minutes

97545 Work hardening/conditioning; initial 2 hours

+ 97546 each additional hour (List separately in addition to code for primary procedure)

(Use 97546 in conjunction with 97545)

Active Wound Care Management

Active wound care procedures are performed to ▶remove devitalized and/or necrotic tissue and◀ promote healing. ▶Provider is required to have direct (one-on-one) patient contact.◀

(Do not report ▶97597◀-97602 in conjunction with 11040-11044)

● **97597** Removal of devitalized tissue from wound(s), selective debridement, without anesthesia (eg, high pressure waterjet with/without suction, sharp selective debridement with scissors, scalpel and forceps), with or without topical application(s), wound assessment, and instruction(s) for ongoing care, may include use of a whirlpool, per session; total wound(s) surface area less than or equal to 20 square centimeters

● **97598**   total wound(s) surface area greater than 20 square centimeters

►(97601 has been deleted. To report, use 97597, 97598)◄

97602   Removal of devitalized tissue from wound(s), non-selective debridement, without anesthesia (eg, wet-to-moist dressings, enzymatic, abrasion), including topical application(s), wound assessment, and instruction(s) for ongoing care, per session

● **97605**   Negative pressure wound therapy (eg, vacuum assisted drainage collection), including topical application(s), wound assessment, and instruction(s) for ongoing care, per session; total wound(s) surface area less than or equal to 50 square centimeters

● **97606**   total wound(s) surface area greater than 50 square centimeters

Tests and Measurements

Requires direct one-on-one patient contact.

(For muscle testing, manual or electrical, joint range of motion, electromyography or nerve velocity determination, see 95831-95904)

97703   Checkout for orthotic/prosthetic use, established patient, each 15 minutes

97750   Physical performance test or measurement (eg, musculoskeletal, functional capacity), with written report, each 15 minutes

97755   Assistive technology assessment (eg, to restore, augment or compensate for existing function, optimize functional tasks and/or maximize environmental accessibility), direct one-on-one contact by provider, with written report, each 15 minutes

(To report augmentative and alternative communication devices, use 92605 or 92607)

Other Procedures

(For extracorporeal shock wave musculoskeletal therapy, use Category III code 0019T)

►(97780 has been deleted. To report, see 97810, 97811)◄

►(97781 has been deleted. To report, see 97813, 97814)◄

97799   Unlisted physical medicine/rehabilitation service or procedure

Medical Nutrition Therapy

97802   Medical nutrition therapy; initial assessment and intervention, individual, face-to-face with the patient, each 15 minutes

97803   re-assessment and intervention, individual, face-to-face with the patient, each 15 minutes

97804   group (2 or more individual(s)), each 30 minutes

(For medical nutrition therapy assessment and/or intervention performed by a physician, see **Evaluation and Management** or **Preventive Medicine** service codes)

►Acupuncture◄

►Acupuncture is reported based on 15 minute increments of personal (face-to-face) contact with the patient, not the duration of acupuncture needle(s) placement.◄

►If no electrical stimulation is used during a 15 minute increment, use 97810, 97811. If electrical stimulation of any needle is used during a 15 minute increment, use 97813, 97814.◄

● **97810**   Acupuncture, one or more needles; without electrical stimulation, initial 15 minutes of personal one-on-one contact with the patient

+● **97811**   each additional 15 minutes of personal one-on-one contact with the patient, with re-insertion of needle(s) (List separately in addition to code for primary procedure)

►(Use 97811 in conjunction with 97810)◄

►(Do not report 97810, 97811 in conjunction with 97813 or 97814)◄

►(Evaluation and Management services may be reported separately, using modifier 25, if the patient's condition requires a significant separately identifiable E/M service, above and beyond the usual preservice and postservice work associated with the acupuncture services. The time of the E/M service is not included in the time of the acupuncture service.)◄

● **97813**   Acupuncture, one or more needles; with electrical stimulation, initial 15 minutes of personal one-on-one contact with the patient

+● **97814**   each additional 15 minutes of personal one-on-one contact with the patient, with re-insertion of needle(s) (List separately in addition to code for primary procedure)

►(Use 97814 in conjunction with 97813)◄

► (Do not report 97813, 97814 in conjunction with 97810 or 97811)◄

Medicine

►(Evaluation and Management services may be reported separately, using modifier 25, if the patient's condition requires a significant separately identifiable E/M service, above and beyond the usual preservice and postservice work associated with the acupuncture services. The time of the E/M service is not included in the time of the acupuncture service.)◄

Osteopathic Manipulative Treatment

Osteopathic manipulative treatment is a form of manual treatment applied by a physician to eliminate or alleviate somatic dysfunction and related disorders. This treatment may be accomplished by a variety of techniques.

Evaluation and Management services may be reported separately if, using modifier 25, the patient's condition requires a significant separately identifiable E/M service, above and beyond the usual preservice and postservice work associated with the procedure. The E/M service may be caused or prompted by the same symptoms or condition for which the OMT service was provided. As such, different diagnoses are not required for the reporting of the OMT and E/M service on the same date.

Body regions referred to are: head region; cervical region; thoracic region; lumbar region; sacral region; pelvic region; lower extremities; upper extremities; rib cage region; abdomen and viscera region.

98925 Osteopathic manipulative treatment (OMT); one to two body regions involved

98926 three to four body regions involved

98927 five to six body regions involved

98928 seven to eight body regions involved

98929 nine to ten body regions involved

Chiropractic Manipulative Treatment

Chiropractic manipulative treatment (CMT) is a form of manual treatment to influence joint and neurophysiological function. This treatment may be accomplished using a variety of techniques.

The chiropractic manipulative treatment codes include a pre-manipulation patient assessment. Additional Evaluation and Management services may be reported separately using modifier 25, if the patient's condition requires a significant separately identifiable E/M service, above and beyond the usual preservice and postservice work associated with the procedure. The E/M service may be caused or prompted by the same symptoms or condition for which the CMT service was provided. As such, different diagnoses are not required for the reporting of the CMT and E/M service on the same date.

For purposes of CMT, the five spinal regions referred to are: cervical region (includes atlanto-occipital joint); thoracic region (includes costovertebral and costotransverse joints); lumbar region; sacral region; and pelvic (sacro-iliac joint) region. The five extraspinal regions referred to are: head (including temporomandibular joint, excluding atlanto-occipital) region; lower extremities; upper extremities; rib cage (excluding costotransverse and costovertebral joints) and abdomen.

98940 Chiropractic manipulative treatment (CMT); spinal, one to two regions

98941 spinal, three to four regions

98942 spinal, five regions

98943 extraspinal, one or more regions

Special Services, Procedures and Reports

The procedures with code numbers 99000 through 99091 provide the reporting physician or other qualified healthcare professional with the means of identifying the completion of special reports and services that are an adjunct to the basic services rendered. The specific number assigned indicates the special circumstances under which a basic procedure is performed.

Code 99091 should be reported no more than once in a 30-day period to include the physician or health care provider time involved with data accession, review and interpretation, modification of care plan as necessary (including communication to patient and/or caregiver), and associated documentation.

If the services described by 99091 are provided on the same day the patient presents for an E/M service, these services should be considered part of the E/M service and not separately reported.

Do not report 99091 if it occurs within 30 days of care plan oversight services 99374-99380. Do not report 99091 if other more specific CPT codes exist (eg, 93014, 93227, 93233, 93272 for cardiographic services; 95250 for continuous glucose monitoring). Do not report 99091 for transfer and interpretation of data from hospital or clinical laboratory computers.

Miscellaneous Services

99000 Handling and/or conveyance of specimen for transfer from the physician's office to a laboratory

99001 Handling and/or conveyance of specimen for transfer from the patient in other than a physician's office to a laboratory (distance may be indicated)

99002 Handling, conveyance, and/or any other service in connection with the implementation of an order involving devices (eg, designing, fitting, packaging, handling, delivery or mailing) when devices such as orthotics, protectives, prosthetics are fabricated by an outside laboratory or shop but which items have been designed, and are to be fitted and adjusted by the attending physician

(For routine collection of venous blood, use 36415)

99024 Postoperative follow-up visit, normally included in the surgical package, to indicate that an evaluation and management service was performed during a postoperative period for a reason(s) related to the original procedure

(As a component of a surgical "package," see **Surgery Guidelines**)

(99025 has been deleted)

99026 Hospital mandated on call service; in-hospital, each hour

99027 out-of-hospital, each hour

(For physician standby services requiring prolonged physician attendance, use 99360, as appropriate. Time spent performing separately reportable procedure(s) or service(s) should not be included in the time reported as mandated on call service)

99050 Services requested after posted office hours in addition to basic service

99052 Services requested between 10:00 PM and 8:00 AM in addition to basic service

99054 Services requested on Sundays and holidays in addition to basic service

99056 Services provided at request of patient in a location other than physician's office which are normally provided in the office

99058 Office services provided on an emergency basis

99070 Supplies and materials (except spectacles), provided by the physician over and above those usually included with the office visit or other services rendered (list drugs, trays, supplies, or materials provided)

(For spectacles, see 92390-92395)

99071 Educational supplies, such as books, tapes, and pamphlets, provided by the physician for the patient's education at cost to physician

99075 Medical testimony

99078 Physician educational services rendered to patients in a group setting (eg, prenatal, obesity, or diabetic instructions)

99080 Special reports such as insurance forms, more than the information conveyed in the usual medical communications or standard reporting form

(Do not report 99080 in conjunction with 99455, 99456 for the completion of Workmen's Compensation forms)

99082 Unusual travel (eg, transportation and escort of patient)

99090 Analysis of clinical data stored in computers (eg, ECGs, blood pressures, hematologic data)

(For physician/health care professional collection and interpretation of physiologic data stored/transmitted by patient/caregiver, see 99091)

(Do not report 99090 if other more specific CPT codes exist, eg, 93014, 93227, 93233, 93272 for cardiographic services; 95250 for continuous glucose monitoring, 97750 for musculoskeletal function testing)

99091 Collection and interpretation of physiologic data (eg, ECG, blood pressure, glucose monitoring) digitally stored and/or transmitted by the patient and/or caregiver to the physician or other qualified health care professional, requiring a minimum of 30 minutes of time

Qualifying Circumstances for Anesthesia

(For explanation of these services, see **Anesthesia Guidelines**)

+ 99100 Anesthesia for patient of extreme age, under 1 year and over 70 (List separately in addition to code for primary anesthesia procedure)

(For procedure performed on infants less than 1 year of age at time of surgery, see 00326, 00834, 00836)

+ 99116 Anesthesia complicated by utilization of total body hypothermia (List separately in addition to code for primary anesthesia procedure)

+ 99135 Anesthesia complicated by utilization of controlled hypotension (List separately in addition to code for primary anesthesia procedure)

+ 99140 Anesthesia complicated by emergency conditions (specify) (List separately in addition to code for primary anesthesia procedure)

(An emergency is defined as existing when delay in treatment of the patient would lead to a significant increase in the threat to life or body part.)

Sedation With or Without Analgesia (Conscious Sedation)

Sedation with or without analgesia (conscious sedation) is used to achieve a medically controlled state of depressed consciousness while maintaining the patient's airway, protective reflexes and ability to respond to stimulation or verbal commands. Conscious sedation includes performance and documentation of pre- and post-sedation evaluations of the patient, administration of the sedation and/or analgesic agent(s), and monitoring of cardiorespiratory function (ie, pulse oximetry, cardiorespiratory monitor, and blood pressure). The use of these codes requires the presence of an independent trained observer to assist the physician in monitoring the patient's level of consciousness and physiological status.

(If the sedation with or without analgesia (conscious sedation) is administered in support of a procedure provided by another physician, see **Anesthesia** section)

⊘ **99141** Sedation with or without analgesia (conscious sedation); intravenous, intramuscular or inhalation

(94760-94762 may not be reported in addition to 99141)

⊘ **99142** oral, rectal and/or intranasal

(94760-94762 may not be reported in addition to 99142)

Other Services and Procedures

99170 Anogenital examination with colposcopic magnification in childhood for suspected trauma

(For conscious sedation, use 99141, 99142)

99172 Visual function screening, automated or semi-automated bilateral quantitative determination of visual acuity, ocular alignment, color vision by pseudoisochromatic plates, and field of vision (may include all or some screening of the determination(s) for contrast sensitivity, vision under glare)

(This service must employ graduated visual acuity stimuli that allow a quantitative determination of visual acuity (eg, Snellen chart). This service may not be used in addition to a general ophthalmological service or an E/M service)

(Do not report 99172 in conjunction with 99173)

99173 Screening test of visual acuity, quantitative, bilateral

(The screening test used must employ graduated visual acuity stimuli that allow a quantitative estimate of visual acuity (eg, Snellen chart). Other identifiable services unrelated to this screening test provided at the same time may be reported separately (eg, preventive medicine services). When acuity is measured as part of a general ophthalmological service or of an E/M service of the eye, it is a diagnostic examination and not a screening test.)

(Do not report 99173 in conjunction with 99172)

99175 Ipecac or similar administration for individual emesis and continued observation until stomach adequately emptied of poison

(For diagnostic intubation, see 82926-82928, 89130-89141)

(For gastric lavage for diagnostic purposes, see 91055)

99183 Physician attendance and supervision of hyperbaric oxygen therapy, per session

(Evaluation and Management services and/or procedures (eg, wound debridement) provided in a hyperbaric oxygen treatment facility in conjunction with a hyperbaric oxygen therapy session should be reported separately)

99185 Hypothermia; regional

99186 total body

99190 Assembly and operation of pump with oxygenator or heat exchanger (with or without ECG and/or pressure monitoring); each hour

99191 3/4 hour

99192 1/2 hour

99195 Phlebotomy, therapeutic (separate procedure)

99199 Unlisted special service, procedure or report

Home Health Procedures/Services

These codes are used by non-physician health care professionals. Physicians should utilize the home visit codes 99341-99350, and utilize CPT codes other than 99500-99600 for any additional procedure/service provided to a patient living in a residence.

The following codes are used to report services provided in a patient's residence (including assisted living apartments, group homes, non-traditional private homes, custodial care facilities, or schools).

Health care professionals who are authorized to use Evaluation and Management Home Visit codes (99341-99350) may report 99500-99600 in addition to 99341-99350 if both services are performed. Evaluation and Management services may be reported separately, using modifier 25, if the patient's condition requires a significant separately identifiable E/M service, above and beyond the home health service(s)/procedure(s) codes 99500-99600.

99500 Home visit for prenatal monitoring and assessment to include fetal heart rate, non-stress test, uterine monitoring, and gestational diabetes monitoring

99501 Home visit for postnatal assessment and follow-up care

99502 Home visit for newborn care and assessment

99503 Home visit for respiratory therapy care (eg, bronchodilator, oxygen therapy, respiratory assessment, apnea evaluation)

99504 Home visit for mechanical ventilation care

99505 Home visit for stoma care and maintenance including colostomy and cystostomy

99506 Home visit for intramuscular injections

Medicine

99507   Home visit for care and maintenance of catheter(s) (eg, urinary, drainage, and enteral)

       (99508 has been deleted. To report see 95806-95811)

99509   Home visit for assistance with activities of daily living and personal care

       (To report self-care/home management training, see 97535)

       (To report home medical nutrition assessment and intervention services, see 97802-97804)

       (To report home speech therapy services, see 92507-92508)

99510   Home visit for individual, family, or marriage counseling

99511   Home visit for fecal impaction management and enema administration

99512   Home visit for hemodialysis

       (For home infusion of peritoneal dialysis, use 99601, 99602)

       (99551-99569 have been deleted. To report, see 99601-99602)

99600   Unlisted home visit service or procedure

Home Infusion Procedures/Services

99601   Home infusion/specialty drug administration, per visit (up to 2 hours)

+ 99602   each additional hour (List separately in addition to code for primary procedure)

       (Use 99602 in conjunction with 99601)

Medicine

Notes

⊘=Modifier 51 Exempt ⊙=Conscious Sedation ✚=Add-on Code

Category II Codes

The following section of *Current Procedural Terminology (CPT)* contains a set of supplemental tracking codes that can be used for performance measurement. ►It is anticipated that the use of Category II◄ codes for performance measurement will decrease the need for record abstraction and chart review, and thereby minimize administrative burden on physicians, ►other health care professionals, hospitals, and entities seeking to measure the quality of patient care. These codes are intended to facilitate data collection about the quality of care rendered by coding certain services and test results that support nationally established performance measures and that have an evidence base as contributing to quality patient care.◄

The use of these codes is optional. The codes are not required for correct coding and may not be used as a substitute for Category I codes.

►These codes describe clinical components that may be typically included in evaluation and management services or other clinical services and, therefore, do not have a relative value associated with them. Category II codes may also describe results from laboratory tests and procedures, select processes intended to address patient safety practices, or services reflecting compliance with state or federal law.◄

►Category II codes described in this section make use of an alphabetical character as the 5th character in the string (ie, 4 digits followed by the letter **F**). These digits are not intended to reflect the placement of the code in the regular (Category I) part of *CPT*. To promote understanding of these codes and their associated measures, users are referred to Appendix H, which contains information about the measures and their origins. CPT Category II codes are arranged according to the following categories derived from standard clinical documentation format:◄

►Composite Measures. . . . . To begin with 0001F (no measures at this time)◄

►Patient Management . . . . 0500F-0503F◄

►Patient History . . . . 1000F-1002F◄

►Physical Examination . . . . 2000F◄

►Diagnostic/Screening Processes or Results . . . . 3000F (no codes at this time)◄

►Therapeutic, Preventive or Other Interventions . . . . 4000F-4011F◄

►Follow-up or Other Outcomes. . . . . To begin with 5000F (no codes at this time)◄

►Patient Safety . . . . To begin with 6000F (no codes at this time)◄

►Cross-references to the measures associated with each Category II code and their origins are included for reference in Appendix H. Users should review the complete measure(s) associated with each code prior to implementing its use.◄

►Category II codes are reviewed by the Performance Measures Advisory Group (PMAG), an advisory body to the CPT Editorial Panel and the CPT/HCPAC Advisory Committee. The PMAG is comprised of performance measurement experts representing the Agency for Healthcare Research and Quality (AHRQ), the American Medical Association (AMA), the Centers for Medicare and Medicaid Services (CMS), the Joint Commission on Accreditation of Healthcare Organizations (JCAHO), the National Committee for Quality Assurance (NCQA), and the Physician Consortium for Performance Improvement. The PMAG may seek additional expertise and/or input from other national health care organizations, as necessary, for the development of Category II codes. These may include national medical specialty societies, other national health care professional associations, accrediting bodies, and federal regulatory agencies.◄

►Category II codes are published biannually: January 1 and July 1. The most current listing, along with guidelines and forms for submitting code change proposals for Category II codes, may be accessed on the Internet at http://www.ama-assn.org/go/cpt.◄

►(0001F has been deleted. To report, use 2000F)◄

►(0002F has been deleted. To report, use 1000F)◄

►(0003F has been deleted. To report, use 1001F)◄

►(0004F has been deleted. To report, use 4000F)◄

►(0005F has been deleted. To report, use 4001F)◄

►(0006F has been deleted. To report, use 4002F)◄

►(0007F has been deleted. To report, use 4006F)◄

►(0008F has been deleted. To report, use 4009F)◄

►(0009F has been deleted. To report, use 1002F)◄

►(0010F has been deleted)◄

►(0011F has been deleted. To report, use 4011F)◄

►Composite Measures◄

►Composite measures codes combine several measures grouped within a single code descriptor to facilitate reporting for a clinical condition when all components are met. If only some of the components are met, or if services are provided in addition to those included in the composite code, they may be reported individually using the corresponding CPT Category II codes for those services.◄

►No measures at this time.◄

►Patient Management◄

►Patient management codes describe utilization measures or measures of patient care provided for specific clinical purposes (eg, prenatal care, pre- and post-surgical care).◄

● **0500F** Initial prenatal care visit (report at first prenatal encounter with health care professional providing obstetrical care. Report also date of visit and, in a separate field, the date of the last menstrual period - LMP)[2]

● **0501F** Prenatal flow sheet documented in medical record by first prenatal visit (documentation includes at minimum blood pressure, weight, urine protein, uterine size, fetal heart tones, and estimated date of delivery). Report also: date of visit and, in a separate field, the date of the last menstrual period - LMP (Note: If reporting 0501F Prenatal flow sheet, it is not necessary to report 0500F Initial prenatal care visit)[1]

● **0502F** Subsequent prenatal care visit

[Excludes: patients who are seen for a condition unrelated to pregnancy or prenatal care (eg, an upper respiratory infection; patients seen for consultation only, not for continuing care)]

● **0503F** Postpartum care visit[2]

►Patient History◄

►Patient history codes describe measures for select aspects of patient history or review of systems.◄

● **1000F** Tobacco use, smoking, assessed[1]

● **1001F** Tobacco use, non-smoking, assessed[1]

● **1002F** Anginal symptoms and level of activity, assessed[1]

►Physical Examination◄

►Physical examination codes describe aspects of physical examination or clinical assessment.◄

● **2000F** Blood pressure, measured[1]

►Diagnostic/Screening Processes or Results◄

►Diagnostic/screening processes or results codes describe results of tests ordered (clinical laboratory tests, radiological or other procedural examinations).◄

►No codes at this time.◄

►Therapeutic, Preventive or Other Interventions◄

►Therapeutic, preventive or other interventions codes describe pharmacologic, procedural, or behavioral therapies, including preventive services such as patient education and counseling.◄

● **4000F** Tobacco use cessation intervention, counseling[1]

● **4001F** Tobacco use cessation intervention, pharmacologic therapy[1]

● **4002F** Statin therapy, prescribed[1]

● **4006F** Beta-blocker therapy, prescribed[1]

● **4009F** Angiotensin converting enzyme (ACE) inhibitor therapy, prescribed[1]

● **4011F** Oral antiplatelet therapy, prescribed (eg, aspirin, clopidogrel/Plavix, or combination of aspirin and dipyridamole/Aggrenox)[1]

►Follow-up or Other Outcomes◄

►Follow-up or other outcomes codes describe review and communication of test results to patients, patient satisfaction or experience with care, patient functional status, and patient morbidity and mortality.◄

►No codes at this time.◄

►Patient Safety◄

►Patient safety codes that describe patient safety practices.◄

►No codes at this time.◄

►**Footnotes**◄
►[1] Physician Consortium for Perfomance Improvement, www.ama-assn.org/go/quality◄
►[2] National Committee on Quality Assurance (NCQA), Health Employer Data Information Set (HEDIS®), www.ncqa.org◄

Category II Codes

Category III Codes

The following section contains a set of temporary codes for emerging technology, services, and procedures. Category III codes will allow data collection for these services/procedures. Use of unlisted codes does not offer the opportunity for the collection of specific data. If a Category III code is available, this code must be reported instead of a Category I unlisted code. This is an activity that is critically important in the evaluation of health care delivery and the formation of public and private policy. The use of the codes in this section will allow physicians and other qualified health care professionals, insurers, health services researchers, and health policy experts to identify emerging technology, services, and procedures for clinical efficacy, utilization and outcomes.

The inclusion of a service or procedure in this section neither implies nor endorses clinical efficacy, safety or the applicability to clinical practice. The codes in this section do not conform to the usual requirements for CPT Category I codes established by the Editorial Panel. For Category I codes, the Panel requires that the service/procedure be performed by many health care professionals in clinical practice in multiple locations and that FDA approval, as appropriate, has already been received. The nature of emerging technology, services, and procedures is such that these requirements may not be met. For these reasons, temporary codes for emerging technology, services, and procedures have been placed in a separate section of the *CPT* book and the codes are differentiated from Category I CPT codes by the use of alphanumeric characters.

Services/procedures described in this section make use of alphanumeric characters. These codes have an alpha character as the 5th character in the string, preceded by four digits. The digits are not intended to reflect the placement of the code in the Category I section of CPT nomenclature. Codes in this section may or may not eventually receive a Category I CPT code. In either case, a given Category III code will be archived after five years of its inception unless it is demonstrated that a temporary code is still needed. New codes in this section are released semi-annually via the AMA/CPT internet site, to expedite dissemination for reporting. The full set of temporary codes for emerging technology, services, and procedures are published annually in the *CPT* book. Go to www.ama-assn.org/go/cpt for the most current listing.

▶(0001T has been deleted. To report, use 34803)◀

(0002T has been deleted. To report, use 34805)

0003T   Cervicography

▶(0005T-0007T have been deleted. To report, see 0075T, 0076T)◀

0008T   Upper gastrointestinal endoscopy including esophagus, stomach, and either the duodenum and/or jejunum as appropriate, with suturing of the esophagogastric junction

▶(0009T has been deleted. To report, use 58356)◀

0010T   Tuberculosis test, cell mediated immunity measurement of gamma interferon antigen response

▶(0012T has been deleted. To report, use 29866)◀

▶(0013T has been deleted. To report, see 29867, 27415)◀

▶(0014T has been deleted. To report, use 29868)◀

0016T   Destruction of localized lesion of choroid (eg, choroidal neovascularization), transpupillary thermotherapy

0017T   Destruction of macular drusen, photocoagulation

0018T   Delivery of high power, focal magnetic pulses for direct stimulation to cortical neurons

0019T   Extracorporeal shock wave therapy; involving musculoskeletal system

0020T   involving plantar fascia

0021T   Insertion of transcervical or transvaginal fetal oximetry sensor

0023T   Infectious agent drug susceptibility phenotype prediction using genotypic comparison to known genotypic/phenotypic database, HIV 1

0024T   Non-surgical septal reduction therapy (eg, alcohol ablation), for hypertrophic obstructive cardiomyopathy, with coronary arteriograms, with or without temporary pacemaker

(0025T has been deleted. To report, use 76514)

0026T   Lipoprotein, direct measurement, intermediate density lipoproteins (IDL) (remnant lipoproteins)

0027T   Endoscopic lysis of epidural adhesions with direct visualization using mechanical means (eg, spinal endoscopic catheter system) or solution injection (eg, normal saline) including radiologic localization and epidurography

(For diagnostic epidurography, use 64999)

0028T   Dual energy x-ray absorptiometry (DEXA) body composition study, one or more sites

0029T   Treatment(s) for incontinence, pulsed magnetic neuromodulation, per day

0030T   Antiprothrombin (phospholipid cofactor) antibody, each Ig class

0031T   Speculoscopy;

0032T   with directed sampling

0033T   Endovascular repair of descending thoracic aortic aneurysm, pseudoaneurysm or dissection; involving coverage of left subclavian artery origin, initial endoprosthesis

(For radiological supervision and interpretation, use 0038T)

0034T   not involving coverage of left subclavian artery origin, initial endoprosthesis

(For radiological supervision and interpretation, use 0039T)

0035T   Placement of proximal or distal extension prosthesis for endovascular repair of descending thoracic aortic aneurysm, pseudoaneurysm or dissection; initial extension

(For radiological supervision and interpretation, use 0040T)

(Do not report 0034T and 0035T when placement of extension converts repair to cover left subclavian origin, use only 0033T)

+ **0036T**   each additional extension (List separately in addition to code for primary procedure)

(Use 0036T in conjunction with 0035T)

(For radiological supervision and interpretation, use 0040T)

0037T   Open subclavian to carotid artery transposition performed in conjunction with endovascular thoracic aneurysm repair, by neck incision, unilateral

(For bilateral procedure, use modifier 50)

(Do not report 0037T in addition to 35694)

0038T   Endovascular repair of descending thoracic aortic aneurysm, pseudoaneurysm or dissection involving coverage of left subclavian artery origin, initial endoprosthesis, radiological supervision and interpretation

(For implantation of endovascular graft, use 0033T)

0039T   Endovascular repair of descending thoracic aortic aneurysm, pseudoaneurysm or dissection not involving coverage of left subclavian artery origin, initial endoprosthesis, radiological supervision and interpretation

(For implantation of endovascular graft, use 0034T)

0040T   Placement of proximal or distal extension prosthesis for endovascular repair of descending thoracic aortic aneurysm, pseudoaneurysm or dissection, each extension, radiological supervision and interpretation

(For implantation of endovascular graft extensions, see 0035T, 0036T)

0041T   Urinalysis infectious agent detection, semi-quantitative analysis of volatile compounds

0042T   Cerebral perfusion analysis using computed tomography with contrast administration, including post-processing of parametric maps with determination of cerebral blood flow, cerebral blood volume, and mean transit time

0043T   Carbon monoxide, expired gas analysis (eg, $ETCO_c$/hemolysis breath test)

0044T   Whole body integumentary photography, at request of a physician, for monitoring of high-risk patients; with dysplastic nevus syndrome or familial melanoma

0045T   with history of dysplastic nevi or personal history of melanoma

0046T   Catheter lavage of a mammary duct(s) for collection of cytology specimen(s), in high risk individuals (GAIL risk scoring or prior personal history of breast cancer), each breast; single duct

0047T   each additional duct

0048T   Implantation of a ventricular assist device, extracorporeal, percutaneous transseptal access, single or dual cannulation

+ **0049T**   Prolonged extracorporeal percutaneous transseptal ventricular assist device, greater than 24 hours, each subsequent 24 hour period (List separately in addition to code for primary procedure)

(Use 0049T in conjunction with 0048T)

0050T   Removal of a ventricular assist device, extracorporeal, percutaneous transseptal access, single or dual cannulation

0051T   Implantation of a total replacement heart system (artificial heart) with recipient cardiectomy

(For implantation of heart assist or ventricular assist device, see 33975, 33976)

0052T   Replacement or repair of thoracic unit of a total replacement heart system (artificial heart)

(For replacement or repair of other implantable components in a total replacement heart system (artificial heart), use 0053T)

0053T   Replacement or repair of implantable component or components of total replacement heart system (artificial heart), excluding thoracic unit

(For replacement or repair of a thoracic unit of a total replacement heart system (artificial heart), use 0052T)

+ **0054T**   Computer-assisted musculoskeletal surgical navigational orthopedic procedure, with image-guidance based on fluoroscopic images (List separately in addition to code for primary procedure)

+▲ **0055T**   Computer-assisted musculoskeletal surgical navigational orthopedic procedure, with image-guidance based on CT/MRI images (List separately in addition to code for primary procedure)

▶(When CT and MRI are both performed, report 0055T only once)◀

Category III Codes

+ 0056T Computer assisted musculoskeletal surgical navigational orthopedic procedure, image-less (List separately in addition to code for primary procedure)

▶(0057T has been deleted. To report, use 43257)◀

0058T Cryopreservation; reproductive tissue, ovarian

0059T oocyte(s)

(For cryopreservation of embryo(s), sperm and testicular reproductive tissue, see 89258, 89259, 89335)

0060T Electrical impedance scan of the breast, bilateral (risk assessment device for breast cancer)

0061T Destruction/reduction of malignant breast tumor including breast carcinoma cells in the margins, microwave phased array thermotherapy, disposable catheter with combined temperature monitoring probe and microwave sensor, externally applied microwave energy, including interstitial placement of sensor

(For imaging guidance performed in conjunction with 0061T, see 76942, 76986)

● 0062T Percutaneous intradiscal annuloplasty, any method, unilateral or bilateral including fluoroscopic guidance; single level

+● 0063T one or more additional levels (List separately in addition to 0062T for primary procedure)

▶(For CT or MRI guidance and localization for needle placement and annuloplasty in conjunction with 0062T, 0063T, see 76360, 76393)◀

● 0064T Spectroscopy, expired gas analysis (eg, nitric oxide/carbon dioxide test)

● 0065T Ocular photoscreening, with interpretation and report, bilateral

▶(Do not report 0065T in conjunction with 99172 or 99173)◀

● 0066T Computed tomographic (CT) colonography (ie, virtual colonoscopy); screening

● 0067T diagnostic

▶(Do not report 0066T or 0067T in conjunction with 72192-72194, 74150-74170, 76375)◀

+● 0068T Acoustic heart sound recording and computer analysis; with interpretation and report (List separately in addition to codes for electrocardiography)

▶(Use 0068T in conjunction with 93000)◀

+● 0069T acoustic heart sound recording and computer analysis only (List separately in addition to codes for electrocardiography)

▶(Use 0069T in conjunction with 93005)◀

+● 0070T interpretation and report only (List separately in addition to codes for electrocardiography)

▶(Use 0070T in conjunction with 93010)◀

● 0071T Focused ultrasound ablation of uterine leiomyomata, including MR guidance; total leiomyomata volume less than 200 cc of tissue

● 0072T total leiomyomata volume greater or equal to 200 cc of tissue

▶(Do not report 0071T, 0072T in conjunction with 51702 or 76394)◀

● 0073T Compensator-based beam modulation treatment delivery of inverse planned treatment using three or more high resolution (milled or cast) compensator convergent beam modulated fields, per treatment session

▶(For treatment planning, use 77301)◀

▶(Do not report 0073T in conjunction with 77401-77416, 77418)◀

▶Online Medical Evaluation◀

▶An online medical evaluation is a type of Evaluation and Management (E/M) service provided by a physician or qualified health care professional to a patient using internet resources in response to the patient's online inquiry. Reportable services involve the physician's personal timely response to the patient's inquiry and must involve permanent storage (electronic or hard copy) of the encounter. This service should not be reported for patient contacts (eg, telephone calls) considered to be pre-service or post-service work for other E/M or non E/M services. A reportable service would encompass the sum of communication (eg, related telephone calls, prescription provision, laboratory orders) pertaining to the online patient encounter or problem(s).◀

● 0074T Online evaluation and management service, per encounter, provided by a physician, using the Internet or similar electronic communications network, in response to a patient's request, established patient

● 0075T Transcatheter placement of extracranial vertebral or intrathoracic carotid artery stent(s), including radiologic supervision and interpretation, percutaneous; initial vessel

+● 0076T each additional vessel (List separately in addition to code for primary procedure)

▶(Use 0076T in conjunction with 0075T)◀

▶(When the ipsilateral extracranial vertebral or intrathoracic carotid arteriogram (including imaging and selective catheterization) confirms the need for stenting, then 0075T and 0076T include all ipsilateral extracranial vertebral or intrathoracic selective carotid catheterization, all diagnostic imaging for ipsilateral extracranial vertebral or intrathoracic carotid artery stenting, and all related radiologic supervision and interpretation. If stenting is not indicated, then the appropriate codes for selective catheterization and imaging should be reported in lieu of code 0075T or 0076T.)◀

● **0077T**   Implanting and securing cerebral thermal perfusion probe, including twist drill or burr hole, to measure absolute cerebral tissue perfusion

▶(0078T-0081T should be reported in accordance with the Endovascular Abdominal Aneurysm Repair guidelines established for 34800-34826)◀

● **0078T**   Endovascular repair of abdominal aortic aneurysm, pseudoaneurysm or dissection, abdominal aorta involving visceral vessels (superior mesenteric, celiac or renal), using fenestrated modular bifurcated prosthesis (two docking limbs)

▶(Do not report 0078T in conjunction with 34800-34805, 35081, 35102, 35452, 35454, 35472, 37205-37208)◀

▶(Report 0078T in conjunction with 35454, 37205-37208 when these procedures are performed outside the target zone of the endoprosthesis)◀

+● **0079T**   Placement of visceral extension prosthesis for endovascular repair of abdominal aortic aneurysm involving visceral vessels, each visceral branch (List separately in addition to code for primary procedure)

▶(Use 0079T in conjunction with 0078T)◀

▶(Do not report 0079T in conjunction with 34800-34805, 35081, 35102, 35452, 35454, 35472, 37205-37208)◀

▶(Report 0079T in conjunction with 35454, 37205-37208 when these procedures are performed outside the target zone of the endoprosthesis)◀

● **0080T**   Endovascular repair of abdominal aortic aneurysm, pseudoaneurysm or dissection, abdominal aorta involving visceral vessels (superior mesenteric, celiac or renal), using fenestrated modular bifurcated prosthesis (two docking limbs), radiological supervision and interpretation

▶(Do not report 0080T in conjunction with 34800-34805, 35081, 35102, 35452, 35454, 35472, 37205-37208)◀

▶(Report 0080T in conjunction with 35454, 37205-37208 when these procedures are performed outside the target zone of the endoprosthesis)◀

+● **0081T**   Placement of visceral extension prosthesis for endovascular repair of abdominal aortic aneurysm involving visceral vessels, each visceral branch, radiological supervision and interpretation (List separately in addition to code for primary procedure)

▶(Use 0081T in conjunction with 0080T)◀

▶(Do not report 0081T in conjunction with 34800-34805, 35081, 35102, 35452, 35454, 35472, 37205-37208)◀

▶(Report 0081T in conjunction with 35454, 37205-37208 when these procedures are performed outside the target zone of the endoprosthesis)◀

● **0082T**   Stereotactic body radiation therapy, treatment delivery, one or more treatment areas, per day

▶(Do not report 0082T in conjunction with 77401-77416, 77418)◀

● **0083T**   Stereotactic body radiation therapy, treatment management, per day

▶(Do not report 0083T in conjunction with 77427-77432)◀

● **0084T**   Insertion of a temporary prostatic urethral stent

● **0085T**   Breath test for heart transplant rejection

● **0086T**   Left ventricular filling pressure indirect measurement by computerized calibration of the arterial waveform response to Valsalva maneuver

● **0087T**   Sperm evaluation, Hyaluronan binding assay

● **0088T**   Submucosal radiofrequency tissue volume reduction of tongue base, one or more sites, per session (ie, for treatment of obstructive sleep apnea syndrome)

Category III Codes

Appendix A

Modifiers

This list includes all of the modifiers applicable to *CPT 2005* codes.

21 Prolonged Evaluation and Management Services: When the face-to-face or floor/unit service(s) provided is prolonged or otherwise greater than that usually required for the highest level of evaluation and management service within a given category, it may be identified by adding modifier 21 to the evaluation and management code number. A report may also be appropriate.

22 Unusual Procedural Services: When the service(s) provided is greater than that usually required for the listed procedure, it may be identified by adding modifier 22 to the usual procedure number. A report may also be appropriate.

23 Unusual Anesthesia: Occasionally, a procedure, which usually requires either no anesthesia or local anesthesia, because of unusual circumstances must be done under general anesthesia. This circumstance may be reported by adding modifier 23 to the procedure code of the basic service.

24 Unrelated Evaluation and Management Service by the Same Physician During a Postoperative Period: The physician may need to indicate that an evaluation and management service was performed during a postoperative period for a reason(s) unrelated to the original procedure. This circumstance may be reported by adding modifier 24 to the appropriate level of E/M service.

25 Significant, Separately Identifiable Evaluation and Management Service by the Same Physician on the Same Day of the Procedure or Other Service: The physician may need to indicate that on the day a procedure or service identified by a CPT code was performed, the patient's condition required a significant, separately identifiable E/M service above and beyond the other service provided or beyond the usual preoperative and postoperative care associated with the procedure that was performed. The E/M service may be prompted by the symptom or condition for which the procedure and/or service was provided. As such, different diagnoses are not required for reporting of the E/M services on the same date. This circumstance may be reported by adding modifier 25 to the appropriate level of E/M service. **Note:** This modifier is not used to report an E/M service that resulted in a decision to perform surgery. See modifier 57.

26 Professional Component: Certain procedures are a combination of a physician component and a technical component. When the physician component is reported separately, the service may be identified by adding modifier 26 to the usual procedure number.

32 Mandated Services: Services related to *mandated* consultation and/or related services (eg, PRO, third party payer, governmental, legislative or regulatory requirement) may be identified by adding modifier 32 to the basic procedure.

47 Anesthesia by Surgeon: Regional or general anesthesia provided by the surgeon may be reported by adding modifier 47 to the basic service. (This does not include local anesthesia.) **Note:** Modifier 47 would not be used as a modifier for the anesthesia procedures.

50 Bilateral Procedure: Unless otherwise identified in the listings, bilateral procedures that are performed at the same operative session, should be identified by adding modifier 50 to the appropriate five digit code.

51 Multiple Procedures: When multiple procedures, other than E/M services, are performed at the same session by the same provider, the primary procedure or service may be reported as listed. The additional procedure(s) or service(s) may be identified by appending modifier 51 to the additional procedure or service code(s). **Note:** This modifier should not be appended to designated "add-on" codes (see Appendix D).

52 Reduced Services: Under certain circumstances a service or procedure is partially reduced or eliminated at the physician's discretion. Under these circumstances the service provided can be identified by its usual procedure number and the addition of modifier 52, signifying that the service is reduced. This provides a means of reporting reduced services without disturbing the identification of the basic service. **Note:** For hospital outpatient reporting of a previously scheduled procedure/service that is partially reduced or cancelled as a result of extenuating circumstances or those that threaten the well-being of the patient prior to or after administration of anesthesia, see modifiers 73 and 74 (see modifiers approved for ASC hospital outpatient use).

53 Discontinued Procedure: Under certain circumstances, the physician may elect to terminate a surgical or diagnostic procedure. Due to extenuating circumstances or those that threaten the well being of the patient, it may be necessary to indicate that a surgical or diagnostic procedure was started but discontinued. This circumstance may be reported by adding modifier 53 to the code reported by the physician for the discontinued procedure. **Note:** This modifier is not used to report the elective cancellation of a procedure prior to the patient's anesthesia induction and/or surgical preparation in the operating suite. For outpatient hospital/ambulatory surgery center (ASC) reporting of a previously scheduled procedure/service that is partially reduced or cancelled as a result of extenuating circumstances or those that threaten the well being of the patient prior to or after administration of anesthesia, see modifiers 73 and 74 (see modifiers approved for ASC hospital outpatient use).

54 Surgical Care Only: When one physician performs a surgical procedure and another provides preoperative and/or postoperative management, surgical services may be identified by adding modifier 54 to the usual procedure number.

55 Postoperative Management Only: When one physician performed the postoperative management and another physician performed the surgical procedure, the postoperative component may be identified by adding modifier 55 to the usual procedure number.

56 Preoperative Management Only: When one physician performed the preoperative care and evaluation and another physician performed the surgical procedure, the preoperative component may be identified by adding modifier 56 to the usual procedure number.

57 Decision for Surgery: An evaluation and management service that resulted in the initial decision to perform the surgery may be identified by adding modifier 57 to the appropriate level of E/M service.

58 Staged or Related Procedure or Service by the Same Physician During the Postoperative Period: The physician may need to indicate that the performance of a procedure or service during the postoperative period was: a) planned prospectively at the time of the original procedure (staged); b) more extensive than the original procedure; or c) for therapy following a diagnostic surgical procedure. This circumstance may be reported by adding modifier 58 to the staged or related procedure. **Note:** This modifier is not used to report the treatment of a problem that requires a return to the operating room. See modifier 78.

59 Distinct Procedural Service: Under certain circumstances, the physician may need to indicate that a procedure or service was distinct or independent from other services performed on the same day. Modifier 59 is used to identify procedures/services that are not normally reported together, but are appropriate under the circumstances. This may represent a different session or patient encounter, different procedure or surgery, different site or organ system, separate incision/excision, separate lesion, or separate injury (or area of injury in extensive injuries) not ordinarily encountered or performed on the same day by the same physician. However, when another already established modifier is appropriate it should be used rather than modifier 59. Only if no more descriptive modifier is available, and the use of modifier 59 best explains the circumstances, should modifier 59 be used.

62 Two Surgeons: When two surgeons work together as primary surgeons performing distinct part(s) of a procedure, each surgeon should report his/her distinct operative work by adding modifier 62 to the procedure code and any associated add-on code(s) for that procedure as long as both surgeons continue to work together as primary surgeons. Each surgeon should report the co-surgery once using the same procedure code. If additional procedure(s) (including add-on procedure(s)) are performed during the same surgical session, separate code(s) may also be reported with modifier 62 added. **Note:** If a co-surgeon acts as an assistant in the performance of additional procedure(s) during the same surgical session, those services may be reported using separate procedure code(s) with the modifier 80 or modifier 82 added, as appropriate.

63 Procedure Performed on Infants less than 4 kg: Procedures performed on neonates and infants up to a present body weight of 4 kg may involve significantly increased complexity and physician work commonly associated with these patients. This circumstance may be reported by adding modifier 63 to the procedure number. **Note:** Unless otherwise designated, this modifier may only be appended to procedures/services listed in the 20000-69999 code series. Modifier 63 should not be appended to any CPT codes listed in the **Evaluation and Management Services, Anesthesia, Radiology, Pathology/Laboratory, or Medicine** sections.

66 Surgical Team: Under some circumstances, highly complex procedures (requiring the concomitant services of several physicians, often of different specialties, plus other highly skilled, specially trained personnel, various types of complex equipment) are carried out under the "surgical team" concept. Such circumstances may be identified by each participating physician with the addition of modifier 66 to the basic procedure number used for reporting services.

76 Repeat Procedure by Same Physician: The physician may need to indicate that a procedure or service was repeated subsequent to the original procedure or service. This circumstance may be reported by adding modifier 76 to the repeated procedure/service.

77 Repeat Procedure by Another Physician: The physician may need to indicate that a basic procedure or service performed by another physician had to be repeated. This situation may be reported by adding modifier 77 to the repeated procedure/service.

78 Return to the Operating Room for a Related Procedure During the Postoperative Period: The physician may need to indicate that another procedure was performed during the postoperative period of the initial procedure. When this subsequent procedure is related to the first, and requires the use of the operating room, it may be reported by adding modifier 78 to the related procedure. (For repeat procedures on the same day, see modifier 76.)

79 Unrelated Procedure or Service by the Same Physician During the Postoperative Period: The physician may need to indicate that the performance of a procedure or service during the postoperative period was unrelated to the original procedure. This circumstance may be reported by using modifier 79. (For repeat procedures on the same day, see modifier 76.)

80 **Assistant Surgeon:** Surgical assistant services may be identified by adding modifier 80 to the usual procedure number(s).

81 **Minimum Assistant Surgeon:** Minimum surgical assistant services are identified by adding modifier 81 to the usual procedure number.

82 **Assistant Surgeon (when qualified resident surgeon not available):** The unavailability of a qualified resident surgeon is a prerequisite for use of modifier 82 appended to the usual procedure code number(s).

90 **Reference (Outside) Laboratory:** When laboratory procedures are performed by a party other than the treating or reporting physician, the procedure may be identified by adding modifier 90 to the usual procedure number.

91 **Repeat Clinical Diagnostic Laboratory Test:** In the course of treatment of the patient, it may be necessary to repeat the same laboratory test on the same day to obtain subsequent (multiple) test results. Under these circumstances, the laboratory test performed can be identified by its usual procedure number and the addition of modifier 91. **Note:** This modifier may not be used when tests are rerun to confirm initial results; due to testing problems with specimens or equipment; or for any other reason when a normal, one-time, reportable result is all that is required. This modifier may not be used when other code(s) describe a series of test results (eg, glucose tolerance tests, evocative/suppression testing). This modifier may only be used for laboratory test(s) performed more than once on the same day on the same patient.

99 **Multiple Modifiers:** Under certain circumstances two or more modifiers may be necessary to completely delineate a service. In such situations modifier 99 should be added to the basic procedure, and other applicable modifiers may be listed as part of the description of the service.

Anesthesia Physical Status Modifiers

The Physical Status modifiers are consistent with the American Society of Anesthesiologists ranking of patient physical status, and distinguishing various levels of complexity of the anesthesia service provided. All anesthesia services are reported by use of the anesthesia five-digit procedure code (00100-03108) with the appropriate physical status modifier appended.

Example: 00100-P1

Under certain circumstances, when another established modifier(s) is appropriate, it should be used in addition to the physical status modifier.

Example: 00100-P4-53

Physical Status Modifier P1: A normal healthy patient

Physical Status Modifier P2: A patient with mild systemic disease

Physical Status Modifier P3: A patient with severe systemic disease

Physical Status Modifier P4: A patient with severe systemic disease that is a constant threat to life

Physical Status Modifier P5: A moribund patient who is not expected to survive without the operation

Physical Status Modifier P6: A declared brain-dead patient whose organs are being removed for donor purposes

Modifiers Approved for Ambulatory Surgery Center (ASC) Hospital Outpatient Use

CPT Level I Modifiers

25 **Significant, Separately Identifiable Evaluation and Management Service by the Same Physician on the Same Day of the Procedure or Other Service:** The physician may need to indicate that on the day a procedure or service identified by a CPT code was performed, the patient's condition required a significant, separately identifiable E/M service above and beyond the other service provided or beyond the usual preoperative and postoperative care associated with the procedure that was performed. The E/M service may be prompted by the symptom or condition for which the procedure and/or service was provided. As such, different diagnoses are not required for reporting of the E/M services on the same date. This circumstance may be reported by adding modifier 25 to the appropriate level of E/M service. **Note:** This modifier is not used to report an E/M service that resulted in a decision to perform surgery. See modifier 57.

27 **Multiple Outpatient Hospital E/M Encounters on the Same Date:** For hospital outpatient reporting purposes, utilization of hospital resources related to separate and distinct E/M encounters performed in multiple outpatient hospital settings on the same date may be reported by adding modifier 27 to each appropriate level outpatient and/or emergency department E/M code(s). This modifier provides a means of reporting circumstances involving evaluation and management services provided by physician(s) in more than one (multiple) outpatient hospital setting(s) (eg, hospital emergency department, clinic). **Note:** This modifier is not to be used for physician reporting of multiple E/M services performed by the same physician on the same date. For physician reporting of all outpatient evaluation and management services provided by the same physician on the same date and performed in multiple outpatient setting(s) (eg, hospital emergency department, clinic), see **Evaluation and Management, Emergency Department, or Preventive Medicine Services** codes.

50 **Bilateral Procedure:** Unless otherwise identified in the listings, bilateral procedures that are performed at the same operative session should be identified by adding modifier 50 to the appropriate five digit code.

52 **Reduced Services:** Under certain circumstances a service or procedure is partially reduced or eliminated at the physician's discretion. Under these circumstances the service provided can be identified by its usual procedure number and the addition of modifier 52, signifying that the service is reduced. This provides a means of reporting reduced services without disturbing the identification of the basic service. **Note:** For hospital outpatient reporting of a previously scheduled procedure/service that is partially reduced or cancelled as a result of extenuating circumstances or those that threaten the well-being of the patient prior to or after administration of anesthesia, see modifiers 73 and 74.

58 **Staged or Related Procedure or Service by the Same Physician During the Postoperative Period:** The physician may need to indicate that the performance of a procedure or service during the postoperative period was: a) planned prospectively at the time of the original procedure (staged); b) more extensive than the original procedure; or c) for therapy following a diagnostic surgical procedure. This circumstance may be reported by adding modifier 58 to the staged or related procedure. **Note:** This modifier is not used to report the treatment of a problem that requires a return to the operating room. See modifier 78.

59 **Distinct Procedural Service:** Under certain circumstances, the physician may need to indicate that a procedure or service was distinct or independent from other services performed on the same day. Modifier 59 is used to identify procedures/services that are not normally reported together, but are appropriate under the circumstances. This may represent a different session or patient encounter, different procedure or surgery, different site or organ system, separate incision/excision, separate lesion, or separate injury (or area of injury in extensive injuries) not ordinarily encountered or performed on the same day by the same physician. However, when another already established modifier is appropriate it should be used rather than modifier 59. Only if no more descriptive modifier is available, and the use of modifier 59 best explains the circumstances, should modifier 59 be used.

73 **Discontinued Out-Patient Hospital/Ambulatory Surgery Center (ASC) Procedure Prior to the Administration of Anesthesia:** Due to extenuating circumstances or those that threaten the well being of the patient, the physician may cancel a surgical or diagnostic procedure subsequent to the patient's surgical preparation (including sedation when provided, and being taken to the room where the procedure is to be performed), but prior to the administration of anesthesia (local, regional block(s) or general). Under these circumstances, the intended service that is prepared for but cancelled can be reported by its usual procedure number and the addition of modifier 73. **Note:** The elective cancellation of a service prior to the administration of anesthesia and/or surgical preparation of the patient should not be reported. For physician reporting of a discontinued procedure, see modifier 53.

74 **Discontinued Out-Patient Hospital/Ambulatory Surgery Center (ASC) Procedure After Administration of Anesthesia:** Due to extenuating circumstances or those that threaten the well being of the patient, the physician may terminate a surgical or diagnostic procedure after the administration of anesthesia (local, regional block(s), general) or after the procedure was started (incision made, intubation started, scope inserted, etc). Under these circumstances, the procedure started but terminated can be reported by its usual procedure number and the addition of modifier 74. **Note:** The elective cancellation of a service prior to the administration of anesthesia and/or surgical preparation of the patient should not be reported. For physician reporting of a discontinued procedure, see modifier 53.

76 **Repeat Procedure by Same Physician:** The physician may need to indicate that a procedure or service was repeated subsequent to the original procedure or service. This circumstance may be reported by adding modifier 76 to the repeated procedure/service.

77 **Repeat Procedure by Another Physician:** The physician may need to indicate that a basic procedure or service performed by another physician had to be repeated. This situation may be reported by adding modifier 77 to the repeated procedure/service.

78 **Return to the Operating Room for a Related Procedure During the Postoperative Period:** The physician may need to indicate that another procedure was performed during the postoperative period of the initial procedure. When this subsequent procedure is related to the first, and requires the use of the operating room, it may be reported by adding modifier 78 to the related procedure. (For repeat procedures on the same day, see 76.)

79 **Unrelated Procedure or Service by the Same Physician During the Postoperative Period:** The physician may need to indicate that the performance of a procedure or service during the postoperative period was unrelated to the original procedure. This circumstance may be reported by using modifier 79. (For repeat procedures on the same day, see 76.)

91 **Repeat Clinical Diagnostic Laboratory Test:** In the course of treatment of the patient, it may be necessary to repeat the same laboratory test on the same day to obtain subsequent (multiple) test results. Under these circumstances, the laboratory test performed can be identified by its usual procedure number and the addition of modifier 91. **Note:** This modifier may not be used when tests are rerun to confirm initial results; due to testing problems with specimens or equipment; or for any other reason when a normal, one-time, reportable result is all that is required. This modifier may not be used when other code(s) describe a series of test results (eg, glucose tolerance tests, evocative/suppression testing). This modifier may only be used for laboratory test(s) performed more than once on the same day on the same patient.

Level II (HCPCS/National) Modifiers

E1   Upper left, eyelid

E2   Lower left, eyelid

E3   Upper right, eyelid

E4   Lower right, eyelid

F1   Left hand, second digit

F2   Left hand, third digit

F3   Left hand, fourth digit

F4   Left hand, fifth digit

F5   Right hand, thumb

F6   Right hand, second digit

F7   Right hand, third digit

F8   Right hand, fourth digit

F9   Right hand, fifth digit

FA   Left hand, thumb

LC   Left circumflex coronary artery (Hospitals use with codes 92980-92984, 92995, 92996)

LD   Left anterior descending coronary artery (Hospitals use with codes 92980-92984, 92995, 92996)

LT   Left side (used to identify procedures performed on the left side of the body)

QM   Ambulance service provided under arrangement by a provider of services

QN   Ambulance service furnished directly by a provider of services

RC   Right coronary artery (Hospitals use with codes 92980-92984, 92995, 92996)

RT   Right side (used to identify procedures performed on the right side of the body)

T1   Left foot, second digit

T2   Left foot, third digit

T3   Left foot, fourth digit

T4   Left foot, fifth digit

T5   Right foot, great toe

T6   Right foot, second digit

T7   Right foot, third digit

T8   Right foot, fourth digit

T9   Right foot, fifth digit

TA   Left foot, great toe

Appendix B

Summary of Additions, Deletions, and Revisions

Appendix B shows the actual changes that were made to the code descriptors. New codes appear with a bullet (●) and are indicated as "Code added." Revised codes are preceded with a triangle (▲). Within revised codes, the deleted language appears with a ~~strikethrough~~, while new text appears <u>underlined</u>. Codes with which conscious sedation would not be separately reported when performed at the same session by the same provider are denoted with the bullseye (⊙).

Revisions to the headings, notes, introductory paragraphs, and cross-references are not included in this Appendix, but are identified in the main text of the book with the "► ◄" symbols and presented in green. Codes listed as "Grammatical change" contain minor revisions that do not alter the original intent of the codes, and therefore are not preceded with a triangle (▲).

Evaluation and Management

▲ 99293   **Initial inpatient pediatric critical care,** ~~31 days up through 24 months of age,~~ per day, for the evaluation and management of a critically ill infant or young child, <u>29 days through 24 months of age</u>

▲ 99294   **Subsequent inpatient pediatric critical care,** ~~31 days up through 24 months of age,~~ per day, for the evaluation and management of a critically ill infant or young child, <u>29 days through 24 months of age</u>

▲ 99295   **Initial inpatient neonatal critical care,** per day, for the evaluation and management of a critically ill neonate, <u>28</u> ~~30~~ days of age or less

▲ 99296   **Subsequent inpatient neonatal critical care,** per day, for the evaluation and management of a critically ill neonate, <u>28</u>~~30~~ days of age or less

Anesthesia

● 00561   Code added

Surgery

● 11004   Code added

● 11005   Code added

● 11006   Code added

+● 11008   Code added

▲ 19160   Mastectomy, partial <u>(eg, lumpectomy, tylectomy, quadrantectomy, segmentectomy)</u>;

● 19296   Code added

+● 19297   Code added

⊙● 19298   Code added

● 27412   Code added

● 27415   Code added

● 29866   Code added

● 29867   Code added

● 29868   Code added

● 31545   Code added

● 31546   Code added

+⊙● 31620   Code added

▲ 31630   with tracheal/~~or~~bronchial dilation or closed reduction of fracture

▲ 31631   with ~~tracheal dilation and placement of tracheal stent~~<u>placement of tracheal stent(s) (includes tracheal/bronchial dilation as required)</u>

● 31636   Code added

+● 31637   Code added

● 31638   Code added

⊙● 32019   Code added

▲ 32850   Donor pneumonectomy~~(ies)~~ <u>(including cold preservation), from cadaver donor</u> ~~with preparation and maintenance of allograft (cadaver)~~

● 32855   Code added

● 32856   Code added

▲ 33930   Donor cardiectomy-pneumonectomy <u>(including cold preservation)</u>~~, with preparation and maintenance of allograft~~

● 33933   Code added

▲ 33940   Donor cardiectomy <u>(including cold preservation)</u>~~, with preparation and maintenance of allograft~~

● 33944   Code added

● 34803   Code added

~~35161~~   ~~for aneurysm, pseudoaneurysm, and associated occlusive disease, other arteries~~

~~35162~~   ~~for ruptured aneurysm, other arteries~~

~~35582~~   ~~In-situ vein bypass; aortofemoral-popliteal (only femoral-popliteal portion in-situ)~~

● 36475   Code added

+● 36476   Code added

● 36478   Code added

+● 36479   Code added

● 36818   Code added

▲ 37205   Transcatheter placement of an intravascular stent(s), (except ~~non~~-coronary, ~~non-cervical~~-carotid<u>, and vertebral</u> vessel), percutaneous; initial vessel

⊙● 37215   Code added

⊙● 37216   Code added

⊙● 43257   Code added

● 43644   Code added

● 43645   Code added

● 43845   Code added

▲ 43846   Gastric restrictive procedure, with gastric bypass for morbid obesity; with short limb (~~less than 100~~<u>150</u> cm <u>or less</u>) Roux-en-Y gastroenterostomy

▲ 44132   Donor enterectomy (including cold preservation), open, with preparation and maintenance of allograft; from cadaver donor

● 44137   Code added

● 44715   Code added

● 44720   Code added

● 44721   Code added

⊙● 45391   Code added

⊙● 45392   Code added

● 46947   Code added

▲ 47133   Donor hepatectomy (including cold preservation), with preparation and maintenance of allograft, from cadaver donor

▲ 47140   Donor hepatectomy (including cold preservation), with preparation and maintenance of allograft, from living donor; left lateral segment only (segments II and III)

● 47143   Code added

● 47144   Code added

● 47145   Code added

● 47146   Code added

● 47147   Code added

▲ 48550   Donor pancreatectomy (including cold preservation), with preparation and maintenance of allograft from cadaver donor, with or without duodenal segment for transplantation

● 48551   Code added

● 48552   Code added

▲ 50300   Donor nephrectomy (including cold preservation); with preparation and maintenance of allograft, from cadaver donor, unilateral or bilateral

▲ 50320   Donor nephrectomy, open, from living donor(excluding preparation and maintenance of allograft)

● 50323   Code added

● 50325   Code added

● 50327   Code added

● 50328   Code added

● 50329   Code added

▲ 50360   Renal allotransplantation, implantation of graft; excluding donor andwithout recipient nephrectomy

● 50391   Code added

▲ 50547   donor nephrectomy (including cold preservation), from living donor(excluding preparation and maintenance of allograft)

50559   with insertion of radioactive substance with or without biopsy and/or fulguration

50578   with insertion of radioactive substance, with or without biopsy and/or fulguration

50059   with insertion of radioactive substance, with or without biopsy and/or fulguration (not including provision of material)

50078   with insertion of radioactive substance, with or without biopsy and/or fulguration (not including provision of material)

▲ 52234   Cystourethroscopy, with fulguration (including cryosurgery or laser surgery) and/or resection of; SMALL bladder tumor(s) (0.5 up to 2.0 cm)

52347   Cystourethroscopy with transurethral resection or incision of ejaculatory ducts

● 52402   Code added

+● 57267   Code added

▲ 57282   Sacrospinous ligament fixation for prolapse of vaginaColpopexy, vaginal; extra-peritoneal approach (sacrospinous, iliococcygeus)

● 57283   Code added

● 58356   Code added

● 58565   Code added

● 58956   Code added

▲ 61885   Insertion or replacementIncision and subcutaneous placement of cranial neurostimulator pulse generator or receiver, direct or inductive coupling; with connection to a single electrode arrayInsertion or replacement

● 63050   Code added

● 63051   Code added

+● 63295   Code added

▲ 63685   Insertion or replacement Incision and subcutaneous placementof spinal neurostimulator pulse generator or receiver, direct or inductive coupling

▲ 64590   Insertion or replacement Incision and subcutaneous placementof peripheral neurostimulator pulse generator or receiver, direct or inductive coupling

▲ 66710   cyclophotocoagulation, transscleral

● 66711   Code added

Radiology

▲ 75960   Transcatheter introduction of intravascular stent(s), (except coronary, carotid, and vertebral vessel), percutaneous and/or open, radiological supervision and interpretation, each vessel

▲ 76075   Dual energy x-ray absorptiometry (DEXADXA), bone density study, one or more sites; axial skeleton (eg, hips, pelvis, spine)

● 76077   Code added

● 76510   Code added

▲ 76511   Ophthalmic ultrasound, echography, diagnostic;quantitative A-scan only, with amplitude quantification

▲ 76512   contactB-scan (with or without simultaneoussuperimposed non-quantitative A-scan)

● 76820   Code added

● 76821   Code added

▲ 76827   Doppler echocardiography, fetal, cardiovascular system, pulsed wave and/or continuous wave with spectral display; complete

▲ 77418   Intensity modulated treatment delivery, single or multiple fields/arcs, via narrow spatially and temporally modulated beams, (eg, binary, dynamic MLC), binary, dynamic MLC, per treatment session

▲ 77750   Infusion or instillation of radioelement solution (includes three months follow-up care)

▲ 78267   Urea breath test, C-14 (isotopic); acquisition for analysis

▲ 78464   tomographic (SPECT), single study (including attenuation correction when performed), at rest or stress (exercise and/or pharmacologic), with or without quantification

▲ 78465   tomographic (SPECT), multiple studies (including attenuation correction when performed), at rest and/or stress (exercise and/or pharmacologic) and redistribution and/or rest injection, with or without quantification

~~78810~~   ~~Tumor imaging, positron emission tomography (PET), metabolic evaluation~~

● 78811   Code added

● 78812   Code added

● 78813   Code added

● 78814   Code added

● 78815   Code added

● 78816   Code added

~~78990~~   ~~Provision of diagnostic radiopharmaceutical(s)~~

~~79000~~   ~~Radiopharmaceutical therapy, hyper-thyroidism; initial, including evaluation of patient~~

~~79001~~   ~~subsequent, each therapy~~

● 79005   Code added

~~79020~~   ~~Radiopharmaceutical therapy, thyroid suppression (euthyroid cardiac disease), including evaluation of patient~~

~~79030~~   ~~Radiopharmaceutical ablation of gland for thyroid carcinoma~~

~~79035~~   ~~Radiopharmaceutical therapy for metastases of thyroid carcinoma~~

~~79100~~   ~~Radiopharmaceutical therapy, polycythemia vera, chronic leukemia, each treatment by intravenous injection~~

● 79101   Code added

▲ 79200   Radiopharmaceutical therapy, by ~~i~~Intracavitary ~~radioactive colloid therapy~~administration

▲ 79300   Radiopharmaceutical therapy, by ~~i~~Interstitial radioactive colloid administration~~therapy~~

~~79400~~   ~~Radiopharmaceutical therapy, nonthyroid, nonhematologic by intravenous injection~~

~~79420~~   ~~Intravascular radiopharmaceutical therapy, particulate~~

▲ 79440   Radiopharmaceutical therapy, by ~~i~~Intra-articular ~~radiopharmaceutical therapy~~administration

● 79445   Code added

~~79900~~   ~~Provision of therapeutic radiopharmaceutical(s)~~

▲ 79999   ~~Unlisted r~~Radiopharmaceutical therapy, ~~therapeutic~~unlisted procedure

Pathology and Laboratory

● 82045   Code added

● 82656   Code added

● 83009   Code added

▲ 83013   Helicobacter pylori; breath test analysis for urease activity, non-radioactive isotope (eg, C-13)

▲ 83014   drug administration ~~and sample collection~~

● 83630   Code added

● 84163   Code added

▲ 84165   Protein~~;~~ electrophoretic fractionation and quantitation, serum

● 84166   Code added

▲ 85046   reticulocytes, ~~hemoglobin concentration~~ automated, including one or more cellular parameters (eg, reticulocyte hemoglobin content (CHr), immature reticulocyte fraction (IRF), reticulocyte volume (MRV), RNA content), direct measurement

● 86064   Code added

▲ 86334   Immunofixation electrophoresis; serum

● 86335   Code added

● 86379   Code added

● 86587   Code added

▲ 87046   stool, aerobic, additional pathogens, isolation and presumptive identification of isolates, each plate

● 87807   Code added

~~88180~~   ~~Flow cytometry; each cell surface, cytoplasmic or nuclear marker~~

● 88184   Code added

+● 88185   Code added

● 88187   Code added

● 88188   Code added

● 88189   Code added

● 88360   Code added

▲ 88361   ~~tumor immunohistochemistry (eg, Her-2/neu, estrogen receptor/progesterone receptor), quantitative or semiquantitative~~using computer-assisted technology

▲ 88365   ~~Tissue i~~In situ hybridization (eg, FISH)~~, interpretation and report~~each probe

● 88367   Code added

● 88368   Code added

▲ 89346   oocyte(s)

Medicine

● 90465   Code added

+● 90466   Code added

● 90467   Code added

+● 90468   Code added

▲ 90471   Immunization administration (includes percutaneous, intradermal, subcutaneous, or intramuscular ~~and jet~~ injections); one vaccine (single or combination vaccine/toxoid)

⊘● 90656   Code added

⊘▲ 90700   Diphtheria, tetanus toxoids, and acellular pertussis vaccine (DTaP), for use in individuals younger than ~~seven~~7 years, for intramuscular use

~~91032~~   ~~Esophagus, acid reflux test, with intraluminal pH electrode for detection of gastroesophageal reflux;~~

~~91033~~   ~~prolonged recording~~

● 91034   Code added

● 91035   Code added

● 91037   Code added

● 91038   Code added

● 91040   Code added

▲ 91065   Breath hydrogen test (eg, for detection of lactase deficiency), fructose intolerance, bacterial overgrowth, or oro-cecal gastrointestinal transit)

● 91120   Code added

~~92589~~   ~~Central auditory function test(s) (specify)~~

● 92620   Code added

● 92621   Code added

● 92625   Code added

▲ 93741   Electronic analysis of pacing cardioverter-defibrillator (includes interrogation, evaluation of pulse generator status, evaluation of programmable parameters at rest and during activity where applicable, using electrocardiographic recording and interpretation of recordings at rest and during exercise, analysis of event markers and device response); single chamber <u>or wearable cardioverter-defibrillator system</u>, without reprogramming

▲ 93742   single chamber <u>or wearable cardioverter-defibrillator system</u>, with reprogramming

● 93745   Code added

● 93890   Code added

● 93892   Code added

● 93893   Code added

▲ 94060   ~~Bronchospasm evaluation:~~ <u>Bronchodilation responsiveness</u>, spirometry as in 94010, ~~before and after~~<u>pre- and post-</u>bronchodilator <u>administration</u> ~~(aerosol or parenteral)~~

▲ 94070   ~~Prolonged postexposure evaluation of b~~<u>B</u>ronchospasm ~~with~~ <u>provocation evaluation,</u> multiple spirometric determinations <u>as in 94010,</u> ~~after antigen,~~ <u>with administered agents (eg, antigen(s),</u> cold air, methacholine~~) or other chemical agent, with subsequent spirometries~~

● 94452   Code added

● 94453   Code added

● 95928   Code added

● 95929   Code added

▲ 95971   simple ~~brain,~~spinal cord, or peripheral (ie, peripheral nerve, autonomic nerve, neuromuscular) neurostimulator pulse generator/transmitter, with intraoperative or subsequent programming

▲ 95972   complex ~~brain,~~spinal cord, or peripheral (except cranial nerve) neurostimulator pulse generator/transmitter, with intraoperative or subsequent programming, first hour

+▲ 95973   complex ~~brain,~~spinal cord, or peripheral (except cranial nerve) neurostimulator pulse generator/transmitter, with intraoperative or subsequent programming, each additional 30 minutes after first hour (List separately in addition to code for primary procedure)

● 95978   Code added

+● 95979   Code added

▲ 96111   extended (includes assessment of motor, language, social, adaptive and/or cognitive functioning by standardized developmental instruments~~, eg, Bayley Scales of Infant Development~~) with interpretation and report~~, per hour~~

● 97597   Code added

● 97598   Code added

~~97601~~   ~~Removal of devitalized tissue from wound(s); selective debridement, without anesthesia (eg, high pressure waterjet, sharp selective debridement with scissors, scalpel and tweezers), including topical application(s), wound assessment, and instruction(s) for ongoing care, per session~~

● 97605   Code added

● 97606   Code added

~~97780~~   ~~Acupuncture, one or more needles; without electrical stimulation~~

~~97781~~   ~~with electrical stimulation~~

● 97810   Code added

+● 97811   Code added

● 97813   Code added

+● 97814   Code added

Category II Codes

~~0001F~~   ~~Blood pressure, measured~~

~~0002F~~   ~~Tobacco use, smoking, assessed~~

~~0003F~~   ~~Tobacco use, non-smoking, assessed~~

~~0004F~~   ~~Tobacco use cessation intervention, counseling, performed~~

~~0005F~~   ~~Tobacco use cessation intervention, pharmacologic therapy, prescribed~~

~~0006F~~   ~~Statin therapy, prescribed~~

~~0007F~~   ~~Beta-blocker therapy, prescribed~~

~~0008F~~   ~~ACE inhibitor therapy, prescribed~~

~~0009F~~   ~~Anginal symptoms and level of activity, assessed~~

~~0010F~~   ~~Anginal symptoms and level of activity, assessed using a standardized instrument (eg, Canadian Cardiovascular Society Classification CCSC System, Seattle Angina Questionnaire SAQ)~~

~~0011F~~   ~~Oral antiplatelet therapy; prescribed (eg, aspirin, clopidogrel/Plavix, or combination of aspirin and dipyridamole/Aggrenox)~~

● 0500F   Code added

● 0501F   Code added

● 0502F   Code added

● 0503F   Code added

● 1000F   Code added

● 1001F   Code added

● 1002F   Code added

● 2000F   Code added

● 4000F   Code added

● 4001F   Code added

● 4002F   Code added

● 4006F   Code added

● 4009F   Code added

● 4011F   Code added

Category III Codes

~~0001T~~   ~~Endovascular repair of infrarenal abdominal aortic aneurysm or dissection, modular bifurcated prosthesis (two docking limbs)~~

~~0005T~~   ~~Transcatheter placement of extracranial cerebrovascular artery stent(s), percutaneous; initial vessel~~

+ ~~0006T~~   ~~each additional vessel (List separately in addition to code for primary procedure)~~

~~0007T~~   ~~Transcatheter placement of extracranial cerebrovascular artery stent(s), percutaneous, radiological supervision and interpretation, each vessel~~

	~~0009T~~	~~Endometrial cryoablation with ultrasonic guidance~~
	~~0012T~~	~~Arthroscopy, knee, surgical, implantation of osteochondral graft(s) for treatment of articular surface defect; autografts~~
	~~0013T~~	~~allografts~~
	~~0014T~~	~~Meniscal transplantation, medial or lateral, knee (any method)~~
+▲	0055T	Computer-assisted musculoskeletal surgical navigational orthopedic procedure, with image-guidance based on CT/~~and~~MRI images (List separately in addition to code for primary procedure)
	~~0057T~~	~~Upper gastrointestinal endoscopy, including esophagus, stomach, and either the duodenum and/or jejunum as appropriate, with delivery of thermal energy to the muscle of the lower esophageal sphincter and/or gastric cardia, for treatment of gastroesophageal reflux disease~~
●	0062T	Code added
+●	0063T	Code added
●	0064T	Code added
●	0065T	Code added
●	0066T	Code added
●	0067T	Code added
+●	0068T	Code added
+●	0069T	Code added
+●	0070T	Code added
●	0071T	Code added
●	0072T	Code added
●	0073T	Code added
●	0074T	Code added
●	0075T	Code added
+●	0076T	Code added
●	0077T	Code added
●	0078T	Code added
+●	0079T	Code added
●	0080T	Code added
+●	0081T	Code added
●	0082T	Code added
●	0083T	Code added
●	0084T	Code added
●	0085T	Code added
●	0086T	Code added
●	0087T	Code added
●	0088T	Code added

Appendix C

Clinical Examples

As described in *CPT 2005*, clinical examples of the CPT codes for Evaluation and Management (E/M) services are intended to be an important element of the coding system. The clinical examples, when used with the E/M descriptors contained in the full text of *CPT*, provide a comprehensive and powerful tool for physicians to report the services provided to their patients.

The American Medical Association is pleased to provide you with these clinical examples for *CPT 2005*. The clinical examples that are provided in this supplement are limited to Office or Other Outpatient Services, Hospital Inpatient Services, Consultations, Critical Care, Prolonged Services and Care Plan Oversight.

These clinical examples do not encompass the entire scope of medical practice. Inclusion or exclusion of any particular specialty group does not infer any judgment of importance or lack thereof; nor does it limit the applicability of the example to any particular specialty.

Of utmost importance is that these clinical examples are just that: examples. A particular patient encounter, depending on the specific circumstances, must be judged by the services provided by the physician for that particular patient. Simply because the patient's complaints, symptoms, or diagnoses match those of a particular clinical example, does not automatically assign that patient encounter to that particular level of service. The three key components (history, examination, and medical decision making) must be met and documented in the medical record to report a particular level of service.

Office or Other Outpatient Services

New Patient

99201   Initial office visit for a 50-year-old male from out-of-town who needs a prescription refill for a nonsteroidal anti-inflammatory drug. (Anesthesiology)

Initial office visit for a 40-year-old female, new patient, requesting information about local pain clinics. (Anesthesiology/Pain Medicine)

Initial office visit for a 10-year-old girl for determination of visual acuity as part of a summer camp physical (does not include determination of refractive error). (Ophthalmology)

Initial office visit for an out-of-town patient requiring topical refill. (Dermatology)

Initial office visit for a 65-year-old male for reassurance about an isolated seborrheic keratosis on upper back. (Plastic Surgery)

Initial office visit for an out-of-state visitor who needs refill of topical steroid to treat lichen planus. (Dermatology)

Initial office visit for an 86-year-old male, out-of-town visitor, who needs prescription refilled for an anal skin preparation that he forgot. (General Surgery/Colon & Rectal Surgery)

Initial office visit for a transient patient with alveolar osteitis for repacking. (Oral & Maxillofacial Surgery)

Initial office visit for a patient with a pedunculated lesion of the neck which is unsightly. (Dermatology)

Initial office visit for a 10-year-old male, for limited subungual hematoma not requiring drainage. (Internal Medicine)

Initial office visit with an out-of-town visitor who needs a prescription refilled because she forgot her hay fever medication. (Allergy & Immunology/Internal Medicine)

Initial office visit with a 9-month-old female with diaper rash. (Pediatrics)

Initial office visit with a 10-year-old male with severe rash and itching for the past 24 hours, positive history for contact with poison oak 48 hours prior to the visit. (Family Medicine)

Initial office visit with a 5-year-old female to remove sutures from simple wound placed by another physician. (Plastic Surgery)

Initial office visit for a 22-year-old male with a small area of sunburn requiring first aid. (Dermatology/Family Medicine/Internal Medicine)

Initial office visit for the evaluation and management of a contusion of a finger. (Orthopaedic Surgery)

99202   Initial office visit for a 13-year-old patient with comedopapular acne of the face unresponsive to over-the-counter medications. (Family Medicine)

Initial office visit for a patient with a clinically benign lesion or nodule of the lower leg which has been present for many years. (Dermatology)

Initial office visit for a patient with a circumscribed patch of dermatitis of the leg. (Dermatology)

Initial office visit for a patient with papulosquamous eruption of elbows. (Dermatology)

Initial office visit for a 9-year-old patient with erythematous, grouped, vesicular eruption of the lip of three days' duration. (Pediatrics)

Initial office visit for an 18-year-old male referred by an orthodontist for advice regarding removal of four wisdom teeth. (Oral & Maxillofacial Surgery)

Initial office visit for a 14-year-old male, who was referred by his orthodontist, for advice on the exposure of impacted maxillary cuspids. (Oral & Maxillofacial Surgery)

Initial office visit for a patient presenting with itching patches on the wrists and ankles. (Dermatology)

Initial office visit for a 30-year-old male for evaluation and discussion of treatment of rhinophyma. (Plastic Surgery)

Initial office visit for a 16-year-old male with severe cystic acne, new patient. (Dermatology)

Initial office evaluation for gradual hearing loss, 58-year-old male, history and physical examination, with interpretation of complete audiogram, air bone, etc. (Otolaryngology)

Initial evaluation and management of recurrent urinary infection in female. (Internal Medicine)

Initial office visit with a 10-year-old girl with history of chronic otitis media and a draining ear. (Pediatrics)

Initial office visit for a 10-year-old female with acute maxillary sinusitis. (Family Medicine)

Initial office visit for a patient with recurring episodes of herpes simplex who has developed a clustering of vesicles on the upper lip. (Internal Medicine)

Initial office visit for a 25-year-old patient with single season allergic rhinitis. (Allergy & Immunology)

Initial office visit to plan transient dialysis for a 56-year-old stable dialysis patient who has accompanying records. (Nephrology)

99203 Initial office visit for a 76-year-old male with a stasis ulcer of three months' duration. (Dermatology)

Initial office visit for a 30-year-old female with pain in the lateral aspect of the forearm. (Physical Medicine & Rehabilitation)

Initial office visit for a 15-year-old patient with a four-year history of moderate comedopapular acne of the face, chest, and back with early scarring. Discussion of use of systemic medication. (Dermatology)

Initial office visit for a patient with papulosquamous eruption of the elbow with pitting of nails and itchy scalp. (Dermatology)

Initial office visit for a 57-year-old female who complains of painful parotid swelling for one week's duration. (Oral & Maxillofacial Surgery)

Initial office visit for a patient with an ulcerated non-healing lesion or nodule on the tip of the nose. (Dermatology)

Initial office visit for a patient with dermatitis of the antecubital and popliteal fossae. (Dermatology)

Initial office visit for a 22-year-old female with irregular menses. (Family Medicine)

Initial office visit for a 50-year-old female with dyspepsia and nausea. (Family Medicine)

Initial office visit for a 53-year-old laborer with degenerative joint disease of the knee with no prior treatment. (Orthopaedic Surgery)

Initial office visit for a 60-year-old male with Dupuytren's contracture of one hand with multiple digit involvement. (Orthopaedic Surgery)

Initial office visit for a 33-year-old male with painless gross hematuria without cystoscopy. (Internal Medicine)

Initial office visit for a 55-year-old female with chronic blepharitis. There is a history of use of many medications. (Ophthalmology)

Initial office visit for an 18-year-old female with a two-day history of acute conjunctivitis. Extensive history of possible exposures, prior normal ocular history, and medication use is obtained. (Ophthalmology)

Initial office visit for a 14-year-old male with unilateral anterior knee pain. (Physical Medicine & Rehabilitation)

Initial office visit of an adult who presents with symptoms of an upper-respiratory infection that has progressed to unilateral purulent nasal discharge and discomfort in the right maxillary teeth. (Otolaryngology, Head & Neck Surgery)

Initial office visit of a 40-year-old female with symptoms of atopic allergies including eye and sinus congestion, often associated with infections. She would like to be tested for allergies. (Otolaryngology, Head & Neck Surgery)

Initial office visit of a 65-year-old with nasal stuffiness. (Otolaryngology, Head & Neck Surgery)

Initial office visit for initial evaluation of a 48-year-old man with recurrent low back pain radiating to the leg. (General Surgery)

Initial office visit for evaluation, diagnosis and management of painless gross hematuria in a new patient, without cystoscopy. (Internal Medicine)

Initial office visit with couple for counseling concerning voluntary vasectomy for sterility. Spent 30 minutes discussing procedure, risks and benefits, and answering questions. (Urology)

Initial office visit of a 49-year-old male with nasal obstruction. Detailed exam with topical anesthesia. (Plastic Surgery)

Initial office visit for evaluation of a 13-year-old female with progressive scoliosis. (Physical Medicine & Rehabilitation)

Initial office visit for a 21-year-old female desiring counseling and evaluation of initiation of contraception. (Family Practice/Internal Medicine/Obstetrics & Gynecology)

Initial office visit for a 49-year-old male presenting with painless blood per rectum associated with bowel movement. (Colon & Rectal Surgery)

Initial office visit for a 19-year-old football player with three-day-old acute knee injury; now with swelling and pain. (Orthopaedic Surgery)

99204 Initial office visit for a 13-year-old female with progressive scoliosis. (Orthopaedic Surgery)

Initial office visit for a 34-year-old female with primary infertility for evaluation and counseling. (Obstetrics & Gynecology)

Initial office visit for a 6-year-old male with multiple upper respiratory infections. (Allergy & Immunology)

Initial office visit for a patient with generalized dermatitis of 80 percent of the body surface area. (Dermatology)

Initial office visit for an adolescent who was referred by school counselor because of repeated skipping school. (Psychiatry)

Initial office visit for a 50-year-old machinist with a generalized eruption. (Dermatology)

Initial office visit for a 45-year-old female who has been abstinent from alcohol and benzodiazepines for three months but complains of headaches, insomnia, and anxiety. (Psychiatry)

Initial office visit for a 60-year-old male with recent change in bowel habits, weight loss, and abdominal pain. (Abdominal Surgery/General Surgery)

Initial office visit for a 50-year-old male with an aortic aneurysm who is considering surgery. (General Surgery)

Initial office visit for a 17-year-old female with depression. (Internal Medicine)

Initial office visit of a 40-year-old with chronic draining ear, imbalance, and probable cholesteatoma. (Otolaryngology, Head & Neck Surgery)

Initial office visit for initial evaluation of a 63-year-old male with chest pain on exertion. (Cardiology/Internal Medicine)

Initial office visit for evaluation of a 70-year-old patient with recent onset of episodic confusion. (Internal Medicine)

Initial office visit for a 7-year-old female with juvenile diabetes mellitus, new to area, past history of hospitalization times three. (Pediatrics)

Initial office visit of a 50-year-old female with progressive solid food dysphagia. (Gastroenterology)

Initial office visit for a 34-year-old patient with primary infertility, including counseling. (Obstetrics & Gynecology)

Initial office visit for evaluation of a 70-year-old female with polyarthralgia. (Rheumatology)

Initial office visit for a patient with papulosquamous eruption involving 60 percent of the cutaneous surface with joint pain. Combinations of topical and systemic treatments discussed. (Dermatology)

99205 Initial office visit for a patient with disseminated lupus erythematosus with kidney disease, edema, purpura, and scarring lesions on the extremities plus cardiac symptoms. (Dermatology/General Surgery/Internal Medicine)

Initial office visit for a 25-year-old female with systemic lupus erythematosus, fever, seizures, and profound thrombocytopenia. (Rheumatology/Allergy & Immunology)

Initial office visit for an adult with multiple cutaneous blisters, denuded secondarily infected ulcerations, oral lesions, weight loss, and increasing weakness refractory to high dose corticosteroid. Initiation of new immunosuppressive therapy. (Dermatology)

Initial office visit for a 28-year-old male with systemic vasculitis and compromised circulation to the limbs. (Rheumatology)

Initial office visit for a 41-year-old female new to the area requesting rheumatologic care, on disability due to scleroderma and recent hospitalization for malignant hypertension. (Rheumatology)

Initial office visit for a 52-year-old female with acute four extremity weakness and shortness of breath one week post-flu vaccination. (Physical Medicine & Rehabilitation)

Initial office visit for a 60-year-old male with previous back surgery; now presents with back and pelvic pain, two-month history of bilateral progressive calf and thigh tightness and weakness when walking, causing several falls. (Orthopaedic Surgery)

Initial office visit for an adolescent referred from ER after making suicide gesture. (Psychiatry)

Initial office visit for a 49-year-old female with a history of headaches and dependence on opioids. She reports weight loss, progressive headache, and depression. (Psychiatry)

Initial office visit for a 50-year-old female with symptoms of rash, swellings, recurrent arthritic complaints, and diarrhea and lymphadenopathy. Patient has had a 25 lb. weight loss and was recently camping in the Amazon. (Allergy & Immunology)

Initial office visit for a 34-year-old uremic Type I diabetic patient referred for ESRD modality assessment and planning. (Nephrology)

Initial office visit for a 75-year-old female with neck and bilateral shoulder pain, brisk deep tendon reflexes, and stress incontinence. (Physical Medicine & Rehabilitation)

Initial office visit for an 8-year-old male with cerebral palsy and spastic quadriparesis. (Physical Medicine & Rehabilitation)

Initial office visit for a 73-year-old male with known prostate malignancy, who presents with severe back pain and a recent onset of lower extremity weakness. (Physical Medicine & Rehabilitation)

Initial office visit for a 38-year-old male with paranoid delusions and a history of alcohol abuse. (Psychiatry)

Initial office visit for a 12-week-old with bilateral hip dislocations and bilateral club feet. (Orthopaedic Surgery)

Initial office visit for a 29-year-old female with acute orbital congestion, eyelid retraction, and bilateral visual loss from optic neuropathy. (Ophthalmology)

Initial office visit for a 70-year-old diabetic patient with progressive visual field loss, advanced optic disc cupping and neovascularization of retina. (Ophthalmology)

Initial office visit for a newly diagnosed Type I diabetic patient. (Endocrinology)

Initial office evaluation of a 65-year-old female with exertional chest pain, intermittent claudication, syncope and a murmur of aortic stenosis. (Cardiology)

Initial office visit for a 73-year-old male with an unexplained 20 lb. weight loss. (Hematology/Oncology)

Initial office evaluation, patient with systemic lupus erythematosus, fever, seizures and profound thrombocytopenia. (Allergy & Immunology/Internal Medicine/Rheumatology)

Initial office evaluation and management of patient with systemic vasculitis and compromised circulation to the limbs. (Rheumatology)

Initial office visit for a 24-year-old homosexual male who has a fever, a cough, and shortness of breath. (Infectious Disease)

Initial outpatient evaluation of a 69-year-old male with severe chronic obstructive pulmonary disease, congestive heart failure, and hypertension. (Family Medicine)

Initial office visit for a 17-year-old female, who is having school problems and has told a friend she is considering suicide. The patient and her family are consulted in regard to treatment options. (Psychiatry)

Initial office visit for a female with severe hirsutism, amenorrhea, weight loss and a desire to have children. (Endocrinology/Obstetrics & Gynecology)

Initial office visit for a 42-year-old male on hypertensive medication, newly arrived to the area, with diastolic blood pressure of 110, history of recurrent calculi, episodic headaches, intermittent chest pain and orthopnea. (Internal Medicine)

Established Patient

99211 Office visit for an 82-year-old female, established patient, for a monthly B12 injection with documented Vitamin B12 deficiency. (Geriatrics/Internal Medicine/Family Medicine)

Office visit for a 50-year-old male, established patient, for removal of uncomplicated facial sutures. (Plastic Surgery)

Office visit for an established patient who lost prescription for lichen planus. Returned for new copy. (Dermatology)

Office visit for an established patient undergoing orthodontics who complains of a wire which is irritating his/her cheek and asks you to check it. (Oral & Maxillofacial Surgery)

Office visit for a 50-year-old female, established patient, seen for her gold injection by the nurse. (Rheumatology)

Office visit for a 73-year-old female, established patient, with pernicious anemia for weekly B12 injection. (Gastroenterology)

Office visit for an established patient for dressing change on a skin biopsy. (Dermatology)

Office visit for a 19-year-old, established patient, for removal of sutures from a two cm. laceration of forehead, which you placed four days ago in ER. (Plastic Surgery)

Office visit of a 20-year-old female, established patient, who receives an allergy vaccine injection and is observed for a reaction by the nurse. (Otolaryngology, Head & Neck Surgery)

Office visit for a 45-year-old male, established patient, with chronic renal failure for the administration of erythropoietin. (Nephrology)

Office visit for an established patient, a Peace Corps enlistee, who requests documentation that third molars have been removed. (Oral & Maxillofacial Surgery)

Office visit for a 69-year-old female, established patient, for partial removal of antibiotic gauze from an infected wound site. (Plastic Surgery)

Office visit for a 9-year-old, established patient, successfully treated for impetigo, requiring release to return to school. (Dermatology/Pediatrics)

Office visit for an established patient requesting a return-to-work certificate for resolving contact dermatitis. (Dermatology)

Office visit for an established patient who is performing glucose monitoring and wants to check accuracy of machine with lab blood glucose by technician who checks accuracy and function of patient machine. (Endocrinology)

Follow-up office visit for a 65-year-old female with a chronic indwelling percutaneous nephrostomy catheter seen for routine pericatheter skin care and dressing change. (Interventional Radiology)

Outpatient visit with 19-year-old male, established patient, for supervised drug screen. (Addiction Medicine)

Office visit with 12-year-old male, established patient, for cursory check of hematoma one day after venipuncture. (Internal Medicine)

Office visit with 31-year-old female, established patient, for return to work certificate. (Anesthesiology)

Office visit for a 42-year-old, established patient, to read tuberculin test results. (Allergy & Immunology)

Office visit for 14-year-old, established patient, to re-dress an abrasion. (Orthopaedic Surgery)

Office visit for a 45-year-old female, established patient, for a blood pressure check. (Obstetrics & Gynecology)

Office visit for a 23-year-old, established patient, for instruction in use of peak flow meter. (Allergy & Immunology)

Office visit for prescription refill for a 35-year-old female, established patient, with schizophrenia who is stable but has run out of neuroleptic and is scheduled to be seen in a week. (Psychiatry)

99212 Office visit for an 11-year-old, established patient, seen in follow-up for mild comedonal acne of the cheeks on topical desquamating agents. (Dermatology/Family Medicine/Pediatrics)

Office visit for a 10-year-old female, established patient, who has been swimming in a lake, now presents with a one-day history of left ear pain with purulent drainage. (Family Medicine)

Office visit of a child, established patient, with chronic secretory otitis media. (Otolaryngology, Head & Neck Surgery)

Office visit for an established patient seen in follow-up of clearing patch of localized contact dermatitis. (Family Medicine/Dermatology)

Office visit for an established patient returning for evaluation of response to treatment of lichen planus on wrists and ankles. (Dermatology)

Office visit for an established patient with tinea pedis being treated with topical therapy. (Dermatology)

Office visit for an established patient with localized erythematous plaque of psoriasis with topical hydration. (Dermatology)

Office visit for a 50-year-old male, established patient, recently seen for acute neck pain, diagnosis of spondylosis, responding to physical therapy and intermittent cervical traction. Returns for evaluation for return to work. (Neurology)

Office visit for an established patient with recurring episodes of herpes simplex who has developed a clustering of vesicles on the upper lip. (Oral & Maxillofacial Surgery)

Evaluation for a 50-year-old male, established patient, who has experienced a recurrence of knee pain after he discontinued NSAID. (Anesthesiology/Pain Medicine)

Office visit for an established patient with an irritated skin tag for reassurance. (Dermatology)

Office visit for a 40-year-old, established patient, who has experienced a systemic allergic reaction following administration of immunotherapy. The dose must be readjusted. (Allergy & Immunology)

Office visit for a 33-year-old, established patient, for contusion and abrasion of lower extremity. (Orthopaedic Surgery)

Office visit for a 22-year-old male, established patient, one month after I & D of "wrestler's ear." (Plastic Surgery)

Office visit for a 21-year-old, established patient, who is seen in follow-up after antibiotic therapy for acute bacterial tonsillitis. (Otolaryngology, Head & Neck Surgery)

Office visit for a 4-year-old, established patient, with tympanostomy tubes, check-up. (Otolaryngology, Head & Neck Surgery)

Office visit for an established patient who has had needle aspiration of a peritonsillar abscess. (Otolaryngology, Head & Neck Surgery)

Follow-up office examination for evaluation and treatment of acute draining ear in a 5-year-old with tympanotomy tubes. (Otolaryngology, Head & Neck Surgery)

Office visit, established patient, 6-year-old with sore throat and headache. (Family Medicine/Pediatrics)

Office evaluation for possible purulent bacterial conjunctivitis with one- to two-day history of redness and discharge, 16-year-old female, established patient. (Pediatrics/Internal Medicine/Family Medicine)

Office visit with a 65-year-old female, established patient, returns for three-week follow-up for resolving severe ankle sprain. (Orthopaedic Surgery)

Office visit, sore throat, fever and fatigue in a 19-year-old college student, established patient. (Internal Medicine)

Office visit with a 33-year-old female, established patient, recently started on treatment for hemorrhoidal complaints, for re-evaluation. (Colon & Rectal Surgery)

Office visit with a 36-year-old male, established patient, for follow-up on effectiveness of medicine management of oral candidiasis. (Oral & Maxillofacial Surgery)

Office visit for a 27-year-old female, established patient, with complaints of vaginal itching. (Obstetrics & Gynecology)

Office visit for a 65-year-old male, established patient, with eruptions on both arms from poison oak exposure. (Allergy & Immunology/Internal Medicine)

99213 Office visit for an established patient with new lesions of lichen planus in spite of topical therapies. (Dermatology)

Office visit for the quarterly follow-up of a 45-year-old male with stable chronic asthma requiring regular drug therapy. (Allergy & Immunology)

Office visit for a 13-year-old, established patient, with comedopapular acne of the face which has shown poor response to topical medication. Discussion of use of systemic medication. (Dermatology)

Office visit for a 62-year-old female, established patient, for follow-up for stable cirrhosis of the liver. (Internal Medicine/Family Medicine)

Office visit for a 3-year-old, established patient, with atopic dermatitis and food hypersensitivity for quarterly follow-up evaluation. The patient is on topical lotions and steroid creams as well as oral antihistamines. (Allergy & Immunology)

Office visit for an 80-year-old female, established patient, to evaluate medical management of osteoarthritis of the temporomandibular joint. (Rheumatology)

Office visit for a 70-year-old female, established patient, one year post excision of basal cell carcinoma of nose with nasolabial flap. Now presents with new suspicious recurrent lesion and suspicious lesion of the back. (Plastic Surgery)

Office visit for a 68-year-old female, established patient, with polymyalgia rheumatic, maintained on chronic low-dose corticosteroid, with no new complaints. (Rheumatology)

Office visit for a 3-year-old female, established patient, for earache and dyshidrosis of feet. (Pediatrics/Family Medicine)

Office visit for an established patient for 18 months post-operative follow-up of TMJ repair. (Oral & Maxillofacial Surgery)

Office visit for a 45-year-old male, established patient, being re-evaluated for recurrent acute prostatitis. (Urology)

Office visit for a 43-year-old male, established patient, with known reflex sympathetic dystrophy. (Anesthesiology)

Office visit for an established patient with an evenly pigmented superficial nodule of leg which is symptomatic. (Dermatology)

Office visit for an established patient with psoriasis involvement of the elbows, pitting of the nails, and itchy scalp. (Dermatology)

Office visit for a 27-year-old male, established patient, with deep follicular and perifollicular inflammation unable to tolerate systemic antibiotics due to GI upset, requires change of systemic medication. (Dermatology)

Office visit for a 16-year-old male, established patient, who is on medication for exercise-induced bronchospasm. (Allergy & Immunology)

Office visit for a 60-year-old, established patient, with chronic essential hypertension on multiple drug regimen, for blood pressure check. (Family Medicine)

Office visit for a 20-year-old male, established patient, for removal of sutures in hand. (Family Medicine)

Office visit for a 58-year-old female, established patient, with unilateral painful bunion. (Orthopaedic Surgery)

Office visit for a 45-year-old female, established patient, with known osteoarthritis and painful swollen knees. (Rheumatology)

Office visit for a 25-year-old female, established patient, complaining of bleeding and heavy menses. (Obstetrics & Gynecology)

Office visit for a 55-year-old male, established patient, with hypertension managed by a beta blocker/thiazide regime; now experiencing mild fatigue. (Nephrology)

Office visit for a 65-year-old female, established patient, with primary glaucoma for interval determination of intraocular pressure and possible adjustment of medication. (Ophthalmology)

Office visit for a 56-year-old man, established patient, with stable exertional angina who complains of new onset of calf pain while walking. (Cardiology)

Office visit for a 63-year-old female, established patient, with rheumatoid arthritis on auranofin and ibuprofen, seen for routine follow-up visit. (Rheumatology)

Office visit for an established patient with Graves' disease, three months post I-131 therapy, who presents with lassitude and malaise. (Endocrinology)

Office visit for the quarterly follow-up of a 63-year-old male, established patient, with chronic myofascial pain syndrome, effectively managed by doxepin, who presents with new onset urinary hesitancy. (Pain Medicine)

Office visit for the biannual follow-up of an established patient with migraine variant having infrequent, intermittent, moderate to severe headaches with nausea and vomiting, which are sometimes effectively managed by ergotamine tartrate and an antiemetic, but occasionally requiring visits to an emergency department. (Pain Medicine)

Office visit for an established patient after discharge from a pain rehabilitation program to review and adjust medication dosage. (Pain Medicine)

Office visit with 55-year-old male, established patient, for management of hypertension, mild fatigue, on beta blocker/thiazide regimen. (Family Medicine/Internal Medicine)

Outpatient visit with 37-year-old male, established patient, who is three years post total colectomy for chronic ulcerative colitis, presents for increased irritation at his stoma. (General Surgery)

Office visit for a 70-year-old diabetic hypertensive established patient with recent change in insulin requirement. (Internal Medicine/Nephrology)

Office visit with 80-year-old female, established patient, for follow-up osteoporosis, status-post compression fractures. (Rheumatology)

Office visit for an established patient with stable cirrhosis of the liver. (Gastroenterology)

Routine, follow-up office evaluation at a three-month interval for a 77-year-old female, established patient, with nodular small cleaved-cell lymphoma. (Hematology/Oncology)

Quarterly follow-up office visit for a 45-year-old male, established patient, with stable chronic asthma, on steroid and bronchodilator therapy. (Pulmonary Medicine)

Office visit for a 50-year-old female, established patient, with insulin-dependent diabetes mellitus and stable coronary artery disease, for monitoring. (Family Medicine/Internal Medicine)

99214 Office visit for an established patient now presenting with generalized dermatitis of 80 percent of the body surface area. (Dermatology)

Office visit for a 32-year-old female, established patient, with new onset right lower quadrant pain. (Family Medicine)

Office visit for reassessment and reassurance/counseling of a 40-year-old female, established patient, who is experiencing increased symptoms while on a pain management treatment program. (Pain Medicine)

Office visit for a 30-year-old, established patient, under management for intractable low back pain, who now presents with new onset right posterior thigh pain. (Pain Medicine)

Office visit for an established patient with frequent intermittent, moderate to severe headaches requiring beta blocker or tricyclic antidepressant prophylaxis, as well as four symptomatic treatments, but who is still experiencing headaches at a frequency of several times a month that are unresponsive to treatment. (Pain Medicine)

Office visit for an established patient with psoriasis with extensive involvement of scalp, trunk, palms, and soles with joint pain. Combinations of topical and systemic treatments discussed and instituted. (Dermatology)

Office visit for a 55-year-old male, established patient, with increasing night pain, limp, and progressive varus of both knees. (Orthopaedic Surgery)

Follow-up visit for a 15-year-old withdrawn patient with four-year history of papulocystic acne of the face, chest, and back with early scarring and poor response to past treatment. Discussion of use of systemic medication. (Dermatology)

Office visit for a 28-year-old male, established patient, with regional enteritis, diarrhea, and low-grade fever. (Internal Medicine)

Office visit for a 25-year-old female, established patient, following recent arthrogram and MR imaging for TMJ pain. (Oral & Maxillofacial Surgery)

Office visit for a 32-year-old female, established patient, with large obstructing stone in left mid-ureter, to discuss management options including urethroscopy with extraction or ESWL. (Urology)

Evaluation for a 28-year-old male, established patient, with new onset of low back pain. (Anesthesiology/Pain Medicine)

Office visit for a 28-year-old female, established patient, with right lower quadrant abdominal pain, fever, and anorexia. (Internal Medicine/Family Medicine)

Office visit for a 45-year-old male, established patient, four months follow-up of L4-5 diskectomy, with persistent incapacitating low back and leg pain. (Orthopaedic Surgery)

Outpatient visit for a 77-year-old male, established patient, with hypertension, presenting with a three-month history of episodic substernal chest pain on exertion. (Cardiology)

Office visit for a 25-year-old female, established patient, for evaluation of progressive saddle nose deformity of unknown etiology. (Plastic Surgery)

Office visit for a 65-year-old male, established patient, with BPH and severe bladder outlet obstruction, to discuss management options such as TURP. (Urology)

Office visit for an adult diabetic established patient with a past history of recurrent sinusitis who presents with a one-week history of double vision. (Otolaryngology, Head & Neck Surgery)

Office visit for an established patient with lichen planus and 60 percent of the cutaneous surface involved, not responsive to systemic steroids, as well as developing symptoms of progressive heartburn and paranoid ideation. (Dermatology)

Office visit for a 52-year-old male, established patient, with a 12-year history of bipolar disorder responding to lithium carbonate and brief psychotherapy. Psychotherapy and prescription provided. (Psychiatry)

Office visit for a 63-year-old female, established patient, with a history of familial polyposis, status post-colectomy with sphincter sparing procedure, who now presents with rectal bleeding and increase in stooling frequency. (General Surgery)

Office visit for a 68-year-old male, established patient, with the sudden onset of multiple flashes and floaters in the right eye due to a posterior vitreous detachment. (Ophthalmology)

Office visit for a 55-year-old female, established patient, on cyclosporin for treatment of resistant, small vessel vasculitis. (Rheumatology)

Follow-up office visit for a 55-year-old male, two months after iliac angioplasty with new onset of contralateral extremity claudication. (Interventional Radiology)

Office visit for a 68-year-old male, established patient, with stable angina, two months post myocardial infarction, who is not tolerating one of his medications. (Cardiology)

Weekly office visit for 5FU therapy for an ambulatory established patient with metastatic colon cancer and increasing shortness of breath. (Hematology/Oncology)

Follow-up office visit for a 60-year-old male, established patient, whose post-traumatic seizures have disappeared on medication and who now raises the question of stopping the medication (Neurology)

Office evaluation on new onset RLQ pain in a 32-year-old woman, established patient. (Urology/General Surgery/Internal Medicine/Family Medicine)

Office evaluation of 28-year-old, established patient, with regional enteritis, diarrhea and low-grade fever. (Family Medicine/Internal Medicine)

Office visit with 50-year-old female, established patient, diabetic, blood sugar controlled by diet. She now complains of frequency of urination and weight loss, blood sugar of 320 and negative ketones on dipstick. (Internal Medicine)

Follow-up office visit for a 45-year-old, established patient, with rheumatoid arthritis on gold, methotrexate, or immunosuppressive therapy. (Rheumatology)

Office visit for a 60-year-old male, established patient, two years post-removal of intracranial meningioma, now with new headaches and visual disturbance. (Neurosurgery)

Office visit for a 68-year-old female, established patient, for routine review and follow-up of non-insulin dependent diabetes, obesity, hypertension and congestive heart failure. Complains of vision difficulties and admits dietary noncompliance. Patient is counseled concerning diet and current medications adjusted. (Family Medicine)

99215 Office visit for an established patient who developed persistent cough, rectal bleeding, weakness, and diarrhea plus pustular infection on skin. Patient on immunosuppressive therapy. (Dermatology)

Office visit for an established patient with disseminated lupus erythematosus, extensive edema of extremities kidney disease, and weakness requiring monitored course on azathioprene, corticosteroid and complicated by acute depression. (Dermatology/Internal Medicine/Rheumatology)

Office visit for an established patient with progressive dermatomyositis and recent onset of fever, nasal speech, and regurgitation of fluids through the nose. (Dermatology)

Office visit for a 28-year-old female, established patient, who is abstinent from previous cocaine dependence, but reports progressive panic attacks and chest pains. (Psychiatry)

Office visit for an established adolescent patient with history of bipolar disorder treated with lithium; seen on urgent basis at family's request because of severe depressive symptoms. (Psychiatry)

Office visit for an established patient having acute migraine with new onset neurological symptoms and whose headaches are unresponsive to previous attempts at management with a combination of preventive and abortive medication. (Pain Medicine)

Office visit for an established patient with exfoliative lichen planus with daily fever spikes, disorientation, and shortness of breath. (Dermatology)

Office visit for a 25-year-old, established patient, two years post-burn with bilateral ectropion, hypertrophic facial burn scars, near absence of left breast, and burn syndactyly of both hands. Discussion of treatment options following examination. (Plastic Surgery)

Office visit for a 6-year-old, established patient, to review newly diagnosed immune deficiency with recommendations for therapy including IV immunoglobulin and chronic antibiotics. (Allergy & Immunology)

Office visit for a 36-year-old, established patient, three months status post-transplant, with new onset of peripheral edema, increased blood pressure, and progressive fatigue. (Nephrology)

Office visit for an established patient with Kaposi's sarcoma who presents with fever and widespread vesicles. (Dermatology)

Office visit for a 27-year-old female, established patient, with bipolar disorder who was stable on lithium carbonate and monthly supportive psychotherapy but now has developed symptoms of hypomania. (Psychiatry)

Office visit for a 25-year-old male, established patient with a history of schizophrenia who has been seen bi-monthly but is complaining of auditory hallucinations. (Psychiatry)

Office visit for a 62-year-old male, established patient, three years post-op abdominal perineal resection, now with a rising carcinoembryonic antigen, weight loss, and pelvic pain. (Abdominal Surgery)

Office visit for a 42-year-old male, established patient, nine months post-op emergency vena cava shunt for variceal bleeding, now presents with complaints of one episode of "dark" bowel movement, weight gain, tightness in abdomen, whites of eyes seem "yellow" and occasional drowsiness after eating hamburgers. (Abdominal Surgery)

Office visit for a 68-year-old male, established patient, with biopsy-proven rectal carcinoma, for evaluation and discussion of treatment options. (General Surgery)

Office visit for a 60-year-old, established patient, with diabetic nephropathy with increasing edema and dyspnea. (Endocrinology)

Office visit with 30-year-old male, established patient for three-month history of fatigue, weight loss, intermittent fever, and presenting with diffuse adenopathy and splenomegaly. (Family Medicine)

Office visit for restaging of an established patient with new lymphadenopathy one year post-therapy for lymphoma. (Hematology/Oncology)

Office visit for evaluation of recent onset syncopal attacks in a 70-year-old woman, established patient. (Internal Medicine)

Follow-up visit, 40-year-old mother of three, established patient, with acute rheumatoid arthritis, anatomical Stage 3, ARA function Class 3 rheumatoid arthritis, and deteriorating function. (Rheumatology)

Office evaluation and discussion of treatment options for a 68-year-old male, established patient, with a biopsy-proven rectal carcinoma. (General Surgery)

Follow-up office visit for a 65-year-old male, established patient, with a fever of recent onset while on outpatient antibiotic therapy for endocarditis. (Infectious Disease)

Office visit for a 75-year-old, established patient, with ALS (amyotrophic lateral sclerosis), who is no longer able to swallow. (Neurology)

Office visit for a 70-year-old female, established patient, with diabetes mellitus and hypertension, presenting with a two-month history of increasing confusion, agitation and short-term memory loss. (Family Medicine/Internal Medicine)

Hospital Inpatient Services

Initial Hospital Care

New or Established Patient

99221 Initial hospital visit following admission for a 42-year-old male for observation following an uncomplicated mandible fracture. (Plastic Surgery/Oral & Maxillofacial Surgery)

Initial hospital visit for a 40-year-old patient with a thrombosed synthetic arteriovenous conduit. (Nephrology)

Initial hospital visit for a healthy 24-year-old male with an acute onset of low back pain following a lifting injury. (Internal Medicine/Anesthesiology/Pain Medicine)

Initial hospital visit for a 69-year-old female with controlled hypertension, scheduled for surgery. (Internal Medicine/Cardiology)

Initial hospital visit for a 24-year-old healthy female with benign tumor of palate. (Oral & Maxillofacial Surgery)

Initial hospital visit for a 14-year-old female with infectious mononucleosis and dehydration. (Internal Medicine)

Initial hospital visit for a 62-year-old female with stable rheumatoid arthritis, admitted for total joint replacement. (Rheumatology)

Initial hospital visit for a 12-year-old patient with a laceration of the upper eyelid, involving the lid margin and superior canaliculus, admitted prior to surgery for IV antibiotic therapy. (Plastic Surgery)

Initial hospital visit for a 69-year-old female with controlled hypertension, scheduled for surgery. (Cardiology)

Hospital admission, examination, and initiation of treatment program for a 67-year-old male with uncomplicated pneumonia who requires IV antibiotic therapy. (Internal Medicine)

Hospital admission for an 18-month-old with 10 percent dehydration. (Pediatrics)

Hospital admission for a 12-year-old with a laceration of the upper eyelid involving the lid margin and superior canaliculus, admitted prior to surgery for IV antibiotic therapy. (Ophthalmology)

Hospital admission for a 32-year-old female with severe flank pain, hematuria and presumed diagnosis of ureteral calculus as determined by Emergency Department physician. (Urology)

Initial hospital visit for a patient with several large venous stasis ulcers not responding to outpatient therapy. (Dermatology)

Initial hospital visit for 21-year-old pregnant patient (nine weeks gestation) with hyperemesis gravidarum. (Obstetrics & Gynecology)

Initial hospital visit for a 73-year-old female with acute pyelonephritis who is otherwise generally healthy. (Geriatrics)

Initial hospital visit for 62-year-old patient with cellulitis of the foot requiring bedrest and intravenous antibiotics. (Orthopaedic Surgery)

99222 Initial hospital visit for a 50-year-old patient with lower quadrant abdominal pain and increased temperature, but without septic picture. (General Surgery/Abdominal Surgery/Colon & Rectal Surgery)

Initial hospital visit for airway management, due to a benign laryngeal mass. (Otolaryngology, Head & Neck Surgery)

Initial hospital visit for a 66-year-old female with an L-2 vertebral compression fracture with acute onset of paralytic ileus; seen in the office two days previously. (Orthopaedic Surgery)

Initial hospital visit and evaluation of a 15-year-old male admitted with peritonsillar abscess or cellulitis requiring intravenous antibiotic therapy. (Otolaryngology, Head & Neck Surgery)

Initial hospital visit for a 42-year-old male with vertebral compression fracture following a motor vehicle accident. (Orthopaedic Surgery)

Initial hospital visit for a patient with generalized atopic dermatitis and secondary infection. (Dermatology)

Initial hospital visit for a 3-year-old patient with high temperature, limp, and painful hip motion of 18 hours' duration. (Pediatrics/Orthopaedic Surgery)

Initial hospital visit for a young adult, presenting with an acute asthma attack unresponsive to outpatient therapy. (Allergy & Immunology)

Initial hospital visit for an 18-year-old male who has suppurative sialoadenitis and dehydration. (Oral & Maxillofacial Surgery)

Initial hospital visit for a 65-year-old female for acute onset of thrombotic cerebrovascular accident with contralateral paralysis and aphasia. (Neurology)

Initial hospital visit for a 50-year-old male chronic paraplegic patient with pain and spasm below the lesion. (Anesthesiology)

Partial hospital admission for an adolescent patient from chaotic blended family, transferred from inpatient setting, for continued treatment to control symptomatic expressions of hostility and depression. (Psychiatry)

Initial hospital visit for a 15-year-old male with acute status asthmaticus, unresponsive to outpatient therapy. (Internal Medicine)

Initial hospital visit for a 61-year-old male with history of previous myocardial infarction, who now complains of chest pain. (Internal Medicine)

Initial hospital visit of a 15-year-old on medications for a sore throat over the last two weeks. The sore throat has worsened and patient now has dysphagia. The exam shows large necrotic tonsils with an adequate airway and small palpable nodes. The initial mono test was negative. (Otolaryngology, Head & Neck Surgery)

Initial hospital evaluation of a 23-year-old allergy patient admitted with eyelid edema and pain on fifth day of oral antibiotic therapy. (Otolaryngology, Head & Neck Surgery)

Hospital admission, young adult patient, failed previous therapy and now presents in acute asthmatic attack. (Family Medicine/Allergy & Immunology)

Hospital admission of a 62-year-old smoker, established patient, with bronchitis in acute respiratory distress. (Internal Medicine/Pulmonary Medicine)

Hospital admission, examination, and initiation of a treatment program for a 65-year-old female with new onset of right-sided paralysis and aphasia. (Neurology)

Hospital admission for a 50-year-old with left lower quadrant abdominal pain and increased temperature, but without septic picture. (General Surgery)

Hospital admission, examination, and initiation of treatment program for a 66-year-old chronic hemodialysis patient with fever and a new pulmonary infiltrate. (Nephrology)

Hospital admission for an 8-year-old febrile patient with chronic sinusitis and severe headache, unresponsive to oral antibiotics. (Allergy & Immunology)

Hospital admission for a 40-year-old male with submaxillary cellulitis and trismus from infected lower molar. (Oral & Maxillofacial Surgery)

99223 Initial hospital visit for a 45-year-old female, who has a history of rheumatic fever as a child and now has anemia, fever, and congestive heart failure. (Cardiology)

Initial hospital visit for a 50-year-old male with acute chest pain and diagnostic electrocardiographic changes of an acute anterior myocardial infarction. (Cardiology/Family Medicine/Internal Medicine)

Initial hospital visit of a 75-year-old with progressive stridor and dysphagia with history of cancer of the larynx treated by radiation therapy in the past. Exam shows a large recurrent tumor of the glottis with a mass in the neck. (Otolaryngology, Head & Neck Surgery)

Initial hospital visit for a 70-year-old male admitted with chest pain, complete heart block, and congestive heart failure. (Cardiology)

Initial hospital visit for an 82-year-old male who presents with syncope, chest pain, and ventricular arrhythmias. (Cardiology)

Initial hospital visit for a 75-year-old male with history of arteriosclerotic coronary vascular disease, who is severely dehydrated, disoriented, and experiencing auditory hallucinations. (Psychiatry)

Initial hospital visit for a 70-year-old male with alcohol and sedative-hypnotic dependence, admitted by family for severe withdrawal, hypertension, and diabetes mellitus. (Psychiatry)

Initial hospital visit for a persistently suicidal latency-aged child whose parents have requested admission to provide safety during evaluation, but are anxious about separation from her. (Psychiatry)

Initial psychiatric visit for an adolescent patient without previous psychiatric history, who was transferred from the medical ICU after a significant overdose. (Psychiatry)

Initial hospital visit for a 35-year-old female with severe systemic lupus erythematosus on corticosteroid and cyclophosphamide, with new onset of fever, chills, rash, and chest pain. (Rheumatology)

Initial hospital visit for a 52-year-old male with known rheumatic heart disease who presents with anasarca, hypertension, and history of alcohol abuse. (Cardiology)

Initial hospital visit for a 55-year-old female with a history of congenital heart disease; now presents with cyanosis. (Cardiology)

Initial hospital visit for a psychotic, hostile, violently combative adolescent, involuntarily committed, for seclusion and restraint in order to provide for safety on unit. (Psychiatry)

Initial hospital visit for a now subdued and sullen teenage male with six-month history of declining school performance, increasing self-endangerment, and resistance of parental expectations, including running away past weekend after physical fight with father. (Psychiatry)

Initial partial hospital admission for a 17-year-old female with history of borderline mental retardation who has developed auditory hallucinations. Parents are known to abuse alcohol, and Child Protective Services is investigating allegations of sexual abuse of a younger sibling. (Psychiatry)

Initial hospital visit of a 67-year old male admitted with a large neck mass, dysphagia, and history of myocardial infarction three months before. (Otolaryngology, Head & Neck Surgery)

Initial hospital visit for a patient with suspected cerebrospinal fluid rhinorrhea which developed two weeks after head injury. (Otolaryngology, Head & Neck Surgery)

Initial hospital visit for a 25-year-old female with history of poly-substance abuse and psychiatric disorder. The patient appears to be psychotic with markedly elevated vital signs. (Psychiatry)

Initial hospital visit for a 70-year-old male with cutaneous T-cell lymphoma who has developed fever and lymphadenopathy. (Internal Medicine)

Initial hospital visit for a 62-year-old female with known coronary artery disease, for evaluation of increasing edema, dyspnea on exertion, confusion, and sudden onset of fever with productive cough. (Internal Medicine)

Initial hospital visit for a 3-year-old female with 36-hour history of sore throat and high fever; now with sudden onset of lethargy, irritability, photophobia, and nuchal rigidity. (Pediatrics)

Initial hospital visit for a 26-year-old female for evaluation of severe facial fractures (LeFort's II/III). (Plastic Surgery)

Initial hospital visit for a 55-year-old female for bilateral mandibular fractures resulting in flail mandible and airway obstruction. (Plastic Surgery)

Initial hospital visit for a 71-year-old patient with a red painful eye four days following uncomplicated cataract surgery due to endophthalmitis. (Ophthalmology)

Initial hospital visit for a 45-year-old patient involved in a motor vehicle accident who suffered a perforating corneoscleral laceration with loss of vision. (Ophthalmology)

Initial hospital visit for a 58-year-old male who has Ludwig's angina and progressive airway compromise. (Oral & Maxillofacial Surgery)

Initial hospital visit for a patient with generalized systemic sclerosis, receiving immunosuppressive therapy because of recent onset of cough, fever, and inability to swallow. (Dermatology)

Initial hospital visit for an 82-year-old male who presents with syncope, chest pain, and ventricular arrhythmias. (Cardiology)

Initial hospital visit for a 62-year-old male with history of previous myocardial infarction, comes in with recurrent, sustained ventricular tachycardia. (Cardiology)

Initial hospital visit for a chronic dialysis patient with infected PTFE fistula, septicemia, and shock. (Nephrology)

Initial hospital visit for a 1-year-old male, victim of child abuse, with central nervous system depression, skull fracture, and retinal hemorrhage. (Family Medicine/Neurology)

Initial hospital visit for a 25-year-old female with recent C4-5 quadriplegia, admitted for rehabilitation. (Physical Medicine & Rehabilitation)

Initial hospital visit for an 18-year-old male, post-traumatic brain injury with multiple impairment. (Physical Medicine & Rehabilitation)

Initial partial hospital admission for 16-year-old male, sullen and subdued, with six-month history of declining school performance, increasing self-endangerment, and resistance to parental expectations. (Psychiatry)

Initial hospital visit for a 16-year-old primigravida at 32 weeks gestation with severe hypertension (200/110), thrombocytopenia, and headache. (Obstetrics & Gynecology)

Initial hospital visit for a 49-year-old male with cirrhosis of liver with hematemesis, hepatic encephalopathy, and fever. (Gastroenterology)

Initial hospital visit for a 55-year-old female in chronic pain who has attempted suicide. (Psychiatry)

Initial hospital visit for a 70-year-old male, with multiple organ system disease, admitted with history of being aneuric and septic for 24 hours prior to admission. (Urology)

Initial hospital visit for a 3-year-old female with 36-hour history of sore throat and high fever, now with sudden onset of lethargy, irritability, photophobia, and nuchal rigidity. (Internal Medicine)

Initial hospital visit for a 78-year-old male, transfers from nursing home with dysuria and pyuria, increasing confusion, and high fever. (Internal Medicine)

Initial hospital visit for a 1-day-old male with cyanosis, respiratory distress, and tachypnea. (Cardiology)

Initial hospital visit for a 3-year-old female with recurrent tachycardia and syncope. (Cardiology)

Initial hospital visit for a thyrotoxic patient who presents with fever, atrial fibrillation, and delirium. (Endocrinology)

Initial hospital visit for a 50-year-old Type I diabetic who presents with diabetic ketoacidosis with fever and obtundation. (Endocrinology)

Initial hospital visit for a 40-year-old female with anatomical stage 3, ARA functional class 3 rheumatoid arthritis on methotrexate, corticosteroid, and nonsteroidal anti-inflammatory drugs. Patient presents with severe arthritis flare, new oral ulcers, abdominal pain, and leukopenia. (Rheumatology)

Initial hospital exam of a pediatric patient with high fever and proptosis. (Otolaryngology, Head & Neck Surgery)

Initial hospital visit for a 25-year-old patient admitted for the first time to the rehab unit, with recent C-4-5 quadriplegia. (Physical Medicine & Rehabilitation)

Hospital admission, examination, and initiation of treatment program for a previously unknown 58-year-old male who presents with acute chest pain (Cardiology)

Hospital admission, examination, and initiation of induction chemotherapy for a 42-year-old patient with newly diagnosed acute myelogenous leukemia. (Hematology/Oncology)

Hospital admission following a motor vehicle accident of a 24-year-old male with fracture dislocation of C5-6; neurologically intact. (Neurosurgery)

Hospital admission for a 78-year-old female with left lower lobe pneumonia and a history of coronary artery disease, congestive heart failure, osteoarthritis and gout. (Family Medicine)

Hospital admission, examination, and initiation of treatment program for a 65-year-old immunosuppressed male with confusion, fever, and a headache. (Infectious Disease)

Hospital admission for a 9-year-old with vomiting, dehydration, fever, tachypnea and an admitting diagnosis of diabetic ketoacidosis. (Pediatrics)

Initial hospital visit for a 65-year-old male who presents with acute myocardial infarction, oliguria, hypotension, and altered state of consciousness. (Cardiology)

Initial hospital visit for a hostile/resistant adolescent patient who is severely depressed and involved in poly-substance abuse. Patient is experiencing significant conflict in his chaotic family situation and was suspended from school following an attack on a teacher with a baseball bat. (Psychiatry)

Initial hospital visit for 89-year-old female with fulminant hepatic failure and encephalopathy. (Gastroenterology)

Initial hospital visit for a 42-year-old female with rapidly progressing scleroderma, malignant hypertension, digital infarcts, and oligurea. (Rheumatology)

Subsequent Hospital Care

99231   Subsequent hospital visit for a 65-year-old female, post-open reduction and internal fixation of a fracture. (Physical Medicine & Rehabilitation)

Subsequent hospital visit for a 33-year-old patient with pelvic pain who is responding to pain medication and observation. (Obstetrics & Gynecology)

Subsequent hospital visit for a 21-year-old female with hyperemesis who has responded well to intravenous fluids. (Obstetrics & Gynecology)

Subsequent hospital visit to re-evaluate post-op pain and titrate patient-controlled analgesia for a 27-year-old female. (Anesthesiology)

Follow-up hospital visit for a 35-year-old female, status post-epidural analgesia. (Anesthesiology/Pain Medicine)

Subsequent hospital visit for a 56-year-old male, post-gastrectomy, for maintenance of analgesia using an intravenous dilaudid infusion. (Anesthesiology)

Subsequent hospital visit for a 4-year-old on day three receiving medication for uncomplicated pneumonia. (Allergy & Immunology)

Subsequent hospital visit for a 30-year-old female with urticaria which has stabilized with medication. (Allergy & Immunology)

Subsequent hospital visit for a 76-year-old male with venous stasis ulcers. (Dermatology)

Subsequent hospital visit for a 24-year-old female with otitis externa, seen two days before in consultation, now to have otic wick removal. (Otolaryngology, Head & Neck Surgery)

Subsequent hospital visit for a 27-year-old with acute labyrinthitis. (Otolaryngology, Head & Neck Surgery)

Subsequent hospital visit for a 10-year-old male admitted for lobar pneumonia with vomiting and dehydration; is becoming afebrile and tolerating oral fluids. (Family Medicine/Pediatrics)

Subsequent hospital visit for a 62-year-old patient with resolving cellulitis of the foot. (Orthopaedic Surgery)

Subsequent hospital visit for a 25-year-old male admitted for supra-ventricular tachycardia and converted on medical therapy. (Cardiology)

Subsequent hospital visit for a 27-year-old male two days after open reduction and internal fixation for malar complex fracture. (Plastic Surgery)

Subsequent hospital visit for a 76-year-old male with venous stasis ulcers. (Geriatrics)

Subsequent hospital visit for a 67-year-old female admitted three days ago with bleeding gastric ulcer; now stable. (Gastroenterology)

Subsequent hospital visit for stable 33-year-old male, status post-lower gastrointestinal bleeding. (General Surgery/Gastroenterology)

Subsequent hospital visit for a 29-year-old auto mechanic with effort thrombosis of left upper extremity. (General Surgery)

Subsequent hospital visit for a 14-year-old female in middle phase of inpatient treatment, who is now behaviorally stable and making satisfactory progress in treatment. (Psychiatry)

Subsequent hospital visit for an 18-year-old male with uncomplicated asthma who is clinically stable. (Allergy & Immunology)

Subsequent hospital visit for a 55-year-old male with rheumatoid arthritis, two days following an uncomplicated total joint replacement. (Rheumatology)

Subsequent hospital visit for a 60-year-old dialysis patient with an access infection, now afebrile on antibiotic. (Nephrology)

Subsequent hospital visit for a 36-year-old female with stable post-rhinoplasty epistaxis. (Plastic Surgery)

Subsequent hospital visit for a 66-year-old female with L-2 vertebral compression fracture with resolving ileus. (Orthopaedic Surgery)

Subsequent hospital visit for a patient with peritonsillar abscess. (Otolaryngology, Head & Neck Surgery)

Subsequent hospital visit for an 18-year-old female responding to intravenous antibiotic therapy for ear or sinus infection. (Otolaryngology, Head & Neck Surgery)

Subsequent hospital visit for a 70-year-old male admitted with congestive heart failure who has responded to therapy. (Cardiology)

Follow-up hospital visit for a 32-year-old female with left ureteral calculus; being followed in anticipation of spontaneous passage. (Urology)

Subsequent hospital visit for a 4-year-old female, admitted for acute gastroenteritis and dehydration, requiring IV hydration; now stable. (Family Medicine)

Subsequent hospital visit for a 50-year-old Type II diabetic who is clinically stable and without complications requiring regulation of a single dose of insulin daily. (Endocrinology)

Subsequent hospital visit to reassesses the status of a 65-year-old patient post-open reduction and internal fixation of hip fracture, on the rehab unit. (Physical Medicine & Rehabilitation)

Subsequent hospital visit for a 78-year-old male with cholangiocarcinoma managed by biliary drainage. (Interventional Radiology)

Subsequent hospital visit for a 50-year-old male with uncomplicated myocardial infarction who is clinically stable and without chest pain. (Family Medicine/Cardiology/Internal Medicine)

Subsequent hospital visit for a stable 72-year-old lung cancer patient undergoing a five-day course of infusion chemotherapy. (Hematology/Oncology)

Subsequent hospital visit, two days post admission for a 65-year-old male with a CVA (cerebral vascular accident) and left hemiparesis, who is clinically stable. (Neurology/Physical Medicine and Rehabilitation)

Subsequent hospital visit for now stable, 33-year-old male, status post lower gastrointestinal bleeding. (General Surgery)

Subsequent visit on third day of hospitalization for a 60-year-old female recovering from an uncomplicated pneumonia. (Infectious Disease/Internal Medicine/Pulmonary Medicine)

Subsequent hospital visit for a 3-year-old patient in traction for a congenital dislocation of the hip. (Orthopaedic Surgery)

Subsequent hospital visit for a 4-year-old female, admitted for acute gastroenteritis and dehydration, requiring IV hydration; now stable. (Family Medicine/Internal Medicine)

Subsequent hospital visit for 50-year-old female with resolving uncomplicated acute pancreatitis. (Gastroenterology)

99232 Subsequent hospital visit for a patient with venous stasis ulcers who developed fever and red streaks adjacent to the ulcer. (Dermatology/Internal Medicine/Family Medicine)

Subsequent hospital visit for a 66-year-old male for dressing changes and observation. Patient has had a myocutaneous flap to close a pharyngeal fistula and now has a low-grade fever. (Plastic Surgery)

Subsequent hospital visit for a 54-year-old female admitted for myocardial infarction, but who is now having frequent premature ventricular contractions. (Internal Medicine)

Subsequent hospital visit for an 80-year-old patient with a pelvic rim fracture, inability to walk, and severe pain; now 36 hours post-injury, experiencing urinary retention. (Orthopaedic Surgery)

Subsequent hospital visit for a 17-year-old female with fever, pharyngitis, and airway obstruction, who after 48 hours develops a maculopapular rash. (Pediatrics/Family Medicine)

Follow-up hospital visit for a 32-year-old patient admitted the previous day for corneal ulcer. (Dermatology)

Follow-up visit for a 67-year-old male with congestive heart failure who has responded to antibiotics and diuretics, and has now developed a monoarthropathy. (Internal Medicine)

Follow-up hospital visit for a 58-year-old male receiving continuous opioids who is experiencing severe nausea and vomiting. (Pain Medicine)

Subsequent hospital visit for a patient after an auto accident who is slow to respond to ambulation training. (Physical Medicine & Rehabilitation)

Subsequent hospital visit for a 14-year-old with unstable bronchial asthma complicated by pneumonia. (Allergy & Immunology)

Subsequent hospital visit for a 50-year-old diabetic, hypertensive male with back pain not responding to conservative inpatient management with continued radiation of pain to the lower left extremity. (Orthopaedic Surgery)

Subsequent hospital visit for a 37-year-old female on day five of antibiotics for bacterial endocarditis, who still has low-grade fever. (Cardiology)

Subsequent hospital visit for a 54-year-old patient, post MI (myocardial infarction), who is out of the CCU (coronary care unit) but is now having frequent premature ventricular contractions on telemetry. (Cardiology/Internal Medicine)

Subsequent hospital visit for a patient with neutropenia, a fever responding to antibiotics, and continued slow gastrointestinal bleeding on platelet support. (Hematology/Oncology)

Subsequent hospital visit for a 50-year-old male admitted two days ago for sub-acute renal allograft rejection. (Nephrology)

Subsequent hospital visit for a 35-year-old drug addict, not responding to initial antibiotic therapy for pyelonephritis. (Urology)

Subsequent hospital visit of an 81-year-old male with abdominal distention, nausea, and vomiting. (General Surgery)

Subsequent hospital care for a 62-year-old female with congestive heart failure, who remains dyspneic and febrile. (Internal Medicine)

Subsequent hospital visit for a 73-year-old female with recently diagnosed lung cancer, who complains of unsteady gait. (Pulmonary Medicine)

Subsequent hospital visit for a 20-month-old male with bacterial meningitis treated one week with antibiotic therapy; has now developed a temperature of 101.0. (Pediatrics)

Subsequent hospital visit for 13-year-old male admitted with left lower quadrant abdominal pain and fever, not responding to therapy. (General Surgery)

Subsequent hospital visit for a 65-year-old male with hemiplegia and painful paretic shoulder. (Physical Medicine & Rehabilitation)

99233

Subsequent hospital visit for a 38-year-old male, quadriplegic with acute autonomic hyperreflexia, who is not responsive to initial care. (Physical Medicine & Rehabilitation)

Follow-up hospital visit for a teenage female who continues to experience severely disruptive, violent and life-threatening symptoms in a complicated multi-system illness. Family/social circumstances also a contributing factor. (Psychiatry)

Subsequent hospital visit for a 42-year-old female with progressive systemic sclerosis (scleroderma), renal failure on dialysis, congestive heart failure, cardiac arrhythmias, and digital ulcers. (Allergy & Immunology)

Subsequent hospital visit for a 50-year-old diabetic, hypertensive male with nonresponding back pain and radiating pain to the lower left extremity, who develops chest pain, cough, and bloody sputum. (Orthopaedic Surgery)

Subsequent hospital visit for a 64-year-old female, status post-abdominal aortic aneurysm resection, with non-responsive coagulopathy, who has now developed lower GI bleeding. (Abdominal Surgery/Colon & Rectal Surgery/General Surgery)

Follow-up hospital care of a patient with pansinusitis infection complicated by a brain abscess and asthma; no response to current treatment. (Otolaryngology, Head & Neck Surgery)

Subsequent hospital visit for a patient with a laryngeal neoplasm who develops airway compromise, suspected metastasis. (Otolaryngology, Head & Neck Surgery)

Subsequent hospital visit for a 49-year-old male with significant rectal bleeding, etiology undetermined, not responding to treatment. (Abdominal Surgery/General Surgery/Colon & Rectal Surgery)

Subsequent hospital visit for a 50-year-old male, post-aortocoronary bypass surgery; now develops hypotension and oliguria. (Cardiology)

Subsequent hospital visit for an adolescent patient who is violent, unsafe, and noncompliant, with multiple expectations for participation in treatment plan and behavior on the treatment unit. (Psychiatry)

Subsequent hospital visit for an 18-year-old male being treated for presumed PCP psychosis. Patient is still moderately symptomatic with auditory hallucinations and is insisting on signing out against medical advice. (Psychiatry)

Subsequent hospital visit for an 8-year-old female with caustic ingestion, who now has fever, dyspnea, and dropping hemoglobin. (Gastroenterology)

Follow-up hospital visit for a chronic renal failure patient on dialysis who develops chest pain and shortness of breath and a new onset pericardial friction rub. (Nephrology)

Subsequent hospital visit for a 44-year-old patient with electrical burns to the left arm with ascending infection. (Orthopaedic Surgery)

Subsequent hospital visit for a patient with systemic sclerosis who has aspirated and is short of breath. (Dermatology)

Subsequent hospital visit for a 65-year-old female, status post-op resection of abdominal aortic aneurysm, with suspected ischemic bowel. (General Surgery)

Subsequent hospital visit for a 50-year-old male, post-aortocoronary bypass surgery, now develops hypotension and oliguria. (Cardiology)

Subsequent hospital visit for a 65-year-old male, following an acute myocardial infarction, who complains of shortness of breath and new chest pain. (Cardiology)

Subsequent hospital visit for a 65-year-old female with rheumatoid arthritis (stage 3, class 3) admitted for urosepsis. On the third hospital day, chest pain, dyspnea and fever develop. (Rheumatology)

Follow-up hospital care of a pediatric case with stridor, laryngomalacia, established tracheostomy, complicated by multiple medical problems in PICU. (Otolaryngology, Head & Neck Surgery)

Subsequent hospital visit for a 60-year-old female, four days post uncomplicated inferior myocardial infarction who has developed severe chest pain, dyspnea, diaphoresis and nausea. (Family Medicine)

Subsequent hospital visit for a patient with AML (acute myelogenous leukemia), fever, elevated white count and uric acid undergoing induction chemotherapy. (Hematology/Oncology)

Subsequent hospital visit for a 38-year-old quadriplegic male with acute autonomic hyperreflexia, who is not responsive to initial care. (Physical Medicine & Rehabilitation)

Subsequent hospital visit for a 65-year-old female post-op resection of abdominal aortic aneurysm, with suspected ischemic bowel. (General Surgery)

Subsequent hospital visit for a 60-year-old female with persistent leukocytosis and a fever seven days after a sigmoid colon resection for carcinoma. (Infectious Disease)

Subsequent hospital visit for a chronic renal failure patient on dialysis, who develops chest pain, shortness of breath and new onset of pericardial friction rub. (Nephrology)

Subsequent hospital visit for a 65-year-old male with acute myocardial infarction who now demonstrates complete heart block and congestive heart failure. (Cardiology)

Subsequent hospital visit for a 25-year-old female with hypertension and systemic lupus erythematosus, admitted for fever and respiratory distress. On the third hospital day, the patient presented with purpuric skin lesions and acute renal failure. (Allergy & Immunology)

Subsequent hospital visit for a 55-year-old male with severe chronic obstructive pulmonary disease and bronchospasm; initially admitted for acute respiratory distress requiring ventilatory support in the ICU. The patient was stabilized, extubated and transferred to the floor, but has now developed acute fever, dyspnea, left lower lobe rhonchi and laboratory evidence of carbon dioxide retention and hypoxemia. (Family Medicine/Internal Medicine)

Subsequent hospital visit for 46-year-old female, known liver cirrhosis patient, with recent upper gastrointestinal hemorrhage from varices; now with worsening ascites and encephalopathy. (Gastroenterology)

Subsequent hospital visit for 62-year-old female admitted with acute subarachnoid hemorrhage, negative cerebral arteriogram, increased lethargy and hemiparesis with fever. (Neurosurgery)

Consultations

Office or Other Outpatient Consultations

New or Established Patient

99241   Initial office consultation for a 40-year-old female in pain from blister on lip following a cold. (Oral & Maxillofacial Surgery)

Initial office consultation for a 62-year-old construction worker with olecranon bursitis. (Orthopaedic Surgery)

Office consultation with 25-year-old postpartum female with severe symptomatic hemorrhoids. (Colon & Rectal Surgery)

Office consultation with 58-year-old male, referred for follow-up of creatinine level and evaluation of obstructive uropathy, relieved two months ago. (Nephrology)

Office consultation for 30-year-old female tennis player with sprain or contusion of the forearm. (Orthopaedic Surgery)

Office consultation for a 45-year-old male, requested by his internist, with asymptomatic torus palatinus requiring no further treatment. (Oral & Maxillofacial Surgery)

99242   Initial office consultation for a 20-year-old male with acute upper respiratory tract symptoms. (Allergy & Immunology)

Initial office consultation for a 29-year-old soccer player with painful proximal thigh/groin injury. (Orthopaedic Surgery)

Initial office consultation for a 66-year-old female with wrist and hand pain, numbness of finger tips, suspected median nerve compression by carpal tunnel syndrome. (Plastic Surgery)

Initial office consultation for a patient with a solitary lesion of discoid lupus erythematosus on left cheek to rule out malignancy or self-induced lesion. (Dermatology)

Office consultation for management of systolic hypertension in a 70-year-old male scheduled for elective prostate resection. (Geriatrics)

Office consultation with 27-year-old female, with old amputation, for evaluation of existing above-knee prosthesis. (Physical Medicine & Rehabilitation)

Office consultation with 66-year-old female with wrist and hand pain, and finger numbness, secondary to suspected carpal tunnel syndrome. (Orthopaedic Surgery)

Office consultation for 61-year-old female, recently on antibiotic therapy, now with diarrhea and leukocytosis. (Abdominal Surgery)

Office consultation for a patient with papulosquamous eruption of elbow with pitting of nails and itchy scalp. (Dermatology)

Office consultation for a 30-year-old female with single season allergic rhinitis. (Allergy & Immunology)

99243   Initial office consultation for a 60-year-old male with avascular necrosis of the left femoral head with increasing pain. (Orthopaedic Surgery)

Office consultation for a 31-year-old woman complaining of palpitations and chest pains. Her internist had described a mild systolic click. (Cardiology)

Office consultation for a 65-year-old female with persistent bronchitis. (Infectious Disease)

Office consultation for a 65-year-old man with chronic low-back pain radiating to the leg. (Neurosurgery)

Office consultation for 23-year-old female with Crohn's disease not responding to therapy. (Abdominal Surgery/Colon & Rectal Surgery)

Office consultation for 25-year-old patient with symptomatic knee pain and swelling, with torn anterior cruciate ligament and/or torn meniscus. (Orthopaedic Surgery)

Office consultation for a 67-year-old patient with osteoporosis and mandibular atrophy with regard to reconstructive alternatives. (Oral & Maxillofacial Surgery)

Office consultation for 39-year-old patient referred at a perimenopausal age for irregular menses and menopausal symptoms. (Obstetrics & Gynecology)

99244   Initial office consultation for a 28-year-old male, HIV+, with a recent change in visual acuity. (Ophthalmology)

Initial office consultation for a 15-year-old male with failing grades, suspected drug abuse. (Pediatrics)

Initial office consultation for a 36-year-old factory worker, status four months post-occupational low back injury and requires management of intractable low back pain. (Pain Medicine)

Initial office consultation for a 45-year-old female with a history of chronic arthralgia of TMJ and associated myalgia and sudden progressive symptomatology over last two to three months. (Oral & Maxillofacial Surgery)

Initial office consultation for evaluation of a 70-year-old male with appetite loss and diminished energy. (Psychiatry)

Initial office consultation for an elementary school-aged patient, referred by pediatrician, with multiple systematic complaints and recent onset of behavioral discontrol. (Psychiatry)

Initial office consultation for a 23-year-old female with developmental facial skeletal anomaly and subsequent abnormal relationship of jaw(s) to cranial base. (Oral & Maxillofacial Surgery)

Initial office consultation for a 45-year-old myopic patient with a one-week history of floaters and a partial retinal detachment. (Ophthalmology)

Initial office consultation for a 65-year-old female with moderate dementia, mild unsteadiness, back pain fatigue on ambulation, intermittent urinary incontinence. (Neurosurgery)

Initial office consultation for a 33-year-old female referred by endocrinologist with amenorrhea and galactorrhea, for evaluation of pituitary tumor. (Neurosurgery)

Initial office consultation for a 34-year-old male with new onset nephrotic syndrome. (Nephrology)

Initial office consultation for a 39-year-old female with intractable chest wall pain secondary to metastatic breast cancer. (Anesthesiology/Pain Medicine)

Initial office consultation for a patient with multiple giant tumors of jaws. (Oral & Maxillofacial Surgery)

Initial office consultation for a patient with a failed total hip replacement with loosening and pain upon walking. (Orthopaedic Surgery)

Initial office consultation for a 60-year-old female with three-year history of intermittent tic-like unilateral facial pain; now constant pain for six weeks without relief by adequate carbamazepine dosage. (Neurosurgery)

Initial office consultation for a 45-year-old male heavy construction worker with prior lumbar disk surgery two years earlier; now gradually recurring low back and unilateral leg pain for three months, unable to work for two weeks. (Neurosurgery)

Initial office consultation of a patient who presents with a 30-year history of smoking and right neck mass. (Otolaryngology, Head & Neck Surgery)

Office consultation with 38-year-old female, with inflammatory bowel disease, who now presents with right lower quadrant pain and suspected intra-abdominal abscess. (General Surgery/Colon & Rectal Surgery)

Office consultation with 72-year-old male with esophageal carcinoma, symptoms of dysphagia and reflux. (Thoracic Surgery)

Office consultation for discussion of treatment options for a 40-year-old female with a two-centimeter adenocarcinoma of the breast. (Radiation Oncology)

Office consultation for young patient referred by pediatrician because of patient's short attention span, easy distractibility and hyperactivity. (Psychiatry)

Office consultation for 66-year-old female, history of colon resection for adenocarcinoma six years earlier, now with severe mid-back pain; x-rays showing osteoporosis and multiple vertebral compression fractures. (Neurosurgery)

Office consultation for a patient with chronic pelvic inflammatory disease who now has left lower quadrant pain with a palpable pelvic mass. (Obstetrics & Gynecology)

Office consultation for a patient with long-standing psoriasis with acute onset of erythroderma, pustular lesions, chills and fever. Combinations of topical and systemic treatments discussed and instituted. (Dermatology)

99245   Initial office consultation for a 35-year-old multiple-trauma male patient with complex pelvic fractures, for evaluation and formulation of management plan. (Orthopaedic Surgery)

Initial emergency room consultation for 10-year-old male in status epilepticus, recent closed head injury, information about medication not available. (Neurosurgery)

Initial emergency room consultation for a 23-year-old patient with severe abdominal pain, guarding, febrile, and unstable vital signs. (Obstetrics & Gynecology)

Office consultation for a 67-year-old female longstanding uncontrolled diabetic who presents with retinopathy, nephropathy, and a foot ulcer. (Endocrinology)

Office consultation for a 37-year-old male for initial evaluation and management of Cushing's disease. (Endocrinology)

Office consultation for a 60-year-old male who presents with thyrotoxicosis, exophthalmos, frequent premature ventricular contractions and congestive heart failure. (Endocrinology)

Initial office consultation for a 36-year-old patient, one year status post occupational herniated cervical disk treated by laminectomy, requiring management of multiple sites of intractable pain, depression, and narcotic dependence. (Pain Medicine)

Office consultation for a 58-year-old man with a history of MI and CHF who complains of the recent onset of rest angina and shortness of breath. The patient has a systolic blood pressure of 90mmHG and is in Class IV heart failure. (Cardiology)

Emergency room consultation for a 1-year-old with a three-day history of fever with increasing respiratory distress who is thought to have cardiac tamponade by the ER physician. (Cardiology)

Office consultation in the emergency room for a 25-year-old male with severe, acute, closed head injury. (Neurosurgery)

Office consultation for a 23-year-old female with Stage II A Hodgkins disease with positive supraclavicular and mediastinal nodes. (Radiation Oncology)

Office consultation for a 27-year-old juvenile diabetic patient with severe diabetic retinopathy, gastric atony, nephrotic syndrome and progressive renal failure, now with a serum creatinine of 2.7, and a blood pressure of 170/114. (Nephrology)

Office consultation for independent medical evaluation of a patient with a history of complicated low back and neck problems with previous multiple failed back surgeries. (Orthopaedic Surgery)

Office consultation for an adolescent referred by pediatrician for recent onset of violent and self-injurious behavior. (Psychiatry)

Office consultation for a 6-year-old male for evaluation of severe muscle and joint pain and a diffuse rash. Patient well until 4-6 weeks earlier, when he developed arthralgia, myalgias, and a fever of 102 for one week. (Rheumatology)

Initial Inpatient Consultations

New or Established Patient

99251   Initial hospital consultation for a 27-year-old female with fractured incisor post-intubation. (Oral & Maxillofacial Surgery)

Initial hospital consultation for an orthopaedic patient on IV antibiotics who has developed an apparent candida infection of the oral cavity. (Oral & Maxillofacial Surgery)

Initial inpatient consultation for a 30-year-old female complaining of vaginal itching, post orthopaedic surgery. (Obstetrics & Gynecology)

Initial inpatient consultation for a 36-year-old male on orthopaedic service with complaint of localized dental pain. (Oral & Maxillofacial Surgery)

99252   Initial hospital consultation for a 45-year-old male, previously abstinent alcoholic, who relapsed and was admitted for management of gastritis. The patient readily accepts the need for further treatment. (Addiction Medicine)

Initial hospital consultation for a 35-year-old dialysis patient with episodic oral ulcerations. (Oral & Maxillofacial Surgery)

Initial inpatient preoperative consultation for a 43-year-old woman with cholecystitis and well-controlled hypertension. (Cardiology)

Initial inpatient consultation for recommendation of antibiotic prophylaxis for a patient with a synthetic heart valve who will undergo urologic surgery. (Internal Medicine)

Initial inpatient consultation for possible drug induced skin eruption in 50-year-old male. (Dermatology)

Preoperative inpatient consultation for evaluation of hypertension in a 60-year-old male who will undergo a cholecystectomy. Patient had a normal annual check-up in your office four months ago. (Internal Medicine)

Initial inpatient consultation for 66-year-old patient with wrist and hand pain and finger numbness, secondary to carpal tunnel syndrome. (Orthopaedic Surgery/Plastic Surgery)

Initial inpatient consultation for a 66-year-old male smoker referred for pain management immediately status post-biliary tract surgery done via sub-costal incision. (Anesthesiology/Pain Medicine)

99253 Initial hospital consultation for a 50-year-old female with incapacitating knee pain due to generalized rheumatoid arthritis. (Orthopaedic Surgery)

Initial hospital consultation for a 60-year-old male with avascular necrosis of the left femoral heel with increasing pain. (Orthopaedic Surgery)

Initial hospital consultation for a 45-year-old female with compound mandibular fracture and concurrent head, abdominal and/or orthopaedic injuries. (Oral & Maxillofacial Surgery)

Initial hospital consultation for a 22-year-old female, paraplegic, to evaluate wrist and hand pain. (Orthopaedic Surgery)

Initial hospital consultation for a 40-year-old male with 10-day history of incapacitating unilateral sciatica, unable to walk now, not improved by bed rest. (Neurosurgery)

Initial hospital consultation, requested by pediatrician, for treatment recommendations for a patient admitted with persistent inability to walk following soft tissue injury to ankle. (Physiatry)

Initial hospital consultation for a 27-year-old previously healthy male who vomited during IV sedation and may have aspirated gastric contents. (Anesthesiology)

Initial hospital consultation for a 33-year-old female, post-abdominal surgery, who now has a fever. (Internal Medicine)

Initial inpatient consultation for a 57-year-old male, post lower endoscopy, for evaluation of abdominal pain and fever. (General Surgery)

Initial inpatient consultation for rehabilitation of a 73-year-old female one week after surgical management of a hip fracture. (Physical Medicine & Rehabilitation)

Initial inpatient consultation for diagnosis/management of fever following abdominal surgery. (Internal Medicine)

Initial inpatient consultation for a 35-year-old female with a fever and pulmonary infiltrate following cesarean section. (Pulmonary Medicine)

Initial inpatient consultation for a 42-year-old non-diabetic patient, post-op cholecystectomy, now with an acute urinary tract infection. (Nephrology)

Initial inpatient consultation for 53-year-old female with moderate uncomplicated pancreatitis. (Gastroenterology)

Initial inpatient consultation for 45-year-old patient with chronic neck pain with radicular pain of the left arm. (Orthopaedic Surgery)

Initial inpatient consultation for 8-year-old patient with new onset of seizures who has a normal examination and previous history. (Neurology)

99254 Initial hospital consultation for a 15-year-old patient with painless swelling of proximal humerus with lytic lesion by x-ray. (Orthopaedic Surgery)

Initial hospital consultation for evaluation of a 29-year-old female with a diffusely positive medical review of systems and history of multiple surgeries. (Psychiatry)

Initial hospital consultation for a 70-year-old diabetic female with gangrene of the foot. (Orthopaedic Surgery)

Initial inpatient consultation for a 47-year-old female with progressive pulmonary infiltrate, hypoxemia, and diminished urine output. (Anesthesiology)

Initial hospital consultation for a 13-month-old with spasmodic cough, respiratory distress, and fever. (Allergy & Immunology)

Initial hospital consultation for a patient with failed total hip replacement with loosening and pain upon walking. (Orthopaedic Surgery)

Initial hospital consultation for a 62-year-old female with metastatic breast cancer to the femoral neck and thoracic vertebra. (Orthopaedic Surgery)

Initial hospital consultation for a 39-year-old female with nephrolithiasis requiring extensive opioid analgesics, whose vital signs are now elevated. She initially denied any drug use, but today gives history of multiple substance abuse, including opioids and prior treatment for a personality disorder. (Psychiatry)

Initial hospital consultation for a 70-year-old female without previous psychiatric history, who is now experiencing nocturnal confusion and visual hallucinations following hip replacement surgery. (Psychiatry)

Initial inpatient consultation for evaluation of a 63-year-old in the ICU with diabetes and chronic renal failure who develops acute respiratory distress syndrome 36 hours after a mitral valve replacement. (Anesthesiology)

Initial inpatient consultation for a 66-year-old female with enlarged supraclavicular lymph nodes, found on biopsy to be malignant. (Hematology/Oncology)

Initial inpatient consultation for a 43-year-old female for evaluation of sudden painful visual loss, optic neuritis and episodic paresthesia. (Ophthalmology)

Initial inpatient consultation for evaluation of a 71-year-old male with hyponatremia (serum sodium 114) who was admitted to the hospital with pneumonia. (Nephrology)

Initial inpatient consultation for a 72-year-old male with emergency admission for possible bowel obstruction. (Internal Medicine/General Surgery)

Initial inpatient consultation for a 35-year-old female with fever, swollen joints, and rash of one-week duration. (Rheumatology)

99255 Initial inpatient consultation for a 76-year-old female with massive, life-threatening gastrointestinal hemorrhage and chest pain. (Gastroenterology)

Initial inpatient consultation for a 75-year-old female, admitted to intensive care with acute respiratory distress syndrome, who is hypersensitive, has a moderate metabolic acidosis, and a rising serum creatinine. (Nephrology)

Initial hospital consultation for patient with a history of complicated low back pain and neck problems with previous multiple failed back surgeries. (Orthopaedic Surgery/Neurosurgery)

Initial hospital consultation for a 66-year-old female, two days post-abdominal aneurysm repair, with oliguria and hypertension of one-day duration. (Nephrology/Internal Medicine)

Initial hospital consultation for a patient with shotgun wound to face with massive facial trauma and airway obstruction. (Oral & Maxillofacial Surgery)

Initial hospital consultation for patient with severe pancreatitis complicated by respiratory insufficiency, acute renal failure, and abscess formation. (General Surgery/Colon & Rectal Surgery)

Initial hospital consultation for a 35-year-old multiple-trauma male patient with complex pelvic fractures to evaluate and formulate management plan. (Orthopaedic Surgery)

Initial inpatient consultation for adolescent patient with fractured femur and pelvis who pulled out IVs and disconnected traction in attempt to elope from hospital. (Psychiatry)

Initial hospital consultation for a 16-year-old primigravida at 32 weeks gestation requested by a family practitioner for evaluation of severe hypertension, thrombocytopenia, and headache. (Obstetrics & Gynecology)

Initial hospital consultation for a 58-year-old insulin-dependent diabetic with multiple antibiotic allergies, now with multiple fascial plane abscesses and airway obstruction. (Oral & Maxillofacial Surgery)

Initial inpatient consultation for a 55-year-old male with known cirrhosis and ascites, now with jaundice, encephalopathy, and massive hematemesis. (Gastroenterology)

Initial hospital consultation for a 25-year-old male, seen in emergency room with severe, closed head injury. (Neurosurgery)

Initial hospital consultation for a 2-day-old male with single ventricle physiology and subaortic obstruction. Family counseling following evaluation for multiple, staged surgical procedures. (Thoracic Surgery)

Initial hospital consultation for a 45-year-old male admitted with subarachnoid hemorrhage and intracranial aneurysm on angiogram. (Neurosurgery)

Initial inpatient consultation for myxedematous patient who is hypoventilating and obtunded. (Endocrinology)

Initial hospital consultation for a 45-year-old patient with widely metastatic lung carcinoma, intractable back pain, and a history that includes substance dependence, NSAID allergy, and two prior laminectomies with fusion for low back pain. (Pain Medicine)

Initial hospital consultation for evaluation of treatment options in a 50-year-old patient with cirrhosis, known peptic ulcer disease, hypotension, encephalopathy, and massive acute upper gastrointestinal bleeding which cannot be localized by endoscopy. (Interventional Radiology)

Initial inpatient consultation in the ICU for a 70-year-old male who experienced a cardiac arrest during surgery and was resuscitated. (Cardiology)

Initial inpatient consultation for a patient with severe pancreatitis complicated by respiratory insufficiency, acute renal failure and abscess formation. (Gastroenterology)

Initial inpatient consultation for a 70-year-old cirrhotic male admitted with ascites, jaundice, encephalopathy, and massive hematemesis. (Gastroenterology)

Initial inpatient consultation in the ICU for a 51-year-old patient who is on a ventilator and has a fever two weeks after a renal transplantation. (Infectious Disease)

Initial inpatient consultation for evaluation and formulation of plan for management of multiple trauma patient with complex pelvic fracture, 35-year-old male. (General Surgery/Orthopaedic Surgery)

Initial inpatient consultation for a 50-year-old male with a history of previous myocardial infarction, now with acute pulmonary edema and hypotension. (Cardiology)

Initial inpatient consultation for 45-year-old male with recent, acute subarachnoid hemorrhage, hesitant speech, mildly confused, drowsy. High risk group for HIV+ status. (Neurosurgery)

Initial inpatient consultation for 36-year-old female referred by her internist to evaluate a patient being followed for abdominal pain and fever. The patient has developed diffuse abdominal pain, guarding, rigidity and increased fever. (Obstetrics & Gynecology)

Follow-up Inpatient Consultations

Established Patient

99261   Follow-up consultation for a 78-year-old female nursing home resident for evaluation of medical management of pruritus ani. (Colon & Rectal Surgery/Geriatrics/General Surgery)

Follow-up hospital consultation on first post-op day for a 64-year-old male who has undergone uneventful CABG. (Anesthesiology)

Follow-up inpatient consultation for a 67-year-old female admitted several days ago for bleeding ulcer; now stable. (Gastroenterology)

Follow-up hospital consultation for a 35-year-old female with history of mitral valve prolapse. (Cardiology)

Follow-up inpatient consultation to complete initial consultation for dental pain after review of radiographs. (Oral & Maxillofacial Surgery)

Follow-up inpatient consultation for evaluation of response to therapy for moniliasis. (Oral & Maxillofacial Surgery)

Follow-up inpatient consultation for a 22-year-old female with recurrent aphthous ulcers. (Oral & Maxillofacial Surgery)

Follow-up hospital consultation for a 37-year-old female to complete review of previously unavailable studies. (Therapeutic Radiology & Oncology)

Follow-up consultation for a highly functional 75-year-old female with urinary incontinence to review preliminary results of diagnostic evaluation. (Geriatrics)

Follow-up inpatient consultation for a 1-week-old premature female with patent ductus arteriosus. The murmur has disappeared. (Cardiology)

Follow-up hospital consultation to review the results of an audiogram. (Otolaryngology, Head & Neck Surgery)

Follow-up inpatient consultation with 35-year-old female with pulmonary embolism post-op cesarean section, now stable, for assessment of response to anticoagulation and recommended adjustment of heparin dose. (Pulmonary Medicine)

Follow-up inpatient consultation for a 74-year-old male whose postoperative facial paralysis after a cholecystectomy is now resolving. (Neurology)

Follow-up inpatient consultation with 67-year-old female, established patient, for review of diagnostic studies ordered at time of first contact. (Internal Medicine)

Follow-up inpatient consultation for 78-year-old female nursing home resident for evaluation of medical management of pruritis ani. (General Surgery/Colon & Rectal Surgery)

Follow-up inpatient consultation for a 36-year-old female two days after spontaneous passage of 3mm stone. (Urology)

Follow-up inpatient consultation for a 94-year-old male nursing home resident for re-evaluation of hemorrhoids following conservative therapy. (Colon & Rectal Surgery/General Surgery/Geriatrics)

Follow-up inpatient consultation for a 50-year-old male, asymptomatic with borderline ECG abnormality, needs preoperative opinion after a thallium exercise perfusion scan. (Cardiology)

99262   Follow-up inpatient consultation for a 6-year-old female, established patient, with endocarditis and changing heart murmur. (Cardiology)

Follow-up inpatient consultation on a 2-year-old male, one day postoperative ventricular septal defect closure with signs of tachycardia. (Cardiology)

Follow-up inpatient consultation for a 63-year-old man, established patient, with moderately severe pulmonary insufficiency, 10 days postoperative coronary artery bypass for unstable angina. Patient has developed severe dyspnea, fever, and a new exudative right pleural effusion. (Cardiology)

Follow-up inpatient consultation for a 67-year-old woman with lung cancer and syndrome of inappropriate secretion of antidiuretic hormone (SIADH) who has had a seizure following intravenous saline. (Endocrinology)

Follow-up inpatient consultation for a 22-year-old female, established patient, with steroid-dependent systemic lupus erythematosus, arthritis, and glomerulonephritis. Patient is re-evaluated for loss of consciousness and chest pain. (Rheumatology)

Follow-up inpatient consultation for a 75-year-old diabetic with fever, chills, a gangrenous heel ulcer, rhonchi, and dyspnea who appears lethargic and tachypneic. (Endocrinology)

Follow-up inpatient consultation for a 30-year-old, established patient, with intractable neck and low back pain, who is excessively sedated after institution of methadone therapy. (Pain Medicine)

Follow-up inpatient consultation for a 65-year-old man with a history of hypertension and MI who is five days post uncomplicated GI procedure with an unremarkable postoperative recovery. He has just been resuscitated from a cardiopulmonary arrest. (Cardiology)

Follow-up inpatient consultation with 72-year-old female, established patient with bullous pemphigoid on combined oral therapy steroids and immunosuppressive to evaluate progress of cutaneous care orders and adjustment of oral/parenteral therapy dosages. (Dermatology)

Follow-up inpatient consultation for a 71-year-old male who has developed a maculopapular skin rash while on antibiotics recommended for an uncomplicated pneumonia. (Infectious Disease)

Follow-up inpatient consultation with 68-year-old, incapacitated male with spinal stenosis and failure to respond to bedrest, analgesics, and PT. (Neurosurgery)

Follow-up inpatient consultation with 51-year-old male for evaluation and determination of the etiology of postoperative hyponatremia following TURP. (Family Medicine)

Follow-up inpatient consultation for re-evaluation of a stroke patient, and development of plan for initial rehabilitation services. (Neurology)

Follow-up inpatient consultation with 45-year-old male, established patient for discussion of CT scan which demonstrates a cavernous hemangioma. (Ophthalmology)

Follow-up inpatient consultation for an asymptomatic 35-year-old Type I diabetic patient with hyperkalemic, hyperchloremia acidosis, to review lab results. (Nephrology)

Follow-up inpatient consultation for an elderly male with a perioperative myocardial infarction requiring adjustment of vasoactive medications. (Anesthesiology)

99263   Follow-up hospital consultation of an AIDS patient admitted with a sore throat who now has enlarging neck mass. (Otolaryngology, Head & Neck Surgery)

Follow-up hospital consultation of a pansinusitis patient with sudden onset of proptosis. (Otolaryngology, Head & Neck Surgery)

Follow-up inpatient consultation for a 53-year-old man with known angina who develops crescendo angina post cholecystectomy. (Cardiology)

Follow-up inpatient consultation with 72-year-old male established patient admitted for management of alcohol withdrawal, now confused and febrile. (Addiction Medicine)

Follow-up inpatient consultation for an HIV+ patient with an increasing fever following 10 days of antibiotic therapy for pneumocystis carinii pneumonia. (Infectious Disease)

Follow-up inpatient consultation with 58-year-old diabetic female, with bacterial endocarditis, continued fever after two weeks of intravenous antibiotic therapy, and new onset ventricular ectopia. (Cardiology)

Follow-up inpatient consultation for a 90-year-old female with urinary incontinence who has a complicated medical history requiring reassessment of multiple medical problems, recommendations for placement, further recommendation for management of incontinence and reevaluation of cognitive status because of competency issues. (Geriatrics/Psychiatry)

Follow-up inpatient consultation for 42-year-old male with persistent gastrointestinal bleeding, etiology undetermined, not responding to conservative therapy of transfusions. (General Surgery/Colon & Rectal Surgery)

Follow-up inpatient consultation for a 62-year-old female with steroid-dependent asthma, diabetes mellitus, thyrotoxicosis, abdominal pain and possible vasculitis. (Rheumatology)

Follow-up inpatient consultation for a 62-year-old male, status post-op acute small bowel obstruction; now with acute renal failure. (Family Medicine)

Emergency Department Services

New or Established Patient

99281   Emergency department visit for a patient for removal of sutures from a well-healed, uncomplicated laceration. (Emergency Medicine)

Emergency department visit for a patient for tetanus toxoid immunization. (Emergency Medicine)

Emergency department visit for a patient with several uncomplicated insect bites. (Emergency Medicine)

99282   Emergency department visit for a 20-year-old student who presents with a painful sunburn with blister formation on the back. (Emergency Medicine)

Emergency department visit for a child presenting with impetigo localized to the face. (Emergency Medicine)

Emergency department visit for a patient with a minor traumatic injury of an extremity with localized pain, swelling, and bruising. (Emergency Medicine)

Emergency department visit for an otherwise healthy patient whose chief complaint is a red, swollen cystic lesion on his/her back. (Emergency Medicine)

Emergency department visit for a patient presenting with a rash on both legs after exposure to poison ivy. (Emergency Medicine)

Emergency department visit for a young adult patient with infected sclera and purulent discharge from both eyes without pain, visual disturbance or history of foreign body in either eye. (Emergency Medicine)

99283   Emergency department visit for a sexually active female complaining of vaginal discharge who is afebrile and denies experiencing abdominal or back pain. (Emergency Medicine)

Emergency department visit for a well-appearing 8-year-old who has a fever, diarrhea and abdominal cramps, is tolerating oral fluids and is not vomiting. (Emergency Medicine)

Emergency department visit for a patient with an inversion ankle injury, who is unable to bear weight on the injured foot and ankle. (Emergency Medicine)

Emergency department visit for a patient who has a complaint of acute pain associated with a suspected foreign body in the painful eye. (Emergency Medicine)

Emergency department visit for a healthy, young adult patient who sustained a blunt head injury with local swelling and bruising without subsequent confusion, loss of consciousness or memory deficit. (Emergency Medicine)

99284   Emergency department visit for a 4-year-old who fell off a bike sustaining a head injury with brief loss of consciousness. (Emergency Medicine)

Emergency department visit for an elderly female who has fallen and is now complaining of pain in her right hip and is unable to walk. (Emergency Medicine)

Emergency department visit for a patient with flank pain and hematuria. (Emergency Medicine)

Emergency department visit for a female presenting with lower abdominal pain and a vaginal discharge. (Emergency Medicine)

99285   Emergency department visit for a patient with a complicated overdose requiring aggressive management to prevent side effects from the ingested materials. (Emergency Medicine)

Emergency department visit for a patient with a new onset of rapid heart rate requiring IV drugs. (Emergency Medicine)

Emergency department visit for a patient exhibiting active, upper gastrointestinal bleeding. (Emergency Medicine)

Emergency department visit for a previously healthy young adult patient who is injured in an automobile accident and is brought to the emergency department immobilized and has symptoms compatible with intra-abdominal injuries or multiple extremity injuries. (Emergency Medicine)

Emergency department visit for a patient with an acute onset of chest pain compatible with symptoms of cardiac ischemia and/or pulmonary embolus. (Emergency Medicine)

Emergency department visit for a patient who presents with a sudden onset of "the worst headache of her life," and complains of a stiff neck, nausea, and inability to concentrate. (Emergency Medicine)

Emergency department visit for a patient with a new onset of a cerebral vascular accident. (Emergency Medicine)

Emergency department visit for acute febrile illness in an adult, associated with shortness of breath and an altered level of alertness. (Emergency Medicine)

Critical Care Services

99291   First hour of critical care of a 65-year-old man with septic shock following relief of ureteral obstruction caused by a stone.

First hour of critical care of a 15-year-old with acute respiratory failure from asthma.

First hour of critical care of a 45-year-old who sustained a liver laceration, cerebral hematoma, flailed chest, and pulmonary contusion after being struck by an automobile.

First hour of critical care of a 65-year-old woman who, following a hysterectomy, suffered a cardiac arrest associated with a pulmonary embolus.

First hour of critical care of a 6-month-old with hypovolemic shock secondary to diarrhea and dehydration.

First hour of critical care of a 3-year-old with respiratory failure secondary to pneumocystis carinii pneumonia.

Comprehensive Nursing Facility Assessments

New or Established Patient

99301   Annual nursing facility history and physical and MDS/RAI evaluation for a two-year nursing facility resident who is an 84-year-old female with multiple chronic health problems, including: stable controlled hypertension, chronic constipation, osteoarthritis, and moderated stable dementia.

Nursing facility visit for an assessment of a resident with non-insulin dependent diabetes, stable angina, and chronic obstructive pulmonary disease (COPD) one year after previous MDS/RAI.

99302   Nursing facility visit one year after previous MDS/RAI to assess an 80-year-old woman with Parkinson's disease, chronic hypertension, and degenerative arthritis. Visit reveals Stage II decubitus.

Nursing facility assessment of a 28-year-old diabetic, male resident with a new Stage IV pressure ulcer on his left lateral malleolus that is unresponsive to treatment, thus triggering the need for a new MDS/RAI and new medical plan of care.

Nursing facility assessment of an 88-year-old male resident with a permanent change in status following a new cerebral vascular accident (CVA) that has triggered the need for a new MDS/RAI and medical plan of care.

Nursing facility visit and assessment to take over the primary care of a 75-year-old diabetic, previously stable, who was on oral hypoglycemic agents, but who now requires initiation of insulin therapy, a new MDS/RAI, and medical plan of care.

Nursing facility visit and assessment for an 81-year-old female resident with dementia, who, under structured guidance and intensive nutritional support has regained significant levels of function in three activities of daily living and is now able to feed and dress herself and ambulate with appliance and who now thus requires a new MDS/RAI and medical plan of care.

99303 Initial nursing facility assessment (MDS/RAI and medical plan of care) of a 72-year-old insulin dependent diabetic amputee with hearing and visual impairments and possible dementia seen in the office the day before and judged to require nursing facility care.

Sub-acute nursing facility assessment of a previously independently living 90-year-old male who suffered a recent cerebral vascular accident (CVA) and is transferred to the hospital sub-acute rehabilitation unit for further rehabilitation supportive services.

Initial nursing facility visit to evaluate a 72-year-old woman found confused and wandering, admitted by Adult Protective Services without a qualifying hospital stay or inpatient diagnostic work. The patient lives alone and has no relatives or significant others in the community.

Nursing facility assessment and creation of medical plan of care upon readmission to the nursing facility of an 82-year-old male who was previously discharged. The patient has just been discharged from the hospital where he had been treated for an acute gastric ulcer bleed associated with transient delirium. The patient returns to the nursing facility debilitated, protein depleted, and with a Stage III coccygeal decubitus.

Subsequent Nursing Facility Care

New or Established Patient

99311 Scheduled follow-up visit for a known 70-year-old stable paraplegic with no status change noted during visit.

Scheduled monthly nursing home visit with a patient who has mild senile dementia, Alzheimers' type, with no change in status, stable hypertension, and who is ambulating with a walker one year past stroke.

Follow-up in skilled nursing facility with a 70-year-old patient following a 10-day treatment of a cellulitis of the foot.

99312 Scheduled follow-up visit to a resident with controlled dementia, hypertension, and diabetes. During visit, patient seems to exhibit flu symptoms.

Scheduled nursing facility visit with an afebrile demented resident who also has a mild cough, requiring no change in the medical plan of care.

Subsequent visit in a skilled nursing facility with a patient who is six months post stroke and now has a fever and mild cough.

Scheduled nursing facility visit for an 84-year-old male with chronic renal insufficiency, on digitalis and diuretics, requiring adjustment of medications and revision of medical plan of care.

Nursing facility visit of a resident with multiple chronic health problems who is six months post stroke and now has a fever and mild cough, to evaluate for possible pneumonia. Requires the development of a new medical plan of care, but not a revised MDS/RAI.

99313 Follow-up nursing facility visit to evaluate the reason for frequent falls by a 90-year-old ataxic resident, and to determine possible need for change in medications and medical care plan.

Re-admission of a 75-year-old man with stroke who was hospitalized with pneumonia for his illness and who returns to the nursing facility with no permanent change in status from his condition prior to hospitalization; no new MDS/RAI is required.

Nursing facility visit with a diabetic resident who has developed Stage II decubitus ulcers with cellulitis, requiring a revision in the medical plan of care.

Nursing facility visit to develop a new plan of care for an amputee with atherosclerosis obliterans who has refused to eat for three days and has developed decreased urinary output.

Nursing facility visit for a 78-year-old resident with chronic atrial fibrillation and a history of heart failure to evaluate an acute confusional state and to revise the medical plan of care.

Unscheduled nursing facility visit for evaluation of a patient with fever and obtundation who is determined not to require hospital admission or new MDS, but who does require workup and revision of medical plan of care.

Prolonged Services

Prolonged Physician Service With Direct (Face-to-Face) Patient Contact

Office or Other Outpatient

99354/ 99355 A 20-year-old female with history of asthma presents with acute bronchospasm and moderate respiratory distress. Initial evaluation shows respiratory rate 30, labored breathing and wheezing heard in all lung fields. Office treatment is initiated which includes intermittent bronchial dilation and subcutaneous epinephrine. Requires intermittent physician face-to-face time with patient over a period of 2-3 hours. (Family Medicine/Internal Medicine)

Inpatient

99356 A 34-year-old primigravida presents to hospital in early labor. Admission history and physical reveals severe preeclampsia. Physician supervises management of preeclampsia, IV magnesium initiation and maintenance, labor augmentation with pitocin, and close maternal-fetal monitoring. Physician face-to-face involvement includes 40 minutes of continuous bedside care until the patient is stable, then is intermittent over several hours until the delivery. (Family Medicine/Internal Medicine/Obstetrics & Gynecology)

Prolonged Physician Service Without Direct Patient (Face-to-Face) Contact

99358/
99359   A 65-year-old new patient with multiple problems is seen and evaluated. After the visit, the physician requires extensive time to talk with the patient's daughter, to review complex, detailed medical records transferred from previous physicians and to complete a comprehensive treatment plan. This plan also requires the physician to personally initiate and coordinate the care plan with a local home health agency and a dietician. (Family Medicine/Internal Medicine)

Physician Standby Services

99360   A 24-year-old patient is admitted to OB unit attempting VBAC. Fetal monitoring shows increasing fetal distress. Patient's blood pressure is rising and labor progressing slowly. A primary care physician is requested by the OB/GYN to standby in the unit for possible cesarean delivery and neonatal resuscitation. (Family Medicine/Internal Medicine)

Care Plan Oversight Services

99375   First month of care plan oversight for terminal care of a 58-year-old woman with advanced intraabdominal ovarian cancer. Care plan includes home oxygen, diuretics IV for edema and ascites control and pain control management involving IV morphine infusion when progressive ileus occurred. Physician phone contacts with nurse, family, and MSW. Discussion with MSW concerning plans to withdraw supportive measures per patient wishes. Documentation includes review and modification of care plan and certifications from nursing, MSW, pharmacy, and DME. (Family Medicine/Internal Medicine)

Appendix D

Summary of CPT Add-on Codes

This listing is a summary of CPT add-on codes for *CPT 2005*. The codes listed below are identified in *CPT 2005* with a ✚ symbol.

01953	22226	35686	61610	64859	90472	99356
01968	22328	35697	61611	64872	90474	99357
01969	22522	35700	61612	64874	90781	99358
11001	22534	36218	61795	64876	92547	99359
11008	22585	36248	61864	64901	92608	99602
11101	22614	36476	61868	64902	92973	0036T
11201	22632	36479	62148	66990	92974	0049T
11732	26125	37206	62160	67225	92978	0054T
11922	26861	37208	63035	67320	92979	0055T
13102	26863	37250	63043	67331	92981	0056T
13122	27358	37251	63044	67332	92984	0063T
13133	27692	38102	63048	67334	92996	0068T
13153	31620	38746	63057	67335	92998	0069T
15001	31632	38747	63066	67340	93320	0070T
15101	31633	43635	63076	69990	93321	0076T
15121	31637	44015	63078	74301	93325	0079T
15201	32501	44121	63082	75774	93571	0081T
15221	33141	44128	63086	75946	93572	
15241	33225	44139	63088	75964	93609	
15261	33508	44203	63091	75968	93613	
15343	33530	44701	63103	75993	93621	
15351	33572	44955	63295	75996	93622	
15401	33924	47001	63308	75998	93623	
15787	33961	47550	64472	76082	93662	
16036	34808	48400	64476	76083	95920	
17003	34813	49568	64480	76125	95962	
17310	34826	49905	64484	76802	95967	
19001	35390	56606	64623	76810	95973	
19126	35400	57267	64627	76812	95975	
19291	35500	58611	64727	76937	95979	
19295	35572	59525	64778	78020	96412	
19297	35681	60512	64783	78478	96423	
22103	35682	61316	64787	78480	96570	
22116	35683	61517	64832	78496	96571	
22216	35685	61609	64837	87187	97546	
				87904	97811	
				88141	97814	
				88155	99100	
				88185	99116	
				88311	99135	
				88312	99140	
				88313	99290	
				88314	99292	
				90466	99354	
				90468	99355	

Appendix E

Summary of CPT Codes Exempt from Modifier 51

This listing is a summary of CPT codes that are exempt from the use of modifier 51 but have NOT been designated as CPT add-on procedures/services. The codes listed below are identified in *CPT 2005* with a ⊘ symbol.

			90692	93527
			90693	93528
			90698	93529
			90700	93530
			90701	93531
			90702	93532
			90703	93533
			90704	93539
			90705	93540
			90706	93541
			90707	93542
17004	32000	90378	90708	93543
17304	32002	90379	90710	93544
17305	32020	90384	90712	93545
17306	33517	90385	90713	93555
17307	33518	90386	90715	93556
20660	33519	90389	90716	93600
20690	33521	90393	90717	93602
20692	33522	90396	90718	93603
20900	33523	90399	90719	93610
20902	35600	90476	90720	93612
20910	36620	90477	90721	93615
20912	36660	90581	90723	93616
20920	38792	90585	90725	93618
20922	44500	90586	90727	93619
20924	44720	90632	90732	93620
20926	44721	90633	90733	93624
20930	47146	90634	90734	93631
20931	47147	90636	90735	93640
20936	48552	90645	90740	93641
20937	50327	90646	90743	93642
20938	50328	90647	90744	93650
20974	50329	90648	90746	93651
20975	61107	90655	90747	93652
22840	61210	90656	90748	93660
22841	62284	90657	90749	95900
22842	90281	90658	93501	95903
22843	90283	90660	93503	95904
22844	90287	90665	93505	99141
22845	90288	90669	93508	99142
22846	90291	90675	93510	
22847	90296	90676	93511	
22848	90371	90680	93514	
22851	90375	90690	93524	
31500	90376	90691	93526	

Appendix F

Summary of CPT Codes Exempt from Modifier 63

The listing is a summary of CPT codes that are exempt from the use of modifier 63. The codes listed below are additionally identified in *CPT 2005* with the parenthetical instruction "(Do not report modifier 63 in conjunction with …)"

30545	36460	54000
31520	36510	54150
33401	36660	54160
33403	39503	63700
33450	43313	63702
33472	43314	63704
33502	43520	63706
33503	43831	65820
33505	44055	
33506	44126	
33610	44127	
33611	44128	
33619	46070	
33647	46705	
33670	46715	
33690	46716	
33694	46730	
33730	46735	
33732	46740	
33735	46742	
33736	46744	
33750	47700	
33755	47701	
33762	49215	
33778	49491	
33786	49492	
33918	49495	
33919	49496	
33922	49600	
33960	49605	
33961	49606	
36415	49610	
36420	49611	
36450	53025	

Appendix G

Summary of CPT Codes which Include Conscious Sedation

The following list of procedures for *CPT 2005* includes conscious sedation as an inherent part of providing the procedure. The codes listed below are identified in *CPT 2005* with a ⊙ symbol. Conscious sedation is defined as moderate sedation/analgesia and is a drug-induced depression of consciousness during which patients respond knowingly and intentionally to verbal commands, either alone or accompanied by light tactile stimulation. No interventions are required to maintain a patent airway, spontaneous ventilation is adequate, and cardiovascular function is usually maintained. Conscious or moderate sedation is not the less intense minimal sedation ("anxiolysis") or the more intense deep sedation/analgesia.

Since these services include conscious sedation, it is not appropriate for the same physician to report both the service and one of the conscious sedation codes (99141 or 99142). It is expected that if conscious sedation is provided to the patient as part of one of these services, it is provided by the same physician who is providing the service. The provision of conscious sedation by the operating physician includes the oversight of personnel who are monitoring the patient.

The inclusion of a procedure on this list does not prevent separate reporting of an associated anesthesia procedure/service (CPT codes 00100-01999) when performed by a physician other than the operating physician or a qualified professional under the responsible supervision of a physician other than the operating physician. In such cases the person providing anesthesia services shall be present for the purpose of continuously monitoring the patient and shall not act as a surgical assistant. When clinical conditions of the patient require such anesthesia services, or in the circumstances when the patient does not require sedation, the operating physician is not required to report the procedure as a reduced service using modifier 52.

35474	43241	44382
35475	43242	44383
35476	43243	44385
36555	43244	44386
36557	43245	44388
36558	43246	44389
36560	43247	44390
36561	43248	44391
36563	43249	44392
36565	43250	44393
36566	43251	44394
36568	43255	44397
36570	43256	44500
36571	43257	44901
36576	43258	45303
36578	43259	45305
36581	43260	45307
36582	43261	45308
36583	43262	45309
36585	43263	45315
36590	43264	45317
36870	43265	45320
37203	43267	45327
37215	43268	45332
37216	43269	45333
43200	43271	45334
43201	43272	45337
43202	43453	45338
43204	43456	45339
43205	43458	45340
43215	44360	45341
43216	44361	45342
43217	44363	45345
43219	44364	45355
43220	44365	45378
43226	44366	45379
43227	44369	45380
43228	44370	45381
43231	44372	45382
43232	44373	45383
43234	44376	45384
43235	44377	45385
43236	44378	45386
43239	44379	45387
43240	44380	45391

19298	32019	33218	
20982	32020	33220	
31615	32201	33222	
31620	33010	33223	
31622	33011	33233	
31623	33206	33234	
31624	33207	33235	
31625	33208	33240	
31628	33210	33241	
31629	33211	33244	
31635	33212	33249	
31645	33213	35470	
31646	33214	35471	
31656	33216	35472	
31725	33217	35473	

45392	93528
47011	93529
48511	93530
49021	93539
49041	93540
49061	93541
50021	93542
58823	93543
66720	93544
77600	93545
77605	93555
77610	93556
77615	93561
92953	93562
92960	93571
92961	93572
92973	93609
92974	93613
92975	93615
92978	93616
92979	93618
92980	93619
92981	93620
92982	93621
92984	93622
92986	93624
92987	93640
92995	93641
92996	93642
93312	93650
93313	93651
93314	93652
93315	
93316	
93317	
93318	
93501	
93505	
93508	
93510	
93511	
93514	
93524	
93526	
93527	

Appendix H

Alphabetic Index of Performance Measures by Clinical Condition or Topic

Note: Prior to coding, the user must review the complete description of the code in the Category II section of the CPT coding manual and the complete description of its associated measure by accessing the measure developer's Web site provided in the footnoted reference.

Brief Description of Performance Measure & Source: Title, Numerator, Denominator, Inclusion/Exclusion Criteria	CPT Code(s)	Brief Code Descriptor
Coronary Artery Disease (CAD)		
Blood Pressure Measurement[1]—Percentage of patients who had a blood pressure measurement during the last office visit **Numerator:** Patients who had a blood pressure measurement during the last office visit **Denominator:** All patients with CAD **Inclusion/Exclusion:** None	2000F	Blood pressure measured
Smoking Cessation Evaluation[1]—Percentage of patients evaluated for smoking or other tobacco use **Numerator:** Patients evaluated for smoking or other tobacco use **Denominator:** All patients **Inclusion/Exclusion:** None	1000F 1001F	Tobacco use, smoking, assessed Tobacco use, non-smoking, assessed
Smoking Cessation Intervention[1]—Percentage of patients identified as cigarette smokers who received smoking cessation intervention **Numerator:** Patients identified as smokers or other tobacco users who were offered an intervention for tobacco use cessation, either counseling or pharmacologic therapy during one or more office visits **Denominator:** All patients identified as smokers or other tobacco users **Inclusion/Exclusion:** None	4000F 4001F	Tobacco use cessation counseling Tobacco use cessation intervention, pharmacologic therapy
Drug Therapy for Lowering Cholesterol[1]—Percentage of patients who were prescribed a statin (based on current ACC/AHA guidelines) **Numerator:** Patients who were prescribed a statin **Denominator:** All patients with CAD **Inclusion:** None **Exclusion:** Documentation that a statin was not indicated; documentation of medical or patient reason(s) for not prescribing a statin	4002F	Statin therapy prescribed
Beta-blocker Therapy–Prior Myocardial Infarction (MI)[1]—Percentage of CAD patients who also have prior MI who were prescribed beta-blocker therapy **Numerator:** Patients who were prescribed beta-blocker therapy **Denominator:** All patients with CAD **Inclusion:** Patients with prior MI **Exclusion:** Documentation that a beta-blocker was not indicated; documentation of medical or patient reason(s) for not prescribing a beta-blocker	4006F	Beta-blocker therapy prescribed
Angiotensin Converting Enzyme (ACE) Inhibitor Therapy[1]—Percentage of CAD patients who also have diabetes and/or left ventricular systolic dysfunction (LVSD) who were prescribed ACE inhibitor therapy **Numerator:** Patients who were prescribed ACE inhibitor therapy **Denominator:** All patients with CAD who also have diabetes and/or LVSD **Inclusion:** Patients with CAD who also have diabetes and/or LVSD, left ventricular ejection fraction (LVEF) < 40% or moderately or severely depressed left ventricular systolic function) (continued)	4009F	Angiotensin Converting Enzyme (ACE) inhibitor prescribed

[1]Physician Consortium for Performance Improvement, www.ama-assn.org/go/quality
[2]National Committee on Quality Assurance (NCQA), Health Employer Data Information Set (HEDIS®), www.ncqa.org

Brief Description of Performance Measure & Source: Title, Numerator, Denominator, Inclusion/Exclusion Criteria	CPT Code(s)	Brief Code Descriptor
Exclusion: Documentation that ACE inhibitor was not indicated (eg, patients on angiotensin receptor blockers; documentation of medical or patient reason(s) for not prescribing ACE inhibitor		
Symptom & Activity Assessment[1]—Percentage of CAD patients who were evaluated for both level of activity and anginal symptoms during one or more office visits **Numerator:** Patients who were evaluated for both level of activity and anginal symptoms during one or more office visits **Denominator**—All patients with CAD **Inclusion/Exclusion:** None	1002F	Anginal symptoms and level of activity assessed
Antiplatelet Therapy[1]—Percentage of patients who were prescribed antiplatelet therapy **Numerator:** Patients who were prescribed antiplatelet therapy **Denominator:** All patients with CAD **Inclusion:** None **Exclusion:** Documentation that antiplatelet therapy was not indicated; documentation of medical or patient reason(s) for not prescribing a beta-blocker	4011F	Oral antiplatelet therapy prescribed
Prenatal-Postpartum Care		
Timeliness of Prenatal Care[2]—Percentage of patients in the denominator who received prenatal care **Numerator:** Number of women in the denominator who received a prenatal care visit as a member of the managed care organization (MCO) in the first trimester or within 42 days of enrollment in the MCO **Denominator:** Women who had live births between November 6th of the year prior to the measurement year and November 5th of the measurement year, who were continuously enrolled at least 43 days prior to delivery through 56 days after delivery **Inclusion/Exclusion Criteria:** None	0500F	Initial prenatal care visit
Prenatal Flow Sheet[1]—Percentage of patients in the denominator with a prenatal flow sheet in use by the first physician visit **Numerator:** Percentage of patients in the denominator with a flow sheet in use by the date of the first physician visit, which contains at a minimum: blood pressure, weight, urine protein, uterine size, fetal heart tones, and estimated date of delivery **Denominator:** Pregnant women seen for prenatal care **Exclusion Criteria:** Patients seen for consultation only, not for continuing care	0501F	Prenatal flow sheet documented
Frequency of Ongoing Prenatal Care[2]—Percentage of patients in the denominator with expected number of prenatal visits **Numerator:** Number of women in the denominator who had an unduplicated count of less than 21%, 21%-40%, 41%-60%, 61%-80%, or greater than or equal to 81% of the expected number of prenatal care visits, adjusted for the month of pregnancy at time of enrollment and gestational age **Denominator:** Women who had live births during the measurement year **Inclusion/Exclusion Criteria:** MCOs must exclude members for whom a prenatal visit is not indicated	0502F	Subsequent prenatal care visit
Postpartum Care[2]—Percentage of patients in the denominator who had a postpartum visit between 21 and 56 days after delivery **Numerator:** Number of women in the denominator who had a postpartum visit on or between 21 days and 56 days after delivery **Denominator:** Women who had live births between November 6th of the year prior to the measurement year and November 5th of the measurement year, who were continuously enrolled at least 43 days prior to delivery through 56 days after delivery **Inclusion/Exclusion:** None	0503F	Postpartum care visit

[1]Physician Consortium for Performance Improvement, www.ama-assn.org/go/quality
[2]National Committee on Quality Assurance (NCQA), Health Employer Data Information Set (HEDIS®), www.ncqa.org

Appendix I

Genetic Testing Code Modifiers

This listing of modifiers is intended for reporting with molecular laboratory procedures related to genetic testing. Genetic test modifiers should be used in conjunction with CPT and HCPCS codes to provide diagnostic granularity of service to enable providers to submit complete and precise genetic testing information without altering test descriptors. These modifiers are categorized by mutation. The first (numeric) digit indicates the disease category and the second (alpha) digit denotes gene type. Introductory guidelines in the molecular diagnostic and molecular cytogenetic code sections of CPT provide further guidance in interpretation and application of genetic test modifiers.

Neoplasia (solid tumor)

0A   BRCA1 (Hereditary breast/ovarian cancer)

0B   BRCA2 (Hereditary breast cancer)

0C   Neurofibromin (Neurofibromatosis, type 1)

0D   Merlin (Neurofibromatosis, type 2)

0E   c-RET (Multiple endocrine neoplasia, types 2A/B, familial medullary thyroid carcinoma)

0F   VHL (Von Hippel Lindau disease)

0G   SDHD (Hereditary paraganglioma)

0H   SDHB (Hereditary paraganglioma)

0I   Her-2/neu

0J   MLH1 (HNPCC)

0K   MSH2 (HNPCC)

0L   APC (Hereditary polyposis coli)

0M   Rb (Retinoblastoma)

1Z   Solid tumor, not otherwise specified

Neoplasia (lymphoid/hematopoetic)

2A   AML1 - also ETO (Acute myeloid leukemia)

2B   BCR - also ABL (Chronic myeloid, acute lymphoid leukemia)

2C   CGF1

2D   CBF beta (Leukemia)

2E   MML (Leukemia)

2F   PML/RAR alpha (Promyelocytic leukemia)

2G   TEL (Leukemia)

2H   bcl-2 (Lymphoma)

2I   bcl-1 (Lymphoma)

2J   c-myc (Lymphoma)

2K   IgH (Lymphoma/leukemia)

2Z   Lymphoid/hematopoetic neoplasia, not otherwise specified

Non-neoplastic hematology/coagulation

3A   Factor V (Leiden, others) (Hypercoagulable state)

3B   FACC (Fanconi anemia)

3C   FACD (Fanconi anemia)

3D   Beta globin (Thalassemia)

3E   Alpha globin (Thalassemia)

3F   MTHFR (Elevated homocysteine)

3G   Prothrombin (Factor II, 20210A) (Hypercoagulable state)

3H   Factor VIII (Hemophilia A/VWF)

3I   Factor IX (Hemophilia B)

3J   Beta globin

3Z   Non-neoplastic hematology/coagulation, not otherwise specified

Histocompatibility/blood typing

4A   HLA-A

4B   HLA-B

4C   HLA-C

4D   HLA-D

4E   HLA-DR

4F   HLA-DQ

4G   HLA-DP

4H   Kell

4Z   Histocompatibility/blood typing, not otherwise specified

Neurologic, non-neoplastic

5A   Aspartoacylase A (Canavan disease)

5B   FMR-1 (Fragile X, FRAXA, syndrome)

5C   Frataxin (Freidreich's ataxia)

5D   Huntington (Huntington's disease)

5E   GABRA (Prader Willi-Angelman syndrome)

5F   Connexin-26 (GJB2) (Hereditary deafness)

5G   Connexin-32 (X-linked Charcot-Marie-Tooth disease)

5H   SNRPN (Prader Willi-Angelman syndrome)

5I   Ataxin-1 (Spinocerebellar ataxia, type 1)

5J   Ataxin-2 (Spinocerebellar ataxia, type 2)

5K   Ataxin-3 (Spinocerebellar ataxia, type 3, Machado-Joseph disease)

5L   CACNA1A (Spinocerebellar ataxia, type 6)

5M   Ataxin-7 (Spinocerebellar ataxia, type 7)

5N   PMP-22 (Charcot-Marie-Tooth disease, type 1A)

5O   MECP2 (Rett syndrome)

5Z   Neurologic, non-neoplastic, not otherwise specified

Muscular, non-neoplastic

6A   Dystrophin (Duchenne/Becker muscular dystrophy)

6B   DMPK (Myotonic dystrophy, type 1)

6C   ZNF-9 (Myotonic dystrophy, type 2)

6D   SMN (Autosomal recessive spinal muscular atrophy)

6Z   Muscular, not otherwise specified

Metabolic, other

7A   Apolipoprotein E (Cardiovascular disease, Alzheimer's disease)

7B   Sphingomyelin phosphodiesterase (Nieman-Pick disease)

7C   Acid Beta Glucosidase (Gaucher disease)

7D   HFE (Hemochromatosis)

7E   Hexosaminidase A (Tay-Sachs disease)

7Z   Metabolic, other, not otherwise specified

Metabolic, transport

8A   CFTR (Cystic fibrosis)

8Z   Metabolic, transport, not otherwise specified

Metabolic-pharmacogenetics

9A   TPMT (thiopurine methyltransferase) (patients on antimetabolite therapy)

9L   Metabolic-pharmacogenetics, not otherwise specified

Dysmorphology

9M   FGFR1 (Pfeiffer and Kallmann syndromes)

9N   FGFR2 (Crouzon, Jackson-Weiss, Apert, Saethre-Chotzen syndromes)

9O   FGFR3 (Achondroplasia, Hypochondroplasia, Thanatophoric dysplasia, types I and II, Crouzon syndrome with acanthosis nigricans, Muencke syndromes)

9P   TWIST (Saethre-Chotzen syndrome)

9Q   CATCH-22 (22q11 deletion syndromes)

9Z   Dysmorphology, not otherwise specified

Notes

Index

Instructions for the Use of the CPT Index

Main Terms

The index is organized by main terms. Each main term can stand alone, or be followed by up to three modifying terms. There are four primary classes of main entries:

1. Procedure or service.
   For example: Endoscopy; Anastomosis; Splint

2. Organ or other anatomic site.
   For example: Tibia; Colon; Salivary Gland

3. Condition.
   For example: Abscess; Entropion; Tetralogy of Fallot

4. Synonyms, Eponyms and Abbreviations.
   For example: EEG; Bricker Operation; Clagett Procedure

Modifying Terms

A main term may be followed by a series of up to three indented terms that modify the main term. When modifying terms appear, one should review the list, as these subterms do have an effect on the selection of the appropriate code for the procedure.

Code Ranges

Whenever more than one code applies to a given index entry, a code range is listed. If several non-sequential codes apply, they will be separated by a comma. For example:

Esophagus
    Reconstruction 43300, 43310, 43313

If two or more sequential codes apply, they will be separated by a hyphen. For example:

Debridement
    Burns 01951-01953, 16010-16030

Conventions

As a space saving convention, certain words infer some meaning. This convention is primarily used when a procedure or service is listed as a subterm. For example:

Knee
    Incision (of)

In this example, the word in parentheses (of) does not appear in the index, but it is inferred. As another example:

Pancreas
    Anesthesia (for procedures on)

In this example, as there is no such entity as pancreas anesthesia, the words in parentheses are inferred. That is, anesthesia for procedures on the pancreas.

The alphabetic index is NOT a substitute for the main text of *CPT*. Even if only one code appears, the user must refer to the main text to ensure that the code selection is accurate.

A

A Vitamin
See Vitamin, A

A-II
See Angiotensin II

Abbe-Estlander Procedure
See Reconstruction; Repair, Cleft Lip

Abdomen
Abdominal Wall
  Removal
    Mesh 11008
    Prosthesis 11008
  Repair
    Hernia 49491-49496, 49501, 49507,
                              49521, 49590
  Tumor
    Excision 22900
    Unlisted Services and Procedures 22999
Abscess
    Incision and Drainage 49020, 49040
      Open 49040
      Percutaneous 49021
Angiography 74175, 75635
Artery
    Ligation 37617
Biopsy 49000
Bypass Graft 35907
Cannula/Catheter
    Removal 49422
Celiotomy
    for Staging 49220
CT Scan 74150-74175, 75635
Cyst
    Destruction/Excision 49200-49201
Drainage
    Fluid 49080-49081
Ectopic Pregnancy 59130
Endometrioma
    Destruction/Excision 49200-49201
Exploration 49000-49002
    Blood Vessel 35840
    Staging 58960
Incision 49000
    Staging 58960
Incision and Drainage
    Pancreatitis 48000
Injection
    Air 49400
    Contrast Material 49400
Insertion
    Catheter 49419-49421
    Venous Shunt 49425
Intraperitoneal
    Catheter Removal 49422
    Shunt
      Ligation 49428
      Removal 49429
Laparotomy
    Staging 49220
Magnetic Resonance Imaging
(MRI) 74181-74183

Needle Biopsy
    Mass 49180
Peritoneocentesis 49080-49081
Radical Resection 51597
Repair
    Blood Vessel 35221
      with Other Graft 35281
      with Vein Graft 35251
    Hernia 49491-49525, 49560-49587
    Suture 49900
Revision
    Venous Shunt 49426
Suture 49900
Tumor
    Destruction/Excision 49200-49201
Ultrasound 76700-76705
Unlisted Services and Procedures 49999
Wound Exploration
    Penetrating 20102
X-Ray 74000-74022

Abdominal Aorta
See Aorta, Abdominal

Abdominal Aortic Aneurysm
See Aorta, Abdominal, Aneurysm

Abdominal Deliveries
See Cesarean Delivery

Abdominal Hysterectomy
See Hysterectomy, Abdominal

Abdominal Lymphangiogram
See Lymphangiography, Abdomen

Abdominal Paracentesis
See Abdomen, Drainage

Abdominal Radiographies
See Abdomen, X-Ray

Abdominal Wall
Debridement
    Infected 11005-11006
Reconstruction 49905
Removal
    Mesh 11008
    Prosthesis 11008
Surgery 22999
Tumor
    Excision 22900

Abdominohysterectomy
See Hysterectomy, Abdominal

Abdominopelvic Amputation
See Amputation, Interpelviabdominal

Abdominoplasty 15831

Ablation
Anal
    Polyp 46615
    Tumor 46615
Bone
    Tumor 20982
Colon
    Tumor 45339
CT Scan Guidance 76362
Endometrial 58353-58356, 58563

Endometrium
    Ultrasound Guidance 58356
Heart
    Arrhythmogenic Focus 93650-93652
      See Cardiology; Diagnostic, Intracardiac
      Pacing and Mapping
Liver
    Tumor
      Laparoscopic 47370-47371
      Open 47380-47382
Magnetic Resonance Guidance 76394
Prostate 55873
Renal Cyst 50541
Renal Mass 50542
Turbinate Mucosa 30801-30802
Ultrasound
    Guidance 76940
    Uterine Tumor 0071T-0072T
Uterine Tumor
    Ultrasound, Focused 0071T-0072T
Vein
    Endovenous 36475-36479

Abortion
See Obstetrical Care
Incomplete 59812
Induced
    by Dilation and Curettage 59840
    by Dilation and Evacuation 59841
    by Saline 59850-59851
    by Vaginal Suppositories 59855-59856
    with Hysterectomy 59100, 59852, 59857
Missed
    First Trimester 59820
    Second Trimester 59821
Septic 59830
Spontaneous 59812
Therapeutic
    by Saline 59850
      with Dilation and Curettage 59851
      with Hysterectomy 59852

Abrasion
Skin
    Chemical Peel 15788-15793
    Dermabrasion 15780-15783
    Lesion 15786-15787
    Salabrasion 15810-15811

Abscess
Abdomen 49040-49041
    Incision and Drainage
      Open 49040
      Percutaneous 49021
Anal
    Incision and Drainage 46045-46050
Ankle 27603
Appendix
    Incision and Drainage 44900
      Open 44900
      Percutaneous 44901
Arm, Lower 25028
    Excision 25145
    Incision and Drainage 25035
Arm, Upper
    Incision and Drainage 23930-23935
Auditory Canal, External 69020
Bartholin's Gland
    Incision and Drainage 56420

Bladder
    Incision and Drainage 51080
Brain
    Drainage 61150-61151
    Excision 61514, 61522
    Incision and Drainage 61320-61321
Breast
    Incision and Drainage 19020
Carpals
    Incision, Deep 25035
Clavicle
    Sequestrectomy 23170
Drainage
    with X-Ray 75989
Ear, External
    Complicated .69005
    Simple 69000
Elbow
    Incision and Drainage 23930-23935
Epididymis
    Incision and Drainage 54700
Excision
    Olecranon Process 24138
    Radius 24136
    Ulna 24138
Eyelid
    Incision and Drainage 67700
Facial Bones
    Excision 21026
Finger 26010-26011
    Incision and Drainage 26034
Foot
    Incision 28005
Gums
    Incision and Drainage 41800
Hand
    Incision and Drainage 26034
Hematoma
    Incision and Drainage 27603
Hip
    Incision and Drainage 26990-26992
Humeral Head .23174
Humerus
    Excision 24134
    Incision and Drainage 23935
Kidney
    Incision and Drainage 50020
        Open 50020
        Percutaneous 50021
Leg, Lower
    Incision and Drainage 27603
Liver 47010
    Drainage
        Open 47010
    Injection 47015
    Repair 47300
Localization
    Nuclear Medicine 78806-78807
Lung
    Percutaneous Drainage 32200-32201
Lymph Node
    Incision and Drainage 38300-38305
Lymphocele Drainage 49062
Mandible
    Excision 21025
Mouth
    Incision and Drainage 40800-40801,
             41005-41009, 41015-41018

Nasal Septum
    Incision and Drainage 30020
Neck
    Incision and Drainage 21501-21502
Ovarian
    Incision and Drainage 58820-58822
        Abdominal Approach 58822
        Vaginal Approach 58820
Ovary
    Drainage
        Percutaneous 58823
Palate
    Incision and Drainage 42000
Paraurethral Gland
    Incision and Drainage 53060
Parotid Gland Drainage 42300-42305
Pelvic
    Drainage
        Percutaneous 58823
Pelvis
    Incision and Drainage . .26990-26992, 45000
Pericolic
    Drainage
        Percutaneous 58823
Perineum
    Incision and Drainage 56405
Perirenal or Renal
    Drainage 50020-50021
    Percutaneous 50021
Peritoneum
    Incision and Drainage
        Open 49020
        Percutaneous 49021
Prostate
    Incision and Drainage 55720-55725
    Transurethral Drainage 52700
Radius
    Incision, Deep 25035
Rectum
    Incision and Drainage 45005-45020,
             46040, 46060
Retroperitoneal 49060-49061
    Drainage
        Open 49060
        Percutaneous 49061
Salivary Gland
    Drainage 42300-42320
Scapula
    Sequestrectomy 23172
Scrotum
    Incision and Drainage 54700, 55100
Shoulder
    Drainage 23030
Skene's Gland
    Incision and Drainage 53060
Skin
    Incision and Drainage 10060-10061
    Puncture Aspiration 10160
Soft Tissue
    Incision 20000-20005
Subdiaphragmatic 49040-49041
Sublingual Gland
    Drainage 42310-42320
Submaxillary Gland
    Drainage 42310-42320
Subphrenic 49040-49041
Testis
    Incision and Drainage 54700

Thoracostomy .32020
Thorax
    Incision and Drainage 21501-21502
Throat
    Incision and Drainage 42700-42725
Tongue
    Incision and Drainage 41000-41006
Tonsil
    Incision and Drainage 42700
Ulna
    Incision, Deep 25035
Urethra
    Incision and Drainage 53040
Uvula
    Incision and Drainage 42000
Vagina
    Incision and Drainage 57010
Vulva
    Incision and Drainage 56405
Wrist
    Excision 25145
    Incision and Drainage 25028, 25035
X-Ray 76080

Abscess, Nasal
See Nose, Abscess

Abscess, Parotid Gland
See Parotid Gland, Abscess

Absorptiometry
Dual Energy
    Body Composition 0028T
    Bone 76075
        Appendicular 76076
        Axial Skeleton 76075
        Vertebral 76077
Dual Photon
    Bone 78351
Radiographic
    Photodensity 76078
Single Photon
    Bone 78350

Absorption Spectrophotometry, Atomic
See Atomic Absorption Spectroscopy

Accessory Nerve, Spinal
See Nerves, Spinal Accessory

Accessory, Toes
See Polydactyly, Toes

ACE
See Angiotensin Converting Enzyme (ACE), Performance Measures

Acetabuloplasty 27120-27122

Acetabulum
Fracture
    Closed Treatment 27220-27222
    Open Treatment 27226-27228
    with Manipulation 27222
    without Manipulation 27220
Reconstruction 27120
    with Resection, Femoral Head 27122
Tumor
    Excision 27076

Acetaldehyde
Blood 82000

Acetaminophen
Urine 82003

Acetic Anhydrides 84600

Acetone
Blood or Urine 82009-82010

Acetone Body 82009-82010

Acetylcholinesterase
Blood or Urine 82013

AcG
See Clotting Factor

Achilles Tendon
Incision 27605-27606
Lengthening 27612
Repair 27650-27654

Achillotomy
See Tenotomy, Achilles Tendon

Acid
Gastric 82926-82928

Acid Diethylamide, Lysergic
See Lysergic Acid Diethylamide

Acid Fast Bacilli (AFB)
Culture 87116

Acid Fast Bacillus Culture
See Culture, Acid Fast Bacilli

Acid Fast Stain 88312

Acid Perfusion Test
Esophagus 91012, 91030

Acid Phosphatase 84060-84066

Acid Probes, Nucleic
See Nucleic Acid Probe

Acid Reflux Test
Esophagus 91034-91038

Acid, Adenylic
See Adenosine Monophosphate (AMP)

Acid, Aminolevulinic
See Aminolevulinic Acid (ALA)

Acid, Ascorbic
See Ascorbic Acid

Acid, Deoxyribonucleic
See Deoxyribonucleic Acid

Acid, Folic
See Folic Acid

Acid, Glycocholic
See Cholylglycine

Acid, Lactic
See Lactic Acid

Acid, N-Acetylneuraminic
See Sialic Acid

Acid, Phenylethylbarbituric
See Phenobarbital

Acid, Uric
See Uric Acid

Acidity /Alkalinity
See pH

Acids, Amino
See Amino Acids

Acids, Bile
See Bile Acids

Acids, Fatty
See Fatty Acid

Acids, Guanylic
See Guanosine Monophosphate

Acids, N-Acetylneuraminic
See Sialic Acid

Acne Surgery
Incision and Drainage
    Abscess 10060-10061
    Comedones 10040
    Cyst 10040
    Milia, Multiple 10040
    Pustules 10040

Acne Treatment
Abrasion 15786-15787
Chemical Peel 15788-15793
Cryotherapy 17340
Dermabrasion 15780-15783
Exfoliation
    Chemical 17360
Salabrasion 15810-15811

Acoustic Evoked Brain Stem Potential
See Evoked Potential, Auditory Brainstem

Acoustic Neuroma
See Brain, Tumor, Excision; Brainstem; Mesencephalon; Skull Base Surgery

Acoustic Recording
Heart Sounds
    with Computer Analysis 0068T-0070T

Acromioclavicular Joint
Arthrocentesis 20605
Arthrotomy 23044
    with Biopsy 23101
Dislocation 23540-23552
    Open Treatment 23550-23552
X-Ray 73050

Acromion
Excision
    Shoulder 23130

Acromionectomy
Partial 23130

Acromioplasty 23415-23420
Partial 23130

ACTH
See Adrenocorticotropic Hormone (ACTH)

ACTH Releasing Factor
See Corticotropic Releasing Hormone (CRH)

Actinomyces
Antibody 86602

Actinomycosis 86000

Actinomycotic Infection
See Actinomycosis

Actinotherapy 96900
See Dermatology

Activated Factor X
See Thrombokinase

Activated Partial Thromboplastin Time
See Thromboplastin, Partial, Time

Activation, Lymphocyte
See Blastogenesis

Activities of Daily Living
See Physical Medicine/Therapy/Occupational Therapy

Activity, Glomerular Procoagulant
See Thromboplastin

Acupuncture
    with Electrical Stimulation 97813-97814
    without Electrical Stimulation ..97810-97811

Acute Poliomyelitis
See Polio

Acylcarnitines 82016-82017

Adamantinoma, Pituitary
See Craniopharyngioma

Addam Operation
See Dupuytren's Contracture

Adductor Tenotomy of Hip
See Tenotomy, Hip, Adductor

Adenoidectomy 42820-42821,
                                   42830-42836

Adenoids
Excision 42830-42836
    with Tonsils 42820-42821
Unlisted Services and Procedures 42999

Adenoma
Pancreas
    Excision 48120
Thyroid Gland Excision 60200

Adenosine 3'5' Monophosphate
See Cyclic AMP

Adenosine Diphosphate
Blood 82030

Adenosine Monophosphate (AMP)
Blood 82030

Adenovirus
Antibody 86603
Antigen Detection
    Enzyme Immunoassay 87301
    Immunofluorescense 87260

Adenovirus Vaccine
See Vaccines

Adenylic Acid
See Adenosine Monophosphate (AMP)

ADH
See Antidiuretic Hormone

Adhesions
Epidural 0027T, 62263-62264
Eye
    Corneovitreal 65880
    Incision
        Anterior Segment 65860-65870
        Posterior Segment 65875
Intermarginal
    Construction 67880
        Transposition of Tarsal Plate 67882
Intestinal
    Enterolysis 44005
        Laparoscopic 44200
Intracranial
    Lysis 62161
Intrauterine
    Lysis 58559
Labial
    Lysis 56441
Lungs
    Lysis 32124
Pelvic
    Lysis 58660, 58662, 58740
Penile
    Lysis
        Post-circumcision 54162
Preputial
    Lysis 54450
Urethral
    Lysis 53500

Adipectomy
See Lipectomy

ADL
See Activities of Daily Living

Administration
Immunization
    Each Additional Vaccine/Toxoid 90472, 90474
        with Counseling 90466, 90468
    One Vaccine/Toxoid 90471, 90473
        with Counseling 90465, 90467

ADP
See Adenosine Diphosphate

ADP Phosphocreatine Phosphotransferase
See CPK

Adrenal Cortex Hormone
See Corticosteroids

Adrenal Gland
Biopsy 60540-60545
Excision
    Laparoscopy 60650
    Retroperitoneal Tumor 60545
Exploration 60540-60545
Nuclear Medicine
    Imaging 78075

Adrenal Medulla
See Medulla

Adrenalectomy 60540
Anesthesia 00866
Laparoscopic 50545

Adrenalin
See Catecholamines
Blood 82383
Urine 82384

Adrenaline-Noradrenaline
Testing 82382-82384

Adrenocorticotropic Hormone (ACTH) 80400-80406, 80412, 80418, 82024
Blood or Urine 82024
Stimulation Panel 80400-80406

Adrenogenital Syndrome .56805, 57335

Adult T Cell Leukemia Lymphoma Virus I
See HTLV I

Advanced Life Support
See Emergency Department Services
Physician Direction 99288

Advancement
Genioglossus 21199
Tendon
    Foot 28238

Advancement Flap
See Skin, Adjacent Tissue Transfer

Aerosol Inhalation
See Pulmonology, Therapeutic
Pentamidine 94642

AFB
See Acid Fast Bacilli (AFB)

Afferent Nerve
See Sensory Nerve

AFP
See Alpha-Fetoprotein

After Hours Medical Services 99050-99054

Agents, Anticoagulant
See Clotting Inhibitors

Agglutinin
Cold 86156-86157
Febrile 86000

Aggregation
Platelet 85576

AHG
See Clotting Factor

AICD (Pacing Cardioverter-Defibrillator)
See Defibrillator, Heart; Pacemaker, Heart

Aid, Hearing
See Hearing Aid

AIDS Antibodies
See Antibody, HIV

AIDS Virus
See HIV-1

Akin Operation
See Bunion Repair

ALA
See Aminolevulinic Acid (ALA)

Alanine 2 Oxoglutarate Aminotransferase
See Transaminase, Glutamic Pyruvic

Alanine Amino (ALT) 84460

Alanine Transaminase
See Transaminase, Glutamic Pyruvic

Albarran Test
See Water Load Test

Albumin
Ischemia modified 82045
Serum 82040
Urine 82042-82044

Alcohol
Breath 82075
Ethyl
    Blood 82055
    Urine 82055
Ethylene Glycol 82693

Alcohol Dehydrogenase
See Antidiuretic Hormone

Alcohol, Isopropyl
See Isopropyl Alcohol

Alcohol, Methyl
See Methanol

Aldolase
Blood 82085

Aldosterone
Blood 82088
Suppression Evaluation 80408
Urine 82088

Alimentary Canal
See Gastrointestinal Tract

Alkaline Phosphatase 84075-84080
Leukocyte 85540
WBC 85540

Alkaloids
See Specific Drug
Urine 82101

Allergen Bronchial Provocation Tests
See Allergy Tests; Bronchial Challenge Test

Allergen Challenge, Endobronchial
See Bronchial Challenge Test

Allergen Immunotherapy
Allergen
    Prescription/Supply/Injection . .95120-95125
      with Extract Supply 95144
        Injection 95115-95117
Antigens 95144
IgE 86003-86005
IgG 86001
Insect Venom
    Prescription/Supply 95145-95149
    Prescription/Supply/Injection . .95130-95134
Prescription/Supply 95165
    Insect, Whole Body 95170
Rapid Desensitization 95180

Allergy Services/Procedures
See Office and/or Other Outpatient Services;
Allergen and Immunotherapy
Education and Counseling 99201-99215
Unlisted Services and Procedures 95199

Allergy Tests
Challenge Test
    Bronchial 95070-95071
    Ingestion 95075
Eye Allergy 95060
Food Allergy 95075
Intradermal
    Allergen Extract 95024-95028
    Biologicals 95015
    Drugs 95015
    Incremental .95027
    Venoms 95015
Nasal Mucous Membrane Test 95065
Nose Allergy 95065
Patch
    Application Tests 95044
    Photo Patch .95052
Photosensitivity .95056
Provocative Testing 95078
Skin Tests
    Allergen Extract 95004
    Biologicals 95010
    Drugs 95010
    Venoms 95010

Allogeneic Donor
Lymphocyte Infusion 38242

Allogeneic Transplantation
See Homograft

Allograft
Aortic Valve 33406, 33413
Bone
    Structural 20931
Cartilage
    Knee 27415
Lung Transplant .32850
Skin 15350-15351
Spine Surgery
    Morselized 20930
    Structural 20931

Allograft Preparation
Heart 33933, 33944
Intestines 44715-44721
Kidney 50323-50329
Liver 47143-47147
Lung 32855-32856, 33933
Pancreas 48551-48552
Renal 50323-50329

Alloplastic Dressing
Burns 15000-15001

Allotransplantation
Intestines 44135-44136
Renal 50360-50365
    Removal 50370

Almen Test
See Blood, Feces

Alpha-1 Antitrypsin 82103-82104

Alpha-2 Antiplasmin 85410

Alpha-Fetoprotein
Amniotic Fluid 82106
Serum 82105

Alphatocopherol 84446

ALT
See Transaminase, Glutamic Pyruvic

Altemeier Procedure
See Anus; Rectum, Prolapse, Excision

Aluminum
Blood 82108

Alveola
Fracture
    Closed Treatment 21421
    Open Treatment 21422-21423

Alveolar Cleft
Ungrafted Bilateral 21147
Ungrafted Unilateral 21146

Alveolar Nerve
Avulsion 64738
Incision 64738
Transection 64738

Alveolar Ridge
Fracture
    Closed Treatment 21440
    Open Treatment 21445

Alveolectomy 41830

Alveoloplasty 41874

Alveolus
Excision 41830

Amide, Procaine
See Procainamide

Amikacin
Assay 80150

Amine
Vaginal Fluid 82120

Amino Acids 82127-82139

Aminolevulinic Acid (ALA)
Blood or Urine 82135

Aminotransferase
See Transaminase

Aminotransferase, Alanine
See Transaminase, Glutamic Pyruvic

Aminotransferase, Aspartate
See Transaminase, Glutamic Oxaloacetic

Amitriptyline
Assay 80152

Ammonia
Blood 82140
Urine 82140

Amniocenteses
See Amniocentesis

Amniocentesis 59000
See Chromosome Analysis
    with Amniotic Fluid Reduction 59001
Induced Abortion 59850
    with Dilation and Curettage 59851
    with Dilation and Evacuation 59851
    with Hysterectomy 59852

Amnioinfusion
Transabdominal .59070

Amnion
Amniocentesis .59000
    with Amniotic Fluid Reduction 59001
Amnioinfusion
    Transabdominal 59070

Amniotic Fluid
Alpha-Fetoprotein 82106
Scan 82143
Testing 83661, 83663-83664

Amniotic Membrane
See Amnion

Amobarbital 82205

AMP
See Adenosine Monophosphate (AMP)

AMP, Cyclic
See Cyclic AMP

Amphetamine
Blood or Urine 82145

Amputation
See Radical Resection; Replantation
Ankle 27888
Arm, Lower 25900-25905, 25915
    Revision 25907-25909
Arm, Upper 24900-24920
    and Shoulder 23900-23921
    Revision 24925-24930
    with Implant 24931-24935
Cervix
    Total 57530
Ear
    Partial 69110
    Total 69120

Finger 26910-26952
Foot 28800-28805
Hand at Metacarpal 25927
　　at Wrist .25920
　　　Revision 25922
　　Revision 25924, 25929-25931
Interpelviabdominal 27290
Interthoracoscapular 23900
Leg, Lower 27598, 27880-27882
　　Revision 27884-27886
Leg, Upper 27590-27592
　　at Hip 27290-27295
　　Revision 27594-27596
Metacarpal 26910
Metatarsal 28810
Penis
　　Partial 54120
　　Radical 54130-54135
　　Total 54125
Thumb 26910-26952
Toe 28810-28825
Tuft of Distal Phalanx 11752
Upper Extremity .24940
　　Cineplasty .24940

Amputation through Hand
See Hand, Amputation

Amputation, Nose
See Resection, Nose

Amylase
Blood 82150
Urine 82150

ANA
See Antinuclear Antibodies (ANA)

Anabolic Steroid
See Androstenedione

Anal Abscess
See Abscess, Anal

Anal Bleeding
See Anus, Hemorrhage

Anal Fistula
See Fistula, Anal

Anal Fistulectomy
See Excision, Fistula, Anal

Anal Fistulotomy
See Fistulotomy, Anal

Anal Sphincter
Dilation 45905
Incision 46080

Anal Ulceration
See Anus, Fissure

Analgesia 99141-99142
See Anesthesia; Sedation

Analgesic Cutaneous Electrostimulation
See Application, Neurostimulation

Analysis
Computer Data .99090
Electroencephalogram
　　Digital 95957
Electronic
　　Drug Infusion Pump 62367-62368
　　Pacing Cardioverter-
　　Defibrillator 93741-93744
　　　See Pacemaker, Heart
　　Pulse Generator 95970-95971
Physiologic Data, Remote 99091
Protein
　　Tissue
　　　Western Blot 88372
Semen
　　Sperm Isolation 89260-89261

Analysis, Spectrum
See Spectrophotometry

Anaspadias
See Epispadias

Anastomosis
Arteriovenous Fistula
　　Direct 36821
　　with Bypass Graft 35686
　　with Graft 36825-36830, 36832
Artery
　　to Aorta 33606
　　to Artery
　　　Cranial .61711
Bile Duct
　　to Bile Duct 47800
　　to Intestines 47760, 47780
Bile Duct to Gastrointestinal 47785
Broncho-Bronchial 32486
Caval to Mesenteric 37160
Colorectal 44620
Epididymis
　　to Vas Deferens
　　　Bilateral 54901
　　　Unilateral 54900
Excision
　　Trachea 31780-31781
Fallopian Tube .58750
Gallbladder to Intestines 47720-47740
Hepatic Duct to Intestines 47765, 47802
Ileo-Anal 45113
Intestines
　　Colo-anal .45119
　　Cystectomy 51590
　　Enterocystoplasty 51960
　　Resection
　　　Laparoscopic 44202-44205
Intestine to Intestine 44130
Intrahepatic Portosystemic 37182-37183
Jejunum 43825
Microvascular
　　Free Transfer
　　　Jejunum 43496
Nerve
　　Facial to Hypoglossal 64868
　　Facial to Phrenic 64870
Oviduct 58750
Pancreas to Intestines 48180, 48520-48540
Portocaval 37140
Pulmonary 33606
Renoportal 37145

Splenorenal 37180-37181
Stomach 43825
　　to Duodenum 43810, 43855
　　Revision 43850
　　to Jejunum 43820, 43860-43865
Tubotubal 58750
Ureter
　　to Bladder 50780-50785
　　to Colon 50810-50815
　　Removal 50830
　　to Intestine 50800, 50820-50825
　　Removal 50830
　　to Kidney 50727-50750
　　to Ureter 50727, 50760-50770
Vein
　　Saphenopopliteal 34530
Vein to Vein 37140-37160, 37182-37183

Anastomosis of Lacrimal Sac to Conjunctival Sac
See Conjunctivorhinostomy

Anastomosis of Pancreas
See Pancreas, Anastomosis

Anastomosis, Aorta-Pulmonary Artery
See Aorta, Anastomosis, to Pulmonary Artery

Anastomosis, Bladder, to Intestine
See Enterocystoplasty

Anastomosis, Hepatic Duct
See Hepatic Duct, Anastomosis

Anderson Tibial Lengthening 27715
See Ankle; Tibia, Osteoplasty, Lengthening

Androstanediol Glucuronide . . .82154

Androstanolone
See Dihydrotestosterone

Androstenedione
Blood or Urine .82157

Androstenolone
See Dehydroepiandrosterone

Androsterone
Blood or Urine .82160

Anesthesia
See Analgesia
Abbe-Estlander Procedure 00102
Abdomen
　　Abdominal Wall 00700, 00730,
　　　　　　　　　　　00800-00802, 00820, 00836
　　Halsted Repair 00750-00756
　　Blood Vessels 00770, 00880-00882
　　Endoscopy 00740, 00810
　　Extraperitoneal 00860-00862,
　　　　　　　　　　　　　　　　00866-00870
　　Hernia Repair 00830-00836
　　Halsted Repair 00750-00756
　　Intraperitoneal . . .00790-00797, 00840-00842
Abdominoperineal Resection 00844
Abortion
　　Induced 01964
Achilles Tendon Repair 01472

Removal
    Foreign Body 46608
    Polyp 46610, 46612
    Tumor 46610, 46612
Excision
    Tag 46220, 46230
Exploration
    Endoscopy 46600
Fissure
    Destruction 46940-46942
    Excision .46200
Fistula
    Excision 46270-46285
    Repair 46706
Hemorrhage
    Endoscopic Control 46614
Hemorrhoids
    Clot Excision 46320
    Destruction 46934-46936
    Excision 46250-46262
    Injection 46500
    Ligation 46221, 46945-46946
    Stapling 46947
    Suture 46945-46946
Imperforated
    Repair 46715-46742
Incision
    Septum 46070
Lesion
    Destruction 46900-46917, 46924
    Excision 45108, 46922
Manometry 91122
Placement
    Seton 46020
Reconstruction 46742
    Congenital Absence 46730-46740
    Sphincter 46750-46751, 46760-46762
    with Graft 46753
    with Implant 46762
Removal
    Foreign Body 46608
    Seton 46030
    Suture .46754
    Wire 46754
Repair
    Anovaginal Fistula 46715-46716
    Cloacal Anomaly 46748
    Fistula .46706
    Stricture 46700-46705
Sphincter
    Electromyography 51784-51785
    Needle 51785
Unlisted Services and Procedures 46999

Aorta
Abdominal
    Aneurysm 0078T-0081T, 34800-34805,
      34825-34832, 35081-35103, 75952-75953
    Thromboendarterectomy 35331
Anastomosis
    to Pulmonary Artery 33606
Angiogram
    Radiologic Injection 93544
      See Cardiac Catheterization, Injection
Angioplasty .35452
Aortography 75600-75630
Balloon 33967, 33970

Catheterization
    Catheter 36200
    Intracatheter/Needle 36160
Circulation Assist 33967, 33970
Conduit to Heart 33404
Excision
    Coarctation 33840-33851
Insertion
    Balloon Device 33967
    Graft 33330-33335
    Intracatheter/Needle 36160
Removal
    Balloon Assist Device 33968, 33971
Repair 33320-33322, 33802-33803
    Coarctation 33840-33851
    Graft 33860-33877
    Hypoplastic or Interrupted Aortic Arch
      with Cardiopulmonary Bypass 33853
      without Cardiopulmonary Bypass . . .33852
    Sinus of Valsalva 33702-33720
Suspension 33800
Suture 33320-33322
Thoracic
    Aneurysm 0033T-0040T
Valve
    Incision 33415
    Repair 33400-33403
      Left Ventricle 33414
      Supravalvular Stenosis 33417
    Replacement 33405-33413
X-Ray with Contrast 75600-75630

Aorta-Pulmonary ART Transposition
See Transposition, Great Arteries

Aortic Sinus
See Sinus of Valsalva

Aortic Stenosis
Repair 33415
    Supravalvular 33417

Aortic Valve
See Heart, Aortic Valve

Aortic Valve Replacement
See Replacement, Aortic Valve

Aortocoronary Bypass
See Coronary Artery Bypass Graft (CABG)

Aortocoronary Bypass for Heart Revascularization
See Artery, Coronary, Bypass

Aortography 75600-75605,
                    75630, 93544

See Angiography
Serial 75625
with Iliofemoral Artery 75630

Aortoiliac
Embolectomy 34151-34201
Thrombectomy 34151-34201

Aortopexy .33800

Aortoplasty
Supravalvular Stenosis 33417

AP
See Voiding Pressure Studies

Apert-Gallais Syndrome
See Adrenogenital Syndrome

Aphasia Testing 96105
See Neurology, Diagnostic

Apheresis
Therapeutic 36511-36516

Apical-Aortic Conduit 33404

Apicectomy
with Mastoidectomy 69605
    Petrous 69530

Apoaminotransferase, Aspartate
See Transaminase, Glutamic Oxaloacetic

Apolipoprotein
Blood or Urine 82172

Appendectomy 44950-44960
Laparoscopic 44970

Appendiceal Abscess
See Abscess, Appendix

Appendico-Vesicostomy
Cutaneous 50845

Appendix
Abscess
    Incision and Drainage
      Open 44900
      Percutaneous 44901
Excision 44950-44960

Application
Allergy Tests 95044
Bone Fixation Device
    Multiplane 20692
    Uniplane 20690
Caliper 20660
Cranial Tongs 20660
Fixation Device
    Shoulder 23700
Halo
    Cranial 20661
      Thin Skull Osteology 20664
    Femoral 20663
    Maxillofacial Fixation 21100
    Pelvic 20662
Interdental Fixation Device 21110
Neurostimulation 64550
Radioelement 77761-77778
    Surface 77789
    with Ultrasound 76965
Stereotactic Frame 20660

Application of External Fixation Device
See Fixation Device, Application, External

APPT
See Thromboplastin, Partial, Time

Aquatic Therapy
See Physical Medicine/Therapy/Occupational Therapy

Artery Catheterization, Pulmonary

See Catheterization, Pulmonary Artery

Arthrectomy

Arthrocentesis

Arthrodeses

See Arthrodesis

Arthrodesis

Arthrography

Arthroplasties, Knee Replacement

See Prosthesis, Knee

Arthroplasty

Trapezium 25445
Ulna 25442
with Implant 25441-25445
Wrist (Pseudarthrosis Type) 25332

Arthroplasty, Hip, Total
See Hip, Total Replacement

Arthroplasty, Shoulder
See Repair, Shoulder

Arthropods
Examination 87168

Arthroscopy
Diagnostic
Elbow 29830
Hip 29860
Knee 29870
Metacarpophalangeal Joint 29900
Shoulder 29805
Temporomandibular Joint 29800
Wrist 29840
Surgical
Ankle 29891-29899
Elbow 29834-29838
Hip 29861-29863
Knee 29871-29889
Cartilage Allograft 29867
Cartilage Autograft 29866
Meniscal Transplantation 29868
Metacarpophalangeal Joint 29901-29902
Shoulder 29806-29827
Temporomandibular Joint 29804
Wrist 29843-29848
Unlisted Services and Procedures 29999

Arthroscopy of Ankle
See Ankle, Arthroscopy

Arthrotomy
Acromioclavicular Joint 23044
Ankle 27610-27612, 27620
Ankle Joint 27625-27626
Carpometacarpal Joint 26070
with Biopsy, Synovium
with Synovial Biopsy 26100
Elbow 24000
Capsular Release 24006
with Joint Exploration 24101
with Synovectomy 24102
with Synovial Biopsy 24100
Finger Joint 26075
Interphalangeal
with Synovial Biopsy 26110
Metacarpophalangeal
with Biopsy, Synovium 26105
Glenohumeral Joint 23040
Hip 27033
for Infection
with Drainage 27030
with Synovectomy 27054
Interphalangeal Joint 26080, 26110
Toe 28024, 28054
Intertarsal Joint 28020, 28050
Knee 27310, 27330-27335, 27403, 29868
Metacarpophalangeal Joint 26075, 26105
Metatarsophalangeal Joint 28022, 28052
Shoulder 23044, 23105-23107

Shoulder Joint 23100-23101
Exploration and/or Removal of Loose or
Foreign Body 23107
Sternoclavicular Joint 23044
Tarsometatarsal Joint 28020, 28050
Temporomandibular Joint 21010
with Biopsy
Acromioclavicular Joint 23101
Glenohumeral Joint 23100
Hip Joint 27052
Knee Joint 27330
Sacroiliac Joint
Hip Joint 27050
Sternoclavicular Joint 23101
with Synovectomy
Glenohumeral Joint 23105
Sternoclavicular Joint 23106
Wrist 25040, 25100-25107

Arthrotomy for Removal of Prosthesis of Ankle
See Ankle, Removal, Implant

Arthrotomy for Removal of Prosthesis of Hip
See Hip, Removal, Prosthesis

Arthrotomy for Removal of Prosthesis of Wrist
See Prosthesis, Wrist, Removal

Articular Ligament
See Ligament

Artificial Abortion
See Abortion

Artificial Cardiac Pacemaker
See Heart, Pacemaker

Artificial Eye
See Prosthesis

Artificial Genitourinary Sphincter
See Prosthesis, Urethral Sphincter

Artificial Insemination 58976
See In Vitro Fertilization
Intra-Cervical 58321
Intra-Uterine 58322
Sperm Washing 58323

Artificial Knee Joints
See Prosthesis, Knee

Artificial Penis
See Penile Prosthesis

Artificial Pneumothorax
See Pneumothorax, Therapeutic

Arytenoid
Excision
Endoscopic 31560-31561

Arytenoid Cartilage
Excision 31400
Repair 31400

Arytenoidectomy 31400
Endoscopic 31560

Arytenoidopexy 31400

Ascorbic Acid
Blood 82180

Aspartate Aminotransferase
See Transaminase, Glutamic Oxaloacetic

Aspergillus
Antibody 86606

Aspiration
See Puncture Aspiration
Amniotic Fluid
Diagnostic 59000
Therapeutic 59001
Bladder 51000-51010
Bone Marrow 38220
Brain Lesion
Stereotactic 61750-61751
Bronchi
Endoscopy 31645-31646
Bursa 20600-20610
Catheter
Nasotracheal 31720
Tracheobronchial 31725
Cyst
Bone 20615
Kidney 50390
Pelvis 50390
Spinal Cord 62268
Thyroid 60001
Duodenal 89100-89105
Fetal Fluid 59074
Ganglion Cyst 20612
Hydrocele
Tunica Vaginalis 55000
Joint 20600-20610
Laryngoscopy
Direct 31515
Lens Material 66840
Liver 47015
Lung 32420
Nucleus of Disk
Lumbar 62287
Orbital Contents 67415
Pelvis
Endoscopy 49322
Pericardium 33010-33011
Pleural Cavity 32000-32002
Puncture
Cyst
Breast 19000-19001
Spinal Cord
Stereotaxis 63615
Syrinx
Spinal Cord 62268
Thyroid 60001
Trachea
Nasotracheal 31720
Puncture 31612
Tunica Vaginalis
Hydrocele 55000
Vitreous 67015

Aspiration Lipectomies
See Liposuction

Aspiration of Bone Marrow from Donor for Transplant
See Bone Marrow, Harvesting

Aspiration, Chest
See Thoracentesis

Aspiration, Lung Puncture
See Pneumocentesis

Aspiration, Nail
See Evacuation, Hematoma, Subungual

Aspiration, Spinal Puncture
See Spinal Tap

Assay Tobramycin
See Tobramycin

Assay, Very Long Chain Fatty Acids
See Fatty Acid, Very Long Chain

Assisted Circulation
See Circulation Assist

AST
See Transaminase, Glutamic Oxaloacetic

Astragalectomy 28130

Astragalus
See Talus

Asymmetry, Face
See Hemifacial Microsomia

Ataxia Telangiectasia
Chromosome Analysis 88248

Ataxy, Telangiectasia
See Ataxia Telangiectasia

Atherectomies, Coronary
See Artery, Coronary, Atherectomy

Atherectomy
See X-Ray, Artery
Open
   Aorta 35481
   Brachiocephalic 35484
   Femoral 35483
   Iliac 35482
   Popliteal 35483
   Renal 35480
   Tibioperoneal 35485
   Visceral 35480
Percutaneous
   Aorta 35491
   Brachiocephalic 35494
   Coronary 92995-92996
    See Artery, Coronary
   Femoral 35493
   Iliac 35492
   Popliteal 35493
   Renal 35490
   Tibioperoneal 35495
   Visceral 35490
X-Ray
   Peripheral Artery 75992-75993
   Renal Artery 75994
   Visceral Artery 75995-75996

ATLV
See HTLV I

ATLV Antibodies
See Antibody, HTLV-I

Atomic Absorption Spectroscopy 0064T, 82190

ATP Creatine Phosphotransferase
See CPK

Atresia, Choanal
See Choanal Atresia

Atresia, Congenital
Auditory Canal, External
   Reconstruction 69320

Atria
Reconstruction 33253

Atrial Electrogram
See Cardiology, Diagnostic
Esophageal Recording 93615-93616

Atrial Fibrillation
See Fibrillation, Atrial

Atrioseptopexy
See Heart, Repair, Atrial Septum

Atrioseptoplasty
See Heart, Repair, Atrial Septum

Attachment
See Fixation

Atticotomy 69631, 69635

Audiologic Function Tests
See Ear, Nose and Throat; Hearing Evaluation
Acoustic Reflex 92568
Acoustic Reflex Decay 92569
Audiometry
   Bekesy 92560-92561
   Comprehensive 92557
   Conditioning Play 92582
   Groups 92559
   Pure Tone 92552-92553
   Select Picture 92583
   Speech 92555-92556
   Visual Reinforcement 92579
Central Auditory Function 92620-92621
Electrocochleography 92584
Evoked Otoacoustic Emission 92587-92588
Filtered Speech 92571
Lombard Test 92573
Loudness Balance 92562
Screening 92551
Sensorineural Acuity 92575
Short Increment Sensitivity Index 92564
Staggered Spondaic Word Test 92572
Stenger Test 92565, 92577
Synthetic Sentence Test 92576
Tinnitus Assessment 92625
Tone Decay 92563

Audiometry
Bekesy 92560-92561
Brainstem Evoked Response 92585-92586
Comprehensive 92557

Conditioning Play 92582
Groups 92559
   See Ear, Nose and Throat
Pure Tone 92552-92553
Select Picture 92583
Speech 92555-92556
Tympanometry 92567

Auditory Brain Stem Evoked Response
See Evoked Potential, Auditory Brainstem

Auditory Canal
Decompression 61591
External
   Abscess
    Incision and Drainage 69020
    Biopsy 69105
   Lesion
    Excision 69140-69155
   Reconstruction
    for Congenital Atresia 69320
    for Stenosis 69310
   Removal
    Cerumen 69210
    Ear Wax 69210
    Foreign Body 69200-69205
Internal
   Decompression 69960

Auditory Canal Atresia, External
See Atresia, Congenital, Auditory Canal, External

Auditory Evoked Otoacoustic Emission 92587-92588

Auditory Evoked Potentials 92585-92586
See Audiologic Function Tests

Auditory Labyrinth
See Ear, Inner

Auditory Meatus
X-Ray 70134

Auditory Tube
See Eustachian Tube

Augmentation
Chin 21120, 21123
Malar 21270
Mandibular Body
   with Bone Graft 21127
   with Prosthesis 21125
Osteoplasty
   Facial Bones 21208

Augmentation Mammoplasty
See Breast, Augmentation

Augmented Histamine Test 91052
See Gastric Analysis Test

Aural Rehabilitation 92510

Auricle (Heart)
See Atria

Auricular Fibrillation
See Fibrillation, Atrial

Auricular Prosthesis 21086

Australia Antigen
See Hepatitis Antigen, B Surface

Autograft
Bone
  Local 20936
  Morselized 20937
  Structural 20938
Chondrocytes
  Knee 27412
for Spine Surgery
  Local 20936
  Morselized 20937
  Structural 20938

Autologous Blood Transfusion
See Autotransfusion

Autologous Transplantation
See Autograft

Automated Data
Nuclear Medicine 78890-78891

Autonomic Nervous System Function
See Neurology, Diagnostic; Neurophysiologic Testing

Autoprothrombin C
See Thrombokinase

Autoprothrombin I
See Proconvertin

Autoprothrombin II
See Christmas Factor

Autoprothrombin III
See Stuart-Prower Factor

Autopsy
Coroner's Exam 88045
Forensic Exam 88040
Gross and Micro Exam 88020-88029
Gross Exam 88000-88016
Organ 88037
Regional 88036
Unlisted Services and Procedures 88099

Autotransfusion
Blood 86890-86891

Autotransplant
See Autograft

Autotransplantation
Renal 50380

AV Fistula
See Arteriovenous Fistula

AV Shunt
See Arteriovenous Shunt

Avulsion
Nails 11730-11732
Nerve 64732-64772

Axillary Arteries
See Artery, Axillary

Axillary Nerve
Injection
  Anesthetic 64417

Axis, Dens
See Odontoid Process

B

B Antibodies, Hepatitis
See Antibody, Hepatitis B

B Antigens, Hepatitis
See Hepatitis Antigen, B

B Complex Vitamins
B-12 Absorption 78270-78272

B-DNA
See Deoxyribonucleic Acid

b-Hexosaminidase 83080

B1 Vitamin
See Thiamine

B6 Vitamin
See Vitamin, B-6

B12 Vitamin
See Cyanocobalamin

Babcock Operation
See Ligation, Vein, Saphenous

Bacillus Calmette Guerin Vaccine
See BCG Vaccine

Back/Flank
Biopsy 21920-21925
Repair
  Hernia 49540
  Strapping 29220
Tumor
  Excision 21930
  Radical Resection 21935
Wound Exploration
  Penetrating 20102

Backbone
See Spine

Bacteria Culture
Additional Methods 87077
Aerobic 87040-87071
Anaerobic 87073-87076
Blood 87040
Other Source 87070-87075
Screening 87081
Stool 87045-87046
Urine 87086-87088

Bacterial Endotoxins 87176

Bacterial Overgrowth Breath Test 91065

Bactericidal Titer, Serum 87197

Bacterium
Antibody 86609

BAER
See Evoked Potential, Auditory Brainstem

Baker Tube
Intestine Decompression 44021

Baker's Cyst 27345

Balanoplasty
See Penis, Repair

Baldy-Webster Operation
See Uterus, Repair, Suspension

Balkan Grippe
See Q Fever

Balloon Angioplasties, Coronary
See Percutaneous Transluminal Angioplasty

Balloon Angioplasty
See Angioplasty

Balloon Assisted Device
Aorta 33967-33974, 93727

Band, Pulmonary Artery
See Banding, Artery, Pulmonary

Banding
Artery
  Fistula 37607
  Pulmonary 33690

Bank, Blood
See Blood Banking

Bankart Procedure
See Capsulorrhaphy, Anterior

Barany Caloric Test
See Caloric Vestibular Test

Barbiturates
Blood or Urine 82205

Bardenheurer Operation
See Ligation, Artery, Chest

Bariatric Surgery 43644-43645,
                                43842-43848

Barium 83015

Barium Enema 74270-74280

Barker Operation
See Talus, Excision

Barr Bodies 88130

Barr Procedure
See Tendon, Transfer, Leg, Lower

Bartholin's Gland
Abscess
  Incision and Drainage 56420
Cyst
  Repair 56440
  Excision 56740
  Marsupialization 56440

Bartonella
Antibody 86611

Bartonella Detection 87470-87472

Basic Life Services 99450

Basic Proteins, Myelin
See Myelin Basic Protein

Basilar Arteries
See Artery, Basilar

Batch-Spittler-McFaddin Operation
See Disarticulation, Knee

BCG Vaccine
See Vaccines

Be Antigens, Hepatitis
See Hepatitis Antigen, Be

Bed Sores
See Debridement; Pressure Ulcer (Decubitus);
Skin Graft and Flap

Bekesy Audiometry
See Audiometry, Bekesy

Belsey IV Procedure
See Fundoplasty

Bender-Gestalt Test 96100

Benedict Test for Urea
See Urinalysis, Qualitative

Benign Cystic Mucinous Tumor
See Ganglion

Benign Neoplasm of Cranial Nerves
See Cranial Nerve

Bennett Fracture
See Phalanx; Thumb, Fracture

Bennett Procedure
See Repair, Leg, Upper, Muscle; Revision

Benzidine Test
See Blood, Feces

Benzodiazepine
Assay 80154

Benzoyl Cholinesterase
See Cholinesterase

Bernstein Test
See Acid Perfusion Test, Esophagus

Beryllium .83015

Beta 2 Glycoprotein I Antibody 86146

Beta Blocker Therapy
See Performance Measures

Beta Glucosidase 82963

Beta Hypophamine
See Antidiuretic Hormone

Beta Lipoproteins
See Lipoprotein, LDL

Beta Test .96100
See Psychiatric Diagnosis

Beta-2-Microglobulin
Blood 82232
Urine 82232

Beta-hydroxydehydrogenase . .80406

Bethesda System 88164-88167

Bicarbonate 82374

Biceps Tendon
Insertion 24342

Bichloride, Methylene
See Dichloromethane

Bicuspid Valve
See Mitral Valve

Bifrontal Craniotomy 61557

Bilaminate Skin Substitute/Neodermis
See Tissue
Repair
　See Tissue, Culture
　　Repair; Tissue, Culture, Skin Grafts

Bile Acids 82239
Blood 82240

Bile Duct
See Gallbladder
Anastomosis
　Cyst 47716
　with Intestines 47760, 47780-47785
Biopsy
　Endoscopy 47553
Catheterization 75982
Change Catheter Tube 75984
Cyst
　Excision 47715
　Repair 47716
Destruction
　Calculi (Stone) 43265
Dilation
　Endoscopy 43271, 47555-47556
Drainage
　Transhepatic 75980
Endoscopy
　Biopsy 47553
　Destruction
　　Calculi (Stone) 43265
　　Tumor 43272
　Dilation 43271, 47555-47556
　Exploration 47552
　Intraoperative 47550
　Removal
　　Calculi (Stone) 43264, 47554
　　Foreign Body 43269
　　Stent 43269
　Specimen Collection 43260
　Sphincter Pressure 43263
　Sphincterotomy 43262
　Tube Placement 43267-43268

Exploration
　Atresia 47700
　Endoscopy 47552
Incision
　Sphincter 43262, 47460
Incision and Drainage 47420-47425
Insertion
　Catheter 47510, 47525, 75982
　　Revision 47530
　Stent 47511, 47801
Nuclear Medicine
　Imaging 78223
Reconstruction
　Anastomosis 47800
Removal
　Calculi (Stone) 43264, 47420-47425
　　Percutaneous 47630
　Foreign Body 43269
　Stent 43269
Repair 47701
　Cyst 47716
　Gastrointestinal Tract 47785
　with Intestines 47760, 47780
Tube Placement
　Nasobiliary 43267
　Stent 43268
Tumor
　Destruction 43271
　Excision 47711-47712
Unlisted Services and Procedures 47999
X-Ray
　Guide Dilation 74360
　with Contrast 74300-74320
　　Calculus Removal 74327
　Guide Catheter 74328, 74330

Bile Duct, Common, Cystic Dilatation
See Cyst, Choledochal

Bilirubin
Blood 82247-82248
Feces 82252
Total
　Direct 82247-82248
　Transcutaneous 88400

Billroth I or II
See Gastrectomy, Partial

Bilobectomy 32482

Bimone
See Testosterone

Binding Globulin, Testosterone-Estradiol
See Globulin, Sex Hormone Binding

Binet Test 96100

Binet-Simon Test 96100

Binocular Microscopy 92504

Biofeedback
See Training, Biofeedback
Anorectal 90911
Psychiatric Treatment 90875-90876

Biofeedback Training
See Training, Biofeedback

Bioimpedance
Breast 0060T
Thorax 93701

Biological Skin Grafts
See Allograft, Skin

Biometry
Eye 76516-76519, 92136

Biopsies, Needle
See Needle Biopsy

Biopsy
See Brush Biopsy; Needle Biopsy
Abdomen 49000
Adrenal Gland 60540-60545
Anal
   Endoscopy 46606
Ankle 27613-27614, 27620
Arm, Lower 25065-25066
Arm, Upper 24065-24066
Artery
   Temporal 37609
Auditory Canal, External 69105
Back/Flank 21920-21925
Bile Duct
   Endoscopy 47553
Bladder 52354
   Cystourethroscope 52204
   Cystourethroscopy 52224, 52250
Blood Vessel
   Transcatheter 75970
Bone 20220-20245
Bone Marrow 38221
Brain 61140
   Stereotactic 61750-61751
Brainstem 61575-61576
Breast 19100-19103
   Stereotactic Localization 76095
Bronchi
   Catheterization 31717
   Endoscopic 31625-31629, 31632-31633
Brush
   Bronchi 31717
   Renal Pelvis 52007
   Ureter 52007
   with Cystourethroscopy 52204
Carpometacarpal Joint
   Synovium 26100
Cervix 57454-57455, 57460,
57500, 57520
Chorionic Villus 59015
Colon 44025, 44100
   Endoscopy 44389, 45380, 45391, 45392
   Multiple
     with Colostomy, Cecostomy 44322
Colon-Sigmoid
   Endoscopy 45305, 45331
Conjunctiva 68100
Cornea 65410
Duodenum 44010
Ear
   External 69100
Elbow 24065-24066, 24101
   Synovium 24100
Embryo Blastomere 89290-89291

Endometrium 58100, 58558
Epididymis 54800-54820
Esophagus
   Endoscopy 43202
Eye Muscle 67350
Eyelid 67810
Forearm
   Soft Tissue 25065-25066
Gallbladder
   Endoscopy 43261
Gastrointestinal, Upper
   Endoscopy 43239
Hand Joint
   Synovium 26100
Heart 93505
Hip 27040-27041
   Joint 27052
Hypopharynx 42802
Ileum
   Endoscopy 44382
Interphalangeal Joint
   Finger 26110
   Toe 28054
Intertarsal Joint
   Toe 28050
Intestines, Small 44020, 44100
   Endoscopy 44361, 44377
Kidney 50200-50205
   Endoscopic 50555-50557,
50574-50576, 52354
Knee 27323-27324
   Synovium 27330
Knee Joint
   Synovium 27330
Lacrimal Gland 68510
Lacrimal Sac 68525
Larynx
   Endoscopy 31510, 31576
Leg
   Lower 27613-27614
   Upper 27323-27324
Lip 40490
Liver 47000-47001, 47100
Lung
   Needle 32405
   Thoracotomy 32095-32100
Lymph Nodes 38500-38530
   Injection Procedure
     for Identification of Sentinel Node ..38792
   Laparoscopic 38570-38572
   Needle 38505
   Open 38500, 38510-38530
     Superficial 38500
Mediastinum 39400
   Needle 32405
Metacarpophalangeal Joint 26105
Metatarsophalangeal Joint 28052
Mouth 40808, 41108
Muscle 20200-20206
Nail 11755
Nasopharynx 42804-42806
Neck 21550
Nerve 64795
Nose
   Endoscopic 31237
   Intranasal 30100
Oocyte Polar Body 89290-89291

Orbit 61332
   Exploration 67400, 67450
   Fine Needle Aspiration 67415
Oropharynx 42800
Ovary 58900
Palate 42100
Pancreas 48100
Pelvis 27040-27041
Penis 54100
   Deep Structures 54105
Percutaneous Needle
   Spinal Cord 62269
Perineum 56605-56606
Peritoneum
   Endoscopic 47561
Pharynx 42800-42806
Pleura
   Needle 32400-32402
   Thoracotomy 32095-32100
Pleural
   Open 32402
Prostate 55700-55705
Rectum 45100
Retroperitoneal Area 49010
Sacroiliac Joint 27050
Salivary Gland 42405
Shoulder
   Deep 23066
   Soft Tissue 23065
Shoulder Joint 23100-23101
Sinus
   Sphenoid 31050-31051
Skin Lesion 11100-11101
Spinal Cord 63275-63290
   Percutaneous 62269
   Stereotaxis 63615
Stomach 43600-43605
Tarsometatarsal Joint
   Synovial 28050
Testis 54500-54505
Thorax 21550
Throat 42800-42806
Tongue 41100-41105
Transcatheter 37200
Ureter 52354
   Endoscopic 50955-50957, 50974-50976
Urethra 52204, 52354, 53200
Uterus
   Endometrial 58100
   Endoscopic 58558
Uvula 42100
Vagina 57100-57105, 57421
Vertebral Body 20250-20251
Vulva 56605-56606, 56821
with Arthrotomy
   Acromioclavicular Joint 23101
   Glenohumeral Joint 23100
   Sternoclavicular Joint 23101
with Cystourethroscopy 52354
Wrist 25065-25066, 25100-25101

Biopsy, Skin
See Skin, Biopsy

Biopsy, Vein
See Vein, Biopsy

Biostatistics
See Biometry

Biosterol
See Vitamin, A

Biotinidase 82261

Birthing Room
Newborn Care 99431

Bischof Procedure
See Laminectomy, Surgical

Bismuth 83015

Bizzozero's Corpuscle/Cell
See Blood, Platelet

Bladder
Abscess
   Incision and Drainage 51080
Anastomosis 51960
Aspiration 51000-51010
Biopsy 52204
Catheterization 51045, 51701-51703
Change Tube 51705-51710
Creation
   Stoma 51980
Cyst
   Urachal
      Excision 51500
Destruction
   Endoscopic 52214-52224, 52354
Dilation
   Ureter 52260-52265, 52341-52342,
                    52344-52345
Diverticulum
   Excision 51525
   Incision 52305
   Resection 52305
Endoscopy 52000
   Biopsy 52204, 52354
   Catheterization 52005, 52010
   Destruction 52214-52224, 52400
   Dilation 52260-52265
   Diverticulum 52305
   Evacuation
      Clot 52001
   Excision
      Tumor 52234-52240, 52355
   Exploration 52351
   Injection 52283
   Lithotripsy 52353
   Radiotracer 52250
   Removal
      Calculus 52310-52315, 52352
      Foreign Body 52310-52315
   Sphincter Surgery 52277
   Tumor
      Excision 52355
   Ureter Surgery 52290-52300
   Urethral Syndrome 52285
   with Urethrotomy 52270-52276
Excision
   Partial 51550-51565
   Total 51570, 51580, 51590-51597
      with Nodes 51575, 51585, 51595
   Transurethral 52640
   Tumor 52234-52240
Incision
   Catheter 51045
   with Destruction 51020-51030
   with Radiotracer 51020

Incision and Drainage 51040
Injection
   Radiologic 51600-51610
Insertion
   Stent 51045, 52334
Instillation
   Drugs 51720
Irrigation 51700
Lesion
   Destruction 51030
Neck
   Endoscopy
      Injection of Implant Material 51715
   Excision 51520
Nuclear Medicine
   Residual Study 78730
Radiotracer 52250
Reconstruction
   and Urethra 51800-51820
   with Intestines 51960
Removal
   Calculus 51050, 52310-52315
   Foreign Body 52310-52315
   Urethral Stent 52310-52315
Repair
   Diverticulum 52305
   Exstrophy 51940
   Fistula 44660-44661,
        45800-45805, 51880-51925
   Neck 51845
   Wound 51860-51865
Resection 52500
Sphincter Surgery 52277
Suspension 51990
Suture
   Fistula 44660-44661,
        45800-45805, 51880-51925
   Wound 51860-51865
Tumor
   Excision 51530
Unlisted Services and Procedures 53899
Urethrocystography 74450-74455
Urethrotomy 52270-52276
Urinary Incontinence Procedures
   Laparoscopy 51990-51992
   Pulsed Magnetic Neuromodulation ...0029T
X-Ray 74430
   with Contrast 74450-74455

Bladder Voiding Pressure Studies 51795

Blalock-Hanlon Procedure 33735-33737
See Septostomy, Atrial

Blalock-Taussig Procedure
See Shunt, Great Vessel

Blast Cells
See Stem Cell

Blast Transformation
See Blastogenesis

Blastocyst Implantation
See Implantation

Blastocyst Transfer
See Embryo Transfer

Blastogenesis 86353

Blastomyces
Antibody 86612

Blastomycosis, European
See Cryptococcus

Bleeding
See Hemorrhage

Bleeding Disorder
See Coagulopathy

Bleeding Time 85002

Bleeding Tube
Passage and Placement 91100

Bleeding, Anal
See Anus, Hemorrhage

Bleeding, Uterine
See Hemorrhage, Uterus

Bleeding, Vaginal
See Hemorrhage, Vagina

Blepharoplasty 15820-15823
See Canthoplasty
Anesthesia 00103

Blepharoptosis
Repair 67901-67909
   Frontalis Muscle Technique 67901
      with Fascial Sling 67902
   Superior Rectus Technique with
      Fascial Sling 67906
   Tarso Levator Resection/Advancement
      External Approach 67904
      Internal Approach 67903

Blepharorrhaphy
See Tarsorrhaphy

Blepharospasm
Chemodenervation 64612

Blepharotomy 67700

Blister
See Bulla

Blom-Singer Prosthesis 31611

Blood
See Blood Cell Count, Complete Blood Count
Bleeding Time 85002
Collection, for Autotransfusion
   Intraoperative 86891
   Preoperative 86890
Feces 82270
   by Hemoglobin Immunoassay 82274
Gastric Contents 82273
Hemoglobin Concentration 85046
Nuclear Medicine
   Flow Imaging 78445
   Plasma Iron 78160
   Red Cell 78140
   Red Cell Survival 78130-78135
Osmolality 83930
Other Source 82273

Plasma
  Exchange 36514-36516
Platelet
  Aggregation 85576
  Automated Count 85049
  Count 85008
  Manual Count 85032
Stem Cell
  Count 86587
  Donor Search 38204
  Harvesting 38205-38206
  Transplantation 38240-38242
    Cell Concentration 38215
    Cryopreservation 38207, 88240
    Plasma Depletion 38214
    Platelet Depletion 38213
    Red Blood Cell Depletion 38212
    T-cell Depletion 38210
    Thawing 38208-38209, 88241
    Tumor Cell Depletion 38211
    Washing 38209
Transfusion 36430
  Exchange 36455
    Newborn 36450
  Fetal 36460
  Push
    Infant 36440
Unlisted Services and Procedures 85999
Urine 83491
Viscosity 85810

Blood Banking
Frozen Blood Preparation 86930-86932
Frozen Plasma Preparation 86927
Physician Services 86077-86079

Blood Cell
CD4 and CD8
  Including Ratio 86360
Enzyme Activity 82657
Exchange 36511-36513
Sedimentation Rate
  Automated 85652
  Manual 85651

Blood Cell Count
Automated 85049
B-Cells 86064
Blood Smear 85007-85008
Differential WBC Count ...85004-85007, 85009
Hematocrit 85014
Hemoglobin 85018
Hemogram
  Added Indices 85025-85027
  Automated 85025-85027
  Manual 85032
Microhematocrit.....................85013
Natural Killer (NK) Cells 86379
Red Blood Cells 85032-85041
Reticulocyte 85044-85046
Stem Cells 86587
T-Cells 86359-86361
White Blood Cells 85032, 85048, 89055

Blood Cell Count, Red
See Red Blood Cell (RBC), Count

Blood Cell Count, White
See White Blood Cell, Count

Blood Cell, Red
See Red Blood Cell (RBC)

Blood Cell, White
See Leukocyte

Blood Clot
Assay 85396
Clot Lysis Time 85175
Clot Retraction 85170
Clotting Factor 85250-85293
Clotting Factor Test 85210-85244
Clotting Inhibitors ...85300-85302, 85305, 85307
Coagulation Time 85345-85348

Blood Coagulation Defect
See Coagulopathy

Blood Coagulation Disorders
See Clot

Blood Coagulation Factor
See Clotting Factor

Blood Coagulation Factor I
See Fibrinogen

Blood Coagulation Factor II
See Prothrombin

Blood Coagulation Factor III
See Thromboplastin

Blood Coagulation Factor IV
See Calcium

Blood Coagulation Factor VII
See Proconvertin

Blood Coagulation Factor VIII
See Clotting Factor

Blood Coagulation Factor IX
See Christmas Factor

Blood Coagulation Factor X
See Stuart-Prower Factor

Blood Coagulation Factor X, Activated
See Thrombokinase

Blood Coagulation Factor XI
See Plasma Thromboplastin, Antecedent

Blood Coagulation Factor XIII
See Fibrin Stabilizing Factor

Blood Coagulation Test
See Coagulation

Blood Component Removal
See Apheresis

Blood Count, Complete
See Complete Blood Count (CBC)

Blood Flow Check, Graft 15860, 90939-90940

Blood Gases
CO2 82803
HCO3 82803
O2 Saturation 82805-82810
pCO2 82803
pH 82800-82803
pO2 82803

Blood Letting
See Phlebotomy

Blood Lipoprotein
See Lipoprotein

Blood Occult
See Occult, Blood

Blood Pool Imaging 78472-78473, 78481-78483, 78494-78496

Blood Pressure
See Performance Measures
Left Ventricular Filling 0086T
Monitoring, 24 Hour 93784-93790
Venous 93770

Blood Products
Irradiation 86945
Pooling 86965
Splitting 86985

Blood Sample
Fetal 59030

Blood Serum
See Serum

Blood Smear 85060

Blood Syndrome
Chromosome Analysis 88245-88248

Blood Tests
Nuclear Medicine
  Iron Absorption 78162
  Iron Utilization 78170
  Iron, Chelatable 78172
  Plasma Volume 78110-78111
  Platelet Survival 78190-78191
  Red Cell Volume 78120-78121
  Whole Blood Volume 78122
Panels
  Electrolyte 80051
  General Health Panel 80050
  Hepatic Function 80076
  Hepatitis, Acute.................80074
  Lipid Panel 80061
  Metabolic
    Basic 80048
    Comprehensive 80053
  Obstetric Panel 80055
  Renal Function 80069
Volume Determination 78122

Blood Transfusion, Autologous
See Autotransfusion

Blood Typing
ABO Only 86900
Antigen Screen 86903-86904
Crossmatch 86920-86922
Other RBC Antigens 86905
Paternity Testing 86910-86911
Rh (D) 86901
Rh Phenotype 86906

Blood Urea Nitrogen 84520-84525

Blood Vessels
See Artery; Vein
Angioscopy
　　Non-Coronary 35400
Endoscopy
　　Surgical 37500
Excision
　　Arteriovenous Malformation . . .63250-63252
Exploration
　　Abdomen .35840
　　Chest 35820
　　Extremity .35860
　　Neck 35800
Great
　　Suture 33320-33322
Harvest
　　Endoscopic 33508
　　Lower Extremity Vein 35572
　　Upper Extremity Artery 35600
　　Upper Extremity Vein 35500
Kidney
　　Repair 50100
Repair
　　Abdomen
　　　　See Aneurysm Repair; Fistula, Repair
　　　　with Composite Graft 35681-35683
　　　　with Other Graft 35281
　　　　with Vein Graft 35251
　　Aneurysm 61705-61708
　　Arteriovenous Malformation . . .61680-61692,
　　　　　　　　　　　　61705-61710, 63250-63252
　　Chest
　　　　with Composite Graft 35681-35683
　　　　with Other Graft 35271-35276
　　　　with Vein Graft 35241-35246
　　Direct 35201-35226
　　Finger 35207
　　Graft Defect 35870
　　Hand 35207
　　Lower Extremity 35226
　　　　with Composite Graft 35681-35683
　　　　with Other Graft 35281
　　　　with Vein Graft 35251
　　Neck
　　　　with Composite Graft 35681-35683
　　　　with Other Graft 35261
　　　　with Vein Graft 35231
　　Upper Extremity 35206
　　　　with Composite Graft 35681-35683
　　　　with Other Graft 35266
　　　　with Vein Graft 35236
Shunt Creation
　　Direct 36818, 36821
　　Thomas Shunt 36835
　　with Bypass Graft 35686
　　with Graft 36825-36830
Shunt Revision
　　with Graft 36832

Blood, Occult
See Occult Blood

Bloom Syndrome
Chromosome Analysis 88245

Blot Test, Ink
See Inkblot Test

Blotting, Western
See Western Blot

Blow-Out Fracture
Orbital Floor 21385-21395

Blue, Dome Cyst
See Breast, Cyst

BMT
See Bone Marrow, Transplantation

Boarding Home Care 99321-99333

Bodies, Acetone
See Acetone Body

Bodies, Barr
See Barr Bodies

Bodies, Carotid
See Carotid Body

Bodies, Ciliary
See Ciliary Body

Bodies, Heinz
See Heinz Bodies

Bodies, Inclusion
See Inclusion Bodies

Bodies, Ketone
See Ketone Body

Body Cast
Halo 29000
Removal 29700, 29710-29715
Repair 29720
Risser Jacket 29010-29015
Turnbuckle Jacket 29020-29025
Upper Body and Head 29040
Upper Body and Legs 29046
Upper Body and One Leg 29044
Upper Body Only 29035

Body Composition
Dual Energy X-Ray Absorptiometry 0028T

Body Fluid
Crystal Identification 89060

Body of Vertebra
See Vertebral Body

Body Section
X-Ray 76100
　　Motion 76101-76102

Body System, Neurologic
See Nervous System

Boil
See Furuncle

Boil, Vulva
See Abscess, Vulva

Bone
See Specific Bone
Ablation
　　Tumor 20982
Biopsy 20220-20245

CT Scan
　　Density Study 76070-76071
Cyst
　　Drainage .20615
　　Injection .20615
Dual Energy X-Ray
Absorptiometry 76075-76077
Excision
　　Epyphyseal Bar 20150
　　Facial Bones 21026
　　Mandible .21025
Fixation
　　Caliper 20660
　　Cranial Tong 20660
　　Halo 20661-20663, 21100
　　Interdental 21110
　　Multiplane 20692
　　Pin/Wire .20650
　　Skeletal
　　　　Humeral Epicondyle
　　　　　　Percutaneous 24566
　　Stereotactic Frame 20660
　　Uniplane .20690
Insertion
　　Needle 36680
　　Osseointegrated Implant
　　　　for External Speech Processor/Cochlear
　　　　　　Stimulator 69714-69718
Nuclear Medicine
　　Density Study 78350-78351
　　Imaging 78300-78320
　　SPECT 78320
　　Unlisted Services and Procedures 78399
Protein 83937
Removal
　　Fixation Device 20670-20680
Replacement
　　Osseointegrated Implant
　　　　for External Speech Processor/Cochlear
　　　　　　Stimulator 69717-69718
X-Ray
　　Age Study 76020
　　Dual Energy Absorptiometry . . .76075-76077
　　Length Study 76040
　　Osseous Survey 76061-76065

Bone 4-Carboxyglutamic Protein
See Osteocalcin

**Bone Conduction Hearing Device,
Electromagnetic**
Implantation/Replacement 69710
Removal/Repair 69711

Bone Density Study
Appendicular Skeleton 76071, 76076
Axial Skeleton 76070, 76075
Ultrasound .76977
Vertebral Fracture Assessment 76077

Bone Graft
Augmentation
　　Mandibular Body 21127
Femur 27170
Fracture
　　Orbit 21408
Harvesting 20900-20902
Malar Area .21210
Mandible 21215

Mandibular Ramus 21194
Maxilla 21210
Microvascular Anastomosis
    Fibula 20955
    Other 20962
Nasal Area 21210
Nasomaxillary Complex Fracture 21348
Open Treatment
    Craniofacial Separation 21436
Osteocutaneous Flap 20969-20973
Reconstruction
    Mandibular Rami 21194
    Midface 21145-21160
Skull 61316
    Excision 62148
Spine Surgery
    Allograft
        Morselized 20930
        Structural 20931
    Autograft
        Local 20936
        Morselized 20937
        Structural 20938
Vascular Pedicle 25430

Bone Healing
Electrical Stimulation
    Invasive 20975
    Noninvasive .20974
Ultrasound Stimulation 20979

Bone Infection
See Osteomyelitis

Bone Marrow
Aspiration 38220
Harvesting 38230
Magnetic Resonance Imaging (MRI) 76400
Needle Biopsy 38221
Nuclear Medicine
    Imaging 78102-78104
Smear 85097
T-Cell Transplantation 38240-38242
Trocar Biopsy 38221

Bone Plate
Mandible 21244

Bone Scan
See Bone, Nuclear Medicine; Nuclear Medicine

Bone Spur
See Exostosis

Bone Wedge Reversal
Osteotomy 21122

Bone, Carpal
See Carpal Bone

Bone, Cheek
See Cheekbone

Bone, Facial
See Facial Bone

Bone, Hyoid
See Hyoid Bone

Bone, Metatarsal
See Metatarsal

Bone, Nasal
See Nasal Bone

Bone, Navicular
See Navicular

Bone, Scan
See Bone, Nuclear Medicine; Nuclear Medicine Imaging

Bone, Semilunar
See Lunate

Bone, Sesamoid
See Sesamoid Bone

Bone, Tarsal
See Ankle Bone

Bone, Temporal
See Temporal Bone

Bordetella
Antibody 86615
Antigen Detection
    Direct Fluorescence 87265

Borrelia
Antibody 86618-86619

Borrelia burgdorferi ab
See Antibody, Lyme Disease

Borreliosis, Lyme
See Lyme Disease

Borthen Operation
See Iridotasis

Bost Fusion
See Arthrodesis, Wrist

Bosworth Operation
See Acromioclavicular Joint, Dislocation; Arthrodesis, Vertebrae; Fasciotomy,

Bottle Type Procedure 55060

Botulinum Toxin
See Chemodenervation

Boutonniere Deformity 26426-26428

Bowel
See Intestine

Bowleg Repair 27455-27457

Boyce Operation
See Nephrotomy

Boyd Hip Disarticulation
See Amputation, Leg, Upper; Radical Resection; Replantation

Brace
See Cast
for Leg Cast 29358

Brachial Arteries
See Artery, Brachial

Brachial Plexus
Decompression .64713
Injection
    Anesthetic 64415-64416
Neuroplasty 64713
Release 64713
Repair/Suture 64861

Brachiocephalic Artery
See Artery, Brachiocephalic

Brachycephaly 21175

Brachytherapy 77761-77778, 77789
Dose Plan 77326-77328
Remote Afterloading
    1-4 Positions 77781
    5-8 Positions 77782
    9-12 Positions 77783
    Over 12 Positions 77784
    Over 4 Positions 77781-77784
Unlisted Services and Procedures 77799

Bradykinin
Blood or Urine .82286

Brain
See Brainstem; Mesencephalon; Skull Base Surgery
Abscess
    Drainage 61150-61151
    Excision 61514, 61522
    Incision and Drainage 61320-61321
Adhesions
    Lysis 62161
Anesthesia 00210-00218, 00220-00222
Angiography 70496
Biopsy 61140
    Stereotactic 61750-61751
Catheter
    Irrigation 62194, 62225
    Replacement 62160, 62194, 62225
Cisternography .70015
Computer Assisted
    Surgery 61795
Cortex
    Magnetic Stimulation 0018T
Craniopharyngioma
    Excision 61545
CT Scan 0042T, 70450-70470, 70496
Cyst
    Drainage 61150-61151, 62161-62162
    Excision 61516, 61524, 62162
Doppler, Transcranial 93886-93893
Epileptogenic Focus
    Excision 61534, 61536
Excision
    Amygdala 61566
    Choroid Plexus 61544
    Hemisphere 61542-61543
    Hippocampus 61566
    Other Lobe 61323, 61539-61540
    Temporal Lobe 61537-61538
Exploration
    Infratentorial 61305
    Supratentorial 61304
Hematoma
    Drainage 61154
    Incision and Drainage 61312-61315

Broken, Nose
See Fracture, Nasal Bone

Bronchi
Aspiration
    Endoscopic 31645-31646
Biopsy
    Endoscopic 31625-31629, 31632-31633
Catheterization
    Insertion 31710
    with Bronchial Brush Biopsy 31717
Endoscopy
    Aspiration 31645-31646
    Biopsy 31625-31629, 31632-31633
    Destruction
      Tumor 31641
    Dilation 31630-31631, 31636-31638
    Excision
      Lesion 31640
    Exploration 31622
    Foreign Body Removal 31635
    Fracture 31630
    Injection 31656
    Lesion 31640-31641
    Stenosis 31641
    Tumor 31640-31641
    Ultrasound 31620
Exploration
    Endoscopic 31622
Fracture
    Endoscopy 31630
Injection
    X-Ray 31656, 31715
Instillation
    Contrast Material 31708
Needle Biopsy 31629, 31633
Reconstruction 31770
    Graft Repair 31770
    Stenosis 31775
Removal
    Foreign Body 31635
Repair
    Fistula 32815
Stenosis
    Endoscopic Treatment 31641
Stent
    Placement 31636-31637
    Revision 31638
Tumor
    Excision 31640
Ultrasound 31620
Unlisted Services and Procedures 31899
X-Ray
    with Contrast 71040-71060

Bronchial Allergen Challenge
See Bronchial Challenge Test

Bronchial Alveolar Lavage 31624

Bronchial Brush Biopsy
with Catheterization 31717

Bronchial Brushings/Protected Brushing 31623

Bronchial Challenge Test
See Allergy Tests
with Antigens, Gases 95070
with Chemicals 95071

Bronchial Provocation Tests
See Bronchial Challenge Test

Bronchioalveolar Lavage
See Lung, Lavage

Broncho-Bronchial Anastomosis 32486

Bronchoalveolar Lavage
See Lung, Lavage

Bronchography 71040-71060
Catheterization 31710
Injection
    Transtracheal 31715
Instillation
    Contrast Material 31708
Segmental
    Injection 31656

Bronchoplasty 32501
See Reconstruction, Bronchi
Excision Stenosis and Anastomosis 31775
Graft Repair 31770

Bronchopneumonia, Hiberno-Vernal
See Q Fever

Bronchopulmonary Lavage
See Lung, Lavage

Bronchoscopy
Alveolar Lavage 31624
Aspiration 31645-31646
Biopsy 31625-31629, 31632-31633
Brushing/Protected Brushing 31623
Catheter Placement
    Intracavitary Radioelement 31643
Dilation 31630-31631, 31636-31638
Exploration 31622
Fracture 31630
Injection 31656
Needle Biopsy 31629, 31633
Removal
    Foreign Body 31635
    Tumor 31640-31641
Stenosis 31641
Stent Placement 31631, 31636-31637
Stent Revision 31638
Ultrasound 31620
X-Ray Contrast 31656

Bronchospasm Evaluation
See Pulmonology, Diagnostic, Spirometry

Bronkodyl
See Theophylline

Brow Ptosis
Repair 67900

Brucella 86000
Antibody 86622

Bruise
See Hematoma

Brunschwig Operation 58240
See Hip; Pelvis, Exenteration

Brush Biopsy
See Biopsy; Needle Biopsy
Bronchi 31717

Brush Border ab
See Antibody, Heterophile

Bucca
See Cheek

Buccal Mucosa
See Mouth, Mucosa

Bulbourethral Gland
Excision 53250

Bulla
Incision and Drainage
    Puncture Aspiration 10160
Lung
    Excision-Plication 32141
      Endoscopic 32655

BUN
See Blood Urea Nitrogen; Urea Nitrogen

Bunion Repair 28296-28299
Chevron Procedure 28296
Concentric Procedure 28296
Joplin Procedure 28294
Keller Procedure 28292
Lapidus Procedure 28297
Mayo Procedure 28292
McBride Procedure 28292
Mitchell Procedure 28296
Silver Procedure 28290
with Implant 28293

Burgess Amputation
See Disarticulation, Ankle

Burhenne Procedure
See Bile Duct, Removal, Calculi (Stone); Gallbladder

Burkitt Herpesvirus
See Epstein-Barr Virus

Burns
Allograft 15350-15351
Debridement 01951-01953,
             15000-15001, 16010-16030
Dressings 16010-16030
Escharotomy 16035-16036
Excision 01951-01953, 15000-15001
Initial Treatment 16000
Tissue Culture Skin Grafts 15100-15121,
                 15342-15343
Xenograft 15400-15401

Burr Hole
Anesthesia 00214
Skull
    Biopsy Brain 61140
    Catheterization 61210
    Drainage
      Abscess 61150-61151
      Cyst 61150-61151
      Hematoma 61154-61156

C

Calcitonin
Blood or Urine 82308
Stimulation Panel 80410

Calcium
Blood
  Infusion Test 82331
Deposits
  See Removal, Calculi (Stone); Removal,
  Foreign Bodies
Ionized 82330
Total 82310
Urine 82340

Calcium-Binding Protein, Vitamin K-Dependent
See Osteocalcin

Calcium-Pentagastrin Stimulation 80410

Calculus
Analysis 82355-82370
Destruction
  Bile Duct 43265
  Pancreatic Duct 43265
Removal
  Bile Duct 43264, 47554, 74327
  Bladder .... .51050, 52310-52318, 52352
  Kidney 50060-50081, 50130, 50561,
                          50580, 52352
  Pancreatic Duct 43264
  Ureter 50610-50630, 50961, 50980,
         51060-51065, 52320-52325, 52352
  Urethra 52310-52315, 52352

Calculus of Kidney
See Calculus, Removal, Kidney

Caldwell-Luc Procedure
See Sinus, Maxillary; Sinusotomy; Sternum, Fracture
Orbital Floor Blowout Fracture 21385
Sinusotomy 31030-31032

Caliper
Application/Removal 20660

Callander Knee Disarticulation
See Disarticulation, Knee

Callosum, Corpus
See Corpus Callosum

Calmette Guerin Bacillus Vaccine
See BCG Vaccine

Caloric Vestibular Test 92533

Calycoplasty 50405

Camey Enterocystoplasty 50825

CAMP
See Cyclic AMP

Campbell Procedure 27422

Campylobacter
Antibody 86625

Campylobacter Pylori
See Helicobacter Pylori

Canal, Ear
See Auditory Canal

Canal, Semicircular
See Semicircular Canal

Canaloplasty 69631, 69635

Candida
Antibody 86628
Skin Test 86485

Cannulation 36821
Arterial 36620-36625
Sinus
  Maxillary 31000
  Sphenoid 31002
Thoracic Duct 38794

Cannulation, Renoportal
See Anastomosis, Renoportal

Cannulization
See Catheterization
Arteriovenous 36145, 36810-36815
Declotting 36550, 36860-36861
ECMO 36822
External
  Declotting 36860-36861
Vas Deferens 55200
Vein to Vein 36800

Canthocystostomy
See Conjunctivorhinostomy

Canthopexy
Lateral 21282
Medial 21280

Canthoplasty 67950

Canthorrhaphy 67880-67882

Canthotomy 67715

Canthus
Reconstruction 67950

Cap, Cervical
See Cervical Cap

Capsule
See Capsulodesis
Elbow
  Arthrotomy 24006
  Excision 24006
Foot 28264
Interphalangeal Joint
  Excision 26525
  Incision 26525
Knee 27435
Metacarpophalangeal Joint
  Excision 26520
  Incision 26520
Metatarsophalangeal Joint
  Release 28289
Shoulder
  Incision 23020
Wrist
  Excision 25320

Capsulectomy
Breast
  Periprosthetic 19371

Capsulodesis
Metacarpophalangeal Joint 26516-26518

Capsulorrhaphy
Anterior 23450-23462
Multi-Directional Instability 23466
Posterior 23465
Wrist 25320

Capsulotomy
Breast
  Periprosthetic 19370
Foot 28260-28262
Hip
  with Release, Flexor Muscles 27036
Interphalangeal Joint 28272
Knee 27435
Metacarpophalangeal Joint 26520
Metatarsophalangeal Joint 28270
Toe 28270-28272
Wrist 25085

Captopril 80416-80417

Carbamazepine
Assay 80156-80157

Carbazepin
See Carbamazepine

Carbinol
See Methanol

Carbohydrate Deficient Transferrin 82373

Carbon Dioxide
Blood or Urine 82374

Carbon Monoxide
Blood 82375-82376

Carbon Tetrachloride 84600

Carboxycathepsin
See Angiotensin Converting Enzyme (ACE)

Carboxyhemoglobin 82375-82376

Carbuncle
Incision and Drainage 10060-10061

Carcinoembryonal Antigen
See Antigen, Carcinoembryonic

Carcinoembryonic Antigen 82378

Cardiac
See Coronary

Cardiac Arrhythmia, Tachycardia
See Tachycardia

Cardiac Atria
See Atria

Cervical Cap 57170

Cervical Lymphadenectomy 38720-38724

Cervical Mucus Penetration Test 89330

Cervical Plexus
Injection
    Anesthetic 64413

Cervical Pregnancy 59140

Cervical Puncture 61050-61055

Cervical Smears 88141, 88155,
88164-88167, 88174-88175
See Cytopathology

Cervical Spine
See Vertebra, Cervical

Cervical Sympathectomy
See Sympathectomy, Cervical

Cervicectomy 57530

Cervicography 0003T

Cervicoplasty 15819

Cervicothoracic Ganglia
See Stellate Ganglion

Cervix
See Cytopathology
Amputation
    Total 57530
Biopsy 57500, 57520
    Colposcopy 57454-57455, 57460
Cauterization 57522
    Cryocautery 57511
    Electro or Thermal 57510
    Laser Ablation 57513
Cerclage 57700
    Abdominal 59325
    Removal Under Anesthesia 59871
    Vaginal 59320
Cervicography 0003T
Colposcopy 57452-57461
Conization 57461, 57520-57522
Curettage
    Endocervical 57454, 57456, 57505
Dilation
    Canal 57800
    Stump 57820
Dilation and Curettage 57820
Ectopic Pregnancy 59140
Excision
    Radical 57531
    Stump
        Abdominal Approach 57540-57545
        Vaginal Approach 57550-57556
    Total 57530
Exploration
    Endoscopy 57452
Insertion
    Dilation 59200
    Laminaria 59200
    Prostaglandin 59200
    Sensor, Fetal Oximetry 0021T

Repair
    Cerclage 57700
        Abdominal 59325
        Suture 57720
        Vaginal 59320
Unlisted Services and Procedures 58999

Cesarean Delivery
Antepartum Care 59610, 59618
Delivery
    after Attempted Vaginal Delivery 59618
        Delivery Only 59620
        Postpartum Care 59622
        Routine Care 59610, 59618
Delivery Only 59514
Postpartum Care 59515
Routine Care 59510
Tubal Ligation at Time of 58611
with Hysterectomy 59525

CGMP
See Cyclic GMP

Chalazion
Excision 67805
    Multiple
        Different Lids 67805
        Same Lid 67801
    Single 67800
    Under Anesthesia 67808

Challenge Tests
Bronchial Ingestion 95070-95075

Chambers Procedure 28300

Change
Catheter
    Bile Duct 75984
Fetal Position
    by Manipulation 59412
Tube or Stent
    Endoscopic
        Bile or Pancreatic Duct 43269

Change of, Dressing
See Dressings, Change

Change, Gastrostomy Tube
See Gastrostomy Tube, Change of

Cheek
Bone
    Excision 21030, 21034
    Fracture
        Closed Treatment with
        Manipulation 21355
        Open Treatment 21360-21366
        Reconstruction 21270
Fascia Graft 15840
Muscle Graft 15841-15845
Muscle Transfer 15845

Cheilectomy
Metatarsophalangeal Joint Release 28289

Cheiloplasty
See Lip, Repair

Cheiloschisis
See Cleft Lip

Cheilotomy
See Incision, Lip

Chemical Cauterization
Granulation Tissue 17250

Chemical Exfoliation 17360

Chemical Peel 15788-15793

Chemiluminescent Assay 82397

Chemistry Tests
Clinical
    Unlisted Services and Procedures 84999

Chemocauterization
Corneal Epithelium 65435
    with Chelating Agent 65436

Chemodenervation
Cervical Spinal Muscle 64613
Extraocular Muscle 67345
Extremity Muscle 64614
Facial Muscle 64612
Trunk Muscle 64614

Chemonucleolysis 62292

Chemosurgery
Mohs Technique 17304-17310
Skin Lesion 17004, 17110, 17270, 17280

Chemotaxis Assay 86155

Chemotherapy
Arterial Catheterization 36640
Bladder Instillation 51720
CNS 61517, 96450
Extracorporeal Circulation
    Extremity 36823
Home Infusion Procedures 99601-99602
Intra-Arterial 96420-96425
Intralesional 96405-96406
Intramuscular 96400
Intravenous 96408-96414
Kidney Instillation 50391
Peritoneal Cavity 96445
Pleural Cavity 96440
Pump Services
    Implantable 96530
    Maintenance 95990-95991
    Portable 96520
Reservoir Filling 96542
Subcutaneous 96400
Supply of Agent 96545
Unlisted Services and Procedures 96549
Ureteral Instillation 50391

Chest
See Mediastinum; Thorax
Angiography 71275
Artery
    Ligation 37616
CT Scan 71250-71275
Exploration
    Blood Vessel 35820
Magnetic Resonance Imaging
(MRI) 71550-71552

Repair
　Blood Vessel 35211-35216
　　with Other Graft 35271-35276
　　with Vein Graft 35241-35246
Ultrasound 76604
Wound Exploration
　Penetrating 20101
X-Ray 71010-71035
　Complete (four Views)
　　with Fluoroscopy 71034
　Insertion Pacemaker 71090
　Partial (Two Views)
　　with Fluoroscopy 71023
　Stereo 71015
　with Fluoroscopy 71090

Chest Cavity
Bypass Graft .35905
Endoscopy
　Exploration 32601-32606
　Surgical 32650-32665

Chest Wall
See Pulmonology, Therapeutic
Manipulation 94667-94668
Reconstruction 49904
　Trauma 32820
Repair 32905
　Closure 32810
　Fistula 32906
Tumor
　Excision 19260-19272
Unlisted Services and Procedures 32999

Chest Wall Fistula
See Fistula, Chest Wall

Chest, Funnel
See Pectus Excavatum

Chevron Procedure 28296

Chiari Osteotomy of the Pelvis
See Osteotomy, Pelvis

Chicken Pox Vaccine 90716

Child Procedure
See Excision, Pancreas, Partial

Chin
Repair
　Augmentation 21120
　Osteotomy 21121-21123

Chinidin
See Quinidine

Chiropractic Manipulation
See Manipulation, Chiropractic

Chiropractic Treatment
Spinal
　Extraspinal 98940-98943

Chlamydia
Antibody 86631-86632
Antigen Detection
　Direct Fluorescence 87270
　Enzyme Immunoassay 87320
Culture 87110

Chloramphenicol 82415

Chloride
Blood 82435
Other Source 82438
Spinal Fluid 82438
Urine 82436

Chloride, Methylene
See Dichloromethane

Chlorinated Hydrocarbons 82441

Chlorohydrocarbon
See Chlorinated Hydrocarbons

Chlorpromazine 84022

Choanal Atresia
Repair 30540-30545

Cholangiography
Injection 47500-47505
Intraoperative 74300-74301
Percutaneous 74320
　with Laparoscopy 47560-47561
Postoperative 74305
Repair
　with Bile Duct Exploration 47700
　with Cholecystectomy . .47563, 47605, 47620

Cholangiopancreatography 43260
See Bile Duct; Pancreatic Duct
Repair
　See Bile Duct; Pancreatic Duct
　with Biopsy 43261
　with Surgery 43262-43267, 43269

Cholangiostomy
See Hepaticostomy

Cholangiotomy
See Hepaticostomy

Cholecalciferol
See Vitamin, D-3

Cholecystectomy 47562-47564,
　　　　　　　　　　　　　　　　47600-47620
Any Method 47562-47564
　with Cholangiography . .47563, 47605, 47620
　with Exploration Common
　Duct 47564, 47610

Cholecystenterostomy 47570,
　　　　　　　　　　　　　　　　47720-47741

Cholecystography 74290-74291

Cholecystotomy 47480, 48001
Percutaneous 47490

Choledochoplasty
See Bile Duct, Repair

Choledochoscopy 47550

Choledochostomy 47420-47425

Choledochotomy 47420-47425

Choledochus, Cyst
See Cyst, Choledochal

Cholera Vaccine
Injectable .90725

Cholesterol
Measurement 83721
Serum 82465
Testing 83718-83719

Choline Esterase I
See Acetylcholinesterase

Choline Esterase II
See Cholinesterase

Cholinesterase
Blood 82480-82482

Cholylglycine
Blood 82240

Chondroitin Sulfate 82485

Chondromalacia Patella
Repair 27418

Chondropathia Patellae
See Chondromalacia Patella

Chondrosteoma
See Exostosis

Chopart Procedure 28800-28805
See Amputation, Foot; Radical Resection;
Replantation

Chordotomies
See Cordotomy

Chorioangioma
See Lesion, Skin

Choriogonadotropin
See Chorionic Gonadotropin

Choriomeningitides, Lymphocytic
See Lymphocytic Choriomeningitis

Chorionic Gonadotropin 80414,
　　　　　　　　　　　　　　　　84702-84703
Stimulation 80414-80415

Chorionic Growth Hormone
See Lactogen, Human Placental

Chorionic Tumor
See Hydatidiform Mole

Chorionic Villi
See Biopsy, Chorionic Villus

Chorionic Villus
Biopsy 59015

Choroid
Destruction
　Lesion 0016T, 67220-67225

Choroid Plexus
Excision 61544

Christmas Factor 85250

Chromaffinoma, Medullary
See Pheochromocytoma

Chromatin, Sex
See Barr Bodies

Chromatography
Column/Mass Spectrometry 82541-82544
Gas Liquid or HPLC 82486, 82491-82492
Paper 82487-82488
Thin-Layer 82489

Chromium 82495

Chromogenic Substrate Assay .85130

Chromosome Analysis
See Amniocentesis
Added Study 88280-88289
Amniotic Fluid 88267-88269
    Culture 88235
Biopsy Culture
    Tissue 88233
Bone Marrow Culture 88237
Chorionic Villus .88267
    5 Cells 88261
    15-20 Cells .88262
    20-25 Cells .88264
    45 Cells 88263
    Culture 88235
for Breakage Syndromes 88245-88249
Fragile-X 88248
Lymphocyte Culture 88230
Pregnancy Associated Plasma Protein-A . . .84163
Skin Culture
    Tissue 88233
Tissue Culture 88239
Unlisted Services and Procedures 88299

Chromotubation 58350
Oviduct 58350

Chronic Erection
See Priapism

Chronic Interstitial Cystitides
See Cystitis, Interstitial

Ciliary Body
Cyst
    Destruction
        Cryotherapy 66720
        Cyclodialysis 66740
        Cyclophotocoagulation 66710, 66711
        Diathermy 66700
        Nonexcisional 66770
Destruction
    Cyclophotocoagulation 66710, 66711
    Endoscopic .66711
Lesion
    Destruction .66770
Repair 66680

Cimino Type Procedure 36821

Cinefluorographies
See Cineradiography

Cineplasty
Arm, Lower or Upper 24940

Cineradiography
Esophagus 74230
Pharynx 70371, 74230
Speech Evaluation 70371

Swallowing Evaluation 74230
Unlisted Services and Procedures . .76120-76125

Circulation Assist
Aortic 33967, 33970
Balloon .33967, 33970
External .33960-33961

Circulation, Extracorporeal
See Extracorporeal Circulation

Circulatory Assist
See Circulation Assist

Circumcision
Repair 54163
Surgical Excision 54161
    Newborn 54160
with Clamp or Other Device 54152
    Newborn 54150

Cisternal Puncture 61050-61055

Cisternography 70015
Nuclear 78630

Citrate
Blood or Urine .82507

Clagett Procedure
See Chest Wall, Repair, Closure

Clavicle
Craterization 23180
Cyst
    Excision 23140
        with Allograft 23146
        with Autograft 23145
Diaphysectomy 23180
Dislocation
    Acromioclavicular Joint
        Closed Treatment 23540-23545
        Open Treatment 23550-23552
    Sternoclavicular Joint
        Closed Treatment 23520-23525
        Open Treatment 23530-23532
        without Manipulation 23540
Excision 23170
    Partial 23120, 23180
    Total 23125
Fracture
    Closed Treatment
        with Manipulation 23505
        without Manipulation 23500
    Open Treatment 23515
Pinning, Wiring 23490
Prophylactic Treatment 23490
Repair Osteotomy 23480-23485
Saucerization .23180
Sequestrectomy 23170
Tumor
    Excision 23140, 23146, 23200
        with Autograft 23145
        Radical Resection 23200
X-Ray 73000

Clavicula
See Clavicle

Claviculectomy
Partial 23120
Total 23125

Claw Finger Repair 26499

Cleft Cyst, Branchial
See Branchial Cleft, Cyst

Cleft Foot
Reconstruction .28360

Cleft Hand
Repair 26580

Cleft Lip
Repair .40700-40761
Rhinoplasty 30460-30462

Cleft Palate
Repair .42200-42225
Rhinoplasty 30460-30462

Cleft, Branchial
See Branchial Cleft

Clinical Act of Insertion
See Insertion

Clinical Chemistry Test
See Chemistry Tests, Clinical

Clinical Pathology
See Pathology, Clinical

Clitoroplasty
Intersex State 56805

Closed [Transurethral] Biopsy of Bladder
See Biopsy, Bladder, Cystourethroscopy

Clostridial Tetanus
See Tetanus

Clostridium Botulinum Toxin
See Chemodenervation

Clostridium Difficile
Antigen Detection
    Enzyme Immunoassay 87324
by Immunoassay
    with Direct Optical Observation 87803

Clostridium Tetani ab
See Antibody, Tetanus

Closure 12001-13160
Anal Fistula 46288
Atrioventricular Valve 33600
Cystostomy 51880
Enterostomy 44625-44626
Lacrimal Fistula 68770
Lacrimal Punctum
    Plug 68761
    Thermocauterization, Ligation or Laser
        Surgery .68760
Rectovaginal Fistula 57300-57308
Semilunar Valve 33602
Septal Defect .33615
Sternotomy 21750
Ventricular Tunnel 33722

Closure of Esophagostomy
See Esophagostomy, Closure

Closure of Gastrostomy
See Gastrostomy, Closure

Closure, Atrial Septal Defect
See Heart, Repair, Atrial Septum

Closure, Cranial Sutures, Premature
See Craniosynostosis

Closure, Fistula, Vesicouterine
See Fistula, Vesicouterine, Closure

Closure, Meningocele Spinal
See Meningocele Repair

Closure, Vagina
See Vagina, Closure

Clot 34401-34490, 35875-35876, 50230
See Thrombectomy; Thromboendarterectomy

Clot Lysis Time 85175

Clot Retraction 85170

Clotting Disorder
See Coagulopathy

Clotting Factor 85210-85293

Clotting Inhibitors . . .85300-85305, 85307

Clotting Operation
See Excision, Nail Fold

Clotting Test
Protein C .85303, 85307
Protein S 85306

Clotting Time
See Coagulation Time

Clubfoot Cast 29450
Wedging 29750

CMG
See Cystometrogram

CMRI
See Cardiac Magnetic Resonance Imaging

CMV
See Cytomegalovirus

CNPB
See Continuous Negative Pressure Breathing (CNPB); Pulmonology, Therapeutic

Co-Factor I, Heparin
See Antithrombin III

CO2
See Carbon Dioxide

Coagulation
Unlisted Services and Procedures 85999

Coagulation Defect
See Coagulopathy

Coagulation Factor
See Clotting Factor

Coagulation Factor I
See Fibrinogen

Coagulation Factor II
See Prothrombin

Coagulation Factor III
See Thromboplastin

Coagulation Factor IV
See Calcium

Coagulation Factor VII
See Proconvertin

Coagulation Factor VIII
See Clotting Factor

Coagulation Factor IX
See Christmas Factor

Coagulation Factor X
See Stuart-Prower Factor

Coagulation Factor Xa
See Thrombokinase

Coagulation Factor XI
See Plasma Thromboplastin, Antecedent

Coagulation Factor XII
See Hageman Factor

Coagulation Factor XIII
See Fibrin Stabilizing Factor

Coagulation Time 85345-85348

Coagulation, Blood
See Blood Clot

Coagulation, Light
See Photocoagulation

Coagulin
See Thromboplastin

Coagulopathy 85390
Assay 85130

Cocaine
Blood or Urine .82520
Screen 82486

Coccidioides
Antibody 86635

Coccidioidin Test
See Streptokinase, Antibody

Coccidioidomycosis
Skin Test 86490

Coccygeal Spine Fracture
See Coccyx, Fracture

Coccygectomy 15920-15922, 27080

Coccyx
Excision 27080
Fracture
   Closed Treatment 27200
   Open Treatment 27202
Tumor
   Excision 49215
X-Ray 72220

Cochlear Device
Insertion 69930
Programming 92601-92604

Codeine
Alkaloid Screening 82101

Codeine Screen 82486

Cofactor Protein S
See Protein S

Coffey Operation
See Uterus, Repair, Suspension

Cognitive Function Tests 96115
See Neurology, Diagnostic

Cognitive Skills Development 97532
See Physical Medicine/Therapy/Occupational Therapy

Cold Agglutinin 86156-86157

Cold Pack Treatment 97010

Cold Preservation
See Cryopreservation

Cold Therapies
See Cryotherapy

Colectomy
Partial 44140
   with Anastomosis 44140
     Laparoscopic 44204, 44207-44208
   with Coloproctostomy 44145-44146
   with Colostomy 44141-44144
     Laparoscopic 44206, 44208
   with Ileocolostomy
     Laparoscopic 44205
   with Ileostomy 44144
   with Ileum Removal 44160
   with Transcanal Approach 44147
Total
   Laparoscopic 44210-44212
     with Proctectomy and
     Ileostomy 44210-44212
     without Proctectomy 44210
   Open
     with Anastomosis 44152
     with Complete Proctectomy 45121
     with Ileal Reservoir 44153
     with Ileostomy 44150-44151
     with Proctectomy 44155-44156

Collagen Cross Links 82523

Collagen Injection 11950-11954

Collar Bone
See Clavicle

Collateral Ligament
Ankle
    Repair 27695-27698
Interphalangeal Joint 26545
Knee Joint
    Repair 27409
Knee Repair 27405
Metacarpophalangeal Joint 26540-26542
Repair
    Ankle 27695-27698

Collection and Processing
Allogenic Blood
    Harvesting of Stem Cells 38205
Autologous Blood
    Harvesting of Stem Cells 38206
    Intraoperative 86891
    Preoperative 86890
Specimen
    Capillary Blood 36416
    Venous Blood 36415, 36540
Washings
    Esophagus 91000
    Stomach 91055

Colles Fracture 25600-25620

Colles Fracture Reversed
See Smith Fracture

Collins Syndrome, Treacher
See Treacher-Collins Syndrome

Collis Procedure
See Gastroplasty with Esophagogastric Fundoplasty

Colon
See Colon-Sigmoid
Biopsy 44025, 44100, 44322
    Endoscopic 44389, 45380, 45391, 45392
Colostomy
    Revision 44340-44346
Colotomy 44322
    Colostomy 44320
CT Scan
    Colonography 0066T-0067T
    Virtual Colonoscopy 0066T-0067T
Destruction
    Lesion 44393, 45383
    Tumor 44393, 45383
Endoscopy
    Biopsy 44389, 45380, 45391, 45392
    Destruction
       Lesion 44393
       Tumor 44393, 45383
    Dilation 45386
    Exploration 44388, 45378, 45381, 45386
    Hemorrhage 44391, 45382
    Injection, Submucosal 45381
    Placement
       Stent 45387
    Removal
       Foreign Body 44390, 45379
       Polyp 44392, 45384-45385
       Tumor 45384-45385
    Specimen Collection 45380
    Ultrasound 45391-45392

    via Colotomy 45355
    via Stoma 44388-44397
    Virtual 0066T-0067T
Excision
    Partial 44140-44147, 44160
       Laparoscopic 44204-44208
    Total 44150-44156
       Laparoscopic 44210-44212
Exploration 44025
    Endoscopy 44388, 45378, 45381, 45386
Hemorrhage
    Endoscopic Control 44391, 45382
Hernia 44050
Incision
    Creation
       Stoma 44320-44322
    Exploration 44025
    Revision
       Stoma 44340-44346
Lavage
    Intraoperative 44701
Lesion
    Destruction 45383
    Excision 44110-44111
Lysis
    Adhesions 44005
Obstruction 44025-44050
Reconstruction
    Bladder from 50810
Removal
    Foreign Body 44025, 44390, 45379
    Polyp 44392
Repair
    Diverticula 44605
    Fistula 44650-44661
    Hernia 44050
    Malrotation 44055
    Obstruction 44050
    Ulcer 44605
    Volvulus 44050
    Wound 44605
Stoma Closure 44620-44625
Suture
    Diverticula 44605
    Fistula 44650-44661
    Plication 44680
    Stoma 44620-44625
    Ulcer 44605
    Wound 44605
Tumor
    Destruction 45383
Ultrasound
    Endoscopic 45391-45392
X-Ray with Contrast
    Barium Enema 74270-74280

Colon-Sigmoid
See Colon
Biopsy
    Endoscopy 45331
Dilation
    Endoscopy 45340
Endoscopy
    Ablation
       Polyp 45339
       Tumor 45339
    Biopsy 45331

    Dilation 45340
    Exploration 45330, 45335
    Hemorrhage 45334
    Needle Biopsy 45342
    Placement
       Stent 45327, 45345
    Removal
       Foreign Body 45332
       Polyp 45333, 45338
       Tumor 45333, 45338
       Ultrasound 45341-45342
       Volvulus 45337
Exploration
    Endoscopy 45330, 45335
Hemorrhage
    Endoscopy 45334
Needle Biopsy
    Endoscopy 45342
Removal
    Foreign Body 45332
Repair
    Volvulus
       Endoscopy 45337
Ultrasound
    Endoscopy 45341-45342

Colonna Procedure
See Acetabulum, Reconstruction

Colonography
CT Scan 0066T-0067T

Colonoscopy
Biopsy 45380, 45392
Collection Specimen 45380
    via Colotomy 45355
Destruction
    Lesion 45383
    Tumor 45383
Dilation 45386
Hemorrhage Control 45382
Injection
    Submucosal 45381
Placement
    Stent 45387
Removal
    Foreign Body 45379
    Polyp 45384-45385
    Tumor 45384-45385
Ultrasound 45391-45392
via Stoma 44388-44390
    Biopsy 44389
    Destruction
       of Lesion 44393
       of Tumor 44393
    Exploration 44388
    Hemorrhage 44391
    Placement
       Stent 44397
    Removal
       Foreign Body 44390
       Polyp 44392, 44394
       Tumor 44392, 44394
Virtual 0066T-0067T

Color Vision Examination 92283

Colorrhaphy 44604

Condylectomy
Temporomandibular Joint 21050
with Skull Base Surgery 61596-61597

Condyloma
Destruction 54050-54065

Conference
Medical
    with Interdisciplinary Team 99361-99373

Confirmation
Drug 80102

Confirmatory Consultations
See Consultations
New or Established Patient 99271-99275

Congenital Arteriovenous Malformation
See Arteriovenous Malformation

Congenital Elevation of Scapula
See Sprengel's Deformity

Congenital Heart Septum Defect
See Septal Defect

Congenital Kidney Abnormality
Nephrolithotomy 50070
Pyeloplasty 50405
Pyelotomy 50135

Congenital Laryngocele
See Laryngocele

Congenital Vascular Anomaly
See Vascular Malformation

Conisation
See Cervix, Conization

Conization
Cervix 57461, 57520-57522

Conjoint Psychotherapy 90847
See Psychiatric Treatment, Family

Conjunctiva
Biopsy 68100
Cyst
    Incision and Drainage 68020
Fistulize for Drainage
    with Tube 68750
    without Tube 68745
Graft 65782
    Harvesting 68371
Harvesting 68371
Insertion Stent 68750
Lesion
    Destruction 68135
    Excision 68110-68130
      Over 1 cm 68115
      with Adjacent Sclera 68130
Reconstruction 68320-68335
    Symblepharon
      with Graft 68335
    with Flap
      Bridge or Partial 68360
      Total 68362

Repair
    Symblepharon
      Division 68340
      with Graft 68335
      without Graft 68330
    Wound
      Direct Closure 65270
      Mobilization and
      Rearrangement 65272-65273
Unlisted Services and Procedures 68399

Conjunctivo-Tarso-Muller Resection 67908

Conjunctivocystorhinostomy
See Conjunctivorhinostomy

Conjunctivodacryocystostomy
See Conjunctivorhinostomy

Conjunctivoplasty 68320-68330
Reconstruction Cul de Sac
    with Extensive Rearrangement 68326
    with Graft 68326
      Buccal Mucous Membrane 68328
with Extensive Rearrangement 68320
with Graft 68320
    Buccal Mucous Membrane 68325

Conjunctivorhinostomy
with Tube 68750
without Tube 68745

Conscious Sedation
See Sedation

Construction
Finger
    Toe to Hand Transfer 26551-26556
Neobladder 51596
Vagina
    with Graft 57292
    without Graft 57291

Consultation
See Second Opinion; Third Opinion
Clinical Pathology 80500-80502
Confirmatory 99271-99275
    New or Established Patient 99271-99275
Follow-up Inpatient
    Established Patient 99261-99263
Initial Inpatient 99251-99255
    New or Established Patient 99251-99255
Office and/or Other Outpatient 99241-99245
    New or Established Patient ...99241-99245
Psychiatric, with Family 90887
Radiation Therapy
    Radiation Physics 77336-77370
Surgical Pathology 88321-88325
    Intraoperation 88329-88332
X-Ray 76140

Consumption Test, Antiglobulin
See Coombs Test

Contact Lens Services
Fittings and Prescription 92070, 92310-92313
Modification 92325
Prescription 92314-92317
Replacement 92326
Supply 92391, 92396

Continuous Negative Pressure Breathing (CNPB) 94662

Continuous Positive Airway Pressure (CPAP) 94660
See Pulmonology, Therapeutic

Contouring
Silicone Injections 11950-11954
Tumor
    Facial Bone 21029

Contraception
Cervical Cap
    Fitting 57170
Diaphragm
    Fitting 57170
Intrauterine Device (IUD)
    See Insertion, Intrauterine Device (IUD);
    Intrauterine Device (IUD); Removal,
    Intrauterine Device (IUD)
    Insertion 58300
    Removal 58301

Contraceptive Capsules, Implantable
Insertion 11975
Removal 11976
    with Reinsertion 11977

Contraceptive Device, Intrauterine
See Intrauterine Device (IUD)

Contracture
Elbow
    Release
      with Radical Resection of Capsule ..24149
Palm
    Release 26121-26125
Thumb
    Release 26508

Contracture of Palmar Fascia
See Dupuytren's Contracture

Contralateral Ligament
Repair
    Knee 27405

Contrast Aortogram
See Aortography

Contrast Bath Therapy 97034
See Physical Medicine/Therapy/Occupational Therapy

Contrast Material
Injection
    via Peritoneal Catheter 49424
Instillation
    Bronchography 31708
    Laryngography 31708

Contrast Phlebogram
See Venography

Contusion
See Hematoma

Converting Enzyme, Angiotensin
See Angiotensin Converting Enzyme (ACE)

Count, Blood Platelet
See Blood, Platelet, Count

Count, Cell
See Cell Count

Count, Complete Blood
See Complete Blood Count (CBC)

Count, Erythrocyte
See Red Blood Cell (RBC), Count

Count, Leukocyte
See White Blood Cell, Count

Count, Reticulocyte
See Reticulocyte, Count

Counterimmuno-electrophoresis 86185

Counters, Cell
See Cell Count

Countershock, Electric
See Cardioversion

Coventry Tibial Wedge Osteotomy
See Osteotomy, Tibia

Cowper's Gland
Excision 53250

Coxa
See Hip

Coxiella Burnetii
Antibody 86638

Coxsackie
Antibody 86658

CPAP
See Continuous Positive Airway Pressure

CPK
Blood 82550-82552

CPR (Cardiopulmonary Resuscitation) .92950

Cranial Bone
Halo
    Thin Skull Osteology 20664
Reconstruction
    Extracranial 21181-21184
Tumor
    Excision 61563-61564

Cranial Halo 20661

Cranial Nerve
See Specific Nerve
Avulsion 64732-64760, 64771
Decompression 61458, 64716
Implantation
    Electrode 64553, 64573
Incision 64732-64752, 64760, 65771
Injection
    Anesthetic 64400-64408, 64412
    Neurolytic 64600-64610
Insertion
    Electrode 64553, 64573

Neuroplasty 64716
Release 64716
Repair
    Suture, with or without Graft . . .64864-64865
Section 61460
Transection 64732-64760, 64771
Transposition 64716

Cranial Nerve II
See Optic Nerve

Cranial Nerve V
See Trigeminal Nerve

Cranial Nerve VII
See Facial Nerve

Cranial Nerve X
See Vagus Nerve

Cranial Nerve XI
See Accessory Nerve

Cranial Nerve XII
See Hypoglossal Nerve

Cranial Tongs
Application/Removal 20660
Removal 20665

Craniectomy 61501
See Craniotomy
Decompression 61322-61323, 61340-61343
Exploratory 61304-61305
Extensive, for Multiple Suture Craniosynostosis . .
    61558-61559
for Electrode 61860-61875
Release Stenosis 61550-61552
Surgical 61312-61315, 61320-61323,
    61440-61480, 61500-61516, 61518-61522

Craniofacial Procedures
Unlisted Services and Procedures 21299

Craniofacial Separation
Closed Treatment 21431
Open Treatment 21432-21436
Wire Fixation 21431

Craniomegalic Skull
Reduction 62115-62117

Craniopharyngioma
Excision 61545

Cranioplasty 62120
Encephalocele Repair 62120
for Defect 62140-62141, 62145
with Autograft 62146-62147
with Bone Graft 61316, 62146-62147

Craniostenosis
See Craniosynostosis

Craniosynostosis
Bifrontal Craniotomy 61557
Extensive Craniectomy 61558-61559

Craniotomy
See Burr Hole; Craniectomy; Drill Hole; Puncture
Bifrontal 61557
Decompression 61322-61323
Exploratory 61304-61305

for Craniosynostosis 61556-61557
for Encephalocele 62121
for Implant of Neurostimulators 61850-61875
Frontal 61556
Parietal 61556
Surgery 61312-61315, 61320-61323, 61440,
    61490, 61546, 61570-61571, 61582-61583,
        61590, 61592, 61760, 62120
with Bone Flap 61510-61516, 61526-61530,
        61533-61545, 61566-61567

Cranium
See Skull

Craterization
Calcaneus 28120
Clavicle 23180
Femur 27070-27071, 27360
Fibula 27360, 27641
Hip 27070
Humerus 23184, 24140
Ileum 27070
Metacarpal 26230
Metatarsal 28122
Olecranon Process 24147
Phalanges
    Finger 26235-26236
    Toe 28124
Pubis 27070
Radius .24145, 25151
Scapula 23182
Talus 28120
Tarsal 28122
Tibia 27360, 27640
Ulna 24147, 25150

Creatine 82553-82554
Blood or Urine 82540

Creatine Kinase
Total 82550

Creatine Phosphokinase
Blood 82552
Total 82550

Creatinine
Blood 82565
Clearance 82575
Other Source 82570
Urine 82570-82575

Creation
Arteriovenous
    Fistula/Autogenous Graft 36825
Colonic Reservoir 45119
Complete Heart Block 93650
Defect 40720
Ileal Reservoir 44153, 45113
Lesion .61790, 63600
Mucofistula 44144
Pericardial Window 32659
Recipient Site 15000
Shunt
    Cerebrospinal Fluid 62200
    Subarachnoid
        Lumbar-Peritoneal 63740
        Subarachnoid-Subdural 62190
    Ventriculo 62220

Culture

Curettage

See Dilation and Curettage

Curettage and Dilatation

See Dilation and Curettage

Curettage, Uterus

See Uterus, Curettage

Curettement

Curietherapy

See Brachytherapy

Custodial Care

See Domiciliary Services; Nursing Facility Services

Cutaneolipectomy

See Lipectomy

Cutaneous Electrostimulation, Analgesic

See Application, Neurostimulation

Cutaneous Tag

See Skin, Tags

Cutaneous Tissue

See Integumentary System

Cutaneous-Vesicostomy

See Vesicostomy, Cutaneous

CVS

See Biopsy, Chorionic Villus

Cyanacobalamin

See Cyanocobalamin

Cyanide

Cyanocobalamin 82607-82608

Cyclic AMP 82030

Cyclic GMP 83008

Cyclic Somatostatin

See Somatostatin

Cyclocryotherapy

See Cryotherapy, Destruction, Ciliary Body

Cyclodialysis

Cyclophotocoagulation

Cyclosporine

Cyst

Ureteral Guide Wire 52334
Urethral Stent 52282
Lithotripsy 52353
Manipulation of Ureteral Calculus 52330
Meatotomy
    Ureteral 52290-52305
Removal
    Calculus ..52310-52315, 52320-52325, 52352
    Foreign Body 52310-52315
    Urethral Stent 52310-52315
Resection
    Ejaculatory Duct 52402
    External Sphincter 52277
    Tumor 52355
Urethral Syndrome 52285
Vasectomy
    Transurethral 52402
Vasotomy
    Transurethral 52402
with Direct Vision Internal Urethrotomy ...52276
with Ejaculatory Duct Catheterization 52010
with Fulguration 52214, 52354
    Lesion 52224
    Tumor 52234-52240
with Internal Urethrotomy
    Female 52270
    Male 52275
with Steroid Injection 52283
with Ureteral Catheterization 52005
with Ureteral Meatotomy 52290-52305

Cytochrome Reductase, Lactic
See Lactic Dehydrogenase

Cytogenetic Study
Molecular
    DNA Probe 88271-88275, 88291, 88365
Unlisted Services and Procedures 88299

Cytomegalovirus
Antibody 86644-86645
Antigen Detection
    Direct Fluorescence 87271
    Enzyme Immunoassay 87332
    Nucleic Acid 87495-87497

Cytometries, Flow
See Flow Cytometry

Cytopathology
Cervical or Vaginal
    Requiring Interpretation by Physician ..88141
    Thin Layer Prep 88142-88143,
                         88174-88175
Concentration Technique 88108
    See Saccomonno Technique
Evaluation 88172
Fluids, Washings, Brushings 88104-88108
Forensic 88125
Other Source 88160-88162
Selective Cellular Enhancement Technique .88112
Smears
    Cervical or Vaginal 88141-88167,
                         88174-88175
Unlisted Services and Procedures 88199

Cytoscopy
See Bladder, Endoscopy

Cytosol Aminopeptidase
See Leucine Aminopeptidase

Cytotoxic Screen
Lymphocyte 86805-86806
Percent Reactive Antibody (PRA) ..86807-86808
Serum Antibodies 86807-86808

D

D & C Yellow No. 7
See Fluorescein

D 2, Vitamin
See Calciferol

D and C
See Dilation and Curettage

D and E
See Dilation and Evacuation

D Galactose
See Galactose

D Glucose
See Glucose

D Vitamin
See Vitamin, D

D-Xylose Absorption Test 84620

Dacryoadenectomy
Partial 68505
Total 68500

Dacryocystectomy 68520

Dacryocystogram
See Dacryocystography

Dacryocystography 68850, 70170
Nuclear Imaging 78660

Dacryocystorhinostomy 68720
Total
    with Nasal/Sinus Endoscopy 31239

Dacryocystostomies
See Dacryocystotomy

Dacryocystotomy 68420

Daily Living Activities
See Activities of Daily Living

Damus-Kaye-Stansel Procedure
See Anastomosis, Pulmonary

Dana Operation
See Rhizotomy

Dandy Operation
See Ventriculocisternostomy

Dark Adaptation Examination ..92284

Dark Field Examination ...87164-87166

Darkroom Test
See Glaucoma, Provocative Test

Darrach Procedure
See Excision, Ulna, Partial

Day Test
See Blood, Feces

de Quervain's Disease
Treatment 25000

Death, Brain
See Brain Death

Debridement
Brain 62010
Burns 01951-01953, 16010-16030
Mastoid Cavity
    Complex 69222
    Simple 69220
Metatarsophalangeal Joint 28289
Muscle
    Infected 11004-11006
Nails 11720-11721
Nose
    Endoscopic 31237
Pancreatic Tissue 48005
Skin
    Eczematous 11000-11001
    Full Thickness 11041
    Infected 11000-11006
    Partial Thickness 11040
    Subcutaneous Tissue 11042-11044
        Infected 11004-11006
    with Open Fracture and/or
        Dislocation 11010-11012
Sternum 21627
Wound
    Non-Selective 97602
    Selective 97597-97598

Debulking Procedure
Ovary/Pelvis 58952-58954

Decompression
See Section
Arm, Lower 24495, 25020-25025
Auditory Canal, Internal 69960
Brainstem 61575-61576
Cauda Equina 63011, 63017, 63047-63048,
                 63056-63057, 63087-63091
Cranial Nerve 61458
Esophagogastric Varices 37181
Facial Nerve 61590
    Intratemporal
        Lateral to Geniculate Ganglion 69720,
                          69740
        Medial to Geniculate Ganglion 69725,
                          69745
    Total 69955
Finger 26035
Gasserian Ganglion
    Sensory Root 61450
Hand 26035-26037
Intestines
    Small 44021

Jejunostomy
    Laparoscopic 44201
Leg
    Fasciotomy 27600-27602
Nerve 64702-64727
    Root 63020-63048, 63055-63103
Nucleus of Disk
    Lumbar 62287
Optic Nerve 67570
Orbit 61330
    Removal of Bone 67414, 67445
Skull 61322-61323, 61340-61345
Spinal Cord 63001-63017, 63045-63103
    Cauda Equina 63005
Tarsal Tunnel Release 28035
Volvulus 45321, 45337
with Nasal/Sinus Endoscopy
    Optic Nerve 31294
    Orbit Wall 31292-31293
Wrist 25020-25025

Decortication
Lung
    Endoscopic 32651-32652
    Partial 32225
    Total 32220
    with Parietal Pleurectomy 32320

Decubiti
See Pressure Ulcer (Decubitus)

Decubitus Ulcers
See Debridement; Pressure Ulcer (Decubitus);
Skin Graft and Flap

Deetjeen's Body
See Blood, Platelet

Defect, Coagulation
See Coagulopathy

Defect, Heart Septal
See Septal Defect

Defect, Septal Closure, Atrial
See Heart, Repair, Atrial Septum

Deferens, Ductus
See Vas Deferens

Defibrillation
See Cardioversion

Defibrillator, Heart
See Pacemaker, Heart
Evaluation and Testing 93640-93642,
                      93741-93744
Insertion Single/Dual Chamber
    Electrodes 33216-33217,
         33224-33225, 33245-33249
    Pulse Generator 33240, 33246
Removal Single/Dual Chamber
    Electrodes 33243-33244
    Pulse Generator 33241
Repair .33218-33220
Repositioning Single/Dual Chamber
    Electrodes 33215, 33226
Revise Pocket Chest 33223
Wearable Device 93741-93742, 93745

Deformity, Boutonniere
See Boutonniere Deformity

Deformity, Sprengel's
See Sprengel's Deformity

Degenerative, Articular Cartilage, Patella
See Chondromalacia Patella

Degradation Products, Fibrin
See Fibrin Degradation Products

Dehydroepiandrosterone 82626

Dehydroepiandrosterone Sulfate .82627

Dehydrogenase, 6-Phosphogluconate
See Phosphogluconate-6, Dehydrogenase

Dehydrogenase, Alcohol
See Antidiuretic Hormone

Dehydrogenase, Glucose-6-Phosphate
See Glucose-6-Phosphate, Dehydrogenase

Dehydrogenase, Glutamate
See Glutamate Dehydrogenase

Dehydrogenase, Isocitrate
See Isocitric Dehydrogenase

Dehydrogenase, Lactate
See Lactic Dehydrogenase

Dehydrogenase, Malate
See Malate Dehydrogenase

Dehydroisoandrosterone Sulfate
See Dehydroepiandrosterone Sulfate

Delay of Flap
Skin Graft 15600-15630

Deligation
Ureter 50940

Deliveries, Abdominal
See Cesarean Delivery

Delivery
See Cesarean Delivery; Vaginal Delivery

Delorme Operation
See Pericardiectomy

Denervation
Hip
    Femoral .27035
    Obturator 27035
    Sciatic 27035

Denervation, Sympathetic
See Excision, Nerve, Sympathetic

Denis-Browne Splint 29590

Dens Axis
See Odontoid Process

Denver Developmental Screening Test 96100

Denver Krupic Procedure
See Aqueous Shunt, to Extraocular Reservoir

Denver Shunt
Patency Test .78291

Denver-Krupin Procedure 66180

Deoxycorticosterone
See Desoxycorticosterone

Deoxycortisol 80436, 82634

Deoxyephedrine
See Methamphetamine

Deoxyribonuclease
Antibody 86215

Deoxyribonuclease I
See DNAse

Deoxyribonucleic Acid
Antibody 86225-86226

Depilation
See Removal, Hair

Depletion
Plasma 38214
Platelet 38213
T-Cell 38210
Tumor Cell 38211

Deposit Calcium
See Calcium, Deposits

Depth Electrode
Insertion 61760

Derma-Fat-Fascia Graft 15770

Dermabrasion 15780-15783

Dermatology
Actinotherapy 96900
Examination of Hair
    Microscopic 96902
Ultraviolet A Treatment 96912
Ultraviolet B Treatment 96910-96913
Ultraviolet Light Treatment 96900-96913
Unlisted Services and Procedures 96999

Dermatoplasty
Septal 30620

Dermoid
See Cyst, Dermoid

Derrick-Burnet Disease
See Q Fever

Descending Abdominal Aorta
See Aorta, Abdominal

Desipramine
Assay 80160

Desmotomy
See Ligament, Release

Desoxycorticosterone 82633

Desoxycortone
See Desoxycorticosterone

Diagnostic Aspiration of Anterior Chamber of Eye
See Eye, Paracentesis, Anterior Chamber, with Diagnostic Aspiration of Aqueous

Diagnostic Radiologic Examination
See Radiology, Diagnostic

Diagnostic Skin and Sensitization Tests
See Allergy Tests

Diagnostic Ultrasound
See Echography

Diagnostic Ultrasound of Heart
See Echocardiography

Dialyses, Peritoneal
See Dialysis, Peritoneal

Dialysis
Arteriovenous Fistula
    Revision
        without Thrombectomy 36832
Arteriovenous Shunt 36145
    Revision
        with Thrombectomy 36833
    Thrombectomy 36831
End Stage Renal Disease 90918-90925
Hemodialysis 90935-90937
    Blood Flow Study 90939-90940
Hemoperfusion 90997
Patient Training
    Completed Course 90989
    Per Session 90993
Peritoneal 90945-90947
Unlisted Services and Procedures 90999

Dialysis, Extracorporeal
See Hemodialysis

Diaphragm
Repair
    for Eventration 39545
    Hernia 39502-39541
    Laceration 39501
Resection 39560-39561
Unlisted Procedures 39599
Vagina
    Fitting 57170

Diaphragm Contraception
See Contraception, Diaphragm

Diaphysectomy
Calcaneus 28120
Clavicle 23180
Femur 27360
Fibula 27360, 27641
Humerus 23184, 24140
Metacarpal 26230
Metatarsal 28122
Olecranon Process 24147
Phalanges
    Finger 26235-26236
    Toe 28124
Radius 24145, 25151
Scapula 23182
Talus 28120

Tarsal 28122
Tibia 27360, 27640
Ulna 24147, 25150

Diastase
See Amylase

Diastasis
See Separation

Diathermy 97024
See Physical Medicine/Therapy/Occupational Therapy
Destruction
    Ciliary Body 66700
Lesion
    Retina 67208, 67227
Retinal Detachment
    Prophylaxis 67141
    Repair 67101

Diathermy, Surgical
See Electrocautery

Dibucaine Number 82638

Dichloride, Methylene
See Dichloromethane

Dichlorides, Ethylene
See Dichloroethane

Dichloroethane 84600

Dichloromethane 84600

Diethylamide, Lysergic Acid
See Lysergic Acid Diethylamide

Diethylether 84600

Differential Count
See White Blood Cell Count

Differentiation Reversal Factor
See Prothrombin

Diffusion Test, Gel
See Immunodiffusion

Digestive Tract
See Gastrointestinal Tract

Digit
See Finger; Toe
Replantation 20816-20822

Digital Artery Sympathectomy 64820

Digital Slit-Beam Radiograph
See Scanogram

Digits
Pinch Graft 15050

Digoxin
Assay 80162

Dihydrocodeinone 82646

Dihydrocodeinone Screen 82486

Dihydroepitestosterone
See Dihydrotestosterone

Dihydrohydroxycodeinone
See Oxycodinone

Dihydromorphinone 82486, 82649

Dihydrotestosterone 82651

Dihydroxyethanes
See Ethylene Glycol

Dihydroxyvitamin D 82652

Dilatation, Transluminal Arterial
See Angioplasty, Transluminal

Dilation
See Dilation and Curettage
Anal
    Endoscopy 46604
    Sphincter 45905
Bile Duct
    Endoscopy 43271, 47555-47556
    Stricture 74363
Bladder
    Cystourethroscopy 52260-52265
Bronchi
    Endoscopy 31630, 31636-31638
Cervix
    Canal 57800
    Stump 57820
Colon
    Endoscopy 45386
Colon-Sigmoid
    Endoscopy 45340
Esophagus 43450-43458
    Balloon 43220, 43249
    Endoscopy 43220-43226, 43249
    Surgical 43510
Intestines, Small
    Endoscopy 44370
Kidney 50395
    Intra-Renal Stricture 52343, 52346
Lacrimal Punctum 68801
Larynx
    Endoscopy 31528-31529
Pancreatic Duct
    Endoscopy 43271
Rectum
    Endoscopy 45303
    Sphincter 45910
Salivary Duct 42650-42660
Trachea
    Endoscopy 31630-31631, 31636-31638
Ureter 50395, 52341-52342, 52344-52345
    Endoscopy 50553, 50572, 50953, 50972
Urethra 52260-52265
    General 53665
    Suppository and/or Instillation .53660-53661
Urethral
    Stenosis 52281
    Stricture 52281, 53600-53621
Vagina 57400

Dilation and Curettage 59840
See Curettage; Dilation
Cervix 57800-57820
Corpus Uteri 58120

Radius
  Closed Treatment 24640
  with Fracture
    Closed Treatment 24620
    Open Treatment 24635
Shoulder
  Closed Treatment with
  Manipulation 23650-23655
  Open Treatment 23660
  with Greater Tuberosity Fracture
    Closed Treatment 23665
    Open Treatment 23670
  with Surgical or Anatomical Neck
  Fracture
    Closed Treatment 23675
    Open Treatment 23680
Skin
  Debridement 11010-11012
Sternoclavicular Joint
  Closed Treatment
    with Manipulation 23525
    without Manipulation 23520
  Open Treatment 23530-23532
Talotarsal Joint
  Closed Treatment 28570-28575
  Open Treatment 28546
  Percutaneous Fixation 28576
Tarsal
  Closed Treatment 28540-28545
  Open Treatment 28555
  Percutaneous Fixation 28546
Tarsometatarsal Joint
  Closed Treatment 28600-28605
  Open Treatment 28615
  Percutaneous Fixation 28606
Temporomandibular Joint
  Closed Treatment 21480-21485
  Open Treatment 21490
Thumb
  Closed Treatment 26641-26645
  Open Treatment 26665
  Percutaneous Fixation 26650
  with Fracture 26645
    Open Treatment 26665
    Percutaneous Fixation 26650-26665
  with Manipulation 26641-26650
Tibiofibular Joint
  Closed Treatment 27830-27831
  Open Treatment 27832
Vertebra
  Additional Segment
    Open Treatment 22328
  Cervical
    Open Treatment 22326
  Closed Treatment 22305
    with Manipulation, Casting
    and/or Bracing 22315
    without Manipulation 22310
  Lumbar
    Open Treatment 22325
  Thoracic
    Open Treatment 22327
Wrist
  Closed Treatment 25660, 25675, 25680
  Intercarpal .25660
  Open Treatment 25670
  Open Treatment 25670, 25685
  Percutaneous Fixation 25671

Radiocarpal .25660
  Open Treatment 25670
Radioulnar
  Closed Treatment 25675
  Open Treatment 25676
  Percutaneous Fixation 25671
  with Fracture
    Closed Treatment 25680
    Open Treatment 25685
  with Manipulation 25660, 25675, 25680

Dislocation, Radiocarpal Joint
See Radiocarpal Joint, Dislocation

Disorder
Blood Coagulation
  See Coagulopathy
Penis
  See Penis
Retinal
  See Retina

Displacement Therapy
Nose 30210

Dissection
Hygroma, Cystic
  Axillary/Cervical 38550-38555
Lymph Nodes 38542

Dissection, Neck, Radical
See Radical Neck Dissection

Distention
See Dilation

Diverticula, Meckel's
See Diverticulum, Meckel's

Diverticulectomy 44800
Esophagus 43130-43135

Diverticulectomy, Meckel's
See Meckel's Diverticulum, Excision

Diverticulum
Bladder
  See Bladder, Diverticulum
Meckel's
  Excision .44800
Repair
  Urethra 53400-53405

Division
Muscle
  Foot 28250
Plantar Fascia
  Foot 28250

Division, Isthmus, Horseshoe Kidney
See Symphysiotomy, Horseshoe Kidney

Division, Scalenus Anticus Muscle
See Muscle Division, Scalenus Anticus

DI-Amphetamine
See Amphetamine

DMO
See Dimethadione

DNA
Antibody 86225-86226

DNA Endonuclease
See DNAse

DNA Probe
See Cytogenetics Studies; Nucleic Acid Probe

DNAse
Antibody 86215

Domiciliary Services
See Nursing Facility Services
Discharge Services 99315-99316
Established Patient 99331-99333
New Patient 99321-99323

Donor Procedures
Conjunctival Graft 68371
Heart Excision 33940
Heart/Lung Excision 33930
Liver Segment 47140-47142
Stem Cells
  Donor Search 38204

Dopamine
See Catecholamines
Blood .82383-82384
Urine .82382, 82384

Doppler Echocardiography 76827-
                                  76828, 93307-93308, 93320-93350
Extracranial .93875
Intracardiac .93662
Transesophageal 93318
Transthoracic 93303-93317

Doppler Scan
Arterial Studies
  Extremities 93922-93924
  Fetal
    Middle Cerebral Artery 76821
    Umbilical Artery 76820
Extremities .93965
Intracranial Arteries 93886-93893

Dorsal Vertebra
See Vertebra, Thoracic

Dose Plan
See Dosimetry

Dosimetry
Radiation Therapy 77300, 77331
  Brachytherapy 77326-77328
  Intensity Modulation 77301
  Teletherapy 77305-77321

Double-Stranded DNA
See Deoxyribonucleic Acid

Doxepin
Assay 80166

DPH
See Phenytoin

Drainage
See Excision; Incision; Incision and Drainage
Abdomen
  Abdomen Fluid 49080-49081

Abscess
  Appendix 44900-44901
    Percutaneous 44901
  Brain 61150-61151
  Eyelid 67700
  Liver 47010-47011
  Ovary
    Percutaneous 58823
  Pelvic
    Percutaneous 58823
  Pericolic
    Percutaneous 58823
  Perirenal or Renal 50020-50021
    Percutaneous 50021
  Prostate 52700
  Retroperitoneal 49060-49061
    Percutaneous 49061
  Subdiaphragmatic or
  Subphrenic 49040-49041
    Percutaneous 49040-49041
    with X-Ray 75989
Amniotic Fluid
  Diagnostic Aspiration 59000
  Therapeutic Aspiration 59001
Bile Duct
  Transhepatic 75980
Brain Fluid 61070
Bursa 20600-20610
Cerebrospinal Fluid 61000-61020, 61050,
                              61070, 62272
Cervical Fluid 61050
Cisternal Fluid 61050
Cyst
  Bone 20615
  Brain 61150-61151, 62161-62162
  Breast 19000-19001
  Ganglion 20612
  Liver 47010-47011
    Percutaneous 47011
  Salivary Gland 42409
  Sublingual Gland 42409
  with Fistula 42325-42326
Extraperitoneal Lymphocele
  Laparoscopic 49323
  Open 49062
Eye
  Anterior Chamber Paracentesis
    with Diagnostic Aspiration of
    Aqueous 65800
    with Therapeutic Release of
    Aqueous 65805
  Removal Blood 65815
  Removal of Vitreous and/or Discission
  Anterior Hyaloid Membrane 65810
Fetal Fluid 59074
Ganglion Cyst 20612
Hematoma
  Brain 61154-61156
  Vagina 57022-57023
Hematoma, Subungual 11740
Joint 20600-20610
Liver
  Abscess or Cyst 47010-47011
    Percutaneous 47011
Lymphocele
  Endoscopic 49323

Onychia 10060-10061
Orbit 67405, 67440
Pancreas
  See Anastomosis, Pancreas to Intestines
  Pseudocyst 48510-48511
    Percutaneous 48511
Paronychia 10060-10061
Pericardial Sac 32659
Pericardium
  See Aspiration, Pericardium
Pseudocyst
  Gastrointestinal, Upper
    Transmural Endoscopic 43240
  Pancreas 48510
  Open 48510
  Percutaneous 48511
Puncture
  Chest 32000-32002
Skin 10040-10180
Spinal Cord
  Cerebrospinal Fluid 62272
Subdural Fluid 61000-61001
Urethra
  Extravasation 53080-53085
Ventricular Fluid 61020

Drainage Implant, Glaucoma
See Aqueous Shunt

Dressings
Burns 16010-16030
Change
  Anesthesia 15852

DREZ Procedure
See Incision, Spinal Cord; Incision and Drainage

DRIL
See Revascularization, Distal

Drill Hole
Skull
  Catheter 61107
  Drain Hematoma 61108
  Exploration 61105
  Implant Electrode 61850, 61863-61868

Drinking Test for Glaucoma
See Glaucoma, Provocative Test

Drug
See Drug Assay; Specific Drug
Analysis
  Tissue Preparation 80103
Confirmation 80102
Infusion 62360-62362

Drug Assay
Amikacin 80150
Amitriptyline 80152
Benzodiazepine 80154
Carbamazepine 80156-80157
Cyclosporine 80158
Desipramine 80160
Digoxin 80162
Dipropylacetic Acid 80164
Doxepin 80166
Ethosuximide 80168
Gentamicin 80170

Gold 80172
Haloperidol 80173
Imipramine 80174
Lidocaine 80176
Lithium 80178
Nortriptyline 80182
Phenobarbital 80184
Phenytoin 80185-80186
Primidone 80188
Procainamide 80190-80192
Quantitative
  Other 80299
Quinidine 80194
Salicylate 80196
Tacrolimus 80197
Theophylline 80198
Tobramycin 80200
Topiramate 80201
Vancomycin 80202

Drug Delivery Implant
Insertion 11981
Maintenance and Refill
  Brain 95990
  Epidural 95990-95991
  Intra-arterial 96530
  Intrathecal 95990-95991
  Intravenous 96530
  Intraventricular 95990-95991
Removal 11982-11983
  with Reinsertion 11983

Drug Instillation
See Instillation, Drugs

Drug Management
Psychiatric 90862

Drug Screen 80100-80101, 82486

Drugs, Anticoagulant
See Clotting Inhibitors

DST
See Dexamethasone, Suppression Test

DT Shots 90702

DTaP Immunization 90721

DTaP-HepB-IPV Immunization
.........................90723

DTP Immunization 90701, 90720

Dual Photon Absorptiometry
See Absorptiometry, Dual Photon

Dual X-Ray Absorptiometry (DXA)
Appendicular 76076
Axial Skeleton 76075
Body Composition 0028T
Vertebral Fracture 76077

Duct, Bile
See Bile Duct

Duct, Hepatic
See Hepatic Duct

Duct, Mammary
Lavage 0046T-0047T

Duct, Nasolacrimal
See Nasolacrimal Duct

Duct, Omphalomesenteric
See Omphalomesenteric Duct

Duct, Pancreatic
See Pancreatic Duct

Duct, Salivary
See Salivary Duct

Duct, Stensen's
See Parotid Duct

Duct, Thoracic
See Thoracic Duct

Ductogram, Mammary
See Galactogram

Ductus Arteriosus
Repair 33820-33824

Ductus Deferens
See Vas Deferens

Duhamel Procedure
See Proctectomy, Total

Dunn Operation
See Arthrodesis, Foot Joint

Duodenotomy 44010

Duodenum
Biopsy 44010
Exclusion 48547
Exploration 44010
Incision 44010
Removal
  Foreign Body 44010
X-Ray 74260

Duplex Scan
See Vascular Studies
Arterial Studies
  Aorta 93978-93979
  Extracranial 93880-93882
  Lower Extremity 93925-93926
  Penile 93980-93981
  Upper Extremity 93930-93931
  Visceral 93975-93979
Hemodialysis Access 93990
Venous Studies
  Extremity 93970-93971
  Penile 93980-93981

Dupuy-Dutemp Operation
See Reconstruction, Eyelid; Revision

Dupuytren's
Contracture 26040-26045

Durand-Nicolas-Favre Disease
See Lymphogranuloma Venereum

Dust, Angel
See Phencyclidine

Duvries Operation
See Tenoplasty

Dwyer Procedure
See Osteotomy, Calcaneus

DXA
See Dual X-Ray Absorptiometry (DXA)

Dynamometry
See Osteotomy, Calcaneus
Venous Studies
  See Osteotomy, Calcaneus
  with Ophthalmoscopy 92260

E

E Antigens
See Hepatitis Antigen, Be

E B Virus
See Epstein-Barr Virus

E Vitamin
See Tocopherol

E1
See Estrone

E2
See Estradiol

E3
See Estriol

Ear
Collection of Blood 36415-36416
Drum 69420-69421, 69433-69436,
                    69450, 69610-69620
  See Tympanic Membrane
External
  Abscess Incision and Drainage
    Complicated 69005
    Simple 69000
  Biopsy 69100
  Excision
    Partial 69110
    Total 69120
  Hematoma
    Incision and Drainage 69000-69005
  Reconstruction 69300
  Unlisted Services and Procedures 69399
Inner
  CT Scan 70480-70482
  Excision
    Labyrinth 69905-69910
  Exploration
    Endolymphatic Sac 69805-69806
  Incision 69820
    Labyrinth 69801-69802
    Semicircular Canal 69840
  Insertion
    Cochlear Device 69930
  Semicircular Canal 69820
  Unlisted Services and Procedures 69949

Middle
  Catheterization 69405
  CT Scan 70480-70482
  Exploration 69440
  Inflation
    with Catheterization 69400
    without Catheterization 69401
  Insertion
    Baffle 69410
    Catheter 69405
  Lesion
    Excision 69540
  Reconstruction
    Tympanoplasty with Antrotomy
      or Mastoidotomy 69635-69637
    Tympanoplasty with
      Mastoidectomy 69641-69646
    Tympanoplasty without
      Mastoidectomy 69631-69633
  Removal
    Ventilating Tube 69424
  Repair
    Oval Window 69666
    Round Window 69667
  Revision
    Stapes 69662
  Tumor
    Excision 69550-69554
  Unlisted Services and Procedures 69799
Outer
  CT Scan 70480-70482

Ear Canal
See Auditory Canal

Ear Cartilage
Graft
  to Face 21235

Ear Lobes
Pierce 69090

Ear Protector Attenuation 92596
See Hearing Aid Services

Ear Wax
See Cerumen

Ear, Nose, and Throat
See Hearing Aid Services; Otorhinolaryngology,
Diagnostic
Audiologic Function Tests
  Acoustic Reflex 92568
  Acoustic Reflex Decay 92569
  Audiometry
    Bekesy 92560-92561
    Comprehensive 92557
    Conditioning Play 92582
    Evoked Response 92585-92586
    Groups 92559
    Pure Tone 92552-92553
    Select Picture 92583
    Speech 92555-92556
  Brainstem Evoked Response ..92585-92586
  Central Auditory Function 92620-92621
  Ear Protector Evaluation 92596
  Electrocochleography 92584
  Filtered Speech 92571
  Hearing Aid Evaluation 92590-92595

Embryo/Fetus Monitoring
See Monitoring, Fetal

Embryonated Eggs
Inoculation 87250

Emergency Department Services 99281-99288
See Critical Care; Emergency Department Services
Anesthesia 99140
Physician Direction of Advanced
Life Support 99288

Emesis Induction 99175

EMG
See Electromyography, Needle

EMI Scan
See CT Scan

Emission Computerized Tomography 78607

Emission-Computed Tomography, Single-Photon
See SPECT

Emmet Operation
See Vagina, Repair, Obstetric

Empyema
Closure
   Chest Wall 32810
Thoracostomy 32020-32036

Empyema, Lung
See Abscess, Thorax

Empyemectomy 32540

Encephalitis
Antibody 86651-86654

Encephalitis Virus Vaccine 90735

Encephalocele
Repair 62120
   Craniotomy 62121

Encephalon
See Brain

End Stage Renal Disease Services 90918-90925

End-Expiratory Pressure, Positive
See Pressure Breathing, Positive

Endarterectomy
Coronary Artery 33572
Pulmonary 33916

Endemic Flea-Borne Typhus
See Murine Typhus

Endobronchial Challenge Tests
See Bronchial Challenge Test

Endocavitary Fulguration
See Electrocautery

Endocrine System
Unlisted Services and Procedures ..60699, 78099

Endocrine, Pancreas
See Islet Cell

Endolymphatic Sac
Exploration
   with Shunt 69806
   without Shunt 69805

Endometrial Ablation 58353
Curettage 58356
Exploration
   via Hysteroscopy 58563

Endometrioma
Abdomen
   Destruction/Excision 49200-49201
Retroperitoneal
   Destruction/Excision 49200-49201

Endometriosis, Adhesive
See Adhesions, Intrauterine

Endometrium
Ablation 58356
Biopsy 58100, 58558

Endonuclease, DNA
See DNAse

Endoscopic Retrograde Cannulation of Pancreatic Duct (ERCP)
See Cholangiopancreatography

Endoscopies, Pleural
See Thoracoscopy

Endoscopy
See Arthroscopy; Thoracoscopy
Adrenal Gland
   Biopsy 60650
   Excision 60650
Anus
   Biopsy 46606
   Dilation 46604
   Exploration 46600
   Hemorrhage 46614
   Removal
      Foreign Body 46608
      Polyp 46610, 46612
      Tumor 46610, 46612
Bile Duct
   Biopsy 47553
   Destruction
      Calculi (Stone) 43265
      Tumor 43272
   Dilation 43271, 47555-47556
   Exploration 47552
   Intraoperative 47550
   Percutaneous 47552-47555
   Removal
      Calculi (Stone) 43264, 47554
      Foreign Body 43269
      Stent 43269
   Specimen Collection 43260
   Sphincter Pressure 43263
   Sphincterotomy 43262
   Tube Placement 43267-43268

Bladder 52000
   Biopsy 52204, 52354
   Catheterization 52005, 52010
   Destruction 52354
      Lesion 52400
   Evacuation
      Clot 52001
   Excision
      Tumor 52355
   Exploration 52351
   Lithotripsy 52353
   Removal
      Calculus 52352
   Urethral Stent 52282
Bladder Neck
   Injection of Implant Material 51715
Brain
   Shunt
      Creation 62201
Bronchi
   Aspiration 31645-31646
   Biopsy 31625-31629, 31632-31633
   Destruction
      Lesion 31641
      Tumor 31641
   Dilation 31630-31631, 31636-31638
   Exploration 31622
   Injection 31656
   Lesion
      Destruction 31641
   Needle Biopsy 31629, 31633
   Placement
      Stent 31631, 31636-31637
   Revision
      Stent 31638
   Specimen Collection 31623-31624
   Stenosis 31641
   Tumor
      Destruction 31641
   Ultrasound 31620
Cervix
   Biopsy 57454-57455, 57460
   Curettage 57454, 57456
   Exploration 57452
   Loop Electrode Biopsy 57460
   Loop Electrode Conization 57461
Chest Cavity
   Exploration 32601-32606
   Surgical 32650-32665
Colon
   Biopsy 44389, 45380, 45392
   Destruction
      Lesion 44393, 45383
      Tumor 44393, 45383
   Exploration 45378
   Hemorrhage 44391, 45382
   Injection 45381
   Placement
      Stent 45387
   Removal
      Foreign Body 44390, 45379
      Polyp 44392, 45384-45385
      Tumor 44392, 45384-45385
   Specimen Collection 45380
   Ultrasound 45391-45392
   via Colotomy 45355
   via Stoma 44388-44393, 44397
   Virtual 0066T-0067T

Uterus
Anesthesia 00952
Hysteroscopy
  Diagnostic 58555
  with Division/Resection Intrauterine
  Septum 58560
  with Lysis of Intrauterine
  Adhesions 58559
Placement
  Fallopian Tube 58565
Removal
  Endometrial 58563
  Impacted Foreign Body 58562
  Leiomyomata 58561
  Surgical with Biopsy 58558
Vagina
Anesthesia 00950
Biopsy 57454
Exploration 57452
Vascular
Surgical 33508, 37500-37501
Virtual
Colon 0066T-0067T

Endosteal Implant
Reconstruction
  Mandible 21248-21249
  Maxilla 21248-21249

Endothelioma, Dural
See Meningioma

Endotracheal Intubation
See Insertion, Endotracheal Tube

Endotracheal Tube
Intubation 31500

Endovascular Repair 0033T-0040T,
  0078T-0081T, 34800-34805,
  34812-34826, 34833-34900
Angiography 75952-75954
Imaging Neck 0037T

Endovascular Therapy
Ablation
  Vein 36475-36479
Occlusion 61623

Enema
Home Visit for Fecal Impaction 99511
Intussusception 74283
Therapeutic
  for Intussusception 74283

Energies, Electromagnetic
See Irradiation

ENT
See Ear, Nose, and Throat; Otorhinolaryngology,
Diagnostic
Therapeutic
  See Otorhinolaryngology

Entamoeba Histolytica
Antigen Detection
  Enzyme Immunoassay 87336-87337

Enterectomy 44120-44121,
  44126-44128, 44137, 44202
Donor .44132-44133
with Enterostomy 44125

Enterocele
Repair 57556
Hysterectomy
  with Colpectomy 58280

Enterocystoplasty 51960
Camey 50825

Enteroenterostomy
See Anastomosis, Intestines

Enterolysis 44005
Laparoscopic 44200

Enteropancreatostomy
See Anastomosis, Pancreas to Intestines

Enterorrhaphy 44602-44603, 44615

Enterostomy 44300
Closure 44625-44626
with Enterectomy
  Intestine, Small 44125

Enterotomy 44615

Enterovirus
Antibody 86658

Entropion
Repair 67921-67924
  Excision Tarsal Wedge 67923
  Suture 67921
  Thermocauterization 67922

Enucleation
Eye
  with Implant 65103
    Muscles Attached 65105
  without Implant 65101
Pleural 32540

Enucleation, Cyst, Ovarian
See Cystectomy, Ovarian

Environmental Intervention
for Psychiatric Patients 90882

Enzyme Activity 82657
Radioactive Substrate 82658

Enzyme, Angiotensin Converting
See Angiotensin Converting Enzyme (ACE)

Enzyme, Angiotensin-Forming
See Renin

EOG
See Electro-oculography

Eosinocyte
See Eosinophils

Eosinophils
Nasal Smear 89190

Epiandrosterone 82666

Epicondylitides, Lateral Humeral
See Tennis Elbow

Epicondylitis, Radiohumeral
See Tennis Elbow

Epidemic Parotitis
See Mumps

Epididymectomy
Bilateral 54861
Unilateral 54860

Epididymis
Abscess
  Incision and Drainage 54700
Anastomosis
  to Vas Deferens
    Bilateral 54901
    Unilateral 54900
Biopsy 54800-54820
Epididymography 74440
Excision
  Bilateral .54861
  Unilateral 54860
Exploration
  Biopsy 54820
Hematoma
  Incision and Drainage 54700
Lesion
  Excision
    Local 54830
    Spermatocele 54840
Needle Biopsy 54800
Spermatocele
  Excision .54840
Unlisted Services and Procedures 55899
X-Ray with Contrast 74440

Epididymograms 55300

Epididymography 74440

Epididymoplasty
See Repair, Epididymis

Epididymovasostomy
Bilateral 54901
Unilateral 54900

Epidural
Electrode
  Insertion .61531
  Removal .61535
Injection 62281-62282, 62310-62319,
  64479-64484
Lysis 0027T, 62263-62264

Epidural Anesthesia
See Anesthesia, Epidural

Epidurography 72275

Epigastric
Hernia Repair 49572

Epiglottidectomy 31420

Epiglottis
Excision 31420

Esophagus, Varix
See Esophageal Varices

Established Patient
Confirmatory Consultations 99271-99275
Domiciliary or Rest Home Visit 99331-99333
Emergency Department Services ... 99281-99285
Home Services 99347-99350
Hospital Inpatient Services 99221-99239
Hospital Observation Services 99217-99220
Initial Inpatient Consultations 99251-99255
Office and/or Other Outpatient
  Consultations 99241-99245
Office Visit 99211-99215
Online Evaluation and Management
  Services 0074T
Outpatient Visit 99211-99215

Establishment
Colostomy
  Abdominal 50810
  Perineal 50810

Estes Operation
See Ovary, Transposition

Estlander Procedure 40525

Estradiol 82670
Response 80414

Estriol
Blood or Urine 82677

Estrogen
Blood or Urine 82671-82672
Receptor 84233

Estrone
Blood or Urine 82679

Ethanediols
See Ethylene Glycol

Ethanol
Blood 82055
Breath 82075
Urine 82055

Ethchlorovynol
See Ethchlorvynol

Ethchlorvinol
See Ethchlorvynol

Ethchlorvynol
Blood 82690
Urine 82690

Ethmoid
Fracture
  with Fixation 21340

Ethmoid, Sinus
See Sinus, Ethmoid

Ethmoidectomy 31200-31205
Endoscopic 31254-31255
Skull Base Surgery 61580-61581
with Nasal/Sinus Endoscopy 31254-31255

Ethosuccimid
See Ethosuximide

Ethosuximide 80168
Assay 80168

Ethyl Alcohol
See Ethanol

Ethylene Dichlorides
See Dichloroethane

Ethylene Glycol 82693

Ethylmethylsuccimide
See Ethosuximide

Etiocholanalone Measurement
See Etiocholanolone

Etiocholanolone 82696

ETOH
See Alcohol, Ethyl

Euglobulin Lysis 85360

European Blastomycosis
See Cryptococcus

Eustachian Tube
Catheterization 69405
Inflation
  Myringotomy 69420
    Anesthesia 69421
  with Catheterization 69400
  without Catheterization 69401
Insertion
  Catheter 69405

Eutelegenesis
See Artificial Insemination

Evacuation
Cervical Pregnancy 59140
Hematoma
  Brain 61312-61315
  Subungual 11740
Hydatidiform Mole 59870

Evaluation and Management
Assistive Technology
  Assessment 97755
Athletic Training
  Evaluation 97005
  Re-evaluation 97006
Basic Life and/or Disability
Evaluation Services 99450
Care Plan Oversight Services 99374-99380
  Home Health Agency Care 99374
  Hospice 99377-99378
  Nursing Facility 99379-99380
Case Management Services 99361-99373
Consultation 99241-99275
Critical Care 99291-99292
  Interfacility Pediatric Transport .99289-99290
Domiciliary or Rest Home 99321-99333
Emergency Department 99281-99288
Health Behavior
  Assessment 96150
  Family Intervention 96154-96155
  Group Intervention 96153
  Individual Intervention 96152
  Re-assessment 96151

Home Services 99341-99350
Hospital 99221-99233
  Discharge 99238-99239
Hospital Services
  Observation Care 99217-99220
Insurance Exam 99455-99456
Internet Communication 0074T
Low Birthweight Infant 99298-99299
Medical
  with Individual Psychotherapy
    Hospital or Residential Care 90817,
      90819, 90822, 90824, 90827, 90829
    Office or Outpatient . .90805, 90807, 90809
  with Individual Psychotherapy, Interactive
    Office or Outpatient . .90811, 90813, 90815
Neonatal Critical Care 99295-99296
Newborn Care 99431-99440
Nursing Facility 99301-99313
  See Nursing Facility Services
Occupation Therapy Evaluation 97003
  Re-evaluation 97004
Office and Other Outpatient 99201-99215
Online 0074T
Pediatric Critical Care 99293-99294
Pediatric Interfacility Transport 99289-99290
Physical Therapy Evaluation 97001
  Re-evaluation 97002
Physician Standby Services 99360
Preventive Services 99381-99429
Prolonged Services 99356-99357
Psychiatric
  Records or Reports 90885
Psychiatric Residential Treatment
Facility Care 99301-99313
Unlisted Services and Procedures 99499
Work-Related and/or Medical Disability
Evaluation 99450

Evaluation Studies, Drug, Pre-Clinical
See Drug Screen

Evisceration
Ocular Contents
  with Implant 65093
  without Implant 65091

Evisceration, Pelvic
See Exenteration, Pelvis

Evocative/Suppression Test 80400-80440
Stimulation Panel 80410

Evoked Potential
See Audiologic Function Tests
Auditory Brainstem 92585-92586
Central Motor
  Transcranial Motor Stimulation .95928-95929
Somatosensory Testing 95925-95927
Visual, CNS 95930

Evoked Potential, Auditory
See Auditory Evoked Potentials

Ewart Procedure
See Palate, Reconstruction, Lengthening

Excavatum, Pectus
See Pectus Excavatum

Exchange
Arterial Catheter 37209, 75900
Drainage Catheter
    Under Radiologic Guidance 49423
Intraocular Lens .66986

Exchange Transfusion
See Blood, Transfusion, Exchange

Excision
See Debridement; Destruction
Abscess
    Brain .61514, 61522
    Olecranon Process 24138
    Radius 24136
    Ulna 24138
Acromion
    Shoulder 23130
Adenoids 42830-42836
Adenoma
    Thyroid Gland 60200
Adrenal Gland .60540
    Laparoscopic 60650
    with Excision Retroperitoneal Tumor . .60545
Alveolus 41830
Anal Crypt 46210-46211
Anal Fissure 46200
Anal Tag 46220, 46230
Aorta
    Coarctation 33840-33851
Appendix 44950-44960
Arteriovenous Malformation
    Spinal 63250-63252
Arytenoid Cartilage 31400
    Endoscopic 31560-31561
Atrial Septum 33735-33737
Bartholin's Gland 56740
Bladder
    Diverticulum 51525
    Neck 51520
    Partial 51550-51565
    Total 51570, 51580, 51590-51597
      with Nodes 51575, 51585, 51595
    Transurethral 52640
    Tumor 51530
Bladder Neck Contracture
    Postoperative 52640
Bone
    Facial 21026
    Mandible 21025
    Postoperative
      Femur 20150
      Fibula 20150
      Radius 20150
      Tibia 20150
      Ulna 20150
Bone Abscess
    Facial 21026
    Mandible 21025
Brain
    Amygdala 61566
    Epileptogenic Focus 61536
    Hemisphere 61542-61543
    Hippocampus 61566
    Other Lobe 61323, 61539-61540
    Temporal Lobe 61537-61538

Brain Lobe
    See Lobectomy, Brain
Breast
    Biopsy 19100-19103
    Chest Wall Tumor 19260-19272
    Cyst .19120-19126
    Lactiferous Duct Fistula 19112
    Lesion 19120-19126
      by Needle Localization 19125-19126
    Mastectomy 19140-19240
    Nipple Exploration 19110
Bulbourethral Gland 53250
Bullae
    Lung 32141
      Endoscopic 32655
Burns 01951-01953, 15000-15001
Bursa
    Elbow 24105
    Femur 27062
    Ischial 27060
    Knee 27340
    Wrist .25115-25116
Bypass Graft 35901-35907
Calcaneus 28118-28120
Calculi (Stone)
    Parotid Gland 42330, 42340
    Salivary Gland 42330-42340
    Sublingual Gland 42330
    Submandibular Gland 42330-42335
Carotid Artery .60605
Carpal 25145, 25210-25215
Cartilage
    Knee Joint 27332-27333
    Shoulder Joint 23101
    Temporomandibular Joint 21060
    Wrist 25107
Caruncle
    Urethra 53265
Cataract
    Secondary 66830
Cervix
    Radical 57531
    Stump
      Abdominal Approach 57540-57545
      Vaginal Approach 57550-57556
    Total 57530
Chalazion
    Multiple
      Different Lids 67805
      Same Lid 67801
    Single 67800
    with Anesthesia 67808
Chest Wall
    Tumor 19260-19272
Choroid Plexus 61544
Clavicle
    Partial 23120, 23180
    Sequestrectomy 23170
    Total 23125
    Tumor
      Radical Resection 23200
Coccyx 27080
Colon
    Excision
      Partial 44140-44147, 44160
        with Anastomosis 44140
      Total 44150-44156

Laparoscopic
    with Anastomosis 44204, 44207-44208
    with Colostomy 44206, 44208
    with Ileocolostomy 44205
Condyle
    Temporomandibular Joint 21050
Constricting Ring
    Finger 26596
Cornea
    Epithelium 65435
      with Chelating Agent 65436
    Scraping 65430
Coronoidectomy 21070
Cowper's Gland 53250
Cranial Bone
    Tumor 61563-61564
Cyst
    See Ganglion Cyst
    Bile Duct 47715
    Bladder 51500
    Brain 61516, 61524, 62162
    Branchial 42810-42815
    Calcaneus 28100-28103
    Carpal 25130-25136
    Cheekbone .21030
    Clavicle 23140
      with Allograft 23146
      with Autograft 23145
    Facial Bones 21030
    Femur 27065-27067, 27355-27358
    Fibula 27635-27638
    Finger 26160
    Foot 28090
    Hand 26160
    Hip 27065-27067
    Humerus 23150, 24110
      with Allograft 23156, 24116
      with Autograft 23155, 24115
    Ileum 27065-27067
    Kidney 50280-50290
    Knee 27345-27347
    Lung 32140
    Mandible 21040, 21046-21047
    Maxilla 21030, 21048-21049
    Mediastinal .39200
    Mediastinum 32662
    Metacarpal 26200-26205
    Metatarsal 28104-28107
    Mullerian Duct 55680
    Nose 30124-30125
    Olecranon 24120
    Olecranon Process
      with Allograft 24126
      with Autograft 24125
    Ovarian 58925
      See Cystectomy, Ovarian
    Pericardial 33050
      Endoscopic 32661
    Phalanges 26210-26215
      Toe 28108
    Pilonidal 11770-11772
    Pubis 27066-27067
    Radius 24120, 25120-25126
      with Allograft 24126
      with Autograft 24125
    Salivary Gland 42408

Scapula 23140
   with Allograft 23146
   with Autograft 23145
Seminal Vesicle 55680
Sublingual Gland 42408
Talus 28100-28103
Tarsal 28104-28107
Thyroglossal Duct 60280-60281
Thyroid Gland 60200
Tibia 27635-27638
Toe 28092
Ulna 24120, 25120-25126
   with Allograft 24126
   with Autograft 24125
Urachal
   Bladder 51500
Vaginal 57135
Destruction of the Vestibule of the Mouth
   See Mouth, Vestibule of, Excision, Destruction
Diverticulum, Meckel's
   See Meckel's Diverticulum, Excision
Ear, External
   Partial 69110
   Total 69120
Elbow Joint 24155
Electrode 57522
Embolectomy/Thrombectomy
   Aortoiliac Artery 34151-34201
   Axillary Artery 34101
   Brachial Artery 34101
   Carotid Artery 34001
   Celiac Artery 34151
   Femoral Artery 34201
   Heart 33310-33315
   Iliac Artery 34151-34201
   Innominate Artery 34001-34101
   Mesentery Artery 34151
   Peroneal Artery 34203
   Popliteal Artery 34203
   Radial Artery 34111
   Renal Artery 34151
   Subclavian Artery 34001-34101
   Tibial Artery 34203
   Ulnar Artery 34111
Embolism
   Pulmonary Artery 33910-33916
Empyema
   Lung 32540
   Pleural 32540
Epididymis
   Bilateral 54861
   Unilateral 54860
Epiglottis 31420
Esophagus
   Diverticula 43130-43135
   Partial 43116-43124
   Total 43107-43113, 43124
Eye
   See Enucleation, Eye
Fallopian Tube
   Salpingectomy 58700
   Salpingo-Oophorectomy 58720
Fascia
   See Fasciectomy
Femur 27360
   Partial 27070-27071
Fibula 27360, 27455-27457, 27641

Fistula
   Anal 46270-46285
Foot
   Fasciectomy 28060
     Radical 28060-28062
Gallbladder 47600-47620
   Cholecystectomy 47562-47564
     with Cholangiography 47563
     with Exploration Common Duct 47564
Ganglion Cyst
   Knee 27347
   Wrist 25111-25112
Gingiva 41820
Gums 41820
   Alveolus 41830
   Operculum 41821
Heart
   Donor 33940
Heart/Lung
   Donor 33930
Hemangioma 11400-11446
Hemorrhoids 46221, 46250
   Clot 46320
   Complex 46260-46262
   Simple 46255
   with Fissurectomy 46257-46258
Hip
   Partial 27070-27071
Hippocampus 61566
Humeral Head
   Resection 23195
   Sequestrectomy 23174
Humerus 23184, 23220-23222, 24134, 24140,
                           24150-24151
Hydrocele
   Spermatic Cord 55500
   Tunica Vaginalis 55040-55041
     Bilateral 55041
     Unilateral 55040
Hygroma, Cystic
   Axillary/Cervical 38550-38555
Hymenotomy 56700
   See Hymen, Excision
Ileum
   Ileoanal Reservoir 45136
   Partial 27070-27071
Inner Ear
   See Ear, Inner, Excision
Interphalangeal Joint
   Toe 28160
Intervertebral Disk
   Decompression 63075-63078
   Hemilaminectomy 63040, 63043-63044
   Herniated 63020-63044, 63055-63066
Intestine
   Laparoscopic
     with Anastomosis 44202-44203
Intestines
   Donor 44132-44133
Intestines, Small 44120-44128
   Transplantation 44137
Iris
   Iridectomy
     Optical 66635
     Peripheral 66625
     Sector 66630

   with Corneoscleral or
     Corneal Section 66600
   with Cyclectomy 66605
Kidney
   Donor 50300-50320, 50547
   Partial 50240
   Recipient 50340
   Transplantation 50370
   with Ureters 50220-50236
Kneecap 27350
Labyrinth
   Transcanal 69905
   with Mastoidectomy 69910
Lacrimal Gland
   Partial 68505
   Total 68500
Lacrimal Sac 68520
Larynx
   Partial 31367-31382
   Total 31360-31365
   with Pharynx 31390-31395
Lesion
   Anal 45108, 46922
   Ankle 27630
     Arthroscopic 29891
   Auditory Canal, External
     Exostosis 69140
     Radical with Neck Dissection 69155
     Radical without Neck Dissection 69150
     Soft Tissue 69145
   Bladder 52224
   Brain 61534, 61536-61540
   Brainstem 61575-61576
   Carotid Body 60600-60605
   Colon 44110-44111
   Conjunctiva 68110-68130
     Over 1 cm 68115
     with Adjacent Sclera 68130
   Cornea 65400
     without Graft 65420
   Ear, Middle 69540
   Epididymis
     Local 54830
     Spermatocele 54840
   Esophagus 43100-43101
   Eye 65900
   Eyelid
     Multiple, Different Lids 67805
     Multiple, Same Lid 67801
     Single 67800
     Under Anesthesia 67808
     without Closure 67840
   Femur 27062
   Finger 26160
   Foot 28080, 28090
   Gums 41822-41828
   Hand 26160
   Intestines 44110
     Small 43250, 44111
   Intraspinal 63265-63273
   Knee 27347
   Larynx
     Endoscopic 31545-31546
   Leg, Lower 27630
   Meniscus 27347
   Mesentery 44820
   Mouth 40810-40816, 41116

Scapula
  Ostectomy 23190
  Partial 23182
  Sequestrectomy 23172
  Tumor
    Radical Resection 23210
Sclera 66160
Scrotum 55150
Semilunar Cartilage of Knee
  See Knee, Meniscectomy
Seminal Vesicle 55650
Sesamoid Bone
  Foot 28315
Sinus
  Ethmoid 31200-31205
  Maxillary 31225-31230
Skene's Gland 53270
Skin
  Excess 15831-15839
  Lesion
    Benign 11400-11471
    Malignant 11600-11646
  Nose 30120
Skin Graft
  Preparation of Site 15000
Skull 61501
Spermatic Veins 55530-55540
  Abdominal Approach 55535
  Hernia Repair 55540
Spleen 38100-38102
  Laparoscopic 38120
Stapes
  with Footplate Drill Out 69661
  without Foreign Material 69660
Sternum 21620, 21630-21632
Stomach
  Partial 43631-43639, 43845
  Total 43620-43622
Sublingual Gland 42450
Submandibular Gland 42440, 42508
Sweat Glands
  Axillary 11450-11451
  Inguinal 11462-11463
  Perianal 11470-11471
  Perineal 11470-11471
  Umbilical 11470-11471
Synovium
  Ankle 27625-27626
  Carpometacarpal Joint 26130
  Elbow 24102
  Hip Joint 27054
  Interphalangeal Joint 26140
  Intertarsal Joint 28070
  Knee Joint 27334-27335
  Metacarpophalangeal Joint 26135
  Metatarsophalangeal Joint 28072
  Shoulder 23105-23106
  Tarsometatarsal Joint 28070
  Wrist 25105, 25118-25119
Talus 28120, 28130
Tarsal 28116, 28122
Temporal Bone 69535
Temporal, Petrous
  Apex 69530
Tendon
  Finger 26180, 26390, 26415
  Hand 26390, 26415
  Palm 26170

Tendon Sheath
  Finger 26145
  Foot 28086-28088
  Palm 26145
  Wrist 25115-25116
Testis
  Laparoscopic 54690
  Partial 54522
  Radical 54530-54535
  Simple 54520
  Tumor 54530-54535
Thrombectomy
  Axillary Vein 34490
  Bypass Graft 35875-35876
  Femoropopliteal Vein 34401-34451
  Iliac Vein 34401-34451
  Subclavian Vein 34471-34490
  Vena Cava 34401-34451
Thromboendarterectomy
  Aorta, Abdominal 35331
  Aortoiliofemoral 35363
  Axillary Artery 35321
  Brachial Artery 35321
  Carotid Artery 35301, 35390
  Celiac Artery 35341
  Femoral Artery 35371-35381
  Iliac 35361-35363
  Iliac Artery 35351
  Iliofemoral Artery 35355, 35363
  Innominate Artery 35311
  Mesenteric Artery 35341
  Peroneal Artery 35381
  Popliteal Artery 35381
  Renal Artery 35341
  Subclavian Artery 35301-35311
  Tibial Artery 35381
  Vertebral Artery 35301
Thymus Gland 60521
Thyroid Gland for Malignancy
  Partial 60210-60225
  Removal All Thyroid Tissue 60260
  Secondary 60260
  Total 60240
    Cervical Approach 60271
    Limited Neck Dissection 60252
    Radical Neck Dissection 60254
    Sternal Split/Transthoracic
    Approach 60270
Tibia 27360, 27640
Tongue
  Complete 41140-41155
  Frenum 41115
  Partial 41120-41135
  with Mouth Resection 41150-41153
  with Radical Neck 41135, 41145-41155
Tonsils 42825-42826
  Lingual 42870
  Radical 42842-42845
  Tag 42860
  with Adenoids 42820-42821
Torus Mandibularis 21031
Trachea
  Stenosis 31780-31781
Transcervical Approach 60520
Tricuspid Valve 33460
Tumor
  Abdominal Wall 22900
  Acetabulum 27076

Ankle 27615-27619
Arm, Lower 25075-25077
Arm, Upper 24075-24077
Back/Flank 21930
Bile Duct 47711-47712
Bladder 51530, 52234-52240, 52355
Brain 61510, 61518, 61520-61521,
              61526-61530, 61545, 62164
Bronchi 31640
Calcaneus 27647, 28100-28103
Carpal 25130-25136
Cheekbone ...21030, 21034, 21048-21049
Clavicle 23140
  with Allograft 23146
  with Autograft 23145
Ear, Middle
  Extended 69554
  Transcanal 69550
  Transmastoid 69552
Elbow 24075-24077
Esophagus
  Endoscopic Ablation 43228
Facial Bones 21029-21030,
              21034-21040, 21046-21049
Facial Tissue 21015
Femur ...27065-27067, 27355-27358, 27365
Fibula 27635-27638, 27646
Finger 26115-26117
Foot 28043-28046
Gums 41825-41827
Hand 26115-26117
Heart 33120-33130
Hip 27047-27049, 27065-27067
  Radical 27075-27076
Humerus 23150, 23220-23222,
              24110-24115
  with Allograft 23156, 24116
  with Autograft 23155, 24116
Ileum 27065-27067
Innominate 27077
Intestines
  Small 43250
Ischial 27078-27079
Kidney 52355
Knee 27327-27329, 27365
Lacrimal Gland
  Frontal Approach 68540
  Involving Osteotomy 68550
Larynx 31300
  Endoscopic 31540-31541, 31578
Leg, Lower 27615-27619
Leg, Upper 27327-27329
Mandible 21040-21047
Maxilla 21030, 21034, 21048-21049
Mediastinal 39220
Mediastinum 32662
Metacarpal 26200-26205
  Radical 26250-26255
Metatarsal 28104-28107, 28173
Neck 21555-21557
Olecranon Process 24120
  with Allograft 24126
  with Autograft 24125
Parotid Gland 42410-42426
Pelvis 27047-27049
Pericardial 33050
Pericardium 32661

Exploration, Larynx by Incision

Exploratory Laparotomy

Expression

Exteriorization, Small Intestine

External Auditory Canal

External Cephalic Version 59412

External Ear

External Extoses

External Fixation

Extirpation, Lacrimal Sac

Extracorporeal Circulation 33960-33961

Extracorporeal Dialyses

Extracorporeal Membrane Oxygenation

Extracorporeal Photochemotherapies

Extracorporeal Shock Wave Therapy

Extracranial

Extraction

Extraction, Cataract

Extradural Anesthesia

Extradural Injection

Extraocular Muscle

Extrauterine Pregnancy

Extravasation Blood

Extremity

Eye

Repair with Graft
Retraction .67911
Skin Graft
Full Thickness 67961
Split 67961
Suture 67880
with Transposition of Tarsal Plate 67882
Tissue Transfer, Adjacent 67961
Unlisted Services and Procedures 67999

Eyelid Ptoses
See Blepharoptosis

F

Face
CT Scan 70486-70488
Lesion
Destruction 17000-17004, 17280-17286
Magnetic Resonance Imaging
(MRI) 70540-70543
Tumor Resection .21015

Face Lift 15824-15828

Facial Asymmetries
See Hemifacial Microsomia

Facial Bone
See Mandible; Maxilla
Tumor
Excision 21034

Facial Bones
Abscess
Excision 21026
Reconstruction
Secondary .21275
Repair 21208-21209
Tumor
Excision 21029-21030
Resection
Radical .21015
X-Ray 70140-70150

Facial Nerve
Anastomosis
to Hypoglossal 64868
to Phrenic Nerve 64870
to Spinal Accessory 64866
Avulsion 64742
Decompression 61590, 61596
Intratemporal
Lateral to Geniculate
Ganglion 69720, 69740
Medial to Geniculate
Ganglion 69725, 69745
Total 69955
Function Study .92516
Incision 64742
Injection
Anesthetic 64402
Mobilization 61590

Repair
Lateral to Geniculate Ganglion 69740
Medial to Geniculate Ganglion 69745
Repair/Suture
with or without Graft 64864-64865
Suture
Lateral to Geniculate Ganglion 69740
Medial to Geniculate Ganglion 69745
Transection 64742

Facial Nerve Paralysis
Graft .15840-15845
Repair 15840-15845

Facial Prosthesis
Impression 21088

Facial Rhytidectomy
See Face Lift

Factor I
See Fibrinogen

Factor II
See Prothrombin

Factor III
See Thromboplastin

Factor IV
See Calcium

Factor VII
See Proconvertin

Factor VIII
See Clotting Factor

Factor IX
See Christmas Factor

Factor X
See Stuart-Prower Factor

Factor X, Activated
See Thrombokinase

Factor Xa Inhibitor
See Antithrombin III

Factor XI
See Plasma Thromboplastin, Antecedent

Factor XII
See Hageman Factor

Factor XIII
See Fibrin Stabilizing Factor

Factor, ACTH-Releasing
See Corticotropic Releasing Hormone (CRH)

Factor, Antinuclear
See Antinuclear Antibodies (ANA)

Factor, Blood Coagulation
See Clotting Factor

Factor, Fitzgerald
See Fitzgerald Factor

Factor, Fletcher
See Fletcher Factor

Factor, Hyperglycemic-Glycogenolytic
See Glucagon

Factor Inhibitor Test 85335

Factor, Intrinsic
See Intrinsic Factor

Factor, Rheumatoid
See Rheumatoid Factor

Factor, Sulfation
See Somatomedin

Fallopian Tube
Anastomosis 58750
Catheterization 58345, 74742
Destruction
Endoscopy .58670
Ectopic Pregnancy 59121
with Salpingectomy and/or
Oophorectomy 59120
Excision 58700-58720
Ligation 58600-58611
Lysis
Adhesions .58740
Occlusion 58615
Endoscopy .58671
Placement
Implant for Occlusion 58565
Repair 58752
Anastomosis 58750
Create Stoma 58770
Tumor
Resection 58950, 58952-58956
Unlisted Services and Procedures 58999
X-Ray 74742

Fallopian Tube Pregnancy
See Ectopic Pregnancy, Tubal

Fallot, Tetralogy of
See Tetralogy of Fallot

Family Psychotherapy
See Psychotherapy, Family

Fanconi Anemia
Chromosome Analysis 88248

Farnsworth-Munsell Color Test
See Color Vision Examination

Farr Test
See Gammaglobulin, Blood

Fasanella-Servat Procedure . . .67908

Fascia Graft 15840

Fascia Lata Graft
Harvesting 20920-20922

Fascial Defect
Repair 50728

Fascial Graft
Free
Microvascular Anastomosis 15758
Open Treatment
Sternoclavicular Dislocation 23532

Fluid Drainage 59074
Shunt Placement 59076
Unlisted 59897

Fetal Testing
Amniotic Fluid
    Lung Maturity 83661, 83663-83664
Heart 76825-76826
    Doppler
        Complete 76827
        Follow-up or Repeat Study 76828
Hemoglobin 83030-83033, 85460
Ultrasound 76801-76828
    Heart 76825
    Middle Cerebral Artery 76821
    Umbilical Artery 76820

Fetuin
See Alpha-Fetoprotein

Fever, Australian Q
See Q Fever

Fever, Japanese River
See Scrub Typhus

Fibrillation
Atrial 33253

Fibrillation, Heart
See Heart, Fibrillation

Fibrin Degradation Products 85362-85380

Fibrin Deposit
Removal 32150

Fibrin Stabilizing Factor 85290-85291

Fibrinase
See Plasmin

Fibrinogen 85384-85385

Fibrinolysin
See Plasmin

Fibrinolysins 85390

Fibrinolysis
Alpha-2 Antiplasmin 85410
Assay 85396
Plasmin 85400
Plasminogen 85420-85421
Plasminogen Activator 85415

Fibroadenoma
Excision 19120-19126

Fibroblastoma, Arachnoidal
See Meningioma

Fibrocutaneous Tags 11200-11201

Fibromatosis, Dupuytren's
See Dupuytren's Contracture

Fibromatosis, Penile
See Peyronie Disease

Fibromyoma
See Leiomyomata

Fibronectin, Fetal 82731

Fibrosis, Penile
See Peyronie Disease

Fibrosis, Retroperitoneal
See Retroperitoneal Fibrosis

Fibrous Cavernitides
See Peyronie Disease

Fibrous Dysplasia ...21029, 21181-21184

Fibula
See Ankle; Knee; Tibia
Bone Graft with Microvascular
Anastomosis 20955
Craterization 27360, 27641
Cyst
    Excision 27635-27638
Diaphysectomy 27360, 27641
Excision 27360, 27641
    Epiphyseal Bar 20150
Fracture
    Malleolus 27786-27814
    Shaft 27780-27784
Incision 27607
Osteoplasty
    Lengthening 27715
Repair
    Epiphysis 27477-27485, 27730-27742
    Osteotomy 27707-27712
Saucerization 27360, 27641
Tumor
    Excision 27635-27638, 27646
X-Ray 73590

Figure of Eight Cast 29049

Filariasis 86280

Filtering Operation
See Incision, Sclera, Fistulization; Incision and Drainage

Filtration Implant, Glaucoma
See Aqueous Shunt

Fimbrioplasty 58760
Laparoscopic 58672

Fine Needle Aspiration ...10021-10022
Evaluation 88172-88173

Finger
See Phalanx, Finger
Abscess
    Bone
        Incision and Drainage 26034
        Incision and Drainage 26010-26011
Amputation 26951-26952
    with Exploration or Removal 26910
Arthrocentesis 20600
Arthrodesis
    Interphalangeal Joint 26860-26863
    Metacarpophalangeal Joint 26850-26852
Bone
    Incision and Drainage 26034
Cast 29086
Collection of Blood 36415-36416
Decompression 26035

Excision
    Constricting Ring 26596
    Tendon 26180, 26390, 26415
Insertion
    Tendon Graft 26392
Magnetic Resonance Imaging (MRI) 73221
Reconstruction
    Extra Digit 26587
    Toe to Hand Transfer 26551-26556
Removal
    Implantation 26320
    Tube 26392, 26416
Repair
    Blood Vessel 35207
    Claw Finger 26499
    Extra Digit 26587
    Macrodactylia 26590
    Tendon
        Extensor 26415-26434,
            26445-26449, 26460
        Flexor 26356-26358,
            26440-26442, 26455
        Volar Plate 26548
        Web Finger 26560-26562
Replantation 20816-20822
Reposition 26555
Sesamoidectomy 26185
Splint 29130-29131
Strapping 29280
Tendon Sheath
    Excision 26145
    Incision 26055
    Incision and Drainage 26020
Tenotomy 26060, 26460
    Flexor 26455
Tumor
    Excision 26115-26117
Unlisted Services and Procedures 26989
X-Ray 73140

Finger Flap
Tissue Transfer 14350

Finger Joint
See Intercarpal Joint

Finney Operation
See Gastroduodenostomy

FISH
See Fluorescent In Situ Hybridization

Fishberg Concentration Test
See Water Load Test

Fissure in Ano
See Anus, Fissure

Fissurectomy 46200

Fissurectomy, Anal
See Anus, Fissure, Excision

Fistula
Anal
    Repair 46288, 46706
Autogenous Graft 36825
Bronchi
    Repair 32815

Spine/Paraspinous
　　Guide Catheter/Needle 76005
Unlisted Services and Procedures 76496
Ureter
　　Guide Catheter 74480
Venous Access Device 75998
Vertebra
　　Osteoplasty 76012

Flurazepam
Blood or Urine 82742

Flush Aortogram 75722-75724

FNA
See Fine Needle Aspiration

Foam Stability Test 83662

Fold, Vocal
See Vocal Cords

Foley Operation Pyeloplasty
See Pyeloplasty

Foley Y-Pyeloplasty 50400-50405

Folic Acid 82747
Blood 82746

Follicle Stimulating Hormone
(FSH) 80418, 80426, 83001

Folliculin
See Estrone

Follitropin
See Follicle Stimulating Hormone (FSH)

Follow-up Inpatient Consultations
See Consultation, Follow-up Inpatient

Follow-up Services
See Hospital Services; Office and/or Other
Outpatient Services
Inpatient Consultations 99261-99263
Post-Op 99024

Fontan Procedure
See Repair, Heart, Anomaly; Revision

Food Allergy Test 95075
See Allergy Tests

Foot
See Metatarsal; Tarsal
Amputation 28800-28805
Bursa
　　Incision and Drainage 28001
Capsulotomy 28260-28264
Cast 29450
Fasciectomy .28060
　　Radical 28060-28062
Fasciotomy .28008
　　Endoscopic 29893
Incision 28002-28005
Joint
　　See Talotarsal Joint; Tarsometatarsal Joint
　　Magnetic Resonance Imaging
　　(MRI) 73721-73723
Lesion
　　Excision 28080, 28090

Magnetic Resonance Imaging
(MRI) 73718-73720
Nerve
　　Excision .28030
　　Incision .28035
Neuroma
　　Excision .28080
Reconstruction
　　Cleft Foot 28360
Removal
　　Foreign Body 28190-28193
Repair
　　Muscle .28250
　　Tendon 28200-28230, 28234-28238
Replantation 20838
Sesamoid
　　Excision .28315
Splint 29590
Strapping 29540, 29590
Suture
　　Tendon 28200-28210
Tendon Sheath
　　Excision 28086-28088
Tenotomy 28230, 28234
Tumor
　　Excision 28043-28046
Unlisted Services and Procedures 28899
X-Ray 73620-73630

Foot Abscess
See Abscess, Foot

Foot Navicular Bone
See Navicular

Forearm 20805
See Arm, Lower

Forehead
Reconstruction 21179-21180, 21182-21184
　　Midface 21159-21160
Reduction 21137-21139

Forehead and Orbital Rim
Reconstruction 21172-21180

Foreign Body Removal
Pharynx 42809
Shoulder 23331

Forensic Exam 88040
Cytopathology 88125
Phosphatase, Acid 84061

Foreskin of Penis
See Penis, Prepuce

Formycin Diphosphate
See Fibrin Degradation Products

Fournier's Gangrene
See Debridement, Skin, Subcutaneous Tissue,
Infected

Fowler-Stephens Orchiopexy
See Orchiopexy

Fowler-Stephens Procedure . . .54650

Fox Operation
See Entropion, Repair

Fraction, Factor IX
See Christmas Factor

Fracture
Acetabulum
　　Closed Treatment 27220-27222
　　Open Treatment 27226-27228
　　with Manipulation 27222
　　without Manipulation 27220
Alveola
　　Closed Treatment 21421
　　Open Treatment 21422-21423
Alveolar Ridge
　　Closed Treatment 21440
　　Open Treatment 21445
Ankle
　　Closed Treatment 27816-27818
　　Lateral 27786-27814
　　Medial 27760-27766, 27808-27814
　　Open Treatment 27822-27823
　　Trimalleolar 27816-27823
　　with Manipulation 27818
　　without Manipulation 27816
Ankle Bone
　　Medial 27760-27762
Bennett's
　　See Thumb, Fracture
Bronchi
　　Endoscopy 31630
Calcaneus
　　Closed Treatment 28400-28405
　　Open Treatment 28415-28420
　　Percutaneous Fixation 28436
　　with Manipulation 28405-28406
　　without Manipulation 28400
Carpal
　　Closed Treatment
　　　with Manipulation 25624, 25635
　　　without Manipulation 25622, 25630
　　Open Treatment 25628, 25645
Carpal Scaphoid
　　Closed Treatment 25622
Cheekbone
　　Open Treatment 21360-21366
　　with Manipulation 21355
Clavicle
　　Closed Treatment
　　　with Manipulation 23505
　　　without Manipulation 23500
　　Open Treatment 23515
Closed Treatment 27520
Coccyx
　　Closed Treatment 27200
　　Open Treatment 27202
Colles
　　See Colles Fracture
Colles-Reversed
　　See Smith Fracture
Elbow
　　Monteggia
　　　Closed Treatment 24620
　　　Open Treatment 24635
　　Open Treatment 24586-24587
Femur 27244
Femur
　　Closed Treatment 27230, 27238-27240,
　　　　　　　　27246, 27500-27503, 27508,
　　　　　　　　27510, 27516-27517
　　with Manipulation 27232

Finger/Thumb
  Closed Treatment 26720-26725
    Shaft 26720, 26727
    with Manipulation 26725-26727
Great Toe 28490
  Closed Treatment 28495
  Open Treatment 28505
  Percutaneous Fixation 28496
  with Manipulation 28495-28496
Open Treatment 26735, 26746
  Distal 26765
Shaft
  Closed Treatment 26725
  Open Treatment 26735
  Percutaneous Fixation 26727
Toe
  Closed Treatment 28515
  Open Treatment 28525
  with Manipulation 28515
  without Manipulation 28510
  with Manipulation 26742, 26755
  without Manipulation 26740, 26750
Radius
  Closed Treatment 25560-25565
  Colles 25600-25605
  Distal 25600-25611
    Open Treatment 25620
    Smith 25600-25620
  Head/Neck
    Closed Treatment 24650-24655
    Open Treatment 24665-24666
  Open Treatment 25515, 25620
  Percutaneous Fixation 25611
  Shaft 25500, 25525-25526
    Closed Treatment 25500-25505, 25520
    Open Treatment 25515, 25525-25526,
                      25574
  with Manipulation 25565, 25605
  with Ulna 25560-25565
    Open Treatment 25575
  without Manipulation 25560, 25600
Rib
  Closed Treatment 21800
  External Fixation 21810
  Open Treatment 21805
Scaphoid
  Closed Treatment 25622
  Open Treatment 25628
  with Dislocation
    Closed Treatment 25680
    Open Treatment 25685
  with Manipulation 25624
Scapula
  Closed Treatment
    with Manipulation 23575
    without Manipulation 23570
  Open Treatment 23585
Sesamoid
  Closed Treatment 28530
  Foot 28530-28531
  Open Treatment 28531
Skin
  Debridement 11010-11012
Skull 62000-62010
  Closed Treatment 21300
Sternum
  Closed Treatment 21820
  Open Treatment 21825

Talus
  Closed Treatment 28430-28435
  Open Treatment 28445
  with Manipulation 28435-28436
  without Manipulation 28430
Tarsal
  Open Treatment 28465
  Percutaneous Fixation 28456
  with Manipulation 28455-28456
Thumb
  with Dislocation 26645-26650
    Open Treatment 26665
Tibia 27759
Tibia
  Arthroscopic Treatment 29855-29856
  Closed Treatment 27530-27532, 27538,
              27750-27752, 27760-27762,
              27808-27810, 27824-27825
  Distal 27824-27828
  Intercondylar 27538-27540
  Malleolus 27760-27766, 27808-27814
  Open Treatment 27535-27536, 27540,
             27758, 27766, 27814, 27826-27828
  Percutaneous Fixation 27756
  Plateau 27530-27536, 29855-29856
  Shaft 27750-27759
  with Manipulation 27752, 27760-27762,
                         27810
  without Manipulation 27530, 27750,
             27760-27762, 27808, 27825
Trachea
  Endoscopy 31630
Ulna
  See Elbow; Humerus; Radius
  Closed Treatment 25560-25565
  Olecranon
    Closed Treatment 24670-24675
    Open Treatment 24685
  Open Treatment 25574-25575
  Shaft
    Closed Treatment 25530-25535
    Open Treatment 25545, 25574
  Styloid Process
    Closed Treatment 25650
    Open Treatment 25652
    Percutaneous Fixation 25651
  with Dislocation
    Closed Treatment 24620
    Monteggia 24620-24635
    Open Treatment 24635
  with Manipulation 25535, 25565
  with Radius 25560-25565
    Open Treatment 25575
  without Manipulation 25530, 25560
Vertebra
  Additional Segment
    Open Treatment 22328
  Cervical
    Open Treatment 22326
  Closed Treatment
    with Manipulation, Casting and/or
      Bracing 22315
    without Manipulation 22310
  Lumbar
    Open Treatment 22325
  Posterior
    Open Treatment 22325-22327

Thoracic
  Open Treatment 22327
  with Shoulder Dislocation
    Closed Treatment 23675
    Open Treatment 23680
Vertebral Process
  Closed Treatment 22305
Wrist
  with Dislocation
    Closed Treatment 25680
    Open Treatment 25685
Zygomatic Arch
  Open Treatment 21356-21366
  with Manipulation 21355

Fragile-X
Chromosome Analysis 88248

Fragility
Red Blood Cell
  Mechanical 85547
  Osmotic 85555-85557

Frames, Stereotactic
See Stereotactic Frame

Francisella 86000
Antibody 86668

Fredet-Ramstedt Procedure 43520

Free E3
See Estriol

Free Skin Graft
See Skin, Grafts, Free

Free T4
See Thyroxine, Free

Frei Disease
See Lymphogranuloma Venereum

Frenectomy 40819, 41115

Frenectomy, Lingual
See Excision, Tongue, Frenum

Frenotomy 40806, 41010

Frenulectomy 40819

Frenuloplasty 41520

Frenum
Lip
  Incision 40806
    See Lip

Frenumectomy 40819

Frickman Operation
See Proctopexy

Frontal Craniotomy 61556

Frontal Sinus
See Sinus, Frontal

Frontal Sinusotomy
See Exploration, Sinus, Frontal

Frost Suture 67875

Frozen Blood Preparation 86930-86932

Fructose 84375
Semen 82757

Fructose Intolerance Breath Test 91065

Fruit Sugar
See Fructose

FSF 85290-85291

FSH
See Follicle Stimulating Hormone (FSH)

FSP
See Fibrin Degradation Products

FT-4 84439

Fulguration
See Destruction
Bladder 51020
Cystourethroscopy with 52214
    Lesion 52224
    Tumor 52234-52240
Ureter 50957, 50976
Ureterocele
    Ectopic 52301
    Orthotopic 52300

Fulguration, Endocavitary
See Electrocautery

Full Thickness Graft 15200-15261

Function Test, Lung
See Pulmonology, Diagnostic

Function Test, Vestibular
See Vestibular Function Tests

Function, Study, Nasal
See Nasal Function Study

Functional Ability
See Activities of Daily Living

Fundoplasty
Esophagogastric 43324-43325
    Laparoscopic 43280
    with Gastroplasty 43326

Fundoplication
See Fundoplasty, Esophagogastric

Fungus
Antibody 86671
Culture
    Blood 87103
    Hair 87101
    Identification 87106
    Nail 87101
    Other 87102
    Skin 87101
Tissue Exam 87220

Funnel Chest
See Pectus Excavatum

Furuncle
Incision and Drainage 10060-10061

Furuncle, Vulva
See Abscess, Vulva

Fusion
See Arthrodesis
Pleural Cavity 32005
Thumb
    in Opposition 26820

Fusion, Epiphyseal-Diaphyseal
See Epiphyseal Arrest

Fusion, Joint
See Arthrodesis

Fusion, Joint, Ankle
See Ankle, Arthrodesis

Fusion, Joint, Interphalangeal, Finger
See Arthrodesis, Finger Joint, Interphalangeal

G

Gago Procedure
See Repair, Tricuspid Valve; Revision

Gait Training 97116
See Physical Medicine/Therapy/Occupational Therapy

Galactogram 76086-76088
Injection 19030

Galactokinase
Blood 82759

Galactose
Blood 82760
Urine 82760

Galactose-1-Phosphate
Uridyl Transferase 82775-82776

Gall Bladder
See Gallbladder

Gallbladder
See Bile Duct
Anastomosis
    with Intestines 47720-47741
Excision 47562-47564, 47600-47620
Exploration 47480
Incision 47490
Incision and Drainage 47480
Nuclear Medicine
    Imaging 78223
Removal
    Calculi (Stone) 47480
Repair
    with Gastroenterostomy 47741
    with Intestines 47720-47740
Unlisted Services and Procedures 47999
X-Ray with Contrast 74290-74291

Galvanocautery
See Electrocautery

Galvanoionization
See Iontophoresis

Gamete Intrafallopian Transfer (GIFT) 58976

Gamete Transfer
In Vitro Fertilization 58976

Gamma Camera Imaging
See Nuclear Medicine

Gamma Glutamyl Transferase 82977

Gamma Seminoprotein
See Antigen, Prostate Specific

Gammacorten
See Dexamethasone

Gammaglobulin
Blood 82784-82787

Gamulin Rh
See Immune Globulins, Rho (D)

Ganglia, Trigeminal
See Gasserian Ganglion

Ganglion
See Gasserian Ganglion
Cyst
    Aspiration/Injection 20612
    Drainage 20612
    Wrist
        Excision 25111-25112
Injection
    Anesthetic 64505, 64510

Ganglion Cervicothoracicum
See Stellate Ganglion

Ganglion Pterygopalatinum
See Sphenopalatine Ganglion

Ganglion, Gasser's
See Gasserian Ganglion

Gardner Operation
See Meningocele Repair

Gardnerella Vaginalis Detection 87510-87512

Gasser Ganglion
See Gasserian Ganglion

Gasserian Ganglion
Sensory Root
    Decompression 61450
    Section 61450
Stereotactic 61790

Gastrectomy
Partial 43631-43639, 43845
    with Gastrojejunostomy 43632
Total 43621-43622
    with Esophagoenterostomy 43620
with Gastroduodenostomy 43631

Gastric Acid 82926-82928

GI Tract
See Gastrointestinal Tract

Giardia
Antigen Detection
    Enzyme Immunoassay 87329
    Immunofluorescence 87269

Giardia Lamblia
Antibody 86674

Gibbons Stent 52332

GIF
See Somatostatin

GIFT
See Gamete Intrafallopian Transfer

Gill Operation 63012

Gillies Approach
Fracture
    Zygomatic Arch 21356

Gingiva
See Gums

Gingiva, Abcess
See Abscess
Fracture
    See Abscess, Gums; Gums
    Zygomatic Arch
        See Abscess, Gums; Gums, Abscess

Gingivectomy 41820

Gingivoplasty 41872

Girdlestone Laminectomy
See Laminectomy

Girdlestone Procedure
See Acetabulum, Reconstruction

Gla Protein (Bone)
See Osteocalcin

Gland
See Specific Gland

Gland, Adrenal
See Adrenal Gland

Gland, Bartholin's
See Bartholin's Gland

Gland, Bulbourethral
See Bulbourethral Gland

Gland, Lacrimal
See Lacrimal Gland

Gland, Mammary
See Breast

Gland, Parathyroid
See Parathyroid Gland

Gland, Parotid
See Parotid Gland

Gland, Pituitary
See Pituitary Gland

Gland, Salivary
See Salivary Glands

Gland, Sublingual
See Sublingual Gland

Gland, Sweat
See Sweat Glands

Gland, Thymus
See Thymus Gland

Gland, Thyroid
See Thyroid Gland

Glasses
See Spectacle Services

Glaucoma
Cryotherapy 66720
Cyclophotocoagulation 66710, 66711
Diathermy 66700
Fistulization of Sclera 66150
Provocative Test 92140

Glaucoma Drainage Implant
See Aqueous Shunt

Glenn Procedure 33766-33767

Glenohumeral Joint
Arthrotomy 23040
    with Biopsy 23100
    with Synovectomy 23105
Exploration 23107
Removal
    Foreign or Loose Body 23107

Glenoid Fossa
Reconstruction 21255

GLN
See Glutamine

Globulin
Antihuman 86880-86886
Immune .90281-90399
Sex Hormone Binding 84270

Globulin, Corticosteroid-Binding
See Transcortin

Globulin, Rh Immune
See Immune Globulins, Rho (D)

Globulin, Thyroxine-Binding
See Thyroxine Binding Globulin

Glomerular Procoagulant Activity
See Thromboplastin

Glomus Caroticum
See Carotid Body

Glossectomies
See Excision, Tongue

Glossopexy
See Tongue, Fixation

Glossorrhaphy
See Suture, Tongue

Glucagon 82943
Tolerance Panel 80422-80424
Tolerance Test 82946

Glucose . . .80422-80424, 80430-80435, 95250
Blood Test 82947-82950, 82962
Body Fluid 82945
Interstitial Fluid
    Continuous Monitoring 95250
Tolerance Test 82951-82952
    with Tolbutamide 82953

Glucose Phosphate Isomerase
See Phosphohexose Isomerase

Glucose Phosphate Isomerase Measurement
See Phosphohexose Isomerase

Glucose-6-Phosphate
Dehydrogenase 82955-82960

Glucosidase 82963

Glucuronide Androstanediol . . .82154

Glue
Cornea Wound 65286
Sclera Wound .65286

Glukagon
See Glucagon

Glutamate Dehydrogenase
Blood 82965

Glutamate Pyruvate Transaminase
See Transaminase, Glutamic Pyruvic

Glutamic Alanine Transaminase
See Transaminase, Glutamic Pyruvic

Glutamic Aspartic Transaminase
See Transaminase, Glutamic Oxaloacetic

Glutamic Dehydrogenase
See Glutamate Dehydrogenase

Glutamine .82975

Glutamyltransferase, Gamma . .82977

Glutathione 82978

Glutathione Reductase 82979

Glutethimide 82980

Glycanhydrolase, N-Acetylmuramide
See Lysozyme

Glycated Hemoglobins
See Glycohemoglobin

Glycated Protein 82985

Glycerol Phosphoglycerides
See Phosphatidylglycerol

Glycerol, Phosphatidyl
See Phosphatidylglycerol

Glycerophosphatase
See Alkaline Phosphatase

Glycinate, Theophylline Sodium
See Theophylline

Glycocholic Acid
See Cholylglycine

Glycohemoglobin 83036

Glycol, Ethylene
See Ethylene Glycol

Glycols, Ethylene
See Ethylene Glycol

Glycosaminoglycan
See Mucopolysaccharides

GMP
See Guanosine Monophosphate

GMP, Cyclic
See Cyclic GMP

Goeckerman Treatment ...96910-96913

Gol-Vernet Operation
See Pyelotomy, Exploration

Gold
Assay 80172

Goldwaite Procedure 27422

Golfer's Elbow
See Tennis Elbow

Gonadectomy, Female
See Oophorectomy

Gonadectomy, Male
See Excision, Testis

Gonadotropin
Chorionic 84702-84703
FSH 83001
ICSH 83002
LH 83002

Gonadotropin Panel 80426

Gonioscopy 92020

Goniotomy 65820

Gonococcus
See Neisseria Gonorrhoeae

Goodenough Harris Drawing Test 96100

GOTT
See Transaminase, Glutamic Oxaloacetic

GPUT
See Galactose-1-Phosphate, Uridyl Transferase

Graft
See Bone Graft; Bypass Graft
Anal 46753
Aorta 33840-33851, 33860-33877
Artery
   Coronary 33503-33505
Bone
  See Bone Marrow, Transplantation
   Harvesting 20900-20902
   Microvascular Anastomosis 20955-20962

Osteocutaneous Flap with Microvascular
   Anastomosis 20969-20973
   Vascular Pedicle 25430
Bone and Skin 20969-20973
Cartilage
   Ear to Face 21235
   Harvesting 20910-20912
    See Cartilage Graft
   Rib to Face 21230
Conjunctiva 65782
   Harvesting 68371
Cornea
   with Lesion Excision 65426
Cornea Transplant
   in Aphakia 65750
   in Pseudophakia 65755
   Lamellar 65710
   Penetrating 65730
Dura
   Spinal Cord 63710
Endovascular 34900
Eye
   Amniotic Membrane 65780
   Conjunctiva 65782
   Stem Cell 65781
Facial Nerve Paralysis 15840-15845
Fascia
   Cheek 15840
Fascia Lata
   Harvesting 20920-20922
Gum Mucosa 41870
Heart
  See Heart, Transplantation
Heart Lung
  See Transplantation, Heart-Lung
Kidney
  See Kidney, Transplantation
Liver
  See Liver, Transplantation
Lung
  See Lung, Transplantation
Muscle
   Cheek 15841-15845
Nail Bed
   Reconstruction 11762
Nerve 64885-64907
Oral Mucosa 40818
Organ
  See Transplantation
Pancreas
  See Pancreas, Transplantation
Skin
   Biological
    See Allograft, Skin
   Blood Flow Check, Graft 15860
    See Skin Graft and Flap
   Vascular Flow Check, Graft 15860
Tendon
   Finger 26392
   Hand 26392
   Harvesting 20924
Tissue
   Harvesting 20926
Vein
   Cross-Over 34520

Grain Alcohol
See Alcohol, Ethyl

Granulation Tissue
Cauterization, Chemical 17250

Gravi, Myasthenia
See Myasthenia Gravis

Gravities, Specific
See Specific Gravity

Great Toe
Free Osteocutaneous Flap with
Microvascular Anastomosis 20973

Great Vessels
Shunt
   Aorta to Pulmonary Artery
    Ascending 33755
    Descending 33762
    Central 33764
   Subclavian to Pulmonary Artery 33750
   Vena Cava to Pulmonary Artery .33766-33767
Unlisted Services and Procedures 33999

Great Vessels Transposition
See Transposition, Great Arteries

Greater Tuberosity Fracture
with Shoulder Dislocation
   Closed Treatment 23665
   Open Treatment 23670

Greater Vestibular Gland
See Bartholin's Gland

Green Operation
See Scapulopexy

Gridley Stain 88312

Grippe, Balkan
See Q Fever

Gritti Operation
See Amputation, Leg, Upper; Radical Resection;
Replantation

Groin Area
Repair
   Hernia 49550-49557

Group Health Education 99078

Grouping, Blood
See Blood Typing

Growth Factors, Insulin-Like
See Somatomedin

Growth Hormone 83003
Human 80418, 80428-80430, 86277

Growth Hormone Release Inhibiting Factor
See Somatostatin

GTT
See Hydatidiform Mole

Guaiac Test
See Blood, Feces

Guanosine Monophosphate 83008

Guanosine Monophosphate, Cyclic
See Cyclic GMP

Guanylic Acids
See Guanosine Monophosphate

Guard Stain 88313

Gullet
See Esophagus

Gums
Abscess
   Incision and Drainage 41800
Alveolus
   Excision 41830
Cyst
   Incision and Drainage 41800
Excision
   Gingiva 41820
   Operculum 41821
Graft
   Mucosa 41870
Hematoma
   Incision and Drainage 41800
Lesion
   Destruction 41850
   Excision 41822-41828
Mucosa
   Excision 41828
Reconstruction
   Alveolus 41874
   Gingiva 41872
Removal
   Foreign Body 41805
Tumor
   Excision 41825-41827
Unlisted Services and Procedures 41899

Gunning-Lieben Test
See Acetone, Blood or Urine

Guthrie Test 84030

H

H Flu
See Hemophilus Influenza

H-Reflex Study 95934-95936

HAA (Hepatitis Associated Antigen)
See Hepatitis Antigen, B Surface

HAAb
See Antibody, Hepatitis

Haemoglobin F
See Fetal Hemoglobin

Haemorrhage
See Hemorrhage

Haemorrhage Rectum
See Hemorrhage, Rectum

Hageman Factor 85280

HAI Test
See Hemagglutination Inhibition Test

Hair
Electrolysis 17380
KOH Examination 87220
Microscopic Evaluation 96902
Transplant
   Punch Graft 15775-15776
   Strip Graft 15220-15221

Hair Removal
See Removal, Hair

Hallux
See Great Toe

Halo
Body Cast 29000
Cranial 20661
   for Thin Skull Osteology 20664
Femur 20663
Maxillofacial 21100
Pelvic 20662
Removal 20665

Haloperidol
Assay 80173

Halsted Mastectomy
See Mastectomy, Radical

Halsted Repair
See Hernia, Repair, Inguinal

Ham Test
See Hemolysins

Hammertoe Repair 28285-28286

Hamster Penetration Test 89329

Hand
See Carpometacarpal Joint; Intercarpal Joint
Amputation
   at Metacarpal 25927
   at Wrist 25920
    Revision 25922
   Revision 25924, 25929-25931
Arthrodesis
   Carpometacarpal Joint 26843-26844
   Intercarpal Joint 25820-25825
Bone
   Incision and Drainage 26034
Cast 29085
Decompression 26035-26037
Fracture
   Metacarpal 26600
Insertion
   Tendon Graft 26392
Magnetic Resonance Imaging
(MRI) 73218-73223
Reconstruction
   Tendon Pulley 26500-26504
Removal
   Implantation 26320
   Tube/Rod 26390-26392, 26416
Repair
   Blood Vessel 35207
   Cleft Hand 26580
   Muscle 26591-26593

Tendon
   Extensor 26410-26416, 26426-26428,
     26433-26437
   Flexor 26350-26358, 26440
   Profundus 26370-26373
Replantation 20808
Strapping 29280
Tendon
   Excision 26390
   Extensor 26415
Tenotomy 26450, 26460
Tumor
   Excision 26115-26117
Unlisted Services and Procedures 26989
X-Ray 73120-73130

Hand Abscess
See Abscess, Hand

Hand Phalange
See Finger, Bone

Hand(s) Dupuytrens Contracture(s)
See Dupuytren's Contracture

Handling
Device 99002
Radioelement 77790
Specimen 99000-99001

Hanganutziu Deicher Antibodies
See Antibody, Heterophile

Haptoglobin 83010-83012

Hard Palate
See Palate

Harelip Operation
See Cleft Lip, Repair

Harii Procedure 25430

Harrington Rod
Insertion 22840
Removal 22850

Hartmann Procedure
Laparoscopic 44206
Open 44143

Harvesting
Bone Graft 20900-20902
Bone Marrow 38230
Cartilage Graft 20910-20912
Conjunctival Graft 68371
Eggs
   In Vitro Fertilization 58970
Endoscopic
   Vein for Bypass Graft 33508
Fascia Lata Graft 20920-20922
Intestines 44132-44133
Kidney 50300-50320, 50547
Liver 47133, 47140-47142
Lower Extremity Vein
   for Vascular Reconstruction 35572
Stem Cell 38205-38206
Tendon Graft 20924
Tissue Grafts 20926

Ear, External
    Complicated 69005
    Simple 69000
Elbow
    Incision and Drainage 23930
Epididymis
    Incision and Drainage 54700
Gums
    Incision and Drainage 41800
Hip 26990
Incision and Drainage
    Neck 21501-21502
    Skin 10140
    Thorax 21501-21502
Knee 27301
Leg, Lower 27603
Leg, Upper 27301
Mouth 41005-41009, 41015-41018
    Incision and Drainage 40800-40801
Nasal Septum
    Incision and Drainage 30020
Nose
    Incision and Drainage 30000-30020
Pelvis 26990
Scrotum
    Incision and Drainage 54700
Shoulder
    Drainage 23030
Skin
    Incision and Drainage 10140
    Puncture Aspiration 10160
Subdural 61108
Subungual
    Evacuation .11740
Testis
    Incision and Drainage 54700
Tongue 41000-41006, 41015
Vagina
    Incision and Drainage 57022-57023
Wrist 25028

Hematopoietic Stem Cell Transplantation
See Stem Cell, Transplantation

Hematopoietin
See Erythropoietin

Hematuria
See Blood, Urine

Hemic System
Unlisted Procedure 38999

Hemiepiphyseal Arrest
Elbow 24470

Hemifacial Microsomia
Reconstruction
    Mandibular Condyle 21247

Hemilaminectomy 63020-63044

Hemilaryngectomy 31370-31382

Hemipelvectomies
See Amputation, Interpelviabdominal

Hemiphalangectomy
Toe 28160

Hemispherectomy
Partial 61543
Total 61542

Hemocytoblast
See Stem Cell

Hemodialyses
See Hemodialysis

Hemodialysis 90935-90937
Blood Flow Study 90939-90940
Duplex Scan of Access 93990

Hemodynamic Monitoring
Non-invasive Left Ventricular 0086T

Hemofiltration 90945-90947

Hemoglobin
Analysis
    O2 Affinity .82820
Carboxyhemoglobin 82375-82376
Chromatography 83021
Concentration 85046
Electrophoresis .83020
Fetal 83030-83033, 85460-85461
Fractionation and Quantitation 83020
Glycated 83036
Methemoglobin 83045-83050
Non-Automated 83026
Plasma 83051
Sulfhemoglobin 83055-83060
Thermolabile 83065-83068
Urine 83069

Hemoglobin F
Fetal
    Chemical 83030
    Qualitative 83033

Hemoglobin, Glycosylated
See Glycohemoglobin

Hemogram
Added Indices 85025-85027
Automated 85025-85027
Manual 85014-85018, 85032

Hemolysins 85475
with Agglutinins 86940-86941

Hemolytic Complement
See Complement, Hemolytic

Hemolytic Complement, Total
See Complement, Hemolytic, Total

Hemoperfusion 90997

Hemophil
See Clotting Factor

Hemophilus Influenza
Antibody 86684

Hemorrhage
Abdomen 49002
Anal
    Endoscopic Control 46614
Bladder
    Postoperative 52606
Chest Cavity
    Endoscopic Control 32654

Colon
    Endoscopic Control 44391, 45382
Colon-Sigmoid
    Endoscopic Control 45334
Esophagus
    Endoscopic Control 43227
Gastrointestinal, Upper
    Endoscopic Control 43255
Intestines, Small
    Endoscopic Control 44366, 44378
Liver
    Control 47350
Lung 32110
Nasal
    Cauterization 30901-30906
    Endoscopic Control 31238
Nasopharynx 42970-42972
Oropharynx 42960-42962
Rectum
    Endoscopic Control 45317
Throat .42960-42962
Uterus
    Postpartum .59160
Vagina 57180

Hemorrhoidectomy
Complex 46260
    with Fissurectomy 46261-46262
External Complete 46250
Ligature 46221
Simple 46255
    with Fissurectomy 46257-46258

Hemorrhoidopexy 46947

Hemorrhoids
Destruction 46934-46936
Incision
    External 46083
Injection
    Sclerosing Solution 46500
Ligation 46945-46946
Stapling 46947
Suture .46945-46946

Hemosiderin 83070-83071

Hemothorax
Thoracostomy .32020

Heparin 85520
See Clotting Inhibitors
Neutralization .85525
Protamine Tolerance Test 85530

Heparin Cofactor I
See Antithrombin III

Hepatectomy
Extensive 47122
Left Lobe 47125
Partial
    Donor 47140-47142
    Lobe 47120
Right Lobe 47130
Total
    Donor 47133

Hepatic Abscess
See Abscess, Liver

Hepatic Arteries
See Artery, Hepatic

Hepatic Artery Aneurysm
See Artery, Hepatic, Aneurysm

Hepatic Duct
Anastomosis
    with Intestines 47765, 47802
Exploration 47400
Incision and Drainage 47400
Nuclear Medicine
    Imaging 78223
Removal
    Calculi (Stone) 47400
Repair
    with Intestines 47765, 47802
Unlisted Services and Procedures 47999

Hepatic Haemorrhage
See Hemorrhage, Liver

Hepatic Portal Vein
See Vein, Hepatic Portal

Hepatic Portoenterostomies
See Hepaticoenterostomy

Hepatic Transplantation
See Liver, Transplantation

Hepaticodochotomy
See Hepaticostomy

Hepaticoenterostomy 47802

Hepaticostomy 47400

Hepaticotomy 47400

Hepatitis A and Hepatitis B 90636

Hepatitis A Vaccine
Adolescent/Pediatric
    2 Dose Schedule 90633
    3 Dose Schedule 90634
Adult Dosage 90632

Hepatitis Antibody
A 86708-86709
B
    B Core 86704-86705
    B Surface 86706
    Be 86707
C 86803-86804
Delta Agent 86692
IgG 86704, 86708
IgM 86704-86705, 86708-86709

Hepatitis Antigen
B 87515-87517
B Surface .87340-87341
Be 87350
C 87520-87522
Delta Agent 87380
G 87525-87527

Hepatitis B and Hib 90748

Hepatitis B Vaccine
Dosage
    Adolescent 90743
    Adult 90746
    Immunosuppressed 90740, 90747
    Pediatric/Adolescent 90744

Hepatitis B Virus E Antibody
See Antibody, Hepatitis

Hepatitis B Virus Surface ab
See Antibody, Hepatitis B, Surface

Hepatorrhaphy
See Liver, Repair

Hepatotomy
Abscess .47010-47011
    Percutaneous 47011
Cyst 47010-47011
    Percutaneous 47011

Hernia Repair
Abdominal 49590
    Incisional 49560
    Recurrent 49565
Diaphragmatic 39502-39541
Epigastric 49570
    Incarcerated 49572
Femoral 49550
    Incarcerated 49553
    Recurrent 49555
    Recurrent Incarcerated 49557
Incisional
    Incarcerated 49561
Inguinal 49491, 49495-49500, 49505
    Incarcerated 49492, 49496, 49501,
                        49507, 49521
    Laparoscopic 49650-49651
    Recurrent 49520
    Sliding 49525
    Strangulated 49492
Lumbar 49540
Lung 32800
Orchiopexy 54640
Recurrent Incisional
    Incarcerated 49566
    Reducible 49565
Umbilicus
    Incarcerated 49582, 49587
    Reducible 49580, 49585
with Spermatic Cord 55540
    Spigelian 49590

Hernia, Cerebral
See Encephalocele

Hernia, Rectovaginal
See Rectocele

Hernia, Umbilical
See Omphalocele

Heroin Screen 82486

Heroin, Alkaloid Screening 82101

Herpes Simplex
Antibody 86696
Antigen Detection
    Immunofluorescence 87273-87274
    Nucleic Acid 87528-87530
Identification
    Smear and Stain 87207

Herpes Smear and Stain 87207

Herpes Virus-4 (Gamma), Human
See Epstein-Barr Virus

Herpes Virus-6
Detection 87531-87533

Herpetic Vesicle
Destruction 54050-54065

Heteroantibodies
See Antibody, Heterophile

Heterograft
Skin 15400

Heterologous Transplant
See Xenograft

Heterologous Transplantation
See Heterograft

Heterophile Antibody 86308-86310

Heterotropia
See Strabismus

Hex B
See b-Hexosaminidase

Hexadecadrol
See Dexamethasone

Hexosephosphate Isomerase
See Phosphohexose Isomerase

Heyman Procedure 27179, 28264

Hg Factor
See Glucagon

HGB
See Hemoglobin, Concentration

HGH
See Growth Hormone, Human

HHV-4
See Epstein-Barr Virus

HIAA
See Hydroxyindolacetic Acid, Urine

Hib Vaccine
4 Dose Schedule
    HbOC 90645
    PRP-T 90648
PRP-D
    Booster 90646
PRP-OMP
    3 Dose Schedule 90647

Hibb Operation
See Spinal Cord; Spine, Fusion; Vertebra;
Vertebral Body; Vertebral Process

Hickmann Catheterization
See Cannulization; Catheterization, Venous,
Central Line; Venipuncture

Hidradenitis
See Sweat Gland
Excision 11450-11471
Suppurative
    Incision and Drainage 10060-10061

High Altitude Simulation Test 94452-94453

High Density Lipoprotein
See Lipoprotein

High Molecular Weight Kininogen
See Fitzgerald Factor

Highly Selective Vagotomy
See Vagotomy, Highly Selective

Highmore Antrum
See Sinus, Maxillary

Hill Procedure 43324
Laparoscopic 43280

Hinton Positive
See RPR

Hip
See Femur; Pelvis
Abscess
   Incision and Drainage 26990
Arthrocentesis 20610
Arthrodesis 27284-27286
Arthrography 73525
Arthroplasty 27130-27132
Arthroscopy 29860-29863
Arthrotomy 27030-27033
Biopsy 27040-27041
Bone
   Drainage 26992
Bursa
   Incision and Drainage 26991
Capsulectomy
   with Release, Flexor Muscles 27036
Cast 29305-29325
Craterization 27070
Cyst
   Excision 27065-27067
Denervation 27035
Echography
   Infant 76885-76886
Endoprosthesis
   See Prosthesis, Hip
Excision 27070
Exploration 27033
Fasciotomy 27025
Fusion 27284-27286
Hematoma
   Incision and Drainage 26990
Injection
   Radiologic 27093-27096
Reconstruction
   Total Replacement 27130
Removal
   Cast 29710
   Foreign Body 27033, 27086-27087
     Arthroscopic 29861
   Loose Body
     Arthroscopic 29861
   Prosthesis 27090-27091
Repair
   Muscle Transfer 27100-27105, 27111
   Osteotomy 27146-27156
   Tendon 27097
Saucerization 27070

Stem Prostheses
   See Arthroplasty, Hip
Strapping 29520
Tenotomy
   Abductor Tendon 27006
   Adductor Tendon 27000-27003
   Iliopsoas 27005
Total Replacement 27130-27132
Tumor
   Excision 27047-27049, 27065-27067
     Radical 27075-27076
Ultrasound
   Infant 76885-76886
X-Ray 73500-73520, 73540
   Intraoperative 73530
   with Contrast 73525

Hip Joint
Arthroplasty 27132
   Revision 27134-27138
Arthrotomy 27052
Biopsy 27052
Capsulotomy
   with Release, Flexor Muscles 27036
Dislocation 27250-27252
   Congenital 27256-27259
   Open Treatment 27253-27254
   without Trauma 27265-27266
Manipulation 27275
Reconstruction
   Revision 27134-27138
Synovium
   Excision 27054
     Arthroscopic 29863
Total Replacement 27132

Hip Stem Prostheses
See Arthroplasty, Hip

Hippocampus
Excision 61566

Histamine 83088

Histamine Release Test 86343

Histochemistry 88318-88319

Histocompatibility Testing
See Tissue Typing

Histoplasma
Antibody 86698
Antigen 87385

Histoplasma capsulatum
Antigen Detection
   Enzyme Immunoassay 87385

Histoplasmin Test
See Histoplasmosis, Skin Test

Histoplasmoses
See Histoplasmosis

Histoplasmosis
Skin Test 86510

History and Physical
See Evaluation and Management, Office and/or Other Outpatient Services
Pelvic Exam 57410

HIV
Antibody 86701-86703
   Confirmation Test 86689

HIV-1
Antigen Detection
   Enzyme Immunoassay 87390

HIV-2
Antigen Detection
   Enzyme Immunoassay 87391

HK3 Kallikrein
See Antigen, Prostate Specific

HLA Typing 86812-86817

HMRK
See Fitzgerald Factor

HMW Kininogen
See Fitzgerald Factor

Hoffman Apparatus 20690

Hofmeister Operation
See Gastrectomy, Total

Holographic Imaging 76375

Holten Test
See Creatinine, Urine, Clearance

Home Services
Activities of Daily Living 99509
Catheter Care 99507
Enema Administration 99511
Established Patient 99347-99350
Hemodialysis 99512
Home Infusion Procedures 99601-99602
Individual or Family Counseling 99510
Intramuscular Injections 99506
Mechanical Ventilation 99504
New Patient 99341-99345
Newborn Care 99502
Postnatal Assessment 99501
Prenatal Monitoring 99500
Respiratory Therapy 99503
Sleep Studies 95805-95811
Stoma Care 99505
Unlisted Services and Procedures 99600

Home Visit
See House Calls

Homocystine 83090
Urine 82615

Homogenization, Tissue 87176

Homograft
Skin 15350

Homologous Grafts
See Graft

Homologous Transplantation
See Homograft

Homovanillic Acid
Urine 83150

Supracondylar
Closed Treatment 24530-24535
Open Treatment 24545-24546
Percutaneous Fixation 24538
Transcondylar
Closed Treatment 24530-24535
Open Treatment 24545-24546
Percutaneous Fixation 24538
with Dislocation 23665-23670
Osteomyelitis 24134
Pinning, Wiring 23491, 24498
Prophylactic Treatment 23491, 24498
Radical Resection 23220-23222
Repair 24430
Nonunion, Malunion 24430-24435
Osteoplasty 24420
Osteotomy 24400-24410
with Graft 24435
Resection Head 23195
Saucerization 23184, 24140
Sequestrectomy 23174, 24134
Tumor
Excision 23150, 23220-23222, 24110
with Allograft 23156, 24116
with Autograft 23155, 24115
X-Ray 73060

Hummelshein Operation
See Strabismus, Repair

Humor Shunt, Aqueous
See Aqueous Shunt

HVA
See Homovanillic Acid

Hyaluron Binding Assay 0087T

Hybridization Probes, DNA
See Nucleic Acid Probe

Hydatid Disease
See Echinococcosis

Hydatid Mole
See Hydatidiform Mole

Hydatidiform Mole
Evacuation and Curettage 59870
Excision 59100

Hydrocarbons, Chlorinated
See Chlorinated Hydrocarbons

Hydrocele
Aspiration 55000
Excision
Bilateral
Tunica Vaginalis 55041
Unilateral
Spermatic Cord 55500
Tunica Vaginalis 55040
Repair 55060

Hydrochloric Acid, Gastric
See Acid, Gastric

Hydrochloride, Vancomycin
See Vancomycin

Hydrocodon
See Dihydrocodeinone

Hydrogen Ion Concentration
See pH

Hydrolase, Acetylcholine
See Acetylcholinesterase

Hydrolase, Triacylglycerol
See Lipase

Hydrolases, Phosphoric Monoester
See Phosphatase

Hydrotherapy (Hubbard Tank) 97036
See Physical Medicine/Therapy/Occupational Therapy

Hydrotubation 58350

Hydroxyacetanilide
See Acetaminophen

Hydroxycorticosteroid 83491

Hydroxyindolacetic Acid 83497
Urine 83497

Hydroxypregnenolone 80406, 84143

Hydroxyprogesterone . . .80402-80406, 83498-83499

Hydroxyproline 83500-83505

Hydroxytyramine
See Dopamine

Hygroma
Cystic
Axillary/Cervical
Excision 38550-38555

Hymen
Excision 56700
Incision 56720

Hymenal Ring
Revision 56700

Hymenectomy 56700

Hymenotomy 56720

Hyoid
Bone
Fracture
Closed Treatment
with Manipulation 21494
without Manipulation 21493
Open Treatment 21495
Muscle
Incision and Suspension 21685

Hyperbaric Oxygen Pressurization 99183

Hypercycloidal X-Ray 76101-76102

Hyperdactylies
See Supernumerary Digit

Hyperglycemic Glycogenolytic Factor
See Glucagon

Hypertelorism of Orbit
See Orbital Hypertelorism

Hyperthermia Therapy
See Thermotherapy

Hyperthermia Treatment . .77600-77620

Hypnotherapy 90880

Hypodermis
See Subcutaneous Tissue

Hypogastric Plexus
Destruction 64681
Injection
Anesthetic .64517
Neurolytic .64681

Hypoglossal Nerve
Anastomosis
to Facial Nerve 64868

Hypoglossal-Facial Anastomosis
See Anastomosis, Nerve, Facial to Hypoglossal

Hypopharynges
See Hypopharynx

Hypopharynx
Biopsy 42802

Hypophysectomy 61546-61548, 62165

Hypophysis
See Pituitary Gland

Hypopyrexia
See Hypothermia

Hypospadias
Repair 54300, 54352
Complications 54340-54348
First Stage 54304
Proximal Penile or Penoscrotal 54332
One Stage
Meatal Advancement 54322
Perineal 54336
Urethroplasty
Local Skin Flaps 54324
Local Skin Flaps and Mobilization of
Urethra 54326
Local Skin Flaps, Skin Graft Patch
and/or Island Flap 54328
Urethroplasty for Second Stage .54308-54316
Free Skin Graft 54316
Urethroplasty for Third Stage 54318

Hypothermia 99185-99186

Hypoxia
Breathing Response 94450
High Altitude Simulation Test 94452-94453

Hysterectomy
Abdominal
Radical 58210
Resection of Ovarian Malignancy 58951, 58953-58956
Supracervical 58180
Total 58150, 58200, 58956
with Colpo-Urethrocystopexy 58152
with Partial Vaginectomy 58200
with Omentectomy 58956

Immunoblotting, Western
See Western Blot

Immunochemical, Lysozyme (Muramidase)
See Lysozyme

Immunocytochemistry 88342

Immunodeficiency Virus Type 1, Human
See HIV 1

Immunodeficiency Virus Type 2, Human
See HIV 2

Immunodeficiency Virus, Human
See HIV

Immunodiffusion 86329-86331

Immunoelectrophoresis 86320-86327, 86334-86335

Immunofixation Electrophoresis 86334-86335

Immunofluorescent Study 88346-88347

Immunogen
See Antigen

Immunoglobulin 82787
Platelet Associated 86023
Thyroid Stimulating 84445

Immunoglobulin E
See IgE

Immunoglobulin Receptor Assay 86243

Immunologic Skin Test
See Skin, Tests

Immunology
Unlisted Services and Procedures 86849

Immunotherapies, Allergen
See Allergen Immunotherapy

Impedance Testing.............92567
See Audiologic Function Tests

Imperfectly Descended Testis
See Testis, Undescended

Implant Removal
See Specific Anatomical Site

Implant, Breast
See Breast, Implants

Implant, Glaucoma Drainage
See Aqueous Shunt

Implant, Orbital
See Orbital Implant

Implant, Penile
See Penile Prosthesis

Implant, Penile Prosthesis, Inflatable
See Penile Prosthesis, Insertion, Inflatable

Implant, Subperiosteal
See Subperiosteal Implant

Implant, Ureters into, Bladder
See Anastomosis, Ureter, to Bladder

Implantation
Artificial Heart
   Intracorporeal 0051T
Bone
   for External Speech Processor/Cochlear
   Stimulator 69714-69718
Brain
   Chemotherapy 61517
   Thermal Perfusion Probe 0077T
Cardiac Event Recorder 33282
Contraceptive Capsules 11975, 11977
Drug Delivery Device 11981, 11983, 61517
Electrode
   Brain 61850-61875
   Nerve 64553-64581
   Spinal Cord 63650-63655
Eye
   Anterior Segment 65920
   Aqueous Shunt to Extraocular Placement or
   Replacement of Pegs 65125
   Posterior Segment
      Extraocular 67120
      Intraocular 67121
   Reservoir 66180
   Vitreous
      Drug Delivery System 67027
Fallopian Tube 58565
Hearing Aid Hormone Pellet(s)
   Bone Conduction 69710
Hip Prosthesis
   See Arthroplasty, Hip
Hormone Pellet.....................11980
Intraocular Lens
   See Insertion, Intraocular Lens
Joint
   See Arthroplasty
Mesh
   Hernia Repair 49568
   Vaginal Repair 57267
Nerve
   into Bone 64787
   into Muscle 64787
Neurostimulators
   Pulse Generator 61885
   Receiver 61886
Ovum 58976
Pulse Generator
   Brain 61885-61886
   Spinal Cord Electrode Array 63685
Receiver
   Brain 61885-61886
   Spinal Cord 63685
Removal 20670-20680
   Elbow 24164
   Radius 24164
Reservoir Vascular Access Device
   Declotting 36550
Total Replacement Heart System
   Intracorporeal 0051T

Tubouterine 58752
Ventricular Assist Device 33976
   Extracorporeal 0048T
   Intracorporeal 33979

Impression, Maxillofacial
Auricular Prosthesis 21086
Definitive Obturator Prosthesis 21080
Facial Prosthesis 21088
Interim Obturator 21079
Mandibular Resection Prosthesis 21081
Nasal Prosthesis 21087
Oral Surgical Splint 21085
Orbital Prosthesis 21077
Palatal Augmentation Prosthesis 21082
Palatal Lift Prosthesis 21083
Speech Aid Prosthesis 21084
Surgical Obturator 21076

In Situ Hybridization
See Nucleic Acid Probe, Cytogenetic Studies, Morphometric Analysis

In Vitro Fertilization 58321-58322

In Vivo NMR Spectroscopy
See Magnetic Resonance Spectroscopy

Incision
See Incision and Drainage
Abdomen 49000
   Exploration 58960
Abscess
   Soft Tissue 20000-20005
Accessory Nerve 63191
Anal
   Fistula 46270, 46280
   Septum 46070
   Sphincter 46080
Ankle 27607
   Tendon 27605-27606
Anus
   See Anus, Incision
Aortic Valve
   for Stenosis 33415
Artery
   Nose 30915-30920
Atrial Septum 33735-33737
Bile Duct
   Sphincter 43262, 47460
Bladder
   Catheterization 51045
   with Destruction 51020-51030
   with Radiotracer 51020
Bladder Diverticulum 52305
Brachial Artery
   Exposure 34834
Brain
   Amygdalohippocampectomy 61566
   Subpial 61567
Breast
   Capsules 19370
Burn Scab 16035-16036
Cataract
   Secondary
      Laser Surgery 66821
      Stab Incision Technique 66820
Chest
   Biopsy 32095-32100

Incisional Hernia Repair
See Hernia, Repair, Incisional

Inclusion Bodies

Incomplete Abortion
See Abortion, Incomplete

Indicator Dilution Studies

Induced Abortion
See Abortion

Induced Hyperthermia
See Thermotherapy

Induced Hypothermia
See Hypothermia

Induratio Penis Plastica
See Peyronie Disease

Infant, Newborn, Intensive Care
See Intensive Care, Neonatal

Infantile Paralysis
See Polio

Infection

Infection, Actinomyces
See Actinomycosis

Infection, Bone
See Osteomyelitis

Infection, Filarioidea
See Filariasis

Infection, Postoperative Wound
See Postoperative Wound Infection

Infection, Wound
See Wound, Infection

Infectious Agent

Phenotype Analysis
  by Nucleic acid
    HIV-1 Drug Resistance 87903-87904
Phenotype Prediction
  by Genetic Database
    HIV-1 Drug Resistance 0023T

Infectious Mononucleosis Virus
See Epstein-Barr Virus

Inflammatory Process
Localization
  Nuclear Medicine 78805-78807

Inflation
Ear, Middle
  Eustachian Tube
    with Catheterization 69400
    without Catheterization 69401
Eustachian Tube
  Myringotomy 69420
  Anesthesia 69424

Influenza A
Antigen Detection
  Direct Fluorescence 87276
  Enzyme Immunoassay 87400

Influenza B
Antigen Detection
  Enzyme Immunoassay 87400
  Immunofluorescence 87275

Influenza Vaccine
See Vaccines

Influenza Virus
Antibody 86710
by Immunoassay
  with Direct Optical Observation 87804

Infraorbital Nerve
Avulsion 64734
Incision 64734
Transection 64734

Infrared Light Treatment 97026
See Physical Medicine/Therapy/Occupational Therapy

Infratentorial Craniectomy 61520-61521

Infusion
Amnion
  Transabdominal 59072
Cerebral
  Intravenous
    for Thrombolysis 37195
Intraosseous 36680
Radioelement 77750
Transcatheter Therapy 37201-37202

Infusion Pump
Electronic Analysis
  Spinal Cord 62367-62368
Insertion
  Intra-arterial 36260
Intraarterial
  Removal 36262
  Revision 36261

Intravenous
  Insertion 36563
  Repair 36576
  Replacement 36583
Maintenance 95990-95991, 96520-96530
  See Chemotherapy, Pump Services
Spinal Cord 62361-62362
Ventricular Catheter 61215

Infusion Therapy 62350-62351, 62360-62362
See Injection, Chemotherapy
Arterial Catheterization 36640
Chemotherapy 96410-96414, 96422-96425
Home Infusion Procedures 99601-99602
Intravenous 90780-90781
Pain 62360-62362, 62367-62368
Transcatheter Therapy 75896

Ingestion Challenge Test 95075
See Allergy Tests

Inguinal Hernia Repair
See Hernia, Repair, Inguinal

INH
See Drug Assay

Inhalation
Pentamidine 94642

Inhalation Provocation Tests
See Bronchial Challenge Test

Inhalation Treatment 94640, 94664, 99503
See Pulmonology, Therapeutic

Inhibin A 86336

Inhibition Test, Hemagglutination
See Hemagglutination Inhibition Test

Inhibition, Fertilization
See Contraception

Inhibitor, Alpha 1-Protease
See Alpha-1 Antitrypsin

Inhibitor, Alpha 2-Plasmin
See Alpha-2 Antiplasmin

Inhibitory Concentration, Minimum
See Minimum Inhibitory Concentration

Initial Inpatient Consultations
See Consultation, Initial Inpatient

Injection
See Allergen Immunotherapy; Infusion
Abdomen
  Air 49400
  Contrast Material 49400
Angiography
  Pulmonary 75746
Ankle
  Radial 27648
Antibiotic
  See Antibiotic Administration
Antigen (Allergen) 95115-95125
Aorta (Aortography)
  Radiologic 93544

Aponeurosis 20550
Bladder
  Radiologic 51600-51610
Brain Canal 61070
Bronchography
  Segmental 31656
Bursa 20600-20610
Cardiac Catheterization 93539-93545
Carpal Tunnel
  Therapeutic 20526
Chemotherapy 96400-96450, 96542
Cistern
  Medication or Other 61055
Contrast
  via Catheter 49424
Corpora Cavernosa 54235
Cyst
  Bone 20615
  Kidney 50390
  Pelvis 50390
  Thyroid 60001
Elbow
  Arthrography
    Radiologic 24220
Epidural
  See Epidural, Injection
Esophageal Varices
  Endoscopy 43243
Esophagus
  Sclerosing Agent 43204
  Submucosal 43201
Extremity
  Pseudoaneurysm 36002
Eye
  Air 66020
  Medication 66030
Eyelid
  Subconjunctival 68200
Ganglion
  Anesthetic 64505, 64510
Ganglion Cyst 20612
Gastric Secretion Stimulant 91052
Gastric Varices
  Endoscopy 43243
Heart Vessels
  Cardiac Catheterization 93539-93545
    See Catheterization, Cardiac
  Radiologic 93545
Hemorrhoids
  Sclerosing Solution 46500
Hip
  Radiologic 27093-27095
Insect Venom 95130-95134
Intervertebral Disk
  Chemonucleolysis Agent 62292
  Radiological 62290-62291
Intraamniotic 59852
Intraarterial
  Diagnostic 90783
  Therapeutic 90783
Intradermal
  for Tattooing 11920-11922
Intralesional
  Skin 11900-11901
Intramuscular
  Antibiotic 90788
  Diagnostic 90782
  Therapeutic 90782, 99506

Inkblot Test 96100

Inner Ear
See Ear, Inner

Innominate

Innominate Arteries
See Artery, Brachiocephalic

Inorganic Sulfates
See Sulfate

Insemination

Insertion
See Implantation; Intubation; Transplantation

Heart 33210-33211, 33216-33217,
33224-33225, 93620-93622
Nerve 64553-64581
Sphenoidal 95830
Spinal Cord 63650-63655
Endotracheal Tube 31500
Gastrostomy Tube
Laparoscopic 43653
Percutaneous 43750
Graft
Aorta 33330-33335
Heart Vessel 33330-33335
Guide
Kidney Pelvis 50395
Guide Wire
Endoscopy 43248
Esophagoscopy 43248
with Dilation 43226
Heyman Capsule
Uterus
for Brachytherapy 58346
Iliac Artery
Occlusion Device 34808
Implant
Bone
for External Speech Processor/Cochlear
Stimulator 69714-69718
Infusion Pump
Intraarterial 36260
Intravenous 36563
Spinal Cord 62361-62362
Intracatheter/Needle
Aorta 36160
Arteriovenous Shunt 36145
Intraarterial 36100-36140
Intravenous 36000
Kidney 50392
Intraocular Lens 66983
Manual or Mechanical
Technique 66982, 66984
Not Associated with Concurrent Cataract
Removal 66985
Intrauterine Device (IUD) 58300
IVC Filter 75940
Jejunostomy Tube
Endoscopy 44372
Keel
Laryngoplasty 31580
Laminaria 59200
Mesh
Pelvic Floor 57267
Nasobiliary Tube
Endoscopy 43267
Nasopancreatic Tube
Endoscopy 43267
Needle
Bone 36680
Intraosseous 36680
Prostate 55859
Needle Wire
Trachea 31730
Neurostimulator
Pulse Generator 64590
Receiver 64590
Nose
Septal Prosthesis 30220
Obturator
Larynx 31527

Ocular Implant
in Scleral Shell 65130
Muscles Attached 65140
Muscles, Not Attached 65135
with Foreign Material 65155
with/without Conjunctival Graft 65150
Orbital Transplant 67550
Oviduct
Chromotubation 58350
Hydrotubation 58350
Ovoid
Vagina
for Brachytherapy 57155
Pacemaker
Fluoroscopy/Radiography 71090
Heart 33200-33208, 33212-33213
Pacing Cardio-Defibrillator
Electrodes 33245-33246
Leads 33216-33220, 33224-33225,
33243-33245
Pulse Generator only 33240-33241
Packing
Vagina 57180
Penile Prosthesis, Inflatable
See Penile Prosthesis, Insertion, Inflatable
Pessary
Vagina 57160
Pin
Skeletal Traction 20650
Probe
Brain 61770
Prostaglandin 59200
Prostate
Radioactive Substance 55860
Prosthesis
Knee 27438, 27445
Nasal Septal 30220
Palate 42281
Pelvic Floor 57267
Penis
Inflatable 54401-54405
Noninflatable 54400
Speech 31611
Testis 54660
Urethral Sphincter 53444-53445
Pulse Generator
Brain 61885-61886
Heart 33212-33213
Spinal Cord 63685
Radioactive Material
Bladder 51020
Cystourethroscopy 52250
Receiver
Brain 61885-61886
Spinal Cord 63685
Reservoir
Brain 61210-61215
Spinal Cord 62360
Subcutaneous 49419
Sensor, Fetal Oximetry
Cervix 0021T
Vagina 0021T
Shunt 36835
Abdomen
Vein 49425
Venous 49426
Intrahepatic Portosystemic 37182

Spinal Instrument 22849
Spinous Process 22841
Spinal Instrumentation
Anterior 22845-22847
Internal Spinal Fixation 22841
Pelvic Fixation 22848
Posterior Nonsegmental
Harrington Rod Technique 22840
Posterior Segmental 22842-22844
Prosthetic Device 22851
Stent
Bile Duct 43268, 47801
Percutaneous 47511
Bladder 51045
Conjunctiva 68750
Coronary 92980-92981
Esophagus 43219
Gastrointestinal, Upper 43256
Ileum 44383
Indwelling 50605
Lacrimal Duct 68815
Pancreatic Duct 43268
Small Intestines 44370, 44379
Ureter via Kidney 50393
Ureteral 50947, 52332
Urethral 0084T, 52282
Tamponade
Esophagus 43460
Tandem
Uterus
for Brachytherapy 57155
Tendon Graft
Finger 26392
Hand 26392
Testicular Prosthesis
See Prosthesis, Testicular, Insertion
Tissue Expanders
Skin 11960-11971
Tube
Bile Duct 43268
Esophagus 43510
Gastrointestinal, Upper 43241
Ileum 44383
Kidney 50398
Pancreatic Duct 43268
Small Intestines 44379
Trachea 31730
Ureter 50688
Ureteral Guide Wire 52334
Vascular Pedicle
Carpal Bone 25430
Venous Access Device
Central 36560-36566
Peripheral 36570-36571
Ventilating Tube 69433
Ventricular Assist Device 33975
Wire
Skeletal Traction 20650

Inspiratory Positive Pressure Breathing

See Intermittent Positive Pressure Breathing (IPPB)

Instillation

Contrast Material
Bronchography 31708
Laryngography 31708

Intracranial Neoplasm, Acoustic Neuroma
See Brain, Tumor, Excision

Intracranial Neoplasm, Craniopharyngioma
See Craniopharyngioma

Intracranial Neoplasm, Meningioma
See Meningioma

Intrafallopian Transfer, Gamete
See GIFT

Intraluminal Angioplasty
See Angioplasty

Intramuscular Injection
See Injection, Intramuscular

Intraocular Lens
Exchange 66986
Insertion 66983
   Manual or Mechanical
   Technique 66982, 66984
   Not Associated with Concurrent Cataract
   Removal 66985

Intratracheal Intubation
See Insertion, Endotracheal Tube

Intrauterine Contraceptive Device
See Intrauterine Device (IUD)

Intrauterine Device (IUD)
Insertion 58300
Removal 58301

Intrauterine Synechiae
See Adhesions, Intrauterine

Intravascular Stent
See Transcatheter, Placement, Intravascular
Stents
X-Ray 75960

Intravascular Ultrasound
Intraoperative 37250-37251

Intravenous Injection
See Injection, Intravenous

Intravenous Pyelogram
See Urography, Intravenous

Intravenous Therapy 90780-90781
See Injection, Chemotherapy
Pain Management 90783-90784

Intravesical Instillation
See Bladder, Instillation

Intravitreal Injection
Pharmacologic Agent 67028

Intrinsic Factor 83528
Antibody 86340

Introduction
Breast
   Metallic Localization Clip Placement ..19295
   Preoperative Placement, Needle 19290-19291

Contraceptive Capsules
   Implantable 11975-11977
Drug Delivery Implant 11981, 11983
Gastrointestinal Tube 44500
   with Fluoroscopic Guidance 74340
Tissue Expanders
   Skin 11960-11971

Intubation
See Insertion
Endotracheal Tube 31500
Eustachian Tube
   See Catheterization, Eustachian Tube
Gastric 89130-89141, 91105
Specimen Collection
   Esophagus 91000
   Stomach 91055

Intubation Tube
See Endotracheal Tube

Intussusception
Barium Enema 74283
Reduction
   Laparotomy 44050

Invagination, Intestinal
See Intussusception

Inversion, Nipple
See Nipples, Inverted

Iodide Test
See Nuclear Medicine, Thyroid, Uptake

Iodine Test
See Starch Granules, Feces

Ionization, Medical
See Iontophoresis

Iontophoreses
See Iontophoresis

Iontophoresis 97033
Sweat Collection 89230

IP
See Allergen Immunotherapy

Ipecac Administration 99175

IPPB
See Intermittent Positive Pressure Breathing;
Pulmonology, Therapeutic

Iridectomy
by Laser Surgery 66761
Peripheral for Glaucoma 66625
with Corneoscleral or Corneal Section ...66600
with Sclerectomy with Punch or Scissors ..66160
with Thermocauterization 66155
with Transfixion as for Iris Bombe 66605
with Trephination 66150

Iridencleisis 66165

Iridodialysis 66680

Iridoplasty 66762

Iridotasis 66165

Iridotomy
by Laser Surgery 66761
by Stab Incision 66500
Excision
   Optical 66635
   Peripheral 66625
   with Corneoscleral or Corneal
   Section 66600
   with Cyclectomy 66605
Incision
   Stab 66500
   with Transfixion as for Iris Bombe 66505
Optical 66635
Peripheral 66625
Sector 66630

Iris
Cyst
   Destruction 66770
Excision
   Iridectomy
      Optical 66635
      Peripheral 66625
      Sector 66630
      with Corneoscleral or
      Corneal Section 66600
      with Cyclectomy 66605
Incision
   Iridotomy
      Stab 66500
      with Transfixion as for Iris Bombe ...66505
Lesion
   Destruction 66770
Repair
   with Ciliary Body 66680
      Suture 66682
Revision
   Laser Surgery 66761
   Photocoagulation 66762
Suture
   with Ciliary Body 66682

Iron 83540
Absorption 78162
Chelatable
   Total Body Iron 78172
Turnover Rate 78160
Utilization 78170

Iron Binding Capacity 83550

Iron Hematoxylin Stain 88312

Iron Stain 85536, 88313

Irradiation
Blood Products 86945

Irrigation
Bladder 51700
Catheter
   Brain 62194, 62225
Corpora Cavernosa
   Priapism 54220
Penis
   Priapism 54220
Peritoneal
   See Peritoneal Lavage
Rectum
   for Fecal Impaction 91123

Meniscectomy 27332-27333
Reconstruction 27437-27438
    Ligament 27427-27429
    with Prosthesis 27445
Removal
    Foreign Body 27310, 27331, 27372
    Loose Body 27331
    Prosthesis 27488
Repair
    Ligament 27405-27409
       Collateral 27405
       Collateral and Cruciate 27409
       Cruciate 27407-27409
    Meniscus 27403
    Tendon 27380-27381
Replacement 27447
Retinacular
    Release .27425
Strapping 29530
Suture
    Tendon 27380-27381
Transplantation
    Chondrocytes 27412
    Meniscus 29868
    Osteochondral
       Allograft 27415, 29867
       Autograft 27412, 29866
Tumor
    Excision 27327-27329, 27365
Unlisted Services and Procedures 27599
X-Ray 73560-73564
    Arthrography 73580
    Bilateral .73565
X-Ray with Contrast
    Arthrography 73580

Knee Joint
Arthroplasty 27446

Knee Prosthesis
See Prosthesis, Knee

Kneecap
Excision .27350
Repair
    Instability 27420-27424

Knock-Knee Repair 27455-27457

Kocher Operation 23650-23680
See Clavicle; Scapula; Shoulder, Dislocation, Closed Treatment

Kocher Pylorectomy
See Gastrectomy, Partial

Kock Pouch 44316
Formation 50825

Kock Procedure 44316

KOH
See Hair, Nails, Tissue, Examination for Fungi

Kraske Procedure 45116

Krause Operation
See Gasserian Ganglion, Sensory Root, Decompression

Kroenlein Procedure 67420

Krukenberg Procedure 25915

Kuhlmann Test 96100

Kyphectomy
More than Two Segments 22819
Up to Two Segments 22818

L

L Ascorbic Acid
See Ascorbic Acid

L Aspartate 2 Oxoglutarate Aminotransferase
See Transaminase, Glutamic Oxaloacetic

L Glutamine
See Glutamine

L-Alanine
See Aminolevulinic Acid (ALA)

L-Leucylnaphthylamidase
See Leucine Aminopeptidase

L/S Ratio
Amniotic Fluid 83661

Labial Adhesions
Lysis 56441

Labyrinth
See Ear, Inner

Labyrinthectomy 69905
with Mastoidectomy 69910
with Skull Base Surgery 61596

Labyrinthotomy
with Mastoidectomy 69802
with/without Cryosurgery 69801

Laceration Repair
See Specific Site

Lacrimal Duct
Canaliculi
    Repair 68700
Exploration 68810
    Canaliculi 68840
    Stent .68815
    with Anesthesia 68811
Insertion
    Stent .68815
Removal
    Dacryolith 68530
    Foreign Body 68530
X-Ray with Contrast 70170

Lacrimal Gland
Biopsy .68510
Close Fistula 68770
Excision
    Partial 68505
    Total .68500
Fistulization 68720

Incision and Drainage 68400
Injection
    X-Ray 68850
Nuclear Medicine
    Tear Flow 78660
Removal
    Dacryolith 68530
    Foreign Body 68530
Repair
    Fistula 68770
Tumor
    Excision
       with Osteotomy 68550
       without Closure 68540

Lacrimal Punctum
Closure
    by Plug 68761
    by Thermocauterization, Ligation or Laser
       Surgery 68760
Dilation .68801
Incision .68440
Repair .68705

Lacrimal Sac
Biopsy .68525
Excision 68520
Incision and Drainage 68420

Lacrimal System
Unlisted Services and Procedures 68899

Lactase Deficiency Breath Test 91065

Lactate 83605

Lactate Dehydrogenase
See Lactic Dehydrogenase

Lactic Acid 83605

Lactic Acid Measurement
See Lactate

Lactic Cytochrome Reductase
See Lactic Dehydrogenase

Lactic Dehydrogenase 83615-83625

Lactiferous Duct
Excision 19112
Exploration 19110

Lactoferrin
Fecal 83630

Lactogen, Human Placental 83632

Lactogenic Hormone
See Prolactin

Lactose
Urine 83633-83634

Ladd Procedure 44055

Lagophthalmos
Repair .67912

Laki Lorand Factor
See Fibrin Stabilizing Factor

Lamblia Intestinalis
See Giardia Lamblia

Lambrinudi Operation
See Arthrodesis, Foot Joint

Lamellar Keratoplasties
See Keratoplasty, Lamellar

Laminaria
Insertion 59200

Laminectomy .. 62351, 63001, 63005-63011,
63015-63044, 63180-63200,
63265-63290, 63300-63655
Lumbar 22630, 63012
Surgical 63170-63172
with Facetectomy 63045-63048

Laminoplasty
Cervical 63050-63051

Langerhans Islands
See Islet Cell

Language Evaluation 92506

Language Therapy 92507-92508

LAP
See Leucine Aminopeptidase

Laparoscopic Appendectomy
See Appendectomy, Laparoscopic

Laparoscopic Biopsy of Ovary
See Biopsy, Ovary, Laparoscopic

Laparoscopy
Abdominal 49320-49329
Adrenal Gland
  Biopsy 60650
  Excision 60650
Adrenalectomy 50545
Appendectomy 44970
Aspiration 49322
Biopsy 47561, 49321
  Lymph Nodes 38570
Cholangiography 47560-47561
Cholecystectomy 47562-47564
Cholecystenterostomy 47570
Colectomy
  Partial 44204-44208
  Total 44210-44212
Destruction
  Lesion 58662
Diagnostic 49320
Drainage
  Extraperitoneal Lymphocele 49323
Ectopic Pregnancy 59150
  with Salpingectomy and/or
  Oophorectomy 59151
Enterolysis 44200
Esophagogastric Fundoplasty 43280
Fimbrioplasty 58672
Gastric Restrictive Procedures 43644-43645
Gastrostomy
  Temporary 43653
Hernia Repair
  Initial 49650
  Recurrent 49651

In Vitro Fertilization 58976
  Retrieve Oocyte 58970
  Transfer Embryo 58974
  Transfer Gamete 58976
Incontinence Repair 51990-51992
Jejunostomy 44201
Kidney
  Ablation 50541-50542
Ligation
  Veins, Spermatic 55550
Liver
  Ablation
    Tumor 47370-47371
Lymphadenectomy 38571-38572
Lymphatic 38570-38589
Lysis of Adhesions 58660
Lysis of Intestinal Adhesions 44200
Nephrectomy 50545-50548
  Partial 50543
Orchiectomy 54690
Orchiopexy 54692
Oviduct Surgery 58670-58671, 58679
Pelvis 49320
Prostatectomy 55866
Pyeloplasty 50544
Removal
  Fallopian Tube 58661
  Leiomyomata 58545-58546
  Ovaries 58661
  Spleen 38120
  Testis 54690
Resection
  Intestines
    with Anastomosis 44202-44203
Salpingostomy 58673
Splenectomy 38120-38129
Stomach 43651-43659
  Gastric Bypass 43644-43645
  Gastroenterostomy 43644-43645
  Roux-En-Y 43644
Unlisted Services and Procedures 38129,
  38589, 43289, 43659, 44238-44239, 44979,
  47379, 47579, 49329, 49659, 50549, 50949,
  54699, 55559, 58578-58579, 58679, 59898
Ureterolithotomy 50945
Ureteroneocystostomy 50947-50948
Urethral Suspension 51990
Vaginal Hysterectomy 58550-58554
Vaginal Suspension 57425
Vagus Nerves
  Transection 43651-43652
with X-Ray 47560

Laparotomy
Exploration 47015, 49000-49002, 58960
for Staging 49220
Hemorrhage Control 49002
Second Look 58960
Staging 58960
with Biopsy 49000

Laparotomy, Exploratory
See Abdomen, Exploration

Lapidus Procedure 28297

Large Bowel
See Anus; Cecum; Rectum

Laroyenne Operation
See Vagina, Abscess, Incision and Drainage

Laryngeal Function Study 92520

Laryngeal Sensory
Testing 92614-92617

Laryngectomy 31360-31382
Partial 31367-31382
Subtotal 31367-31368

Laryngocele
Removal 31300

Laryngofissure 31300

Laryngography 70373
Instillation
  Contrast Material 31708

Laryngopharyngectomy
See Excision, Larynx, with Pharynx

Laryngopharynx
See Hypopharynx

Laryngoplasty
Burns 31588
Cricoid Split 31587
Laryngeal Stenosis 31582
Laryngeal Web 31580
Open Reduction of Fracture 31584

Laryngoscopy
Diagnostic 31505
Direct 31515-31571
Exploration 31505, 31520-31526, 31575
Fiberoptic 31575-31579
  with Stroboscopy 31579
Indirect 31505-31513
Newborn 31520
Operative 31530-31561

Laryngotomy 31300
Diagnostic 31320
Total 31360-31368

Larynx
Aspiration
  Endoscopy 31515
Biopsy
  Endoscopy 31510, 31535-31536, 31576
Dilation
  Endoscopic 31528-31529
Endoscopy
  Direct 31515-31571
  Excision 31545-31546
  Exploration 31505, 31520-31526, 31575
  Fiberoptic 31575-31579
    with Stroboscopy 31579
  Indirect 31505-31513
  Operative 31530-31561
Excision
  Lesion 31512, 31578
    Endoscopic 31545-31546
  Partial 31367-31382

Sclera
Excision 66130
Skin
Abrasion 15786-15787
Biopsy 11100-11101
Destruction
Benign 17000-17250
Malignant 17260-17286
by Photodynamic Therapy 96567
Excision
Benign 11400-11471
Malignant 11600-11646
Injection 11900-11901
Paring or Curettement 11055-11057
Shaving 11300-11313
Skin Tags
Removal 11200-11201
Skull
Excision ..61500, 61600-61608, 61615-61616
Spermatic Cord
Excision 55520
Spinal Cord
Destruction 62280-62282
Excision 63265-63273
Stomach
Excision 43611
Testis
Excision 54512
Toe
Excision 28092
Tongue
Excision 41110-41114
Uvula
Destruction 42145
Excision 42104-42107
Vagina
Destruction 57061-57065
Vulva
Destruction
Extensive 56515
Simple 56501
Wrist Tendon
Excision 25110

Lesion of Sciatic Nerve
See Sciatic Nerve, Lesion

Leu 2 Antigens
See CD8

Leucine Aminopeptidase 83670

**Leukemia Lymphoma Virus I
Antibodies, Human T Cell**
See Antibody, HTLV-I

**Leukemia Lymphoma Virus I,
Adult T Cell**
See HTLV I

**Leukemia Lymphoma Virus II
Antibodies, Human T Cell**
See Antibody, HTLV-II

**Leukemia Virus II, Hairy Cell
Associated, Human T Cell**
See HTLV II

Leukoagglutinins 86021

Leukocyte
See White Blood Cell
Alkaline Phosphatase 85540
Antibody 86021
Histamine Release Test 86343
Phagocytosis 86344
Transfusion 86950

Leukocyte Count
See White Blood Cell, Count

Levarterenol
See Noradrenalin

Levator Muscle Rep
See Blepharoptosis, Repair

LeVeen Shunt
Insertion 49425
Patency Test 78291
Revision 49426

Levulose
See Fructose

LGV
See Lymphogranuloma Venereum

LH
See Luteinizing Hormone (LH)

LHR
See Leukocyte Histamine Release Test

Lid Suture
See Blepharoptosis, Repair

Lidocaine
Assay 80176

Lift, Face
See Face Lift

Ligament
See Specific Site
Collateral
Repair
Knee
with Cruciate Ligament 27409
Dentate
Incision 63180-63182
Section 63180-63182
Injection 20550
Release
Coracoacromial 23415
Transverse Carpal 29848
Repair
Elbow 24343-24346
Knee Joint 27405-27409

Ligation
Artery
Abdomen 37617
Carotid 37600-37606
Chest 37616
Coronary 33502
Coronary Artery 33502
Ethmoidal 30915
Extremity 37618
Fistula 37607

Maxillary 30920
Neck 37615
Temporal 37609
Esophageal Varices 43204, 43400
Fallopian Tube
Oviduct 58600-58611, 58670
Gastroesophageal 43405
Hemorrhoids 46945-46946
Oviducts 59100
Salivary Duct 42665
Shunt
Aorta
Pulmonary 33924
Peritoneal
Venous 49428
Thoracic Duct 38380
Abdominal Approach 38382
Thoracic Approach 38381
Vas Deferens 55450
Vein
Clusters 37785
Esophagus 43205, 43244, 43400
Femoral 37650
Gastric 43244
Iliac 37660
Jugular, Internal 37565
Perforate 37760
Saphenous 37700-37735, 37780
Vena Cava 37620

Ligature Strangulation
Skin Tags 11200-11201

Light Coagulation
See Photocoagulation

Light Scattering Measurement
See Nephelometry

Light Therapy, UV
See Actinotherapy

Limb
See Extremity

**Limited Lymphadenectomy for
Staging**
See Lymphadenectomy, Limited, for Staging

Limited Neck Dissection
with Thyroidectomy 60252

Limited Resection Mastectomies
See Breast, Excision, Lesion

Lindholm Operation
See Tenoplasty

Lingual Bone
See Hyoid Bone

Lingual Frenectomy
See Excision, Tongue, Frenum

Lingual Nerve
Avulsion 64740
Incision 64740
Transection 64740

Lingual Tonsil
See Tonsils, Lingual

Lumbar
See Spine
Aspiration, Disk
   Percutaneous 62287

Lumbar Plexus
Decompression 64714
Injection
   Anesthetic 64449
Neuroplasty 64714
Release 64714
Repair/Suture 64862

Lumbar Puncture
See Spinal Tap

Lumbar Spine Fracture
See Fracture, Vertebra, Lumbar

Lumbar Sympathectomy
See Sympathectomy, Lumbar

Lumbar Vertebra
See Vertebra, Lumbar

Lumen Dilation 74360

Lumpectomy 19160-19162

Lunate
Arthroplasty
   with Implant 25444
Dislocation
   Closed Treatment 25690
   Open Treatment 25695

Lung
Abscess
  Incision and Drainage
   Open .32200
   Percutaneous 32200-32201
Aspiration 32420
Biopsy 32095-32100
Bullae
  Excision .32141
   Endoscopic 32655
Cyst
  Incision and Drainage
   Open .32200
  Removal 32140
Decortication
  Endoscopic 32651-32652
  Partial .32225
  Total 32220
  with Parietal Pleurectomy 32320
Empyema
  Excision .32540
Excision
  Bronchus Resection 32486
  Chest Resection 32520-32525
  Completion 32488
  Donor
   Heart-Lung 33930
   Lung .32850
  Emphysematous 32491
  Lobe 32480-32482
  Segment 32484
  Total 32440-32445
  Wedge Resection 32500
   Endoscopic 32657

Foreign Body
  Removal 32151
Hemorrhage .32110
Lavage
  Bronchial 31624
  Total 32997
Lysis
  Adhesions 32124
Needle Biopsy 32405
Nuclear Medicine
  Imaging, Perfusion 78580-78585
  Imaging, Ventilation 78586-78594
  Unlisted Services and Procedures 78599
Pneumocentesis 32420
Pneumolysis .32940
Pneumothorax 32960
Puncture 32420
Removal
  Bronchoplasty 32501
  Completion Pneumonectomy 32488
  Extrapleural 32445
  Single Lobe 32480
  Single Segment 32484
  Sleeve Lobectomy 32486
  Sleeve Pneumonectomy 32442
  Total Pneumonectomy 32440-32445
  Two Lobes 32482
  Volume Reduction 32491
  Wedge Resection 32500
Repair
  Hernia .32800
Segmentectomy 32484
Tear
  Repair .32110
Thoracotomy
  Biopsy 32095-32100
  Cardiac Massage 32160
  for Post-Op Complications 32120
  Removal
   Bullae 32141
   Cyst .32140
   Intrapleural Foreign Body 32150
   Intrapulmonary Foreign Body 32151
  Repair .32110
  with Excision-Plication of Bullae 32141
  with Open Intrapleural
   Pneumonolysis 32124
Transplantation 32851-32854, 33935
  Allograft Preparation . . .32855-32856, 33933
  Donor Pneumonectomy
   Heart-Lung 33930
   Lung .32850
Unlisted Services and Procedures 32999

Lung Function Tests
See Pulmonology, Diagnostic

Lung Volume Reduction
Emphysematous 32491

Lupus Anticoagulant Assay 85705

Lupus Band Test
See Immunofluorescent Study

Luteinizing Hormone (LH) 80418,
                           80426, 83002

Luteinizing Releasing Factor . . .83727

Lutenizing Hormone
See Luteinizing Hormone (LH)

Luteotropic Hormone
See Prolactin

Luteotropin
See Prolactin

Luteotropin, Placental
See Lactogen, Human Placental

Lyme Disease 86617-86618

Lyme Disease ab
See Antibody, Lyme Disease

Lyme Disease Vaccine
See Vaccination

Lymph Duct
Injection 38790

Lymph Nodes
Abscess
  Incision and Drainage 38300-38305
Biopsy 38500, 38510-38530, 38570
  Needle .38505
Dissection 38542
Excision 38500, 38510-38530
  Abdominal 38747
  Inguinofemoral 38760-38765
  Laparoscopic 38571-38572
  Limited, for Staging
   Para-Aortic 38562
   Pelvic 38562
   Retroperitoneal 38564
  Pelvic 38770
  Radical
   Axillary 38740-38745
   Cervical 38720-38724
   Suprahyoid 38720-38724
  Retroperitoneal Transabdominal 38780
  Thoracic 38746
Exploration .38542
Hygroma, Cystic
  Axillary/Cervical
   Excision 38550-38555
Nuclear Medicine
  Imaging 78195
Removal
  Abdominal 38747
  Inguinofemoral 38760-38765
  Pelvic 38770
  Retroperitoneal Transabdominal 38780
  Thoracic 38746

Lymph Vessels
Abdomen
  Lymphangiography 75805-75807
Arm
  Lymphangiography 75801-75803
Leg
  Lymphangiography 75801-75803
Nuclear Medicine
  Imaging 78195
Pelvis
  Lymphangiography 75805-75807

Lymphadenectomy
Abdominal 38747
Bilateral Inguinofemoral . . .54130, 56632, 56637
Bilateral Pelvic 51575, 51585, 51595, 54135,
55845, 55865
    Total 38571-38572, 57531, 58210
Diaphragmatic Assessment 58960
Gastric 38747
Inguinofemoral 38760-38765
Inguinofemoral, Iliac and Pelvic 56640
Injection
    Sentinel Node 38792
Limited Para-Aortic, Resection of Ovarian
Malignancy 58951, 58954
Limited Pelvic 55842, 55862, 58954
Limited, for Staging
    Para-Aortic 38562
    Pelvic 38562
    Retroperitoneal 38564
Mediastinal 21632
Peripancreatic 38747
Portal 38747
Radical
    Axillary 38740-38745
    Cervical 38720-38724
    Pelvic 54135, 55845
    Suprahyoid 38700
Regional 50230
Retroperitoneal Transabdominal 38780
Thoracic 38746
Unilateral Inguinofemoral 56631, 56634

Lymphadenitis
Incision and Drainage 38300-38305

Lymphadenopathy Associated Antibodies
See Antibody, HIV

Lymphadenopathy Associated Virus
See HIV

Lymphangiogram, Abdominal
See Lymphangiography, Abdomen

Lymphangiography
Abdomen 75805-75807
Arm 75801-75803
Injection 38790
Leg 75801-75803
Pelvis 75805-75807

Lymphangioma, Cystic
See Hygroma

Lymphangiotomy 38308

Lymphatic Channels
Incision 38308

Lymphatic Cyst
See Lymphocele

Lymphatic System
Unlisted Procedure 38999

Lymphatics
See Specific Procedure

Lymphoblast Transformation
See Blastogenesis

Lymphocele
Drainage
    Laparoscopic 49323
Extraperitoneal
    Open Drainage 49062

Lymphocoele
See Lymphocele

Lymphocyte
Culture .86821-86822
Toxicity Assay 86805-86806
Transformation .86353

Lymphocyte, Thymus-Dependent
See T-Cells

Lymphocytes, CD4
See CD4

Lymphocytes, CD8
See CD8

Lymphocytic Choriomeningitis
Antibody 86727

Lymphocytotoxicity 86805-86806

Lymphogranuloma Venereum
Antibody 86729

Lymphoma Virus, Burkitt
See Epstein-Barr Virus

Lynch Procedure 31075

Lysergic Acid Diethylamide . . .80102-80103, 80299

Lysergide
See Lysergic Acid Diethylamide

Lysis
Adhesions
    Epidural 0027T, 62263-62264
    Fallopian Tube 58740
    Foreskin 54450
    Intestinal 44005
    Labial 56441
    Lung 32124
    Nose 30560
    Ovary 58740
    Oviduct 58740
    Penile
      Post-circumcision 54162
    Ureter 50715-50725
    Urethra 53500
    Uterus 58559
Euglobulin 85360
Labial
    Adhesions 56441
Nose
    Intranasal Synechia 30560

Lysozyme 85549

M

MacEwen Operation
See Hernia, Repair, Inguinal

Machado Test
See Complement, Fixation Test

MacLean-De Wesselow Test
See Blood Urea Nitrogen; Urea Nitrogen, Clearance

Macrodactylia
Repair 26590

Madlener Operation
See Tubal Ligation

Magnesium .83735

Magnet Operation
See Ciliary Body; Cornea; Eye, Removal, Foreign Body; Iris; Lens; Retina; Sclera; Vitreous

Magnetic Resonance
Unlisted Services and Procedures 76498

Magnetic Resonance Angiography (MRA)
Abdomen 74185
Arm 73225
Chest 71555
Head 70544-70546
Leg 73725
Neck 70547-70549
Pelvis 72198
Spine 72159

Magnetic Resonance Imaging (MRI)
Abdomen 74181-74183
Ankle 73721-73723
Arm 73218-73220, 73223
Bone Marrow Study 76400
Brain 70551-70553
    Intraoperative 70557-70559
Breast .76093-76094
Chest 71550-71552
Elbow 73221
Face 70540-70543
Finger Joint 73221
Foot 73718-73719
Foot Joints 73721-73723
Guidance
    Needle Placement 76393
    Visceral Tissue Ablation 76394
Hand 73218-73220, 73223
Heart 75552
    Complete Study 75554
    Flow Mapping 75556
    Limited Study 75555
    Morphology .75553
Joint
    Lower Extremity 73721-73723
    Upper Extremity 73221-73223

Knee 73721-73723
Leg 73718-73720
Neck 70540-70543
Orbit 70540-70543
Pelvis 72195-72197
Radiology
    Diagnostic
        Procedures 76499
Spectroscopy .76390
Spine
    Cervical 72141-72142, 72156-72158
    Lumbar 72148-72158
    Thoracic 72146-72147, 72156-72158
Temporomandibular Joint (TMJ) 70336
Toe 73721-73723
Wrist 73221

**Magnetic Resonance
Spectroscopy** 76390

Magnetic Stimulation
Brain Cortex 0018T

**Magnetoencephalography
(MEG)** 95965-95967

Magnuson Procedure 23450

Magpi Operation 54322

MAGPI Procedure
See Hypospadias, Repair

Major Vestibular Gland
See Bartholin's Gland

Malar Area
Augmentation 21270
Bone Graft 21210
Fracture
    Open Treatment 21360-21366
    with Bone Graft 21366
    with Manipulation 21355
Reconstruction 21270

Malar Bone
See Cheekbone

Malaria Antibody 86750

Malaria Smear 87207

Malate Dehydrogenase 83775

Maldescent, Testis
See Testis, Undescended

Male Circumcision
See Circumcision

Malformation, Arteriovenous
See Arteriovenous Malformation

Malic Dehydrogenase
See Malate Dehydrogenase

Malleolus
See Ankle; Fibula; Leg, Lower; Tibia; Tibiofibular
Joint
Metatarsophalangeal Joint 27889

Mallet Finger Repair 26432

Maltose
Tolerance Test 82951-82952

Malunion Repair
Femur
    with Graft 27472
    without Graft 27470
Metatarsal 28322
Tarsal Joint 28320

Mammalian Oviduct
See Fallopian Tube

Mammaplasties
See Breast, Reconstruction

Mammary Abscess
See Abscess, Breast

Mammary Arteries
See Artery, Mammary

Mammary Duct
Catheter Lavage for Cytology 0046T-0047T
X-Ray with Contrast 76086-76088

Mammary Ductogram
Injection 19030

Mammary Stimulating Hormone
See Prolactin

Mammilliplasty
See Nipples, Reconstruction

Mammogram
Breast
    Localization Nodule 76096

Mammography 76090-76092
Screening 76092
with Computer-aided Detection 76082-76083

Mammoplasty
Augmentation 19324-19325
Reduction 19318

Mammotomy
See Mastotomy

Mammotropic Hormone, Pituitary
See Prolactin

Mammotropic Hormone, Placental
See Lactogen, Human Placental

Mammotropin
See Prolactin

Mandated Services
On Call Services 99027

Mandible
See Facial Bones; Maxilla; Temporomandibular
Joint (TMJ)
Abscess
    Excision .21025
Bone Graft 21215
Cyst
    Excision 21040, 21046-21047

Fracture
    Closed Treatment
        with Interdental Fixation 21453
        with Manipulation 21451
        without Manipulation 21450
    Open Treatment 21454-21470
        External Fixation 21454
        with Interdental Fixation 21462
        without Interdental Fixation 21461
    Percutaneous Treatment 21452
Osteotomy 21198-21199
Reconstruction
    with Implant 21244-21246, 21248-21249
Removal
    Foreign Body 41806
Torus Mandibularis
    Excision .21031
Tumor
    Excision 21040-21047
X-Ray 70100-70110

Mandibular Body
Augmentation
    with Bone Graft 21127
    with Prosthesis 21125

Mandibular Condyle
Fracture
    Open Treatment 21465
Reconstruction 21247

Mandibular Condylectomy
See Condylectomy

Mandibular Fracture
See Fracture, Mandible

Mandibular Rami
Reconstruction
    with Bone Graft 21194
    with Internal Rigid Fixation 21196
    without Bone Graft 21193
    without Internal Rigid Fixation 21195

**Mandibular Resection
Prosthesis** 21081

Mandibular Staple Bone Plate
Reconstruction
    Mandible .21244

Manganese 83785

Manipulation
Chest Wall 94667-94668
Chiropractic 98940-98943
Dislocation and/or Fracture 25535
    Acetabulum 27222
    Acromioclavicular 23545
    Ankle 27810, 27818, 27860
    Carpometacarpal 26670-26676
    Clavicular 23505
    Elbow 24300, 24640
    Femoral 27232, 27502, 27510, 27517
        Pertrochanteric 27240
    Fibula 27781, 27788
    Finger 26725-26727, 26742, 26755
    Greater Tuberosity
        Humeral 23625
    Hand 26670-26676

Heel 28405-28406
Hip 27257
Hip Socket 27222
Humeral 23605, 24505, 24535, 24577
   Epicondyle 24565
Hyoid 21494
Intercarpal 25660
Interphalangeal Joint ...26340, 26770-26776
Larynx 31586
Lunate 25690
Malar Area 21355
Mandibular 21451
Metacarpal 26605-26607
Metacarpophalangeal ..26700-26706, 26742
Metacarpophalangeal Joint 26340
Metatarsal 28475-28476
Nasal Bone 21315-21320
Orbit 21401
Phalangeal Shaft 26727
   Distal, Finger or Thumb 26755
   Phalanges, Finger/Thumb 26725
Phalanges
   Finger 26742, 26755, 26770-26776
   Finger/Thumb 26727
   Great Toe 28495-28496
   Toes 28515
Radial 24655, 25565
Radial Shaft 25505
Radiocarpal 25660
Radioulnar 25675
Scapular 23575
Shoulder 23650-23655
   with Greater Tuberosity 23665
Shoulder Dislocation
Sternoclavicular 23525
   with Surgical or Anatomical
   Neck Fracture 23675
Talus 28435-28436
Tarsal 28455-28456
Thumb 26641-26650
Tibial 27532, 27752
Trans-Scaphoperilunar 25680
Ulnar 24675, 25535, 25565
Vertebral 22315
Wrist ...25259, 25624, 25635, 25660, 25675,
                          25680, 25690
Foreskin 54450
Globe 92018-92019
Hip 27275
Interphalangeal Joint, Proximal 26742
Knee 27570
Osteopathic 98925-98929
Shoulder
   Application of Fixation Apparatus 23700
Spine
   with Anesthesia 22505
Tibial, Distal 27762

Manometric Studies

Kidney
   Pressure 50396
Rectum/Anus 91122
Ureter
   Pressure 50686
Ureterostomy 50686

Manometry

Rectum 90911

Mantoux Test

See TB Test, Skin Test

Manual Therapy 97140

Maquet Procedure 27418

Marcellation Operation

See Hysterectomy, Vaginal

Marrow, Bone

See Bone Marrow

Marshall-Marchetti-Krantz
Procedure 51840-51841, 58152,
                          58267, 58293

Marsupialization 10040

Bartholin's Gland Cyst 56440
Cyst
   Sublingual Salivary 42409
Liver
   Cyst or Abscess 47300
Pancreatic Cyst 48500
Urethral Diverticulum 53240

Mass

Kidney
   Ablation 50542

Mass Spectrometry and Tandem
Mass Spectrometry

Analyte
   Qualitative 83788
   Quantitative 83789

Massage

Cardiac 32160
Therapy 97124
   See Physical Medicine/Therapy/Occupational
   Therapy

Masseter Muscle/Bone

Reduction 21295-21296

Mastectomy

Gynecomastia 19140
Modified Radical 19240
Partial 19160-19162
Radical 19200-19220
Simple, Complete 19180
Subcutaneous 19182

Mastectomy, Halsted

See Mastectomy, Radical

Mastoid

Excision
   Complete 69502
   Radical 69511
      Modified 69505
      Petrous Apicectomy 69530
   Simple 69501
Obliteration 69670
Repair
   by Excision 69601-69603
   Fistula 69700
   with Apicectomy 69605
   with Tympanoplasty 69604

Mastoid Cavity

Debridement 69220-69222

Mastoidectomy

Osseointegrated Implant
   for External Speech Processor/Cochlear
   Stimulator 69715, 69718
with Apicectomy 69605
with Skull Base Surgery 61590, 61597
   Decompression 61595
   Facial Nerve 61595
with Tympanoplasty 69604, 69641-69646
   Cochlear Device Implantation 69930
   Complete 69502
      Revision 69601
   Ossicular Chain Reconstruction 69605
   Radical 69511
      Modified 69505
      Revision 69602-69603
   Simple 69501
   with Labyrinthectomy 69910
   with Labyrinthotomy 69802
   with Petrous Apicectomy 69530

Mastoidotomy 69635-69637

with Tympanoplasty 69635
   Ossicular Chain Reconstruction 69636
      and Synthetic Prosthesis 69636

Mastoids

Polytomography 76101-76102
X-Ray 70120-70130

Mastopexy 19316

Mastotomy 19020

Maternity Care

See Abortion; Cesarean Delivery; Ectopic
Pregnancy; Obstetrical Care

Maternity Care and
Delivery 59612-59622, 59898

Maxilla

See Facial Bones; Mandible
Bone Graft 21210
CT Scan 70486-70488
Cyst
   Excision 21048-21049
Excision 21030, 21032-21034
Fracture
   Closed Treatment 21345, 21421
   Open Treatment .21346-21348, 21422-21423
   with Fixation 21345-21347
Osteotomy 21206
Reconstruction
   with Implant ...21245-21246, 21248-21249
Tumor
   Excision 21048-21049

Maxillary Arteries

See Artery, Maxillary

Maxillary Sinus

See Sinus, Maxillary

Maxillary Torus Palatinus

Tumor Excision 21032

Maxillectomy 31225-31230

Maxillofacial Fixation
Application
　Halo Type Appliance 21100

Maxillofacial Impressions
Auricular Prosthesis 21086
Definitive Obturator Prosthesis 21080
Facial Prosthesis .21088
Interim Obturator Prosthesis 21079
Mandibular Resection Prosthesis 21081
Nasal Prosthesis .21087
Oral Surgical Splint 21085
Orbital Prosthesis 21077
Palatal Augmentation Prosthesis 21082
Palatal Lift Prosthesis 21083
Speech Aid Prosthesis 21084
Surgical Obturator Prosthesis 21076

Maxillofacial Procedures
Unlisted Services and Procedures 21299

Maxillofacial Prosthetics 21076-21089
Unlisted Services and Procedures 21089

Maydl Operation 45563, 50810
See Colostomy

Mayo Hernia Repair
See Hernia, Repair, Umbilicus

Mayo Operation
See Varicose Vein, Removal

Mayo Procedure 28292

MBC
See Minimum Bactericidal Concentration

McBride Procedure 28292

McBurney Operation
See Hernia, Repair, Inguinal

McCannel Procedure 66682

McDonald Operation
See Repair, Cervix, Cerclage, Abdominal; Revision

McIndoe Procedure
See Vagina, Construction

McKissock Surgery
See Breast, Reduction

McVay Operation
See Hernia, Repair, Inguinal

Measles Uncomplicated
See Rubeola

Measles Vaccine
See Vaccines

Measles, German
See Rubella

Meat Fibers
Feces 89160

Meatoplasty 69310

Meatotomy 53020-53025
Contact Laser Vaporization with/without
　Transurethral Resection of Prostate . . .52648
　with Cystourethroscopy 52281
Infant 53025
Non-Contact Laser Coagulation Prostate . .52647
Transurethral Electrosurgical Resection
　Prostate 52601
Ureter 52290
Ureteral
　Cystourethroscopy 52290-52305

Meckel's Diverticulum
Excision 44800
Unlisted Services and Procedures 44899

Median Nerve
Decompression .64721
Neuroplasty 64721
Release 64721
Repair/Suture
　Motor 64835
Transposition 64721

Median Nerve Compression
See Carpal Tunnel Syndrome

Mediastinal Cyst
See Cyst, Mediastinal

Mediastinoscopy 39400

Mediastinotomy
Cervical Approach 39000
Transthoracic Approach 39010

Mediastinum
See Chest; Thorax
Cyst
　Excision 32662, 39200
Endoscopy
　Biopsy 39400
　Exploration 39400
Exploration 39000-39010
Incision and Drainage 39000-39010
Needle Biopsy .32405
Removal
　Foreign Body 39000-39010
Tumor
　Excision 32662, 39220
Unlisted Procedures 39499

Medical Disability Evaluation Services 99455-99456

Medical Testimony 99075

Medicine, Preventive
See Preventive Medicine

Medicine, Pulmonary
See Pulmonology

Medulla
Tractotomy 61470

Medullary Tract
Incision 61470
Section 61470

Meibomian Cyst
See Chalazion

Membrane Oxygenation, Extracorporeal
See Extracorporeal Membrane Oxygenation

Membrane, Mucous
See Mucosa

Membrane, Tympanic
See Ear, Drum

Meninges
Tumor
　Excision 61512, 61519

Meningioma
Excision 61512, 61519
Tumor
　Excision 61512, 61519

Meningitis, Lymphocytic Benign
See Lymphocytic Choriomeningitis

Meningocele Repair 63700-63702

Meningococcal
See Vaccines

Meningococcal Vaccine
See Vaccines

Meningococcus
See Neisseria Meningitidis

Meningomyelocele
See Myelomeningocele

Meniscectomy
Knee Joint 27332-27333
Temporomandibular Joint 21060

Meniscus
Knee
　Excision 27332-27333
　Repair 27403
　Transplantation 29868

Mental Nerve
Avulsion 64736
Incision 64736
Transection 64736

Meprobamate 83805

Mercury 83015, 83825

Merskey Test
See Fibrin Degradation Products

Mesencephalic Tract
Incision 61480
Section 61480

Mesencephalon
Tractotomy 61480

Mesenteric Arteries
See Artery, Mesenteric

Mesentery

Lesion
  Excision 44820
Repair 44850
Suture 44850
Unlisted Services and Procedures 44899

Mesh

Implantation
  Hernia 49568
Insertion
  Pelvic Floor 57267
Removal
  Abdominal Infected 11008

Metabisulfite Test
See Red Blood Cell (RBC), Sickling

Metabolite 82520

Metacarpal

Amputation 26910
Craterization 26230
Cyst
  Excision 26200-26205
Diaphysectomy 26230
Excision 26230
  Radical
    for Tumor 26250-26255
Fracture
  Closed Treatment 26605
    with Fixation 26607
  Open Treatment 26615
  Percutaneous Fixation 26608
  with Manipulation 26605-26607
  without Manipulation 26600
Ostectomy
  Radical
    for Tumor 26250-26255
Repair
  Lengthening 26568
  Nonunion 26546
  Osteotomy 26565
Saucerization 26230
Tumor
  Excision 26200-26205

Metacarpophalangeal Joint

Arthrodesis 26850-26852
Arthroplasty 26530-26531
Arthroscopy
  Diagnostic 29900
  Surgical 29901-29902
Arthrotomy 26075
Biopsy
  Synovium 26105
Capsule
  Excision 26520
  Incision 26520
Capsulodesis 26516-26518
Dislocation
  Closed Treatment 26700
  Open Treatment 26715
  Percutaneous Fixation 26705-26706
  with Manipulation 26340
Exploration 26075
Fracture
  Closed Treatment 26740
  Open Treatment 26746
  with Manipulation 26742

Fusion 26516-26518, 26850-26852
Removal of Foreign Body 26075
Repair
  Collateral Ligament 26540-26542
Synovectomy 26135

Metadrenaline
See Metanephrines

Metals, Heavy
See Heavy Metal

Metamfetamine
See Methamphetamine

Metanephrines 83835

Metatarsal
See Foot
Amputation 28810
Condyle
  Excision 28288
Craterization 28122
Cyst
  Excision 28104-28107
Diaphysectomy 28122
Excision 28110-28114, 28122, 28140
Fracture
  Closed Treatment
    with Manipulation 28475-28476
    without Manipulation 28470
  Open Treatment 28485
  Percutaneous Fixation 28476
Free Osteocutaneous Flap with Microvascular
Anastomosis 20972
Repair 28322
  Lengthening 28306-28307
  Osteotomy 28306-28309
Saucerization 28122
Tumor
  Excision 28104-28107, 28173

Metatarsectomy 28140

Metatarsophalangeal Joint

Arthrotomy 28022, 28052
Cheilectomy 28289
Dislocation 28630-28635, 28645
  Percutaneous Fixation 28636
Exploration 28022
Great Toe
  Arthrodesis 28750
  Fusion 28750
Removal
  of Foreign Body 28022
  of Loose Body 28022
Repair
  Hallux Rigidus 28289
Synovial
  Biopsy 28052
  Excision 28072
Toe 28270

Methadone 83840

Methaemoglobin
See Methemoglobin

Methamphetamine

Blood or Urine 82145

Methanol 84600

Methbipyranone
See Metyrapone

Methemalbumin 83857

Methemoglobin 83045-83050

Methenamine Silver Stain 88312

Methopyrapone
See Metyrapone

Methoxyhydroxymandelic Acid
See Vanillylmandelic Acid

Methsuximide 83858

Methyl Alcohol
See Methanol

Methylamphetamine
See Methamphetamine

Methylene Bichloride
See Dichloromethane

Methylfluorprednisolone
See Dexamethasone

Methylmorphine
See Codeine

Metroplasty
See Hysteroplasty

Metyrapone 80436

MIC
See Minimum Inhibitory Concentration

Micro-Ophthalmia
Orbit Reconstruction 21256

Microalbumin
Urine 82043-82044

Microbiology 0023T, 87001-87999

Microdissection 88380

Microfluorometries, Flow
See Flow Cytometry

Microglobulin, Beta 2
Blood 82232
Urine 82232

Micrographic Surgery
Mohs Technique 17304-17310

Micrographic Surgery, Mohs
See Mohs Micrographic Surgery

Micropigmentation
Correction 11920-11922

Microscope, Surgical
See Operating Microscope

Microscopic Evaluation
Hair 96902

Microscopies, Electron
See Electron Microscopy

Microscopy
Ear Exam 92504

Microsomal Antibody 86376

Microsomia, Hemifacial
See Hemifacial Microsomia

Microsurgery
Operating Microscope 69990

Microvascular Anastomosis
Bone Graft
    Fibula 20955
    Other 20962
Fascial Flap, Free 15758
Muscle Flap, Free 15756
Osteocutaneous Flap with 20969-20973
Skin Flap, Free 15757

Microvite A
See Vitamin, A

Microwave Therapy 97020
See Physical Medicine/Therapy/Occupational
Therapy

Midbrain
See Brain; Brainstem; Mesencephalon; Skull
Base Surgery

Midcarpal Medioccipital Joint
Arthrotomy 25040

**Middle Cerebral Artery
Velocimetry** 76821

Middle Ear
See Ear, Middle

Midface
Reconstruction
    Forehead Advancement 21159-21160
    with Bone Graft 21145-21160, 21188
    without Bone Graft 21141-21143

**Migration Inhibitory Factor
(MIF)** 86378

Mile Operation
See Colectomy, Total, with Proctectomy

Milia, Multiple
Removal 10040

Miller Procedure 28737

**Miller-Abbott
Intubation** 44500, 74340

Minerva Cast 29035
Removal 29710

**Minimum Inhibitory
Concentration** 87186

**Minimum Lethal
Concentration** 87187

**Minnesota Multiphasic Personality
Inventory**
See MMPI

Miscarriage
Incomplete Abortion 59812
Missed Abortion
    First Trimester 59820
    Second Trimester 59821
Septic Abortion 59830

Missed Abortion
See Abortion

Mitchell Procedure 28296

Mitogen Blastogenesis 86353

Mitral Valve
Incision 33420-33422
Repair 33420-33427
    Incision 33420-33422
Replacement 33430

Mitrofanoff Operation 50845
See Appendico-Vesicostomy

Miyagawanella
See Chlamydia

MMPI 96100

MMR Shots 90707
See Vaccines

Mobilization
Splenic Flexure 44139
Stapes 69650

Modified Radical Mastectomy
See Mastectomy, Modified Radical

**Mohs Micrographic
Surgery** 17304-17310

Molar Pregnancy
See Hydatidiform Mole

Mold
Culture 87107

Mole, Carneous
See Abortion

Mole, Hydatid
See Hydatidiform Mole

**Molecular
Cytogenetics** 88271-88275
Interpretation and Report 88291

Molecular Diagnostics ...83890-83898
Amplification 83898-83901
Dot/Slot Production 83893
Enzymatic Digestion 83892
Extraction 83890-83891
Interpretation 83912
Molecular Isolation (Extraction) 83890
Mutation Identification 83904-83906
Mutation Scanning 83903
Nucleic Acid Probe 83896
Nucleic Acid Transfer 83897
Polymerase Reaction Chain 83898
Reverse Transcription 83902
Separation 83894

Molecular Oxygen Saturation
See Oxygen Saturation

Molluscum Contagiosum
Destruction 17110-17111, 54050-54065

Molteno Procedure 66180

Monilia
See Candida

Monitoring
Blood Pressure, 24 Hour 93784-93790
Electrocardiogram 93224-93237
    See Electrocardiography
Electroencephalogram 95812-95813,
                95950-95953, 95956
    with Drug Activation 95954
    with Physical Activation 95954
    with WADA Activation 95958
Fetal
    During Labor 59050-59051, 99500
        Interpretation Only 59051
Glucose
    Interstitial Fluid 95250
Interstitial Fluid Pressure 20950
Seizure 61531, 61760

Monitoring, Sleep
See Polysomnography

Monoethylene Glycol
See Ethylene Glycol

Mononucleosis Virus, Infectious
See Epstein-Barr Virus

Monophosphate, Adenosine
See Adenosine Monophosphate (AMP)

Monophosphate, Adenosine Cyclic
See Cyclic AMP

Monophosphate, Guanosine
See Guanosine Monophosphate

Monophosphate, Guanosine Cyclic
See Cyclic GMP

Monospot Test
See Rapid Test for Infection

Monoxide, Carbon
See Carbon Monoxide

Monteggia Fracture 24620-24635

Monticelli Procedure
See Application, Bone Fixation Device

Morbilli
See Rubeola

Morphine Methyl Ether
See Codeine

Morphometric Analysis
Nerve 88356
Skeletal Muscle 88355
Tumor 88358-88361, 88367-88368

Morton's Neuroma
Excision 28080

Moschcowitz Operation
See Repair, Hernia, Femoral; Revision

Mosenthal Test
See Urinalysis, Routine

Mother Cell
See Stem Cell

Motility Study
Esophagus 91010-91012

Motion Analysis
by Video and 3-D Kinematics 96000, 96004
Computer-based 96000, 96004

Mouth
Abscess
    Incision and Drainage 40800-40801,
           41005-41009, 41015-41018
Biopsy 40808, 41108
Cyst
    Incision and Drainage 40800-40801,
           41005-41009, 41015-41018
Excision
    Frenum 40819
Hematoma
    Incision and Drainage 40800-40801,
           41005-41009, 41015-41018
Lesion
    Destruction 40820
    Excision 40810-40816, 41116
    Vestibule of
        Destruction 40820
        Repair 40830
Mucosa
    Excision 40818
Reconstruction 40840-40845
Removal
    Foreign Body 40804-40805
Repair
    Laceration 40830-40831
Unlisted Services and Procedures ..40899, 41599
Vestibule of
    Excision
        Destruction 40808-40820
    Incision 40800-40806
    Other Procedures 40899
    Removal
        Foreign Body 40804
    Repair 40830-40845

Move
See Transfer
Finger 26555
Toe Joint 26556
Toe to Hand 26551-26554

Moynihan Test
See Gastrointestinal Tract, X-Ray, with Contrast

MPD Syndrome
See Temporomandibular Joint (TMJ)

MPR
See Multifetal Pregnancy Reduction

MR Spectroscopy
See Magnetic Resonance Spectroscopy

MRA
See Magnetic Resonance Angiography

MRI
See Magnetic Resonance Imaging (MRI)

MSLT
See Multiple Sleep Latency Testing (MSLT)

Mucin
Synovial Fluid 83872

Mucocele
Sinusotomy
    Frontal 31075

Mucopolysaccharides 83864-83866

Mucormycoses
See Mucormycosis

Mucormycosis
Antibody 86732

Mucosa
Ectopic Gastric Imaging 78290
Excision of Lesion
    Alveolar, Hyperplastic 41828
    Vestibule of Mouth 40810-40818
    via Esophagoscopy 43228
    via Small Intestinal Endoscopy 44369
    via Upper GI Endoscopy 43258
Periodontal Grafting 41870
Urethra, Mucosal Advancement 53450
Vaginal Biopsy 57100-57105

Mucosa, Buccal
See Mouth, Mucosa

Mucous Cyst
Antibody
    Hand or Finger 26160

Mucous Membrane
See Mouth, Mucosa
Cutaneous
    Biopsy 11100-11101
    Excision
        Benign Lesion 11440-11446
        Malignant Lesion 11640-11646
    Layer Closure, Wounds 12051-12057
    Simple Repair, Wounds 12011-12018
Excision
    Sphenoid Sinus 31288
Lid Margin
    Correction of Trichiasis 67835
    Nasal Test 95065
    Ophthalmic Test 95060
Rectum
    Proctoplasty for Prolapse 45505

Mucus Cyst
See Mucous Cyst

MUGA (Multiple Gated Acquisition) 78472-78478, 78483

Muller Procedure
See Sleep Study

Multifetal Pregnancy Reduction 59866

Multiple Sleep Latency Testing (MSLT) 95805

Multiple Valve Procedures
See Valvuloplasty

Mumford Operation
See Claviculectomy, Partial

Mumford Procedure 29824

Mumps
Antibody 86735
Immunization 90704, 90707, 90710
Vaccine 90704
    MMR 90707
    MMRV 90710

Muramidase 85549

Murine Typhus 86000

Muscle
See Specific Muscle
Abdomen
    See Abdominal Wall
Biopsy 20200-20206
Debridement
    Infected 11004-11006
Heart
    See Myocardium
Neck
    See Neck Muscle
Removal
    Foreign Body 20520-20525
Repair
    Forearm 25260-25274
    Wrist 25260-25274
Revision
    Arm, Upper 24330-24331
Transfer
    Arm, Upper 24301, 24320
    Elbow 24301
    Femur 27110
    Hip 27100-27105, 27111
    Shoulder 23395-23397, 24301, 24320

Muscle Compartment Syndrome
Detection 20950

Muscle Denervation
See Denervation

Muscle Division
Scalenus Anticus 21700-21705
Sternocleidomastoid 21720-21725

Muscle Flaps 15732-15738
Free 15756

Muscle Grafts 15841-15845

Muscle Testing
Dynamometry, Eye 92260
Extraocular Multiple Muscles 92265
Manual 95831-95834

Muscle, Oculomotor
See Eye Muscles

Muscles
Repair
    Extraocular .... .65290

Musculo-Skeletal System
See Musculoskeletal System

Musculoplasty
See Muscle, Repair

Musculoskeletal System
Unlisted Services and Procedures 20999,
    24999, 25999, 26989, 27299, 27599, 27899
Unlisted Services and Procedures, Head ...21499

Musculotendinous (Rotator) Cuff
Repair 23410-23412

Mustard Procedure
See Repair, Great Arteries; Revision

Myasthenia Gravis
Tensilon Test 95857-95858

Myasthenic, Gravis
See Myasthenia Gravis

Mycobacteria
Culture .... .87116
    Identification .... .87118
Detection 87550-87562
Sensitivity Studies .... .87190

Mycoplasma
Antibody .... .86738
Culture .... .87109
Detection 87580-87582

Mycota
See Fungus

Myectomy, Anorectal
See Myomectomy, Anorectal

Myelencephalon
See Medulla

Myelin Basic Protein
Cerebrospinal Fluid .... .83873

Myelography
Brain .... .70010
Spine
    Cervical .... .72240
    Lumbosacral .... .72265
    Thoracic .... .72255
    Total .... .72270

Myelomeningocele
Repair 63704-63706

Myelotomy .... .63170

Myocardial
Perfusion Imaging ...78460-78465, 78478-78480
    See Nuclear Medicine
Positron Emission Tomography (PET) ...... .78459

Myocardial Imaging 78466-78469
Positron Emission Tomography
    Perfusion Study 78491-78492
Repair
    Postinfarction .... .33542

Myocutaneous Flaps 15732-15738, 15756

Myofascial Pain Dysfunction Syndrome
See Temporomandibular Joint (TMJ)

Myofibroma
See Leiomyomata

Myoglobin .... .83874

Myomectomy
Anorectal .... .45108
Uterus 58140-58146, 58545-58546

Myoplasty
See Muscle, Repair

Myotomy
Esophagus .... .43030
Hyoid .... .21685

Myringoplasty .... .69620

Myringostomy
See Myringotomy

Myringotomy 69420-69421

Myxoid Cyst
See Ganglion

N

N. Meningitidis
See Neisseria Meningitidis

Naffziger Operation
See Decompression, Orbit; Section

Nagel Test
See Color Vision Examination

Nail Bed
Reconstruction .... .11762
Repair .... .11760

Nail Fold
Excision
    Wedge .... .11765

Nail Plate Separation
See Onychia

Nails
Avulsion 11730-11732
Biopsy .... .11755
Debridement 11720-11721
Evacuation
    Hematoma, Subungual .... .11740
Excision 11750-11752
    Cyst
      Pilonidal 11770-11772
KOH Examination .... .87220
Removal 11730-11732, 11750-11752
Trimming .... .11719

Narcosynthesis
Diagnostic and Therapeutic .... .90865

Nasal Abscess
See Nose, Abscess

Nasal Area
Bone Graft .... .21210

Nasal Bleeding
See Epistaxis

Nasal Bone
Fracture
    Closed Treatment 21310-21320
    Open Treatment 21325-21335
    with Manipulation 21315-21320
    without Manipulation .... .21310
X-Ray .... .70160

Nasal Deformity
Repair 40700-40761

Nasal Function Study .... .92512

Nasal Polyp
See Nose, Polyp

Nasal Prosthesis
Impression .... .21087

Nasal Septum
Abscess
    Incision and Drainage .... .30020
Fracture
    Closed Treatment .... .21337
    Open Treatment .... .21336
Hematoma
    Incision and Drainage .... .30020
Repair .... .30630
Submucous Resection .... .30520

Nasal Sinuses
See Sinus; Sinuses

Nasal Smear
Eosinophils .... .89190

Nasal Turbinate
Fracture
    Therapeutic .... .30930

Nasoethmoid Complex
Fracture
    Open Treatment 21338-21339
    Percutaneous Treatment .... .21340
Reconstruction 21182-21184

Nasogastric Tube
Placement .... .43752

Nasolacrimal Duct
Exploration .... .68810
    with Anesthesia .... .68811
Insertion
    Stent .... .68815
X-Ray
    with Contrast .... .70170

Nasomaxillary

Fracture
    Closed Treatment 21345
    Open Treatment 21346-21348
    with Bone Grafting 21348

Nasopharynges

See Nasopharynx

Nasopharyngoscopy 92511

Nasopharynx

See Pharynx
Biopsy 42804-42806
Hemorrhage 42970-42972
Unlisted Services and Procedures 42999

Natriuretic Peptide 83880

Natural Ostium

Sinus
    Maxillary 31000
    Sphenoid 31002

Navicular

Arthroplasty
    with Implant 25443
Fracture
    Closed Treatment 25622
    Open Treatment 25628
    with Manipulation 25624
Navigation
    Computer Assisted 0054T-0056T
Repair 25440

Neck

Angiography 70498, 70547-70549
Artery
    Ligation 37615
Biopsy 21550
Bypass Graft 35901
CT Scan 70490-70492, 70498
Dissection, Radical
    See Radical Neck Dissection
Exploration
    Blood Vessel 35800
    Lymph Nodes 38542
Incision and Drainage
    Abscess 21501-21502
    Hematoma 21501-21502
Lipectomy, Suction Assisted 15876
Magnetic Resonance Angiography
(MRA) 70547-70549
Magnetic Resonance Imaging
(MRI) 70540-70543
Nerve
    Graft 64885-64886
Repair
    Blood Vessel 35201
      with Other Graft 35261
      with Vein Graft 35231
Skin
    Revision 15819
Tumor
    Excision 21555-21556
    Excision/Resection 21557
Ultrasound Exam 76536
Unlisted Services and Procedures,
Surgery 21899

Urinary Bladder

    See Bladder, Neck
Wound Exploration
    Penetrating 20100
X-Ray 70360

Neck Muscle

Division
    Scalenus Anticus 21700-21705
    Sternocleidomastoid 21720-21725

Necropsy

Coroner's Exam 88045
Forensic Exam 88040
Gross and Micro Exam 88020-88029
Gross Exam 88000-88016
Organ 88037
Regional 88036
Unlisted Services and Procedures 88099

Needle Biopsy

See Biopsy
Abdomen Mass 49180
Bone 20220-20225
Bone Marrow 38221
Breast 19100
Colon
    Endoscopy 45392
Colon-Sigmoid
    Endoscopy 45342
CT Scan Guidance 76360
Epididymis 54800
Esophagus
    Endoscopy 43232
Fluoroscopic Guidance 76003
Gastrointestinal, Upper
    Endoscopy 43238, 43242
Kidney 50200
Liver 47000-47001
Lung 32405
Lymph Nodes 38505
Mediastinum 32405
Muscle 20206
Pancreas 48102
Pleura 32400
Prostate 55700
Retroperitoneal Mass 49180
Salivary Gland 42400
Spinal Cord 62269
Testis 54500
Thyroid Gland 60100
Transbronchial 31629, 31633

Needle Localization

Breast
    Placement 19290-19291
    with Lesion Excision 19125-19126
Magnetic Resonance Guidance 76393

Needle Manometer Technique 20950

Needle Wire

Introduction
    Trachea 31730
Placement
    Breast 19290-19291

Neer Procedure 23470

Neisseria gonorrheae 87590-87592, 87850

Neisseria Meningitidis

Antibody 86741

Neobladder

Construction 51596

Neonatal Critical Care

See Newborn Care
Initial 99295
Subsequent 99296

Neoplasm

Cancer Photoradiation Therapy
    See Photochemotherapy
Cardiac
    See Heart, Tumor
Colon
    See Colon, Tumor
Esophageal
    See Tumor, Esophagus
Spinal Cord
    See Spinal Cord, Neoplasm
Unspecified Nature of Brain
    See Brain, Tumor

Neoplastic Growth

See Tumor

Nephelometry 83883

Nephrectomy

Donor 50300-50320, 50547
Laparoscopic 50545-50548
Partial 50240
    Laparoscopic 50543
Recipient 50340
with Ureters 50220-50236, 50546, 50548

Nephrolith

See Calculus, Removal, Kidney

Nephrolithotomy 50060-50075

Nephropexy 50400-50405

Nephroplasty

See Kidney, Repair

Nephropyeloplasty

See Pyeloplasty

Nephrorrhaphy 50500

Nephroscopy

See Endoscopy, Kidney

Nephrostogram 50394

Nephrostolithotomy

Percutaneous 50080-50081

Nephrostomy 50040

Change Tube 50398
Endoscopic 50562-50570
Percutaneous 52334
with Drainage 50040
X-Ray with Contrast
    Guide Dilation 74485

Nephrostomy Tract
Establishment 50395

Nephrotomogram
See Nephrotomography

Nephrotomography 74415

Nephrotomy 50040-50045
with Exploration 50045

Nerve
Cranial
   See Cranial Nerve
Facial
   See Facial Nerve
Intercostal
   See Intercostal Nerve
Lingual
   See Lingual Nerve
Median
   See Median Nerve
Obturator
   See Obturator Nerve
Peripheral
   See Peripheral Nerve
Phrenic
   See Phrenic Nerve
Sciatic
   See Sciatic Nerve
Spinal
   See Spinal Nerve
Tibial
   See Tibial Nerve
Ulnar
   See Ulnar Nerve
Vestibular
   See Vestibular Nerve

Nerve Conduction
Motor Nerve 95900-95903
Sensory Nerve or Mixed 95904

Nerve II, Cranial
See Optic Nerve

Nerve Root
See Cauda Equina; Spinal Cord
Decompression 63020-63048, 63055-63103
Incision 63185-63190
Section 63185-63190

Nerve Stimulation, Transcutaneous
See Application, Neurostimulation

Nerve Teasing 88362

Nerve V, Cranial
See Trigeminal Nerve

Nerve VII, Cranial
See Facial Nerve

Nerve X, Cranial
See Vagus Nerve

Nerve XI, Cranial
See Accessory Nerve

Nerve XII, Cranial
See Hypoglossal Nerve

Nerves
Anastomosis
   Facial to Hypoglossal 64868
   Facial to Phrenic 64870
   Facial to Spinal Accessory 64866
Avulsion 64732-64772
Biopsy 64795
Decompression 64702-64727
Destruction 64600-64681
   Laryngeal, Recurrent 31595
Foot
   Excision 28030
   Incision 28035
Graft 64885-64907
Implantation
   Electrode 64553-64581
   to Bone 64787
   to Muscle 64787
Incision 43640-43641, 64732-64772
Injection
   Anesthetic 01991-01992, 64400-64530
   Neurolytic Agent 64600-64681
Insertion
   Electrode 64553-64581
Lesion
   Excision 64774-64792
Neurofibroma
   Excision 64788-64792
Neurolemmoma
   Excision 64788-64792
Neurolytic
   Internal 64727
Neuroma
   Excision 64774-64786
Neuroplasty 64702-64721
Removal
   Electrode 64585
Repair
   Graft 64885-64907
   Microdissection 69990
   Suture 64831-64876
Spinal Accessory
   Incision 63191
   Section 63191
Suture 64831-64876
Sympathectomy
   Excision 64802-64818
Transection 43640-43641, 64732-64772
Transposition 64718-64721
Unlisted Services and Procedures 64999

Nervous System
Nuclear Medicine
   Unlisted Services and Procedures 78699

Nesidioblast
See Islet Cell

Neural Conduction
See Nerve Conduction

Neural Ganglion
See Ganglion

Neurectomy
Foot 28030
Gastrocnemius 27320
Hamstring Muscle 27315

Leg, Upper 27315-27320
Popliteal 27320
Tympanic 69676

Neuroendoscopy
Intracranial 62160-62165

Neurofibroma
Cutaneous Nerve
   Excision 64788
Extensive
   Excision 64792
Peripheral Nerve
   Excision 64790

Neurolemmoma
Cutaneous Nerve
   Excision 64788
Extensive
   Excision 64792
Peripheral Nerve
   Excision 64790

Neurologic System
See Nervous System

Neurology
Diagnostic
   Anal Sphincter 51785
   Autonomic Nervous Function
      Heart Rate Response 95921-95923
      Pseudomotor Response 95921-95923
      Sympathetic Function 95921-95923
   Brain Cortex Magnetic Stimulation 0018T
   Brain Surface Electrode
      Stimulation 95961-95962
   Central Motor
      Transcranial Motor
      Stimulation 95928-95929
   Electrocorticogram
      Intraoperative 95829
   Electroencephalogram (EEG) ...95812-95827,
                              95955
      Brain Death 95824
      Electrode Placement 95830
      Intraoperative 95955
      Monitoring ...95812-95813, 95950-95953,
                                95956
      Physical or Drug Activation 95954
      Sleep 95822, 95827
      Standard 95819
      WADA Activation 95958
   Electroencephalography (EEG)
      Digital Analysis 95957
   Electromyography
      See Electromyography
      Fine Wire
         Dynamic 96004
      Ischemic Limb Exercise Test 95875
      Needle 51785, 95860-95872
      Surface
         Dynamic 96002-96004
   Higher Cerebral Function
      Aphasia Test 96105
      Cognitive Function Tests 96115
      Developmental Tests 96110-96111
   Magnetoencephalography
   (MEG) 95965-95967

Norchlorimipramine
See Imipramine

Norepinephrine
See Catecholamines
Blood 82383-82384
Urine 82384

Nortriptyline
Assay 80182

Norwood Procedure 33611-33612,
33619

See Repair, Heart, Ventricle; Revision

Nose
Abscess
   Incision and Drainage 30000-30020
Artery
   Incision 30915-30920
Biopsy
   Intranasal 30100
Dermoid Cyst
   Excision
      Complex 30125
      Simple 30124
Displacement Therapy 30210
Endoscopy
   Diagnostic 31231-31235
   Surgical 31237-31294
Excision
   Rhinectomy 30150-30160
Fracture
   Closed Treatment 21345
   Open Treatment 21325-21336,
        21338-21339, 21346-21347
   Percutaneous Treatment 21340
   with Fixation 21330, 21340, 21345-21347
Hematoma
   Incision and Drainage 30000-30020
Hemorrhage
   Cauterization 30901-30906
Insertion
   Septal Prosthesis 30220
Intranasal
   Lesion
      External Approach 30118
      Internal Approach 30117
Lysis of Adhesions 30560
Polyp
   Excision
      Extensive 30115
      Simple 30110
Reconstruction
   Cleft Lip/Cleft Palate 30460-30462
   Dermatoplasty 30620
   Primary 30400-30420
   Secondary 30430-30450
   Septum 30520
Removal
   Foreign Body 30300
      Anesthesia 30310
      Lateral Rhinotomy 30320
Repair
   Adhesions 30560
   Cleft Lip 40700-40761
   Fistula 30580-30600, 42260
   Rhinophyma 30120

Septum 30540-30545, 30630
Synechia 30560
Vestibular Stenosis 30465
Skin
   Excision 30120
   Surgical Planing 30120
Submucous Resection Turbinate
   Excision 30140
Turbinate
   Excision 30130-30140
   Fracture 30930
   Injection 30200
Turbinate Mucosa
   Cauterization 30801-30802
Unlisted Services and Procedures 30999

Nose Bleed 30901-30906
See Hemorrhage, Nasal

NTD 86384
See Nitroblue Tetrazolium Dye Test

Nuclear Antigen
Antibody 86235

Nuclear Imaging
See Nuclear Medicine

Nuclear Magnetic Resonance Imaging
See Magnetic Resonance Imaging (MRI)

Nuclear Magnetic Resonance Spectroscopy
See Magnetic Resonance Spectroscopy

Nuclear Medicine
Adrenal Gland Imaging 78075
Automated Data 78890-78891
Bile Duct
   Imaging 78223
Bladder
   Residual Study 78730
Blood
   Bone
      Density Study 78350-78351
      Imaging 78300-78320
      SPECT 78320
      Ultrasound 76977
      Unlisted Services and Procedures ... 78399
   Flow Imaging 78445
   Iron
      Absorption 78162
      Chelatable 78172
      Plasma 78160
      Red Cells 78140
      Utilization 78170
   Platelet Survival 78190-78191
   Red Cell Survival 78130-78135
   Red Cells 78120-78121
   Unlisted Services and Procedures 78199
   Whole Blood Volume 78122
Bone Marrow
   Imaging 78102-78104
Brain
   Blood Flow 78610-78615
   Cerebrospinal Fluid 78630-78650
   Imaging 78600-78609
   Vascular Flow 78610

Endocrine System
   Unlisted Services and Procedures 78099
Esophagus
   Imaging (Motility) 78258
   Reflux Study 78262
Gallbladder
   Imaging 78223
Gastric Mucosa
   Imaging 78261
Gastrointestinal
   Blood Loss Study 78278
   Protein Loss Study 78282
   Shunt Testing 78291
   Unlisted Services and Procedures 78299
Genitourinary System
   Unlisted Services and Procedures 78799
Heart
   Blood Flow 78414
   Blood Pool Imaging 78472-78473,
       78481-78483, 78494-78496
   Myocardial Imaging 78459, 78466-78469
   Myocardial Perfusion 78460-78465,
       78478-78480
   Shunt Detection 78428
   Unlisted Services and Procedures 78499
Hepatic Duct
   Imaging 78223
Inflammatory Process 78805-78807
Intestines
   Imaging 78290
Kidney
   Blood Flow 78715
   Function Study 78725
   Imaging 78700-78707, 78710
Lacrimal Gland Tear Flow 78660
Liver
   Function Study 78220
   Imaging 78201-78216
   Vascular Flow 78206
Lung
   Imaging Perfusion 78580-78585
   Imaging Ventilation 78586-78594
   Unlisted Services and Procedures 78599
Lymph Nodes 78195
Lymphatics 78195
   Unlisted Services and Procedures 78199
Musculoskeletal System
   Unlisted Services and Procedures 78399
Nervous System
   Unlisted Services and Procedures 78699
Parathyroid Gland Imaging 78070
Pulmonary Perfusion Imaging 78588
Salivary Gland Function Study 78232
   Imaging 78230-78231
Spleen
   Imaging 78185, 78215-78216
   Unlisted Services and Procedures 78199
Stomach
   Blood Loss Study 78278
   Emptying Study 78264
   Protein Loss Study 78282
   Reflux Study 78262
   Vitamin B-12 Absorption 78270-78272
Testes
   Imaging 78760-78761

Therapeutic
  Interstitial 79300
  Intra-arterial 79445
  Intra-articular 79440
  Intracavitary 79200
  Intravenous 79101
  Intravenous Infusion 79403
  Oral 79005
  Thyroid 79200-79300
  Unlisted Services and Procedures 79999
Thyroid
  Imaging 78010
  Imaging for Metastases 78015-78018
  Imaging with Flow 78011
  Imaging with Uptake 78006
  Metastases Uptake 78020
  Uptake 78000-78003
Tumor Imaging
  Positron Emission Tomography .78811-78816
    with Computed Tomography ..78814-78816
  Tumor Localization 78800-78804
Unlisted Services and Procedures 78999
Urea Breath Test 78267-78268
Ureter
  Reflux Study 78740
Vein
  Thrombosis Imaging 78455-78458

Nucleases, DNA
See DNAse

Nucleic Acid Probe 83896
Amplified Probe Detection
  Infectious Agent
    Bartonella henselae 87471
    Bartonella quintana 87471
    Borrelia burgdorferi 87476
    Candida species 87481
    Chlamydia pneumoniae 87486
    Chlamydia Trachomatis 87491
    Cytomegalovirus 87496
    Gardnerella Vaginalis 87511
    Hepatitis B Virus 87516
    Hepatitis C 87521
    Hepatitis G 87526
    Herpes Simplex Virus 87529
    Herpes Virus-6 87532
    HIV-1 87535
    HIV-2 87538
    Legionella Pneumophila 87541
    Multiple Organisms 87801
    Mycobacteria avium-intracellulare ..87561
    Mycobacteria species 87551
    Mycobacteria tuberculosis 87556
    Mycoplasma pneumoniae 87581
    Neisseria gonorrheae 87591
    Not Otherwise Specified 87798, 87801
    Papillomavirus, Human 87621
    Streptococcus, Group A 87651
Direct Probe Detection
  Infectious Agent
    Bartonella henselae 87470
    Bartonella quintana 87470
    Borrelia burgdorferi 87475
    Candida species 87480
    Chlamydia pneumoniae 87485
    Chlamydia Trachomatis 87490
    Cytomegalovirus 87495
    Gardnerella Vaginalis 87510

Hepatitis B Virus 87515
Hepatitis C 87520
Hepatitis G 87525
Herpes Simplex Virus 87528
Herpes Virus-6 87531
HIV-1 87534
HIV-2 87537
Legionella Pneumophila 87540
Multiple Organisms 87800
Mycobacteria avium-intracellulare ..87560
Mycobacteria species 87550
Mycobacteria tuberculosis 87555
Mycoplasma pneumoniae 87580
Neisseria gonorrheae 87590
Not Otherwise Specified 87797
Papillomavirus, Human 87620
Streptococcus, Group A 87650
Trichomonas vaginalis 87660
Genotype Analysis
  Infectious Agent
    Hepatitis C Virus 87902
    HIV-1 87901
In Situ Hybridization 88365-88368
Phenotype Analysis
  Infectious Agent
    HIV-1 Drug Resistance 87903-87904
Quantification
  Infectious Agent
    Bartonella henselae 87472
    Bartonella quintana 87472
    Borrelia burgdorferi 87477
    Candida species 87482
    Chlamydia pneumoniae 87487
    Chlamydia Trachomatis 87492
    Cytomegalovirus 87497
    Gardnerella Vaginalis 87512
    Hepatitis B Virus 87517
    Hepatitis C 87522
    Hepatitis G 87527
    Herpes Simplex Virus 87530
    Herpes Virus-6 87533
    HIV-1 87536
    HIV-2 87539
    Legionella Pneumophila 87542
    Mycobacteria avium-intracellulare ..87562
    Mycobacteria species 87552
    Mycobacteria tuberculosis 87557
    Mycoplasma pneumoniae 87582
    Neisseria gonorrheae 87592
    Not Otherwise Specified 87799
    Papillomavirus, Human 87622
    Streptococcus, Group A 87652

Nucleolysis, Intervertebral Disk
See Chemonucleolysis

Nucleotidase 83915

Nursemaid Elbow 24640

Nursing Facility Discharge Services
See Discharge Services, Nursing Facility

Nursing Facility Services
Care Plan Oversight Services 99379-99380
Comprehensive Assessments
  New or Established Patient 99301-99303
Discharge Services 99315-99316

Subsequent Care
  New or Established Patient 99311-99313
    See Domiciliary Services

Nuss Procedure
with Thoracoscopy 21743
without Thoracoscopy 21742

Nutrition Therapy
Group 97804
Home Infusion 99601-99602
Initial Assessment 97802
Reassessment 97803

Nystagmus Tests
See Vestibular Function Tests
Optokinetic 92534, 92544
Positional 92532, 92542
Spontaneous 92531, 92541

O

O$_2$ Saturation
See Oxygen Saturation

Ober-Yount Procedure 27025
See Fasciotomy, Hip

Obliteration
  Mastoid 69670
  Vagina
    Total 57110-57112
    Vault 57120

Oblongata, Medulla
See Medulla

Observation 99234-99236
See Evaluation and Management; Hospital
Services

Obstetrical Care
Abortion
  Induced
    by Amniocentesis Injection ..59850-59852
      See Abortion; Cesarean Delivery;
      Ectopic Pregnancy
    by Dilation and Curettage 59840
    by Dilation and Evaluation 59841
  Missed
    First Trimester 59820
    Second Trimester 59821
  Spontaneous 59812
  Therapeutic 59840-59852
Antepartum Care 59425-59426
Cesarean Delivery 59618-59622
  Only 59514
  Postpartum Care 59515
  Routine 59510
  with Hysterectomy 59525
Curettage
  Hydatidiform Mole 59870

Evacuation
Hydatidiform Mole 59870
External Cephalic Version 59412
Miscarriage
Surgical Completion 59812-59821
Placenta Delivery 59414
Postpartum Care 59430, 59514
Septic Abortion 59830
Total (Global) 59400, 59610, 59618
Unlisted Services and Procedures ..59898-59899
Vaginal
after Cesarean 59610-59614
Vaginal Delivery 59409-59410
Delivery after Cesarean 59610-59614

Obstruction
See Occlusion

Obstruction Clearance
Venous Access Device 36595-36596

Obstruction Colon
See Colon, Obstruction

Obturator Nerve
Avulsion 64763-64766
Incision 64763-64766
Transection 64763-64766

Obturator Prosthesis 21076
Definitive 21080
Insertion
Larynx 31527
Interim 21079

Occipital Nerve, Greater
Avulsion 64744
Incision 64744
Injection
Anesthetic 64405
Transection 64744

Occlusion
Extracranial
Intracranial 61623
Fallopian Tube
Oviduct 58565, 58615
Penis
Vein 37790
Umbilical Cord 59072

Occlusive Disease of Artery
See Repair, Artery; Revision

Occult Blood 82270
by Hemoglobin Immunoassay 82274

Occupational Therapy
Evaluation 97003-97004

Ocular Implant
See Orbital Implant
Insertion
in Scleral Shell 65130
Muscles Attached 65140
Muscles, Not Attached 65135
Modification 65125
Reinsertion 65150
with Foreign Material 65155
Removal 65175

Ocular Muscle
See Eye Muscles

Ocular Orbit
See Orbit

Ocular Photoscreening 0065T

Ocular Prostheses
See Prosthesis, Ocular

Oculomotor Muscle
See Eye Muscles

Oddi Sphincter
See Sphincter of Oddi

Odontoid Dislocation
Open Treatment/Reduction 22318
with Grafting 22319

Odontoid Fracture
Open Treatment/Reduction 22318
with Grafting 22319

Odontoid Process
Excision 22548

Oesophageal Neoplasm
See Tumor, Esophagus

Oesophageal Varices
See Esophageal Varices

Oesophagus
See Esophagus

Oestradiol
See Estradiol

Office and/or Other Outpatient Services
See History and Physical
Consultation
Confirmatory Consultations 99271-99275
Established Patient 99211-99215
New Patient 99201-99205
Normal Newborn 99432
Office Visit
Established Patient 99211-99215
New Patient 99201-99205
Outpatient Visit
Established Patient 99211-99215
New Patient 99201-99205
Prolonged Services 99354-99355

Office Medical Services
After Hours 99050-99054
Emergency Care 99058

Office or Other Outpatient Consultations
See Consultation, Office and/or Other Outpatient

Olecranon
See Elbow; Humerus; Radius; Ulna
Bursa
Arthrocentesis 20605
Cyst
Excision 24125-24126
Tumor
Cyst 24120
Excision 24125-24126

Olecranon Process
Craterization 24147
Diaphysectomy 24147
Excision 24147
Abscess 24138
Fracture
See Elbow; Humerus; Radius
Closed Treatment 24670-24675
Open Treatment 24685
Osteomyelitis 24138, 24147
Saucerization 24147
Sequestrectomy 24138

Oligoclonal Immunoglobulins .83916

Omentectomy 49255, 58950-58956
Laparotomy 58960
Oophorectomy 58943
Resection Ovarian Malignancy 58950-58952
Resection Peritoneal Malignancy ...58950-58956
Resection Tubal Malignancy 58950-58956

Omentum
Excision 49255, 58950-58956
Flap 49904-49905
Free
with Microvascular Anastomosis ...49906
Unlisted Services and Procedures 49999

Omphalectomy 49250

Omphalocele
Repair 49600-49611

Omphalomesenteric Duct
Excision 44800

Omphalomesenteric Duct, Persistent
See Diverticulum, Meckel's

Oncoprotein
HER-2/neu 83950

One Stage Prothrombin Time 85610-85611
See Prothrombin Time

Onychectomy
See Excision, Nails

Onychia
Drainage 10060-10061

Oocyte
Assisted Fertilization
Microtechnique 89280-89281
Biopsy 89290-89291
Cryopreservation 0059T
Culture
Extended 89272
Less than 4 Days 89250
with Co-Culture 89251
Identification
Follicular Fluid 89254
Insemination 89268
Retrieval
for In Vitro Fertilization 58970
Storage 89346
Thawing 89356

Orbital Floor
See Orbit; Periorbital Region
Fracture
    Blow Out 21385-21395

Orbital Hypertelorism
Osteotomy
    Periorbital 21260-21263

Orbital Implant
See Ocular Implant
Insertion 67550
Removal 67560

Orbital Prosthesis 21077

Orbital Rim and Forehead
Reconstruction 21172-21180

Orbital Rims
Reconstruction 21182-21184

Orbital Transplant 67560

Orbital Walls
Reconstruction 21182-21184

Orbitocraniofacial Reconstruction
Secondary 21275

Orbitotomy
with Bone Flap
    for Exploration 67450
    Lateral Approach 67420
    with Drainage 67440
    with Removal Foreign Body 67430
    with Removal of Bone for
    Decompression 67445
with Removal Foreign Body 67413
with Removal of Bone for Decompression .67414
without Bone Flap
    for Exploration 67400
    with Drainage Only 67405
    with Removal Lesion 67412

Orchidectomies
See Excision, Testis

Orchidopexy
See Orchiopexy

Orchidoplasty
See Repair, Testis

Orchiectomy
Laparoscopic 54690
Partial 54522
Radical
    Abdominal Exploration 54535
    Inguinal Approach 54530
Simple 54520

Orchiopexy
Abdominal Approach 54650
Inguinal Approach 54640
Intra-Abdominal Testis 54692

Orchioplasty
See Repair, Testis

Organ Grafting
See Transplantation

Organ or Disease-Oriented Panel
Electrolyte 80051
General Health Panel 80050
Hepatic Function Panel 80076
Hepatitis Panel 80074
Lipid Panel 80061
Metabolic
    Basic 80048
    Comprehensive 80053
Obstetric Panel 80055
Renal Function 80069

Organ System, Neurologic
See Nervous System

Organic Acids 83918-83921

Ormond Disease
See Retroperitoneal Fibrosis

Orogastric Tube
Placement 43752

Oropharynx
Biopsy 42800

Orthodontic Cephalogram 70350

Orthomyxoviridae
See Influenza Virus

Orthomyxovirus
See Influenza Virus

Orthopantogram 70355

Orthopedic Cast
See Cast

Orthopedic Surgery
Computer Assisted Navigation 0054T-0056T
Stereotaxis
    Computer Assisted 0054T-0056T

Orthoptic Training 92065

Orthoroentgenogram 76040

Orthosis
See Orthotics

Orthotics
Check-Out 97703
Fitting and Training 97504

Os Calcis Fracture
See Calcaneus, Fracture

Osmolality
Blood 83930
Urine 83935

Osmolality 76061-76065

Osseous Survey 76061-76065

Osseous Tissue
See Bone

Ossicles
Excision
    Stapes
        with Footplate Drill Out 69661
        without Foreign Material 69660-69661

Reconstruction
  Ossicular Chain
    Tympanoplasty with
      Antrotomy or Mastoidotomy .69636-69637
    Tympanoplasty with
      Mastoidectomy 69642, 69644, 69646
    Tympanoplasty without
      Mastoidectomy 69632-69633
Release
  Stapes 69650
Replacement
  with Prosthesis 69633, 69637

Ostectomy
Metacarpal 26250-26255
Metatarsal 28288
Phalanges
  Finger 26260-26262
Pressure Ulcer
  Ischial 15941, 15945
  Sacral 15933, 15935, 15937
  Trochanteric 15951, 15953, 15958
Scapula 23190
Sternum 21620

Osteocalcin 83937

Osteocartilaginous Exostoses
See Exostosis

Osteochondroma
See Exostosis

Osteocutaneous Flap
with Microvascular Anastomosis ...20969-20973

Osteoma
Sinusotomy
  Frontal 31075

Osteomyelitis 20000-20005
Elbow
  Incision and Drainage 23935
Excision
  Clavicle 23180
  Facial 21026
  Humerus, Proximal 23184
  Mandible 21025
  Scapula 23182
Femur/Knee
  Incision and Drainage 27303
Finger
  Incision 26034
Hand Incision 26034
Hip
  Incision, Deep 26992
Humerus 24134
  Incision and Drainage 23935
Incision
  Foot 28005
  Shoulder 23035
  Thorax 21510
Olecranon Process 24138, 24147
Pelvis
  Incision, Deep 26992
Radius 24136, 24145
Sequestrectomy
  Clavicle 23170
  Humeral Head 23174
  Scapula 23172
  Skull 61501

Orbital Floor
See Orbit; Periorbital Region
Fracture
    Blow Out 21385-21395

Orbital Hypertelorism
Osteotomy
    Periorbital 21260-21263

Orbital Implant
See Ocular Implant
Insertion 67550
Removal 67560

Orbital Prosthesis 21077

Orbital Rim and Forehead
Reconstruction 21172-21180

Orbital Rims
Reconstruction 21182-21184

Orbital Transplant 67560

Orbital Walls
Reconstruction 21182-21184

Orbitocraniofacial Reconstruction
Secondary 21275

Orbitotomy
with Bone Flap
    for Exploration 67450
    Lateral Approach 67420
    with Drainage 67440
    with Removal Foreign Body 67430
    with Removal of Bone for
    Decompression 67445
with Removal Foreign Body 67413
with Removal of Bone for Decompression .67414
without Bone Flap
    for Exploration 67400
    with Drainage Only 67405
    with Removal Lesion 67412

Orchidectomies
See Excision, Testis

Orchidopexy
See Orchiopexy

Orchidoplasty
See Repair, Testis

Orchiectomy
Laparoscopic 54690
Partial 54522
Radical
    Abdominal Exploration 54535
    Inguinal Approach 54530
Simple 54520

Orchiopexy
Abdominal Approach 54650
Inguinal Approach 54640
Intra-Abdominal Testis 54692

Orchioplasty
See Repair, Testis

Organ Grafting
See Transplantation

Organ or Disease-Oriented Panel
Electrolyte 80051
General Health Panel 80050
Hepatic Function Panel 80076
Hepatitis Panel 80074
Lipid Panel 80061
Metabolic
    Basic 80048
    Comprehensive 80053
Obstetric Panel 80055
Renal Function 80069

Organ System, Neurologic
See Nervous System

Organic Acids 83918-83921

Ormond Disease
See Retroperitoneal Fibrosis

Orogastric Tube
Placement 43752

Oropharynx
Biopsy 42800

Orthodontic Cephalogram 70350

Orthomyxoviridae
See Influenza Virus

Orthomyxovirus
See Influenza Virus

Orthopantogram 70355

Orthopedic Cast
See Cast

Orthopedic Surgery
Computer Assisted Navigation 0054T-0056T
Stereotaxis
    Computer Assisted 0054T-0056T

Orthoptic Training 92065

Orthoroentgenogram 76040

Orthosis
See Orthotics

Orthotics
Check-Out 97703
Fitting and Training 97504

Os Calcis Fracture
See Calcaneus, Fracture

Osmolality
Blood 83930
Urine 83935

Osseous Survey 76061-76065

Osseous Tissue
See Bone

Ossicles
Excision
    Stapes
      with Footplate Drill Out 69661
      without Foreign Material 69660-69661

Reconstruction
    Ossicular Chain
      Tympanoplasty with
      Antrotomy or Mastoidotomy .69636-69637
      Tympanoplasty with
      Mastoidectomy 69642, 69644, 69646
      Tympanoplasty without
      Mastoidectomy 69632-69633
Release
    Stapes 69650
Replacement
    with Prosthesis 69633, 69637

Ostectomy
Metacarpal 26250-26255
Metatarsal 28288
Phalanges
    Finger 26260-26262
Pressure Ulcer
    Ischial 15941, 15945
    Sacral 15933, 15935, 15937
    Trochanteric 15951, 15953, 15958
Scapula 23190
Sternum 21620

Osteocalcin .83937

Osteocartilaginous Exostoses
See Exostosis

Osteochondroma
See Exostosis

Osteocutaneous Flap
with Microvascular Anastomosis . . .20969-20973

Osteoma
Sinusotomy
    Frontal 31075

Osteomyelitis 20000-20005
Elbow
    Incision and Drainage 23935
Excision
    Clavicle 23180
    Facial 21026
    Humerus, Proximal 23184
    Mandible 21025
    Scapula 23182
Femur/Knee
    Incision and Drainage 27303
Finger
    Incision 26034
Hand Incision 26034
Hip
    Incision, Deep 26992
Humerus 24134
    Incision and Drainage 23935
Incision
    Foot 28005
    Shoulder 23035
    Thorax 21510
Olecranon Process 24138, 24147
Pelvis
    Incision, Deep 26992
Radius .24136, 24145
Sequestrectomy
    Clavicle 23170
    Humeral Head 23174
    Scapula 23172
    Skull 61501

Osteopathic Manipulation 98925-98929

Osteoplasty
Carpal Bone 25394
Facial Bones
    Augmentation 21208
    Reduction 21209
Femoral Neck 27179
Femur 27179
    Lengthening 27466-27468
    Shortening 27465, 27468
Fibula
    Lengthening 27715
Humerus 24420
Metacarpal 26568
Phalanges, Finger 26568
Radius 25390-25393
Tibia
    Lengthening 27715
Ulna 25390-25393
Vertebra 76012-76013
    Lumbar 22521-22522
    Thoracic 22520, 22522

Osteotomy
Calcaneus 28300
Chin 21121-21123
Clavicle 23480-23485
Femur 27140, 27151
    Femoral Neck 27161
    for Slipped Epiphysis 27181
    with Fixation 27165
    with Open Reduction of Hip 27156
    with Realignment 27454
    without Fixation 27448-27450
Fibula 27707-27712
Hip 27146-27151
    Femoral
      with Open Reduction 27156
    Femur 27151
Humerus 24400-24410
Mandible 21198-21199
    Extra-oral 21047
    Intra-oral 21046
Maxilla 21206
    Extra-oral 21049
    Intra-oral 21048
Metacarpal 26565
Metatarsal 28306-28309
Orbit Reconstruction 21256
Pelvis 27158
Periorbital
    Orbital Hypertelorism 21260-21263
    Osteotomy with Graft 21267-21268
Phalanges
    Finger 26567
    Toe 28299, 28310-28312
Radius
    and Ulna 25365, 25375
    Distal Third 25350
    Middle or Proximal Third 25355
    Multiple 25370
Skull Base 61582-61585, 61592
Spine
    Anterior 22220-22226
    Posterior
      Posterolateral 22210-22214

Talus 28302
Tarsal 28304-28305
Tibia 27455-27457, 27705, 27709-27712
Ulna 25360
    and Radius 25365, 25375
    Multiple 25370
Vertebra
    Additional Segment
      Anterior Approach 22226
      Posterior/Posterolateral Approach ..22216
    Cervical
      Anterior Approach 22220
      Posterior/Posterolateral Approach ..22210
    Lumbar
      Anterior Approach 22224
      Posterior/Posterolateral Approach ..22214
    Thoracic
      Anterior Approach 22222
      Posterior/Posterolateral Approach ..22212
    with Graft
      Reconstruction
        Periorbital Region 21267-21268

Otolaryngology
Diagnostic
    Exam Under Anesthesia 92502

Otomy
See Incision

Otoplasty 69300

Otorhinolaryngology
Unlisted Services and Procedures 92700

Ouchterlony Immunodiffusion 86331

Outer Ear
See Ear, Outer

Outpatient Visit
See History and Physical; Office and/or Other Outpatient Services

Output, Cardiac
See Cardiac Output

Ova
Smear 87177

Oval Window
Repair Fistula 69666

Oval Window Fistula
See Fistula, Oval Window

Ovarian Cyst
See Cyst, Ovarian; Ovary, Cyst

Ovarian Vein Syndrome
Ureterolysis 50722

Ovariectomies
See Oophorectomy

Ovariolysis 58740

Ovary
Abscess
    Incision and Drainage 58820-58822
      Abdominal Approach 58822

Biopsy 58900
Cryopreservation 0058T
Cyst
    Incision and Drainage 58800-58805
Excision 58662, 58720
    Cyst 58925
    Partial
      Oophorectomy 58661, 58940
      Ovarian Malignancy 58943
      Peritoneal Malignancy 58943
      Tubal Malignancy 58943
      Wedge Resection 58920
    Total 58940-58943
Laparoscopy 58660-58662, 58679
Lysis
    Adhesions 58660, 58740
Radical Resection 58950-58952
Transposition 58825
Tumor
    Resection 58950-58956
Unlisted Services and Procedures ..58679, 58999
Wedge Resection 58920

Oviduct
Anastomosis 58750
Chromotubation 58350
Ectopic Pregnancy 59120-59121
Excision 58700-58720
Fulguration
    Laparoscopic 58670
Hysterosalpingography 74740
Laparoscopy 58679
Ligation 58600-58611
Lysis
    Adhesions 58740
Occlusion 58615
    Laparoscopic 58671
Repair 58752
    Anastomosis 58750
    Create Stoma 58770
Unlisted Services and Procedures ..58679, 58999
X-Ray with Contrast 74740

Ovocyte
See Oocyte

Ovulation Tests 84830

Ovum Implantation
See Implantation

Ovum Transfer Surgery
See Gamete Intrafallopian Transfer

Oxalate 83945

Oxidase, Ceruloplasmin
See Ceruloplasmin

Oxidoreductase, Alcohol-Nad+
See Antidiuretic Hormone

Oximetry (Noninvasive)
See Pulmonology, Diagnostic
Blood O2 Saturation
    Ear or Pulse 94760-94762

Oxoisomerase
See Phosphohexose Isomerase

Oxosteroids
See Ketosteroids

Oxycodinone 80102-80103, 83925

Oxygen Saturation 82805-82810

Oxygenation, Extracorporeal Membrane
See Extracorporeal Membrane Oxygenation

Oxyproline
See Hydroxyproline

Oxytocin Stress Test, Fetal 59020

P

P & P
See Proconvertin

P B Antibodies
See Antibody, Heterophile

P-Acetamidophenol
See Acetaminophen

Pacemaker, Heart
See Defibrillator, Heart
Conversion 33214
Electronic Analysis 93641-93642
   Antitachycardia System 93724
   Dual Chamber ...93731-93732, 93743-93744
   Single Chamber .93734-93735, 93741-93742
   Wearable Device 93741-93742, 93745
Insertion 33200-33208
   Electrode 33210-33211, 33216-33217,
      33224-33225
   Pulse Generator Only 33212-33213
Removal 33233-33237
   via Thoracotomy 33236-33237
Repair
   Electrode 33218-33220
Replacement
   Catheter 33210
   Electrode 33210-33211
   Insertion 33206-33208
   Pulse Generator 33212-33213
Repositioning
   Electrode 33215, 33226
Revise Pocket
   Chest 33222
Telephonic Analysis 93733, 93736
Upgrade 33214

Pachymetry
Eye 76514

Packing
Nasal Hemorrhage 30901-30906

Pain Management
Epidural/Intrathecal 62350-62351,
      62360-62362, 99601-99602
Intravenous Therapy 90783-90784

Palatal Augmentation Prosthesis 21082

Palatal Lift Prosthesis 21083

Palate
Abscess
   Incision and Drainage 42000
Biopsy 42100
Excision 42120, 42145
Fracture
   Closed Treatment 21421
   Open Treatment 21422-21423
Lesion
   Destruction 42160
   Excision 42104-42120
Prosthesis 42280-42281
Reconstruction
   Lengthening 42226-42227
Repair
   Cleft Palate 42200-42225
   Laceration 42180-42182
   Vomer Flap 42235
Unlisted Services and Procedures 42299

Palate, Cleft
See Cleft Palate

Palatoplasty 42200-42225

Palatoschisis
See Cleft Palate

Palm
Bursa
   Incision and Drainage 26025-26030
Fasciectomy 26121-26125
Fasciotomy 26040-26045
Tendon
   Excision 26170
Tendon Sheath
   Excision 26145
   Incision and Drainage 26020

Palsy, Seventh Nerve
See Facial Nerve Paralysis

Pancreas
Anastomosis
   to Intestines 48180
   with Intestines 48520-48540
Anesthesia 00794
Biopsy 48100
   Needle Biopsy 48102
Cyst
   Anastomosis 48520-48540
   Repair 48500
Debridement
   Peripancreatic Tissue 48005
Excision
   Ampulla of Vater 48148
   Duct 48148
   Partial ...48140-48146, 48150, 48154, 48160
   Peripancreatic Tissue 48005
   Total 48155-48160
Lesion
   Excision 48120
Needle Biopsy 48102
Placement
   Drainage 48000-48001

Pseudocyst
Drainage
   Open 48510
   Percutaneous 48511
Removal
   Calculi (Stone) 48020
Removal Transplanted Allograft 48556
Repair
   Cyst 48500
Suture 48545
Transplantation 48160, 48550, 48554-48556
   Allograft Preparation 48550-48552
Unlisted Services and Procedures 48999
X-Ray with Contrast 74300-74305
   Injection Procedure 48400

Pancreas, Endocrine Only
See Islet Cell

Pancreatectomy
Donor 48550
Partial 48140-48146, 48150-48154, 48160
Total 48155-48160
with Transplantation 48160

Pancreatic DNAse
See DNAse

Pancreatic Duct
Destruction
   Calculi (Stone) 43265
Dilation
   Endoscopy 43271
Endoscopy
   Collection
      Specimen 43260
   Destruction
      Calculi (Stone) 43265
      Tumor 43272
   Dilation 43271
   Removal (Endoscopic)
      Calculi (Stone) 43264
      Foreign Body 43269
      Stent 43269
   Sphincter Pressure 43263
   Sphincterotomy 43262
   Tube Placement 43267-43268
Incision
   Sphincter 43262
Removal
   Calculi (Stone) 43264
   Foreign Body 43269
   Stent 43269
Tube Placement
   Nasopancreatic 43267
   Stent 43268
Tumor
   Destruction 43272
X-Ray with Contrast
   Guide Catheter 74329-74330

Pancreatic Elastase 1 (PE1) 82656

Pancreatic Islet Cell AB
See Antibody, Islet Cell

Pancreaticojejunostomy 48180

Pancreatography
Injection Procedure 48400
Intraoperative 74300-74301
Postoperative 74305

Pancreatojejunostomies
See Pancreaticojejunostomy

Pancreatorrhaphy 48545

Pancreatotomy
See Incision, Pancreas

Pancreozymin-Secretin Test ...82938

Panel
See Organ or Disease Oriented Panel

Panniculectomy
See Lipectomy

Pap Smears 88141-88155,
88164-88167, 88174-88175

Paper Chromatographies
See Chromatography, Paper

Paper, Chromatography
See Chromatography, Paper

Papilla, Interdental
See Gums

Papillectomy 46220

Papilloma
Destruction
Anus 46900-46924
Penis 54050-54065

PAPP D
See Lactogen, Human Placental

Para-Tyrosine
See Tyrosine

Paracentesis
Abdomen 49080-49081
Eye
Anterior Chamber
with Diagnostic Aspiration of
Aqueous 65800
with Removal of Blood 65815
with Removal Vitreous and/or Discission
of Anterior Hyaloid Membrane 65810
with Therapeutic Release of
Aqueous 65805
Thorax 32000-32002

Paracervical Nerve
Injection
Anesthetic 64435

Paraffin Bath Therapy 97018
See Physical Medicine/Therapy/Occupational
Therapy

Paraganglioma, Medullary
See Pheochromocytoma

Parainfluenza Virus
Antigen Detection
Immunofluorescence 87279

Paralysis, Facial Nerve
See Facial Nerve Paralysis

Paralysis, Infantile
See Polio

Paranasal Sinuses
See Sinus; Sinuses

Parasites
Blood 87207
Examination 87169
Smear 87177

Parasitic Worms
See Helminth

Parathormone 83970

Parathyrin
See Parathormone

Parathyroid Autotransplantation 60512

Parathyroid Gland
Autotransplant 60512
Excision 60500-60502
Exploration 60500-60505
Nuclear Medicine
Imaging 78070

Parathyroid Hormone 83970

Parathyroid Hormone Measurement
See Parathormone

Parathyroid Transplantation
See Transplantation, Parathyroid

Parathyroidectomy 60500-60505

Paraurethral Gland
Abscess
Incision and Drainage 53060

Paravertebral Nerve
Destruction 64622-64627
Injection
Anesthetic 64470-64484
Neurolytic 64622-64627

Parietal Cell Vagotomies
See Vagotomy, Highly Selective

Parietal Craniotomy 61556

Paring
Skin Lesion
Benign Hyperkeratotic
More than Four Lesions 11057
Single Lesion 11055
Two to Four Lesions 11056

Paronychia
Incision and Drainage 10060-10061

Parotid Duct
Diversion 42507-42510
Reconstruction 42507-42510

Parotid Gland
Abscess
Incision and Drainage 42300-42305

Calculi (Stone)
Excision 42330, 42340
Excision
Partial 42410-42415
Total 42420-42426
Tumor
Excision 42410-42426

Parotitides, Epidemic
See Mumps

Pars Abdominalis Aortae
See Aorta, Abdominal

Partial Colectomy
See Colectomy, Partial

Partial Cystectomy
See Cystectomy, Partial

Partial Esophagectomy
See Esophagectomy, Partial

Partial Gastrectomy
See Excision, Stomach, Partial

Partial Glossectomy
See Excision, Tongue, Partial

Partial Hepatectomy
See Excision, Liver, Partial

Partial Mastectomies
See Breast, Excision, Lesion

Partial Nephrectomy
See Excision, Kidney, Partial

Partial Pancreatectomy
See Pancreatectomy, Partial

Partial Splenectomy
See Splenectomy, Partial

Partial Thromboplastin Time
See Thromboplastin, Partial, Time

Partial Ureterectomy
See Ureterectomy, Partial

Particle Agglutination 86403-86406

Parvovirus
Antibody 86747

Patch
Allergy Tests 95044
See Allergy Tests

Patella
See Knee
Dislocation 27560-27566
Excision 27350
with Reconstruction 27424
Fracture 27520-27524
Reconstruction 27437-27438
Repair
Chondromalacia 27418
Instability 27420-27424

Patella, Chondromalacia
See Chondromalacia Patella

Patellar Tendon Bearing (PTB) Cast 29435

Incision and Drainage 33025
Puncture Aspiration 33010-33011
Removal
  Clot
    Endoscopic 32658
  Foreign Body
    Endoscopic 32658
Tumor
  Excision 32661, 33050

Peridural Anesthesia
See Anesthesia, Epidural

Peridural Injection
See Epidural, Injection

Perineal Prostatectomy
See Prostatectomy, Perineal

Perineoplasty 56810

Perineorrhaphy
Repair
  Rectocele .57250

Perineum
Abscess
  Incision and Drainage 56405
Colposcopy 99170
Debridement
  Infected 11004, 11006
Removal
  Prosthesis 53442
Repair 56810
X-Ray with Contrast 74775

Perionychia
See Paronychia

Periorbital Region
Reconstruction
  Osteotomy with Graft 21267-21268
Repair-Osteotomy 21260-21263

**Peripheral Artery Disease (PAD)
Rehabilitation** 93668

Peripheral Nerve
Repair/Suture
  Major 64856, 64859

Periprosthetic Capsulectomy
Breast 19371

Peristaltic Pumps
See Infusion Pump

Peritoneal Dialysis 90945-90947

Peritoneal Free Air
See Pneumoperitoneum

Peritoneal Lavage 49080

Peritoneocentesis 49080-49081

Peritoneoscopy
See Endoscopy, Peritoneum

Peritoneum
Abscess
  Incision and Drainage 49020
    Percutaneous 49021

Chemotherapy Administration 96445
  See Chemotherapy
Endoscopy
  Biopsy 47561
  Drainage
    Lymphocele 49323
    X-Ray 47560
  Exchange
    Drainage Catheter 49423
  Injection
    Contrast
      via Catheter 49424
  Ligation
    Shunt 49428
  Removal
    Cannula/Catheter 49422
    Foreign Body 49085
    Shunt 49429
  Tumor
    Resection 58950-58956
  Unlisted Services and Procedures 49999
  Venous Shunt
    Injection 49427
  X-Ray 74190

Persistent Truncus Arteriosus
See Truncus Arteriosus

**Persistent, Omphalomesenteric
Duct**
See Diverticulum, Meckel's

Personal Care
See Self Care

Pessary
Insertion 57160

Pesticides
Chlorinated Hydrocarbons 82441

PET
See Positron Emission Tomography

Petrous Temporal
Excision
  Apex 69530

Peyronie Disease
Injection 54200
Surgical Exposure 54205
with Graft 54110-54112

pH
See Blood
Other Fluid 83986
Urine 83986

Phacoemulsification
Removal
  Extracapsular Cataract 66982, 66984
  Secondary Membranous Cataract 66850

Phagocytosis
White Blood Cells 86344

Phalangectomy
Toe 28150
  Partial 28160

Phalanges (Hand)
See Finger, Bone

Phalanx, Finger
Craterization 26235-26236
Cyst
  Excision 26210-26215
Diaphysectomy 26235-26236
Excision 26235-26236
  Radical
    for Tumor 26260-26262
Fracture
  Articular
    Closed Treatment 26740
    Open Treatment 26746
    with Manipulation 26742
  Distal 26755-26756
    Closed Treatment 26750
    Open Treatment 26765
    Percutaneous Fixation 26756
  Open Treatment 26735
    Distal 26765
  Shaft 26720-26727
    Open Treatment 26735
Incision and Drainage 26034
Ostectomy
  Radical
    for Tumor 26260-26262
Repair
  Lengthening 26568
  Nonunion .26546
  Osteotomy 26567
Saucerization 26235-26236
Thumb
  Fracture
    Shaft 26720-26727
Tumor
  Excision 26210-26215

Phalanx, Great Toe
See Phalanx, Toe
Fracture 28490
  Open Treatment 28505
  with Manipulation 28495-28496
Percutaneous Fixation 28496
without Manipulation 28490

Phalanx, Toe
Condyle
  Excision 28126
Craterization 28124
Cyst
  Excision 28108
Diaphysectomy 28124
Excision 28124, 28150-28160
Fracture
  Open Treatment 28525
  with Manipulation 28515
  without Manipulation 28510
Repair
  Osteotomy 28310-28312
Saucerization 28124
Tumor
  Excision 28108, 28175

Pharmaceutic Preparations
See Drug

Pharmacotherapies
See Chemotherapy

Pharyngeal Tonsil
See Adenoids

Physical Medicine/Therapy/Occupational Therapy

See Neurology, Diagnostic
Activities of Daily Living 97535, 99509
Aquatic Therapy
  with Exercises 97113
Athletic Training
  Evaluation 97005
  Re-evaluation 97006
Check-Out
  Orthotic/Prosthetic 97703
Cognitive Skills Development 97532
Community/Work Reintegration 97537
Evaluation 97001-97002
Kinetic Therapy 97530
Manual Therapy 97140
Modalities
  Contrast Baths 97034
  Diathermy Treatment 97024
  Electric Simulation
    Unattended 97014
  Electric Stimulation
    Attended, Manual 97032
  Hot or Cold Pack 97010
  Hydrotherapy (Hubbard Tank) 97036
  Infrared Light Treatment 97026
  Iontophoresis 97033
  Microwave Therapy 97020
  Paraffin Bath 97018
  Traction 97012
  Ultrasound 97035
  Ultraviolet Light 97028
  Unlisted Services and Procedures 97039
  Vasopneumatic Device 97016
  Whirlpool Therapy 97022
Orthotics Training 97504
Osteopathic Manipulation 98925-98929
Procedures
  Aquatic Therapy 97113
  Gait Training 97116
  Group Therapeutic 97150
  Massage Therapy 97124
  Neuromuscular Reeducation 97112
  Physical Performance Test 97750
  Therapeutic Exercises 97110
  Traction Therapy 97140
  Work Hardening 97545-97546
Prosthetic Training 97520
Sensory Integration 97533
Therapeutic Activities 97530
Unlisted Services and Procedures .. 97139, 97799
Wheelchair Management/Propulsion 97542
Work Reintegration 97537

Physical Therapy
See Physical Medicine/Therapy/Occupational Therapy

Physician Services
Care Plan Oversight Services 99374-99380
  Home Health Agency Care 99374
  Hospice 99377-99378
  Nursing Facility 99379-99380
Direction, Advanced Life Support 99288
Prolonged
  with Direct Patient Contact 99354-99357
    Outpatient/Office 99354-99355

  with Direct Patient Services
    Inpatient 99356-99357
    without Direct Patient Contact .. 99358-99359
Standby 99360
Supervision, Care Plan Oversight
Services 99374-99380

Piercing of Ear Lobe 69090

Piles
See Hemorrhoids

Pilonidal Cyst
Excision 11770-11772
Incision and Drainage 10080-10081

Pin
See Wire
Insertion/Removal
  Skeletal Traction 20650
Prophylactic Treatment
  Femur 27187
  Humerus 24498
  Shoulder 23490-23491

Pinch Graft 15050

Pinna
See Ear, External

Pinworms
Examination 87172

Pirogoff Procedure 27888

Pituitary Epidermoid Tumor
See Craniopharyngioma

Pituitary Gland
Excision 61546-61548
Tumor
  Excision 61546-61548, 62165

Pituitary Growth Hormone
See Growth Hormone

Pituitary Lactogenic Hormone
See Prolactin

Pituitectomy
See Excision, Pituitary Gland

PKU
See Phenylalanine

Placement
Broncheal Stent 31636-31637
Catheter
  Bile Duct 75982
  Breast
    for Interstitial Radioelement
    Application 19296-19298
  Bronchus
    for Intracavitary Radioelement
    Application 31643
    See Catheterization
Catheter, Cardiac 93503
  See Catheterization, Cardiac
Colonic Stent 44397, 45327, 45345, 45387

Drainage
  Pancreas 48001
  IVC Filter 75940
Jejunostomy Tube
  Endoscopic 44372
Metallic Localization Clip
  Breast 19295
Nasogastric Tube 43752
Needle
  Bone 36680
Needle Wire
  Breast 19290-19291
Orogastric Tube 43752
Radiation Delivery Device
  Intracoronary Artery 92974
Seton
  Anal 46020
Tracheal Stent 31631
Ureteral Stent 50947

Placenta
Delivery 59414

Placental Lactogen
See Lactogen, Human Placental

Placental Villi
See Chorionic Villus

Plagiocephaly 21175

Plague Vaccine 90727

Planing
Nose
  Skin 30120

Plantar Digital Nerve
Decompression 64726

Plantar Pressure Measurements
Dynamic 96001, 96004

Plasma
Frozen Preparation 86927

Plasma Prokallikrein
See Fletcher Factor

Plasma Protein-A, Pregnancy-Associated (PAPP-A) 84163

Plasma Test
Volume Determination 78110-78111

Plasma Thromboplastin
Antecedent 85270
Component 85250

Plasmin 85400

Plasmin Antiactivator
See Alpha-2 Antiplasmin

Plasminogen 85420-85421

Plasmodium
Antibody 86750

Plastic Repair of Mouth
See Mouth, Repair

Plate, Bone
See Bone Plate

Platelet
See Blood Cell Count, Complete Blood Count
Aggregation 85576
Antibody 86022-86023
Assay 85055
Blood 85025
Count 85032, 85049
Neutralization 85597

Platelet Cofactor I
See Clotting Factor

Platelet Test
Survival Test 78190-78191

Platysmal Flap 15825

PLC
See Tissue Typing

Pleoptic Training 92065

Plethysmography
See Vascular Studies
Extremities 93922-93923
    Veins 93965
Penis 54240
Total Body 93720-93722

Pleura
Biopsy 32095-32100, 32400-32402
Decortication 32320
Empyema
    Excision 32540
Excision 32310-32320
    Endoscopic 32656
Foreign Body
    Removal 32150-32151
Needle Biopsy 32400
Removal
    Foreign Body 32653
Repair 32215
Thoracotomy 32095-32100
Unlisted Services and Procedures 32999

Pleural Cavity
Aspiration 32000-32002
Catheterization 32019
Chemotherapy Administration 96440
    See Chemotherapy
Fusion 32005
Incision
    Empyema 32035-32036
    Pneumothorax 32020
Puncture and Drainage 32000-32002
Thoracostomy 32035-32036

Pleural Endoscopies
See Thoracoscopy

Pleural Scarification
for Repeat Pneumothorax 32215

Pleural Tap
See Thoracentesis

Pleurectomy
Anesthesia 00542
Parietal 32310-32320
    Endoscopic 32656

Pleuritis, Purulent
See Abscess, Thorax

Pleurocentesis
See Thoracentesis

Pleurodesis
Chemical 32005
Endoscopic 32650

Pleurosclerosis
See Pleurodesis

Pleurosclerosis, Chemical
See Pleurodesis, Chemical

Plexectomy, Choroid
See Choroid Plexus, Excision

Plexus Brachialis
See Brachial Plexus

Plexus Cervicalis
See Cervical Plexus

Plexus Coeliacus
See Celiac Plexus

Plexus Lumbalis
See Lumbar Plexus

Plexus, Choroid
See Choroid Plexus

PLGN
See Plasminogen

Plication, Sphincter, Urinary Bladder
See Bladder, Repair, Neck

Pneumocentesis
Lung 32420

Pneumocisternogram
See Cisternography

Pneumococcal Vaccine
See Vaccines

Pneumocystis Carinii
Antigen Detection
    Immunofluorescence 87281

Pneumogastric Nerve
See Vagus Nerve

Pneumogram
Pediatric 94772

Pneumolysis 32940

Pneumonectomy 32440-32500
Completion 32488
Donor 32850, 33930
Sleeve 32442
Total 32440-32445

Pneumonology
See Pulmonology

Pneumonolysis 32940
Intrapleural 32652
Open Intrapleural 32124

Pneumonostomy 32200-32201

Pneumonotomy
See Incision, Lung

Pneumoperitoneum 49400

Pneumoplethysmography
Ocular 93875

Pneumothorax
Chemical Pleurodesis 32005
Pleural Scarification for Repeat 32215
Therapeutic
    Injection Intrapleural Air 32960
Thoracentesis with Tube Insertion 32002

Polio
Antibody 86658
Vaccine 90712-90713

Poliovirus Vaccine, Inactivated
See Vaccines

Pollicization
Digit 26550

Polya Gastrectomy
See Gastrectomy, Partial

Polydactylism
See Supernumerary Digit

Polydactylous Digit
Reconstruction 26587
Repair 26587

Polydactyly, Toes 28344

Polymerase Chain Reaction ...83898

Polyp
Antrochoanal
    Removal 31032
Esophagus
    Ablation 43228
Nose
    Excision
        Endoscopic 31237-31240
        Extensive 30115
        Simple 30110
Sphenoid Sinus
    Removal 31051
Urethra
    Excision 53260

Polypectomy
Nose
    Endoscopic 31237
Uterus 58558

Polypeptide, Vasoactive Intestinal
See Vasoactive Intestinal Peptide

Polysomnography 95808-95811

Polyuria Test
See Water Load Test

Pomeroy's Operation
See Tubal Ligation

Pooling
Blood Products 86965

Incision and Drainage 33025
Puncture Aspiration 33010-33011
Removal
  Clot
    Endoscopic 32658
  Foreign Body
    Endoscopic 32658
Tumor
  Excision 32661, 33050

Peridural Anesthesia
See Anesthesia, Epidural

Peridural Injection
See Epidural, Injection

Perineal Prostatectomy
See Prostatectomy, Perineal

Perineoplasty 56810

Perineorrhaphy
Repair
  Rectocele 57250

Perineum
Abscess
  Incision and Drainage 56405
Colposcopy 99170
Debridement
  Infected 11004, 11006
Removal
  Prosthesis 53442
Repair 56810
X-Ray with Contrast 74775

Perionychia
See Paronychia

Periorbital Region
Reconstruction
  Osteotomy with Graft 21267-21268
Repair-Osteotomy 21260-21263

Peripheral Artery Disease (PAD) Rehabilitation 93668

Peripheral Nerve
Repair/Suture
  Major 64856, 64859

Periprosthetic Capsulectomy
Breast 19371

Peristaltic Pumps
See Infusion Pump

Peritoneal Dialysis 90945-90947

Peritoneal Free Air
See Pneumoperitoneum

Peritoneal Lavage 49080

Peritoneocentesis 49080-49081

Peritoneoscopy
See Endoscopy, Peritoneum

Peritoneum
Abscess
  Incision and Drainage 49020
    Percutaneous 49021

Chemotherapy Administration 96445
  See Chemotherapy
Endoscopy
  Biopsy 47561
  Drainage
    Lymphocele 49323
    X-Ray 47560
Exchange
  Drainage Catheter 49423
Injection
  Contrast
    via Catheter 49424
Ligation
  Shunt 49428
Removal
  Cannula/Catheter 49422
  Foreign Body 49085
  Shunt 49429
Tumor
  Resection 58950-58956
Unlisted Services and Procedures 49999
Venous Shunt
  Injection 49427
X-Ray 74190

Persistent Truncus Arteriosus
See Truncus Arteriosus

Persistent, Omphalomesenteric Duct
See Diverticulum, Meckel's

Personal Care
See Self Care

Pessary
Insertion 57160

Pesticides
Chlorinated Hydrocarbons 82441

PET
See Positron Emission Tomography

Petrous Temporal
Excision
  Apex 69530

Peyronie Disease
Injection 54200
Surgical Exposure 54205
with Graft 54110-54112

pH
See Blood
Other Fluid 83986
Urine 83986

Phacoemulsification
Removal
  Extracapsular Cataract 66982, 66984
  Secondary Membranous Cataract 66850

Phagocytosis
White Blood Cells 86344

Phalangectomy
Toe 28150
  Partial 28160

Phalanges (Hand)
See Finger, Bone

Phalanx, Finger
Craterization 26235-26236
Cyst
  Excision 26210-26215
Diaphysectomy 26235-26236
Excision 26235-26236
  Radical
    for Tumor 26260-26262
Fracture
  Articular
    Closed Treatment 26740
    Open Treatment 26746
    with Manipulation 26742
  Distal 26755-26756
    Closed Treatment 26750
    Open Treatment 26765
    Percutaneous Fixation 26756
  Open Treatment 26735
    Distal 26765
  Shaft 26720-26727
    Open Treatment 26735
Incision and Drainage 26034
Ostectomy
  Radical
    for Tumor 26260-26262
Repair
  Lengthening 26568
  Nonunion 26546
  Osteotomy 26567
Saucerization 26235-26236
Thumb
  Fracture
    Shaft 26720-26727
Tumor
  Excision 26210-26215

Phalanx, Great Toe
See Phalanx, Toe
Fracture 28490
  Open Treatment 28505
  with Manipulation 28495-28496
Percutaneous Fixation 28496
without Manipulation 28490

Phalanx, Toe
Condyle
  Excision 28126
Craterization 28124
Cyst
  Excision 28108
Diaphysectomy 28124
Excision 28124, 28150-28160
Fracture
  Open Treatment 28525
  with Manipulation 28515
  without Manipulation 28510
Repair
  Osteotomy 28310-28312
Saucerization 28124
Tumor
  Excision 28108, 28175

Pharmaceutic Preparations
See Drug

Pharmacotherapies
See Chemotherapy

Pharyngeal Tonsil
See Adenoids

Popliteal Arteries
See Artery, Popliteal

Popliteal Synovial Cyst
See Baker's Cyst

Poradenitistras
See Lymphogranuloma Venereum

PORP (Partial Ossicular Replacement Prosthesis) 69633, 69637

Porphobilinogen
Urine 84106-84110

Porphyrin Precursors 82135

Porphyrins
Feces 84126-84127
Urine 84119-84120

Port Film 77417

Portal Vein
See Vein, Hepatic Portal

Porter-Silber Test
See Corticosteroid, Blood

Portoenterostomies, Hepatic
See Hepaticoenterostomy

Portoenterostomy 47701

Posadas-Wernicke Disease
See Coccidioidomycosis

Positional Nystagmus Test
See Nystagmus Tests, Positional

Positive End Expiratory Pressure
See Pressure Breathing, Positive

Positive-Pressure Breathing, Inspiratory
See Intermittent Positive Pressure Breathing (IPPB)

Positron Emission Tomography (PET)
Brain 78608-78609
Heart 78459
Myocardial Imaging
    Perfusion Study 78491-78492
Tumor 78811-78813
    with Computed Tomography ...78814-78816

Post-Op Visit 99024

Postauricular Fistula
See Fistula, Postauricular

Postcaval Ureter
See Retrocaval Ureter

Postmortem
See Autopsy

Postop Vas Reconstruction
See Vasovasorrhaphy

Postoperative Wound Infection
Incision and Drainage 10180

Postpartum Care
Cesarean Delivery 59515
    after Attempted Vaginal Delivery 59622
    Previous 59610, 59614-59618, 59622
Vaginal Delivery 59430
    after Previous Cesarean Delivery 59614

Potassium 84132
Urine 84133

Potential, Auditory Evoked
See Auditory Evoked Potentials

Potential, Evoked
See Evoked Potential

Potts-Smith Procedure 33762

Pouch, Kock
See Kock Pouch

PPP
See Fibrin Degradation Products

PRA
See Cytotoxic Screen

Prealbumin 84134

Prebeta Lipoproteins
See Lipoprotein, Blood

Pregl's Test
See Cystourethroscopy, Catheterization, Urethral

Pregnancy
Abortion
    Induced 59855-59857
        by Amniocentesis Injection ..59850-59852
        by Dilation and Curettage 59840
        by Dilation and Evaluation 59841
    Septic 59830
    Therapeutic
        by Dilation and Curettage 59851
        by Hysterectomy 59852
        by Saline 59850
Cesarean Delivery 59618-59622
    Only 59514
    Postpartum Care 59514-59515
    Routine Care 59510
    Vaginal Birth After 59610-59614
    with Hysterectomy 59525
Ectopic
    Abdominal 59130
    Cervix 59140
    Interstitial
        Partial Resection Uterus 59136
        Total Hysterectomy 59135
    Laparoscopy
        with Salpingectomy and/or
        Oophorectomy 59151
        without Salpingectomy and/or
        Oophorectomy 59150
    Tubal 59121
        with Salpingectomy and/or
        Oophorectomy 59120
Miscarriage
    Surgical Completion
        Any Trimester 59812
        First Trimester 59820
        Second Trimester 59821

Molar
    See Hydatidiform Mole
Multifetal Reduction 59866
Placenta Delivery 59414
Vaginal Delivery 59409-59410
    after Cesarean Delivery 59610-59614
    Antepartum Care 59425-59426
    Postpartum Care 59430
    Total Obstetrical Care ..59400, 59610, 59618

Pregnancy Test 84702-84703
Urinalysis 81025

Pregnanediol 84135

Pregnanetriol 84138

Pregnenolone 84140

Prekallikrein
See Fletcher Factor

Prekallikrein Factor 85292

Premature, Closure, Cranial Suture
See Craniosynostosis

Prenatal Procedure 59897
Amnioinfusion
    Transabdominal 59070
Drainage
    Fluid 59074
Occlusion
    Umbilical Cord 59072
Shunt 59076

Prenatal Testing
Amniocentesis 59000
    with Amniotic Fluid Reduction 59001
Chorionic Villus Sampling 59015
Cordocentesis 59012
Fetal Blood Sample 59030
Fetal Monitoring 59050
    Interpretation Only 59051
Non-Stress Test, Fetal 59025, 99500
Oxytocin Stress Test 59020
Stress Test
    Oxytocin 59020
Ultrasound 76801-76817
    Fetal Biophysical Profile 76818-76819
    Fetal Heart 76825

Prentiss Operation
See Orchiopexy, Inguinal Approach

Preparation
for Transfer
    Embryo 89255
for Transplantation
    Heart 33933, 33944
    Heart/Lung 33933
    Intestines 44715-44721
    Kidney 50323-50329
    Liver 47143-47147
    Lung 32855-32856, 33933
    Pancreas 48551-48552
    Renal 50323-50329
Thawing
    Embryo
        Cryopreserved 89352

Oocytes
Cryopreserved 89356
Reproductive Tissue
Cryopreserved 89354
Sperm
Cryopreserved 89353

Presacral Sympathectomy
See Sympathectomy, Presacral

Prescription
Contact Lens 92310-92317
    See Contact Lens Services
Ocular Prosthesis 92330-92335
    See Prosthesis, Ocular

Pressure Breathing
See Pulmonology, Therapeutic
Negative
    Continuous (CNP) 94662
Positive
    Continuous (CPAP) 94660

Pressure Measurement of Sphincter of Oddi
See Sphincter of Oddi, Pressure Measurement

Pressure Ulcer (Decubitus)
See Debridement; Skin Graft and Flap

Pressure Ulcers
Excision 15920-15999

Pressure, Blood
See Blood Pressure

Pressure, Venous
See Blood Pressure, Venous

Pretreatment
Red Blood Cell
    Antibody Identification 86970-86972
Serum
    Antibody Identification 86975-86978

Prevention & Control
See Prophylaxis

Preventive Medicine 99381-99397
See Immunization; Newborn Care, Normal; Office and/or Other Outpatient Services; Performance Measures, Prophylatic Treatment
Administration/Interpretation of Health Risk Assessment 99420
Counseling and/or Risk Factor Reduction
Intervention 99401-99429
    Group Counseling 99411-99412
    Individual Counseling 99401-99404
    Performance Measures 0001F-0014F
Established Patient 99382-99397
New Patient 99381-99387
Newborn Care 99432
Respiratory Pattern Recording 94772
Unlisted Services and Procedures 99429

Priapism
Repair
    Fistulization 54435
    with Shunt 54420-54430

Primidone
Assay 80188

PRL
See Prolactin

Pro-Insulin C Peptide
See C-Peptide

Proalbumin
See Prealbumin

Probes, DNA
See Nucleic Acid Probe

Probes, Nucleic Acid
See Nucleic Acid Probe

Procainamide
Assay 80190-80192

Process
See Anatomic term (eg coracoid, odontoid)

Procidentia
Rectum
    Excision 45130-45135
    Repair 45900

Procoagulant Activity, Glomerular
See Thromboplastin

Proconvertin 85230

Proctectasis
See Dilation, Rectum

Proctectomy
Partial 45111, 45113-45116, 45123
Total 45110, 45112, 45119-45120
    with Colon 45121
with Ileostomy 44212

Proctocele
See Rectocele

Proctopexy 45540-45541
with Sigmoid Excision 45550

Proctoplasty 45500-45505

Proctorrhaphy
See Rectum, Suture

Proctoscopies
See Anoscopy

Proctosigmoidoscopy
Ablation
    Polyp or Lesion 45320
Biopsy 45305
Destruction
    Tumor 45320
Dilation 45303
Exploration 45300
Hemorrhage Control 45317
Placement
    Stent 45327
Removal
    Foreign Body 45307
    Polyp 45308-45315
    Tumor 45315
Volvulus Repair 45321

Products, Gene
See Protein

Proetz Therapy
Nose 30210

Profibrinolysin
See Plasminogen

Progenitor Cell
See Stem Cell

Progesterone 84144

Progesterone Receptors 84234

Progestin Receptors
See Progesterone Receptors

Proinsulin 84206

Projective Test 96100

Prokallikrein
See Fletcher Factor

Prokallikrein, Plasma
See Fletcher Factor

Prokinogenase
See Fletcher Factor

Prolactin 80418, 80440, 84146

Prolapse
See Procidentia

Prolapse, Rectal
See Procidentia, Rectum

Prolastin
See Alpha-1 Antitrypsin

Prolonged Services 99354-99357, 99360
without Direct Patient Contact 99358-99359

Prophylactic Treatment
See Preventive Medicine
Femur 27495
    Nailing 27495
    Pinning 27495
    Wiring 27495
Femoral Neck and Proximal Femur
    Nailing 27187
    Pinning 27187
    Wiring 27187
Humerus
    Pinning, Wiring 24498
Radius 25490, 25492
    Nailing 25490, 25492
    Pinning 25490, 25492
    Plating 25490, 25492
    Wiring 25490, 25492
Shoulder
    Clavicle 23490
    Humerus 23491
Tibia 27745
Ulna 25491-25492
    Nailing 25491-25492
    Pinning 25491-25492
    Plating 25491-25492
    Wiring 25491-25492

Prophylaxis
Retina
  Detachment
    Cryotherapy, Diathermy 67141
    Photocoagulation 67145

Prostaglandin 84150
Insertion 59200

Prostanoids
See Prostaglandin

Prostate
Ablation
  Cryosurgery .55873
Abscess
  Drainage 52700
  Incision and Drainage 55720-55725
Biopsy 55700-55705
Brachytherapy
  Needle Insertion 55859
Coagulation
  Laser 52647
Destruction
  Cryosurgery .55873
  Thermotherapy 53850-53853
    Microwave 53850
    Radio Frequency 53852
Excision
  Partial 55801, 55821-55831
  Perineal 55801-55815
  Radical 55810-55815, 55840-55845
  Retropubic 55831-55845
  Suprapubic 55821
  Transurethral . . .52402, 52601, 52612-52614
Exploration
  Exposure 55860
  with Nodes 55862-55865
Incision
  Exposure 55860-55865
  Transurethral 52450
Insertion
  Radioactive Substance 55860
Needle Biopsy .55700
Thermotherapy
  Transurethral 53850-53853
Ultrasound 76872-76873
Unlisted Services and Procedures 55899
  Urinary System 53899
Urethra
  Stent Insertion 0084T
  Transurethral Balloon Dilation 52510
Vaporization
  Laser 52648

Prostate Specific
Antigen 84152-84154

Prostatectomy 52601
Laparascopic 55866
Perineal
  Partial 55801
  Radical 55810-55815
Retropubic
  Partial 55831
  Radical 55840-55845, 55866
Suprapubic
  Partial 55821
Transurethral 52612-52614

Prostatic Abscess
See Abscess, Prostate

Prostatotomy 55720-55725

Prosthesis
Augmentation
  Mandibular Body 21125
Auricular 21086
Breast
  Insertion 19340-19342
  Removal 19328-19330
  Supply 19396
Check-Out 97703
  See Physical Medicine/Therapy/Occupational
  Therapy
Cornea 65770
Facial 21088
Hernia
  Mesh 49568
Hip
  Removal 27090-27091
Intestines 44700
Knee
  Insertion 27438, 27445
Lens
  Insertion 66982-66985
  Manual or Mechanical
  Technique 66982-66984
  Not Associated with Concurrent Cataract
  Removal 66985
Mandibular Resection 21081
Nasal 21087
Nasal Septum
  Insertion 30220
Obturator 21076
  Definitive 21080
  Interim 21079
Ocular 21077, 65770, 66982-66985,
           92330-92335, 92358, 92393
  Fitting and Prescription 92330
  Loan 92358
  Prescription 92335
  Supply 92393
Orbital 21077
  Partial or Total 69633, 69637
Ossicle Reconstruction
  Chain 69633
Palatal Augmentation 21082
Palatal Lift 21083
Palate 42280-42281
Penile
  Insertion 54400-54405
  Removal 54406, 54410-54417
  Repair 54408
  Replacement 54410-54411, 54416-54417
Perineum
  Removal 53442
Skull Plate
  Removal 62142
  Replacement 62143
Spectacle
  Fitting 92352-92353
  Repair 92371
Speech Aid 21084
Spinal
  Insertion 22851
Synthetic 69633, 69637

Temporomandibular Joint
  Arthroplasty 21243
Testicular
  Insertion 54660
Training 97520
Urethral Sphincter
  Insertion 53444-53445
  Removal 53446-53447
  Repair 53449
  Replacement 53448
Vagina
  Insertion 57267
Wrist
  Removal 25250-25251

Protease F
See Plasmin

Protein
A, Plasma (PAPP-A) 84163
C-Reactive 86140-86141
Electropheresis 84165-84166
Glycated 82985
Myelin Basic 83873
Osteocalcin 83937
Other Fluids 84166
Prealbumin 84134
Serum 84155, 84165
Total .84155-84160
Urine 84156
Western Blot 84181-84182, 88372

Protein Analysis, Tissue
Western Blot 88371

Protein Blotting
See Western Blot

Protein C Activator 85337

Protein C Antigen 85302

Protein C Assay 85303

Protein C Resistance Assay . . .85307

Protein S
Assay 85306
Total 85305

Prothrombase
See Thrombokinase

Prothrombin 85210

Prothrombin Time 85610-85611

Prothrombinase
See Thromboplastin

Prothrombokinase 85230

Protime
See Prothrombin Time

Proton Treatment Delivery
Complex 77525
Intermediate 77523
Simple 77520-77522

Protoporphyrin 84202-84203

Protozoa
Antibody 86753

Unlisted Services and Procedures 94799
    Ventilation Assist 94656-94657, 99504
Unlisted Services and Procedures 94799

Pulse Generator
Electronic Analysis 95970-95971
Heart
    Insertion/Replacement 33212-33213

Pulse Rate Increased
See Tachycardia

Pulsed Magnetic Neuromodulation
Urinary Incontinence 0029T

Pump
See Chemotherapy, Pump Services; Infusion
Pump

Pump Services
Oxygenator/Heat Exchanger 99190-99192

Pump Stomach for Poison 91105

Pump, Infusion
See Infusion Pump

Punch Graft 15775-15776

Puncture
Artery 36600
Chest
    Drainage 32000-32002
Cisternal
    See Cisternal Puncture
Lumbar
    See Spinal Tap
Lung 32420
Pericardium 33010-33011
Pleural Cavity
    Drainage 32000-32002
Skull
    Drain Fluid 61000-61020
        Cistern .61050
        Inject Cistern 61055
        Inject Ventricle 61026
    Shunt
        Drain Fluid 61070
        Injection 61070
Spinal Cord
    Diagnostic .62270
    Drain Fluid .62272
    Lumbar 62270
Tracheal
    Aspiration and/or Injection 31612

Puncture Aspiration
Abscess
    Skin 10160
Bulla 10160
Cyst
    Breast 19000-19001
    Skin 10160
Hematoma 10160

Puncturing
See Puncture

Pure-Tone Audiometry
See Audiometry, Pure Tone

Pustules
Removal 10040

Putti-Platt Procedure 23450

PUVA
See Dermatology; Photochemotherapy;
Ultraviolet Light Therapy

Pyelogram
See Urography, Intravenous; Urography,
Retrograde

Pyelography 74400, 74425
Injection 50394

Pyelolithotomy 50130
Anatrophic 50075
Coagulum 50130

Pyeloplasty 50400-50405, 50544
Repair
    Horseshoe Kidney 50540
Secondary 50405

Pyeloscopy
with Cystourethroscopy 52351
    Biopsy 52354
    Destruction 52354
    Lithotripsy 52353
    Removal
        Calculus 52352
    Tumor Excision 52355

Pyelostogram 50394

Pyelostolithotomy
Percutaneous 50080-50081

Pyelostomy 50125, 50400-50405
Change Tube .50398

Pyelotomy
Complicated 50135
Endoscopic 50570
Exploration 50120
with Drainage 50125
with Removal Calculus 50130

Pyeloureterogram
Antegrade 50394

Pyeloureteroplasty
See Pyeloplasty

Pyloric Sphincter
Incision 43520
Reconstruction 43800

Pyloromyotomy 43520
with Gastrectomy 43639

Pyloroplasty 43800
with Gastrectomy 43639
with Vagotomy 43640

Pyothorax
See Abscess, Thorax

Pyridoxal Phosphate 84207

Pyrophosphate, Adenosine
See Adenosine Diphosphate

Pyrophosphorylase, Udp Galactose
See Galactose-1-Phosphate, Uridyl Transferase

Pyruvate 84210-84220

Q

Q Fever 86000, 86638

Q Fever ab
See Antibody, Coxiella burnetii

Quadrantectomy 19160-19162

Quadriceps Repair 27430

Quick Test
See Prothrombin Time

Quinidine
Assay 80194

Quinine 84228

R

Rabies Vaccine
See Vaccines

Rachicentesis
See Spinal Tap

Radial Arteries
See Artery, Radial

Radial Head, Subluxation
See Nursemaid Elbow

Radial Keratotomy 65771

Radiation
See Irradiation

Radiation Physics
Consultation 77336-77370
Unlisted Services and Procedures 77399

Radiation Therapy 77280-77295
Consultation
    Radiation Physics 77336-77370
CT Scan Guidance 76370
Dose Plan 77300, 77305-77331
    Brachytherapy 77326-77328
    Intensity Modulation 77301
    Teletherapy 77305-77321
Field Set-up 77280-77295
Planning 77261-77263, 77299
Special 77470
Stereotactic
    Body 0082T-0083T
    Cerebral Lesions 77432
Treatment Delivery
    Beam Modulation 0073T

Intensity Modulation 77418
Proton Beam 77520-77525
Single 77402-77406
Stereotactic
    Body 0082T
    Superficial 77401
    Three or More Areas 77412-77416
    Two Areas 77407-77411
    Weekly 77427
Treatment Device 77332-77334
Treatment Management
    One or Two Fractions Only 77431
    Stereotactic
        Body 0083T
        Cerebral 77432
    Unlisted Services and Procedures 77499
    Weekly 77427

Radiation, X
See X-Ray

Radical Excision of Lymph Nodes
See Excision, Lymph Nodes, Radical

Radical Mastectomies, Modified
See Mastectomy, Modified Radical

Radical Neck Dissection
Laryngectomy 31365-31368
Pharyngolaryngectomy 31390-31395
with Auditory Canal Surgery 69155
with Thyroidectomy 60254
with Tongue Excision 41135, 41145,
                                        41153-41155

Radical Resection
See Resection, Radical
Abdomen 51597
Acetabulum .27076
Ankle 27615
Arm, Lower .25077
Calcaneus 27647
Elbow
    Capsule, Soft Tissue, Bone
        with Contracture Release 24149
Face 21015
Fibula 27646
Finger 26117
Foot 28046
Forearm 25077
Hand 26115
Hip
    Soft Tissue 27049
    Tumor or Infection 27075-27076
Humerus 23220-23222
Innominate .27077
Ischial 27078-27079
Knee 27329
Leg
    Lower 27615
    Upper 27329
Metacarpal 26250-26255
Metatarsal 28173
Mouth
    with Tongue Excision 41150, 41155
Ovarian Tumor
    Bilateral Salpingo-Oophorectomy-
    Omentectomy 58950-58956

with Radical Dissection for
Debulking 58952-58954
with Total Abdominal
Hysterectomy 58951, 58953-58956
Pelvis
    Soft Tissue 27049
Peritoneal Tumor
    Bilateral Salpingo-Oophorectomy-
    Omentectomy 58952-58956
    with Radical Dissection for
    Debulking 58952-58954
Phalanges
    Finger 26260-26262
    Toe 28175
Radius 25170
Scalp 21015
Scapula 23210
Shoulder 23077
Sternum 21630-21632
Talus
    Tumor 27647
Tarsal 28171
Tibia 27645
Tonsil 42842-42845
Tumor
    Back/Flank 21935
    Femur 27365
    Knee 27329, 27365
    Leg, Upper 27329
    Neck 21557
    Thorax 21557
Ulna 25170
Wrist 25077

Radical Vaginal Hysterectomy
See Hysterectomy, Vaginal, Radical

Radical Vulvectomy
See Vulvectomy, Radical

Radio-Cobalt B12 Schilling Test
See Vitamin, B12, Absorption Study

Radioactive Colloid Therapy . . .79300

Radioactive Substance
Insertion
    Kidney 50578
    Prostate 55860
    Ureteral Endoscopic 50978
    Urethral Endoscopic 50959

Radiocarpal Joint
Arthrotomy .25040
Dislocation
    Closed Treatment 25660

Radiocinematographies
See Cineradiography

Radioelement
Application 77761-77778
    Surface 77789
    with Ultrasound 76965
Handling 77790
Infusion 77750

Radioelement Substance
Catheter Placement
    Breast 19296-19298
    Bronchus .31643
    Prostate 55859
Needle Placement
    Prostate 55859

Radiography
See Radiology, Diagnostic; X-Ray

Radioimmunosorbent Test
See Gammaglobulin, Blood

Radioisotope Brachytherapy
See Brachytherapy

Radioisotope Scan
See Nuclear Medicine

Radiological Marker
Preoperative Placement
    Excision of Breast Lesion 19125-19126

Radiology
See Nuclear Medicine, Radiation Therapy, X-Ray,
Ultrasound
Diagnostic
    Unlisted Services and Procedures 76499
Stress Views 76006

Radionuclide CT Scan
See Emission Computerized Tomography

Radionuclide Imaging
See Nuclear Medicine

Radionuclide Therapy
See Radiopharmaceutical Therapy

Radionuclide Tomography, Single-Photon Emission-Computed
See SPECT

Radiopharmaceutical Therapy
Interstitial 79300
Intra-arterial .79445
Intra-articular 79440
Intracavitary .79200
Intravenous 79101, 79403
Oral 79005
Unlisted Services and Procedures 79999

Radiotherapeutic
See Radiation Therapy

Radiotherapies
See Irradiation

Radiotherapy, Surface
See Application, Radioelement, Surface

Radioulnar Joint
Arthrodesis
    with Resection of Ulna 25830
Dislocation
    Closed Treatment 25675
    Open Treatment 25676
    Percutaneous Fixation 25671

Radius

See Arm, Lower; Elbow; Ulna
Arthroplasty 24365
    with Implant 24366, 25441
Craterization 24145, 25151
Cyst
    Excision 24125-24126, 25120-25126
Diaphysectomy 24145, 25151
Dislocation
    Partial 24640
    Subluxate 24640
    with Fracture
        Closed Treatment 24620
        Open Treatment 24635
Excision 24130, 24136, 24145, 24152-24153
    Epiphyseal Bar 20150
    Partial 25145
    Styloid Process 25230
Fracture 25605
    Closed Treatment 25500-25505, 25520,
                       25600-25605
        with Manipulation 25605
        without Manipulation 25600
    Distal 25600-25611
        Open Treatment 25620
    Head/Neck
        Closed Treatment 24650-24655
        Open Treatment 24665-24666
    Open Treatment 25515, 25525-25526,
                       25574
    Percutaneous Fixation 25611
    Shaft .25500-25526
        Open Treatment 25574
    with Ulna 25560-25565
        Open Treatment 25575
Implant
    Removal 24164
Incision and Drainage 25035
Osteomyelitis 24136, 24145
Osteoplasty 25390-25393
Prophylactic Treatment 25490, 25492
Repair
    Epiphyseal Arrest 25450-25455
    Epiphyseal Separation
        Closed .25600
        Closed with Manipulation 25605
        Open Treatment 25620
        Percutaneous Fixation 25611
    Malunion or Nonunion 25400, 25415
    Osteotomy 25350-25355, 25370-25375
      and Ulna .25365
    with Graft 25405, 25420-25426
Saucerization 24145, 25151
Sequestrectomy 24136, 25145
Tumor
    Cyst 24120
    Excision . .24125-24126, 25120-25126, 25170

Ramstedt Operation

See Pyloromyotomy

Ramus Anterior, Nervus Thoracicus

See Intercostal Nerve

Range of Motion Test

Extremities or Trunk 95851
Eye 92018-92019
Hand 95852

Rapid Heart Rate

See Tachycardia

Rapid Plasma Reagin Test .86592-86593

Rapid Test for Infection 86308, 86403-86406

Monospot Test .86308

Rapoport Test 52005

Raskind Procedure 33735-33737

Rat Typhus

See Murine Typhus

Rathke Pouch Tumor

See Craniopharyngioma

Rays, Roentgen

See X-Ray

Raz Procedure 51845

See Repair, Bladder, Neck

RBC

See Red Blood Cell (RBC)

RBC ab

See Antibody, Red Blood Cell

Reaction

Lip
    without Reconstruction 40530

Reaction, Polymerase Chain

See Polymerase Chain Reaction

Realignment

Femur
    with Osteotomy 27454
Knee
    Extensor 27422

Receptor

See CD4; Estrogen, Receptor; FC Receptor; Progesterone Receptors

Receptor Assay

Hormone 84233-84235
Non Hormone .84238

Recession

Gastrocnemius
    Leg, Lower .27687

Reconstruction

See Revision
Abdominal Wall
    Omental Flap 49905
Acetabulum 27120-27122
Anal
    Congenital Absence 46730-46740
    Fistula 46742
    Graft 46753
    Sphincter 46750-46751, 46760-46762
    with Implant 46762
Ankle 27700-27703
Apical-Aortic Conduit 33404
Atrial 33253
Auditory Canal, External 69310-69320

Bile Duct
    Anastomosis 47800
Bladder
    and Urethra 51800-51820
    from Colon .50810
    from Intestines 50820, 51960
Breast .19357-19369
    Augmentation 19324-19325
    Mammoplasty 19318-19325
    Nipple 19350-19355
    Revision 19380
    Transverse Rectus Abdominis Myocutaneous
      Flap 19367-19369
    with Free Flap 19364
    with Latissimus Dorsi Flap 19361
    with Other Techniques 19366
    with Tissue Expander 19357
Bronchi 32501
    Graft Repair 31770
    Stenosis 31775
Canthus 67950
Carpal 25443
Carpal Bone 25394, 25430
Cheekbone 21270
Chest Wall
    Omental Flap 49904
    Trauma 32820
Cleft Palate 42200-42225
Conduit
    Apical-Aortic 33404
Conjunctiva 68320-68335
    with Flap
        Bridge or Partial 68360
        Total 68362
Cranial Bone
    Extracranial 21181-21184
Ear, Middle
    Tympanoplasty with Antrotomy or
    Mastoidotomy
        with Ossicular Chain
        Reconstruction 69636-69637
    Tympanoplasty with Mastoidectomy . .69641
        Radical or Complete 69644-69645
        with Intact or Reconstructed
        Wall 69643-69644
        with Ossicular Chain
        Reconstruction 69642
    Tympanoplasty without
    Mastoidectomy 69631
        with Ossicular Chain
        Reconstruction 69632-69633
Elbow 24360
    Total Replacement 24363
    with Implant 24361-24362
Esophagus 43300, 43310, 43313
    Creation
      Stoma 43350-43352
    Esophagostomy 43350
    Fistula 43305, 43312, 43314
    Gastrointestinal 43360-43361
Eye
    Graft
      Conjunctiva 65782
      Stem Cell 65781
    Transplantation
      Amniotic Membrane 65780

Rectal Bleeding
See Hemorrhage, Rectum

Rectal Prolapse
See Procidentia, Rectum

Rectal Sphincter

Rectocele
Repair 45560

Rectopexy
See Proctopexy

Rectoplasty
See Proctoplasty

Rectorrhaphy
See Rectum, Suture

Rectovaginal Fistula
See Fistula, Rectovaginal

Rectovaginal Hernia
See Rectocele

Rectum
See Anus
Abscess
    Incision and Drainage 45005-45020,
                        46040, 46060
Biopsy 45100
Dilation
    Endoscopy 45303
Endoscopy
    Destruction
        Tumor 45320
    Dilation 45303
    Exploration .45300
    Hemorrhage 45317
    Removal
      Foreign Body 45307
      Polyp 45308-45315
      Tumor 45308-45315
    Volvulus 45321
Excision
    Partial 45111, 45113-45116, 45123
    Total 45110, 45112, 45119-45120
    with Colon .45121
Exploration
    Endoscopic .45300
Hemorrhage
    Endoscopic .45317
Injection
    Sclerosing Solution 45520
Lesion
    Excision 45108
Manometry 91122
Prolapse
    Excision 45130-45135
Pulsed Irrigation
    Fecal Impaction 91123
Removal
    Fecal Impaction 45915
      by Pulsed Irrigation 91123
    Foreign Body 45307, 45915
Repair
    Fistula .45800-45825
    Injury .45562-45563
    Prolapse 45505-45541, 45900
    Rectocele 45560
    Stenosis 45500
    with Sigmoid Excision 45550
Sensation, Tone, and Compliance Test 91120
Stricture
    Excision 45150

Suture
    Fistula .45800-45825
    Prolapse 45540-45541
Tumor
    Destruction 45190, 45320, 46937-46938
    Excision 45160-45170
Unlisted Services and Procedures . .44239, 45999

Red Blood Cell (RBC)
Antibody .86850-86870
    Pretreatment 86970-86972
Count 85032-85041
Fragility
    Mechanical .85547
    Osmotic 85555-85557
Hematocrit 85014
Iron Utilization .78170
Morphology 85007
Platelet Estimation 85007
Sedimentation Rate
    Automated .85652
    Manual 85651
Sequestration .78140
Sickling 85660
Survival Test 78130-78135
Volume Determination 78120-78121

Red Blood Cell ab
See Antibody, Red Blood Cell

Reductase, Glutathione
See Glutathione Reductase

Reductase, Lactic Cytochrome
See Lactic Dehydrogenase

Reduction
Forehead 21137-21139
Lung Volume .32491
Mammoplasty 19318
Masseter Muscle/Bone 21295-21296
Osteoplasty
    Facial Bones 21209
Pregnancy
    Multifetal 59866
Skull
    Craniomegalic 62115-62117
Ventricular Septum
    Non-surgical 0024T

Reflex Test
Blink Reflex 95933
H-Reflex 95934-95936

Reflux Study 78262
Gastroesophageal 91034-91038

Refraction 92015

Rehabilitation
Artery
    Occlusive Disease 93668
Aural 92510
Cardiac .93797-93798

Rehabilitative
See Rehabilitation

Rehfuss Test
See Gastroenterology, Diagnostic, Stomach

Reichstein's Substance S
See Deoxycortisol

Reimplantation
Arteries
    Aorta
      Prosthesis 35697
    Carotid 35691, 35694-35695
    Subclavian 35693-35695
    Vertebral 35691-35693
    Visceral 35697
Kidney 50380
Ovary 58825
Pulmonary Artery 33788
Ureter, to Bladder 50780-50785
Ureters 51565

Reinnervation
Larynx
    Neuromuscular Pedicle 31590

Reinsch Test 83015

Reinsertion
Drug Delivery Implant 11983
Implantable Contraceptive Capsules 11977
Spinal Fixation Device 22849

Relative Density
See Specific Gravity

Release
Carpal Tunnel .64721
Elbow Contracture
    with Radical Release of Capsule 24149
Flexor Muscles
    Hip 27036
Muscle
    Knee 27422
Nerve .64702-64726
    Neurolytic .64727
Retina
    Encircling Material 67115
Spinal Cord 63200
Stapes 69650
Tarsal Tunnel .28035
Tendon 24332, 25295

Release-Inhibiting Hormone, Somatotropin
See Somatostatin

Removal
Allograft
    Intestinal 44137
Balloon
    Intra-Aortic .33974
Balloon Assist Device
    Intra-Aortic 33968, 33971
Blood Clot
    Eye 65930
Blood Component
    Apheresis 36511-36516
Breast
    Capsules 19371
    Implants 19328-19330
    Modified Radical 19240
    Partial 19140-19162
    Radical 19200-19220
    Simple, Complete 19180
    Subcutaneous 19182

Renal Abscess
See Abscess, Kidney

Renal Arteries
See Artery, Renal

Renal Autotransplantation
See Autotransplantation, Renal

Renal Calculus
See Calculus, Removal, Kidney

Renal Cyst
See Cyst, Kidney

Renal Dialyses
See Hemodialysis

Renal Disease Services
See Dialysis

Renal Transplantation
See Kidney, Transplantation

Renin 80408, 80416, 84244
Peripheral Vein 80417

Renin-Converting Enzyme 82164

Reoperation

Repair
See Revision

Nephrostomy Tube
　　See Nephrostomy, Change Tube
Nerve 64726
Neurostimulator
　　Pulse Generator/Receiver
　　　　Intracranial 61885
　　　　Peripheral Nerve 64590
　　　　Spinal 63685
Ossicles
　　with Prosthesis 69633, 69637
Ossicular Replacement
　　See TORP (Total Ossicular Replacement
　　Prosthesis)
Pacemaker 33206-33208
　　Catheter 33210
　　Electrode 33210-33211, 33216-33217
Pacing Cardioverter-Defibrillator
　　Leads 33243-33244
　　Pulse Generator Only 33241
Penile
　　Prosthesis 54410-54411, 54416-54417
Prosthesis
　　Skull 62143
　　Urethral Sphincter 53448
Pulmonary Valve 33475
Pulse Generator
　　Brain 61885
　　Peripheral Nerve 64590
　　Spinal Cord 63685
Receiver
　　Brain 61885
　　Peripheral Nerve 64590
　　Spinal Cord 63685
Skull Plate 62143
Spinal Cord
　　Reservoir 62360
Tissue Expanders
　　Skin 11970
Total Replacement
　　See Hip, Total Replacement
Total Replacement Heart System
　　Intracorporeal 0052T-0053T
Tricuspid Valve 33465
Ureter
　　with Intestines 50840
Venous Access Device 36582-36583, 36585
　　Catheter 36578
Venous Catheter
　　Central 36580-36581, 36584

Replantation
Arm, Upper 20802
Digit 20816-20822
Foot 20838
Forearm 20805
Hand 20808
Thumb 20824-20827

Report Preparation
Extended, Medical 99080
Psychiatric 90889

Reposition
Toe to Hand 26551-26556

Repositioning
Central Venous Catheter 36597
Electrode
　　Heart 33215-33217, 33226
Gastrostomy Tube 43761
Heart
　　Defibrillator
　　　　Leads 33215-33216, 33226, 33249
Intraocular Lens 66825
Tricuspid Valve 33468

Reproductive Tissue
Cryopreserved
　　Preparation
　　　　Thawing 89354
Storage 89344

Reprogramming
Shunt
　　Brain 62252

Reptilase Test 85635

Reptilase Time
See Thrombin Time

Resection
Aortic Valve
　　Stenosis 33415
Bladder Diverticulum 52305
Bladder Neck
　　Transurethral 52500
Brain Lobe
　　See Lobectomy, Brain
Chest Wall 19260-19272
Diaphragm 39560-39561
Endaural
　　See Ear, Inner, Excision
Humeral Head 23195
Intestines, Small
　　Laparoscopic 44202-44203
Lung 32520-32525
Mouth
　　with Tongue Excision 41153
Myocardium
　　Aneurysm 33542
　　Septal Defect 33545
Nasal Septum Submucous
　　See Nasal Septum, Submucous Resection
Nose
　　Septum 30520
Ovary, Wedge
　　See Ovary, Wedge Resection
Palate 42120
Phalangeal Head
　　Toe 28153
Prostate Transurethral
　　See Prostatectomy, Transurethral
Radical
　　Arm, Upper 24077
　　Elbow 24077
　　　　with Contracture Release 24149
　　Foot 28046
　　Humerus 24150-24151
　　Radius 24152-24153
Tumor
　　Ankle 27615
　　Calcaneus or Talus 27647

Clavicle 23200
Femur 27365
Fibula 27646
Humerus 23220
Humerus with Autograft 23221
Humerus with Prosthetic
　　Replacement 23222
Knee 27329, 27365
Leg, Lower 27615
Leg, Upper 27329
Metatarsal 28173
Phalanx, Toe 28175
Scapula 23210
Tarsal 28171
Tibia 27645
Ribs 19260-19272, 32900
Synovial Membrane
　　See Synovectomy
Temporal Bone 69535
Ulna
　　Arthrosedis
　　　　Radioulnar Joint 25830
Ureterocele
　　Ectopic 52301
　　Orthotopic 52300
Vena Cava
　　with Reconstruction 37799

Resonance Spectroscopy, Magnetic
See Magnetic Resonance Spectroscopy

Respiration, Positive-Pressure
See Pressure Breathing, Positive

Respiratory Pattern Recording
Preventive
　　Infant 94772

Respiratory Syncytial Virus
Antibody 86756
Antigen Detection
　　Direct Fluorescence 87280
　　Direct Optical Observation 87807
　　Enzyme Immunoassay 87420

Respiratory Syncytial Virus Immune Globulin
See Immune Globulins
Antigen Detection
　　See Immune Globulins, Respiratory Syncytial
　　Virus

Response, Auditory Evoked
See Auditory Evoked Potentials

Rest Home Visit
See Domiciliary Services

Resuscitation
Cardiac
　　See Cardiac Massage
Cardio-Pulmonary
　　See Cardio-Pulmonary Resuscitation
Newborn 99440

Reticulocyte
Count 85044-85045

Retina
Incision
   Encircling Material 67115
Lesion
   Extensive
     Destruction 67227-67228
   Localized
     Destruction 0017T, 67208-67218
Repair
   Detachment
     by Scleral Buckling 67112
     Cryotherapy or Diathermy 67101
     Injection of Air 67110
     Photocoagulation 67105
     Scleral Dissection 67107
     with Vitrectomy 67108, 67112
   Prophylaxis
     Detachment 67141-67145
Retinopathy
   Destruction
     Cryotherapy, Diathermy 67227
     Photocoagulation 67228

Retinacular
Knee
   Release 27425

Retinopathy
Destruction
   Cryotherapy, Diathermy 67227
   Photocoagulation 67228

Retraction, Clot
See Clot Retraction

Retrieval
Transcatheter Foreign Body 37203

Retrocaval Ureter
Ureterolysis 50725

Retrograde Cholangiopancreatographies, Endoscopic
See Cholangiopancreatography

Retrograde Cystourethrogram
See Urethrocystography, Retrograde

Retrograde Pyelogram
See Urography, Retrograde

Retroperitoneal Area
Abscess
   Incision and Drainage
     Open 49060
     Percutaneous 49061
Biopsy 49010
Cyst
   Destruction/Excision 49200-49201
Endometriomas
   Destruction/Excision 49200-49201
Exploration 49010
Needle Biopsy
   Mass 49180
Tumor
   Destruction/Excision 49200-49201

Retroperitoneal Fibrosis
Ureterolysis 50715

Retropubic Prostatectomies
See Prostatectomy, Retropubic

Revascularization
Distal Upper Extremity
   with Interval Ligation 36838
Interval Ligation
   Distal Upper Extremity 36838
Penis 37788
Transmyocardial 33140-33141

Reversal, Vasectomy
See Vasovasorrhaphy

Reverse T3
See Triiodothyronine, Reverse

Reverse Triiodothyronine
See Triiodothyronine, Reverse

Revision
See Reconstruction
Aorta 33404
Atrial 33253
Blepharoplasty 15820-15823
Broncheal Stent 31638
Bronchus 32501
Bypass Graft
   Vein Patch 35685
Cervicoplasty 15819
Colostomy
   See Colostomy, Revision
Cornea
   Prosthesis 65770
   Reshaping
     Epikeratoplasty 65767
     Keratomileusis 65760
     Keratophakia 65765
Defibrillator Site
   Chest 33223
Ear, Middle 69662
External Fixation System 20693
Eye
   Aqueous Shunt 66185
Gastrostomy Tube 44373
Hip Replacement
   See Replacement, Hip, Revision
Hymenal Ring 56700
Ileostomy
   See Ileostomy, Revision
Infusion Pump
   Intraarterial 36261
   Intravenous 36576-36578, 36582-36583
Iris
   Iridoplasty 66762
   Iridotomy 66761
Jejunostomy Tube 44373
Lower Extremity Arterial Bypass ...35879-35881
Pacemaker Site
   Chest 33222
Rhytidectomy 15824-15829
Semicircular Canal
   Fenestration 69840
Shunt
   Intrahepatic Portosystemic 37183
Sling 53442
Stapedectomy
   See Stapedectomy, Revsion

Stomach
   for Obesity 43848
Tracheostomy
   Scar 31830
Urinary-Cutaneous Anastomosis ...50727-50728
Vagina
   Sling
     Stress Incontinence 57287
Venous Access Device 36576-36578,
               36582-36583, 36585
Ventricle
   Ventriculomyectomy 33416
   Ventriculomyotomy 33416

Rh (D)
See Blood Typing

Rh Immune Globulin
See Immune Globulins, Rho (D)

Rheumatoid Factor 86430-86431

Rhinectomy
Partial 30150
Total 30160

Rhinomanometry 92512

Rhinopharynx
See Nasopharynx

Rhinophyma
Repair 30120

Rhinoplasty
Cleft Lip/Cleft Palate 30460-30462
Primary 30400-30420
Secondary 30430-30450

Rhinoscopy
See Endoscopy, Nose

Rhinotomy
Lateral 30118, 30320

Rhizotomy 63185-63190

Rho Variant Du 86905

Rhytidectomy 15824-15829

Rhytidoplasties
See Face Lift

Rib
Antibody 86756
Antigen Detection
   by Immunoassay
     with Direct Optical Observation
     Direct Fluorescense 87280
     Enzyme Immunoassay 87420
Excision 21600-21616, 32900
Fracture
   Closed Treatment 21800
   External Fixation 21810
   Open Treatment 21805
Graft
   to Face 21230
Resection 19260-19272, 32900
X-Ray 71100-71111

Sang-Park Procedure 33735-33737

Sao Paulo Typhus
See Rocky Mountain Spotted Fever

Saucerization
Calcaneus 28120
Clavicle 23180
Femur 27070, 27360
Fibula 27360, 27641
Hip 27070
Humerus 23184, 24140
Ileum 27070
Metacarpal 26230
Metatarsal 28122
Olecranon Process 24147
Phalanges
    Finger 26235-26236
    Toe 28124
Pubis 27070
Radius 24145, 25151
Scapula 23182
Talus 28120
Tarsal 28122
Tibia 27360, 27640
Ulna 24147, 25150

Saundby Test
See Blood, Feces

Scabies
See Tissue, Examination for Ectoparasites

Scalenotomy
See Muscle Division, Scalenus Anticus

Scalenus Anticus
Division 21700-21705

Scaling
See Exfoliation

Scalp
Tumor Resection
    Radical 21015

Scalp Blood Sampling 59030

Scan
See Specific Site, Nuclear Medicine
Abdomen
    See Abdomen, CT Scan
CT
    See CT Scan
MRI
    See Magnetic Resonance Imaging
PET
    See Positron Emission Tomography
Radionuclide
    See Emission Computerized Tomography

Scanning, Radioisotope
See Nuclear Medicine

Scanogram 76040

Scaphoid
Fracture
    Closed Treatment 25622
    Open Treatment 25628
    with Manipulation 25624

Scapula
Craterization .23182
Cyst
    Excision 23140
        with Allograft 23146
        with Autograft 23145
Diaphysectomy 23182
Excision 23172, 23190
    Partial 23182
Fracture
    Closed Treatment
        with Manipulation 23575
        without Manipulation 23570
    Open Treatment 23585
Ostectomy 23190
Repair
    Fixation 23400
    Scapulopexy 23400
Saucerization 23182
Sequestrectomy 23172
Tumor
    Excision 23140, 23210
        with Allograft 23146
        with Autograft 23145
    Radical Resection 23210
X-Ray 73010

Scapulopexy 23400

Scarification
Pleural 32215

Scarification of Pleura
See Pleurodesis

Schanz Operation
See Femur, Osteotomy

Schauta Operation
See Hysterectomy, Vaginal, Radical

Schede Procedure 32905-32906

Scheie Procedure
See Iridectomy

Schilling Test 78270
See Vitamin B-12 Absorption Study

**Schlatter Operation Total
Gastrectomy**
See Excision, Stomach, Total

Schlicter Test 87197
See Bactericidal Titer, Serum

Schocket Procedure 66180
See Aqueous Shunt

Schonbein Test
See Blood, Feces

Schuchard Procedure
Osteotomy
    Maxilla 21206

Schwannoma, Acoustic
See Brain, Tumor, Excision

Sciatic Nerve
Decompression 64712
Injection
    Anesthetic 64445-64446
Lesion
    Excision 64786
Neuroma
    Excision 64786
Neuroplasty .64712
Release 64712
Repair/Suture 64858

Scintigraphy
See Nuclear Medicine
Computed Tomographic
    See Emission Computerized Tomography

Scissoring
Skin Tags 11200-11201

Sclera
Excision
    Sclerectomy with Punch or Scissors . . .66160
Fistulization
    Iridencleisis or Iridotasis 66165
    Sclerectomy with Punch or Scissors with
        Iridectomy 66160
    Thermocauterization with Iridectomy . .66155
    Trabeculectomy ab Externo in Absence of
        Previous Surgery 66170
    Trephination with Iridectomy 66150
Incision
    Fistulization
        Iridencleisis or Iridotasis 66165
        Sclerectomy with Punch or Scissors with
            Iridectomy 66160
        Thermocauterization with Iridectomy 66155
        Trabeculectomy ab Externo in Absence of
            Previous Surgery 66170
        Trephination with Iridectomy 66150
Lesion
    Excision 66130
Repair
    Reinforcement
        with Graft 67255
        without Graft 67250
    Staphyloma
        with Graft 66225
        without Graft 66220
        with Glue 65286
    Wound
        Operative 66250
        Tissue Glue 65286

Scleral Buckling Operation
See Retina, Repair, Detachment

Scleral Ectasia
See Staphyloma, Sclera

Sclerectomy 66160

Sclerotherapy
Venous 36468-36471

Sclerotomy
See Incision, Sclera

Screening, Drug
See Drug Screen

Sesamoid Bone
Excision 28315
Finger
    Excision 26185
Foot
    Fracture 28530-28531
Thumb
    Excision 26185

Sesamoidectomy
Toe 28315

Sever Procedure
See Contracture, Palm, Release

Severing of Blepharorrhaphy
See Tarsorrhaphy, Severing

Sex Change Operation
Female to Male 55980
Male to Female 55970

Sex Chromatin
See Barr Bodies

Sex Chromatin Identification 88130-88140

Sex Hormone Binding Globulin 84270

Sex-Linked Ichthyoses
See Syphilis Test

SGOT 84450

SGPT 84460

Shaving
Skin Lesion 11300-11313

SHBG
See Sex Hormone Binding Globulin

Shelf Procedure
See Osteotomy, Hip

Shiga-like Toxin
Antigen Detection
    Enzyme Immunoassay 87427

Shigella
Antibody 86771

Shirodkar Operation
See Repair, Cervix, Cerclage, Abdominal

Shock Wave (Extracorporeal) Therapy 0019T-0020T

Shock Wave Lithotripsy 50590

Shock Wave, Ultrasonic
See Ultrasound

Shop Typhus of Malaya
See Murine Typhus

Shoulder
See Clavicle; Scapula
Abscess
    Drainage 23030
Amputation 23900-23921
Arthrocentesis 20610

Arthrodesis 23800
    with Autogenous Graft 23802
Arthrography
    Injection
        Radiologic 23350
Arthroscopy
    Diagnostic 29805
    Surgical 29806-29827
Arthrotomy
    with Removal Loose or Foreign Body ..23107
Biopsy
    Deep 23066
    Soft Tissue 23065
Blade
    See Scapula
Bone
    Excision
        Acromion 23130
        Clavicle 23120-23125
    Incision 23035
    Tumor
        Excision 23140-23146
Bursa
    Drainage 23031
Capsular Contracture Release 23020
Cast
    Figure Eight 29049
    Removal 29710
    Spica 29055
    Velpeau 29058
Disarticulation 23920-23921
Dislocation
    Closed Treatment
        with Manipulation 23650-23655
Exploration 23107
Hematoma
    Drainage 23030
Manipulation
    Application of Fixation Apparatus 23700
Prophylactic Treatment 23490-23491
Radical Resection 23077
Removal
    Calcareous Deposits 23000
    Cast 29710
    Foreign Body
        Complicated 23332
        Deep 23331
        Subcutaneous 23330
    Foreign or Loose Body 23107
Repair
    Capsule 23450-23466
    Ligament Release 23415
    Muscle Transfer 23395-23397
    Rotator Cuff 23410-23420
    Tendon 23410-23412, 23430-23440
    Tenomyotomy 23405-23406
Strapping 29240
Surgery
    Unlisted Services and Procedures 23929
Tumor
    Excision 23075-23077
Unlisted Services and Procedures 23929
X-Ray 73020-73030
X-Ray with Contrast 73040

Shoulder Joint
See Clavicle; Scapula
Arthroplasty
    with Implant 23470-23472
Arthrotomy
    with Biopsy 23100-23101
    with Synovectomy 23105-23106
Dislocation
    Open Treatment 23660
    with Greater Tuberosity Fracture
        Closed Treatment 23665
        Open Treatment 23670
    with Surgical or Anatomical Neck Fracture
        Closed Treatment with Manipulation 23675
        Open Treatment 23680
Excision
    Torn Cartilage 23101
Exploration 23040-23044
Incision and Drainage 23040-23044
Removal
    Foreign Body 23040-23044
X-Ray 73050

Shunt(s)
Aqueous
    to Extraocular Reservoir 66180
        Revision 66185
Arteriovenous
    See Arteriovenous Shunt
Brain
    Creation 62180-62223
    Removal 62256-62258
    Replacement 62160, 62194,
        62225-62230, 62258
    Reprogramming 62252
Cerebrospinal Fluid
    See Cerebrospinal Fluid Shunt
Creation
    Arteriovenous
        Direct 36821
        ECMO 36822
        Thomas Shunt 36835
        Transposition 36818-36820
        with Bypass Graft 35686
        with Graft 36825-36830
    Cerebrospinal Fluid 62200
    Thomas Shunt 36835
Fetal 59076
Great Vessel
    Aorta
        Pulmonary 33924
    Aorta to Pulmonary Artery
        Ascending 33755
        Descending 33762
        Central 33764
        Subclavian Pulmonary Artery 33750
        Vena Cava to Pulmonary Artery .33766-33767
    Intra-atrial 33735-33737
LeVeen
    See LeVeen Shunt
Nonvascular
    X-Ray 75809
Peritoneal
    Venous
        Injection 49427
        Ligation 49428
        Removal 49429
        X-Ray 75809

Pulmonary Artery
   See Pulmonary Artery, Shunt
Revision
   Arteriovenous 36832
Spinal Cord
   Creation 63740-63741
   Irrigation 63744
   Removal 63746
   Replacement 63744
Superior Mesenteric-Caval
   See Anastomosis, Caval to Mesenteric
Ureter to Colon 50815
Ventriculocisternal with Valve
   See Ventriculocisternostomy

Shuntogram 75809

Sialic Acid 84275

Sialodochoplasty 42500-42505

Sialogram
See Sialography

Sialography 70390

Sickling
Electrophoresis 83020

Siderocytes 85536

Siderophilin
See Transferrin

Sigmoid
See Colon-Sigmoid

Sigmoid Bladder
Cystectomy 51590

Sigmoidoscopy
Ablation
   Polyp 45339
   Tumor 45339
Biopsy 45331
Collection
   Specimen 45331
Exploration 45330, 45335
Hemorrhage Control 45334
Injection
   Submucosal 45335
Needle Biopsy 45342
Placement
   Stent 45345
Removal
   Foreign Body 45332
   Polyp 45333, 45338
   Tumor 45333, 45338
Repair
   Volvulus 45337
Ultrasound 45341-45342

Signal-Averaged Electrocardiography
See Electrocardiogram

Silica 84285

Silicon Dioxide
See Silica

Silicone
Contouring Injections 11950-11954

Silver Operation
See Keller Procedure

Silver Procedure 28290

Simple Mastectomies
See Mastectomy

Single Photon Absorptiometry
See Absorptiometry, Single Photon

Single Photon Emission Computed Tomography
See SPECT

Sinu, Sphenoid
See Sinuses, Sphenoid

Sinus
Ethmoidectomy
   Excision 31254
Pilonidal
   See Cyst, Pilonidal

Sinus of Valsalva
Repair 33702-33722

Sinus Venosus
Repair 33645

Sinusectomy, Ethmoid
See Ethmoidectomy

Sinuses
Ethmoid
   Excision 31200-31205
     with Nasal/Sinus Endoscopy .31254-31255
   Repair of Cerebrospinal Leak 31290
Frontal
   Destruction 31080-31085
   Exploration 31070-31075
     with Nasal/Sinus Endoscopy 31276
   Fracture
     Open Treatment 21343-21344
   Incision 31070-31087
Injection 20500
   Diagnostic 20501
Maxillary
   Antrostomy 31256-31267
   Excision 31225-31230
   Exploration 31020-31032
     with Nasal/Sinus Endoscopy 31233
   Incision 31020-31032, 31256-31267
   Irrigation 31000
   Skull Base 61581
   Surgery 61581
Multiple
   Incision 31090
Paranasal
   Incision 31090
Sphenoid
   Biopsy 31050-31051
   Exploration 31050-31051
     with Nasal/Sinus Endoscopy 31235
   Incision 31050-31051
     with Nasal/Sinus Endoscopy .31287-31288
   Irrigation 31002
   Repair of Cerebrospinal Leak 31291

Sinusotomy 31050-31051
   Skull Base Surgery 61580-61581
Unlisted Services and Procedures 31299
X-Ray 70210-70220

Sinusoidal Rotational Testing
See Ear, Nose and Throat

Sinusoscopy
Sinus
   Maxillary 31233
   Sphenoid 31235

Sinusotomy
See Sinus, Multiple
Combined 31090
Frontal Sinus
   Exploratory 31070-31075
   Nonobliterative 31086-31087
   Obliterative 31080-31085
Maxillary 31020-31032
Multiple
   Paranasal 31090
Sphenoid Sinus 31050-31051

SISI Test 92564

Sistrunk Operation
See Cyst, Thyroid Gland, Excision

Size Reduction, Breast
See Breast, Reduction

Skeletal Fixation
Humeral Epicondyle
   Percutaneous 24566

Skeletal Traction
Insertion/Removal
   Pin/Wire 20650

Skene's Gland
Abscess
   Incision and Drainage 53060
Destruction 53270
Excision 53270

Skilled Nursing Facilities (SNFs)
See Nursing Facility Services

Skin
Abrasion 15786-15787
   Chemical Peel 15788-15793
   Dermabrasion 15780-15783
   Salabrasion 15810-15811
Abscess
   See Abscess, Skin
Adjacent Tissue Transfer 14000-14350
Allografts
   See Allograft, Skin
Biopsy 11100-11101
Chemical Exfoliation 17360
Cyst
   See Cyst, Skin
Debridement 11000-11006, 11010-11044
   Eczematous 11000-11001
   Full Thickness 11041
   Infected 11000-11006
   Partial Thickness 11040

Sleep Study 95806-95807

Sliding Inlay Graft, Tibia
See Ankle; Tibia, Repair

Sling Operation
Incontinence 53440
    Removal 53442
Stress Incontinence 51992, 57287
Vagina 57287-57288

Small Bowel
See Intestines, Small
Neoplasm
    See Tumor, Intestines, Small

SMAS Flap .... .15829

Smear
Cervical
    See Cervical Smears
Papanicolaou
    See Pap Smears

Smear and Stain
See Cytopathology, Smears
Cornea 65430
Fluorescent 87206
Gram or Giesma 87205
Ova
    Parasites 87177
Parasites 87207
Wet Mount 87210

Smith Fracture 25600-25620

Smith-Robinson Operation
See Arthrodesis, Vertebra

Smithwick Operation
See Excision, Nerve, Sympathetic

SO4
See Sulfate

Soave Procedure .... .45120

Sodium .... .84295, 84302
Urine 84300

Sodium Glycinate, Theophylline
See Theophylline

Sofield Procedure .... .24410

Soft Tissue
See Tissue, Soft

Solar Plexus
See Celiac Plexus

Solitary Cyst
See Bone, Cyst

Somatomammotropin, Chorionic 83632

Somatomedin .... .84305

Somatosensory Testing
Lower Limbs 95926
Trunk or Head 95927
Upper Limbs 95925

Somatostatin .... .84307

Somatotropin .... .83003

Somatotropin Release Inhibiting Hormone
See Somatostatin

Somatropin
See Growth Hormone, Human

Somnographies
See Polysomnography

Somophyllin T
See Theophylline

Sonography
See Echography

Sonohysterography 76831
Saline Infusion
    Injection Procedure 58340

Sore, Bed
See Pressure Ulcer (Decubitus)

Spasm Eyelid
See Blepharospasm

Special Services
After Hours Medical Services 99050-99054
Analysis
    Remote Physiologic Data 99091
Computer Data Analysis 99090
Device Handling 99002
Emergency Care In Office 99058
Group Education 99078
Hyperbaric Oxygen 99183
Hypothermia 99185-99186
Medical Testimony 99075
Non-Office Medical Services 99056
On Call Services 99026-99027
Phlebotomy 99199
Post-Op Visit 99024
Pump Services 99190-99192
Reports and Forms
    Medical, Extended 99080
    Psychiatric 90889
Specimen Handling 99000-99001
Supply of Materials 99070
    Educational 99071
Unlisted Services and Procedures 99199
Unusual Travel 99082

Specific Gravity
Body Fluid 84315

Specimen Collection
Intestines 89100-89105
Stomach 89130-89141

Specimen Concentration ...... .87015

Specimen Handling 99000-99001

SPECT .... .78607
See Emission Computerized Tomography
Abscess Localization 78807
Bone 78320
Cerebrospinal Fluid 78647

Heart
    Multiple 78465
    Single 78464
Kidney 78710
Liver 78205
Tumor Localization 78803

Spectacle Services
Fitting
    Low Vision Aid 92354-92355
    Spectacle Prosthesis 92352-92353
    Spectacles 92340-92342
Repair 92370-92371
Supply
    Low Vision Aids 92392
    Spectacle Prosthesis 92395
    Spectacles 92390

Spectrometry
Mass
    Analyte
        Qualitative 83788
        Quantitative 83789

Spectrophotometry .... .84311
Atomic Absorption
    See Atomic Absorption Spectroscopy

Spectroscopy
Atomic Absorption 82190
Expired Breath Analysis 0064T
Magnetic Resonance 76390

Spectrum Analyses
See Spectrophotometry

Speculoscopy .... .0031T
with Direct Sampling 0032T

Speech Evaluation .... .92506
Cine 70371
for Prosthesis 92597, 92607-92608
Video 70371

Speech Prosthesis 21084, 92609
Creation 31611
Evaluation for Speech 92597, 92607-92608
Insertion 31611

Speech Therapy 92507-92508

Sperm
Cryopreserved
    Preparation
        Thawing 89353
Storage 89343

Sperm Analysis
Antibodies 89325
Cervical Mucus Penetration Test 89330
Cryopreservation 89259
Hamster Penetration Test 89329
Hyaluron Binding Assay 0087T
Identification
    Aspiration 89257
    from Testis Tissue 89264
Isolation 89260-89261

Sperm Evaluation, Cervical Mucus Penetration Test
See Huhner Test

Sperm Washing 58323

Spermatic Cord
Hydrocele
   Excision 55500
Laparoscopy 55559
Lesion
   Excision 55520
Repair
   Veins 55530-55540
      Abdominal Approach 55535
      with Hernia Repair 55540
Varicocele
   Excision 55530-55540

Spermatic Veins
Excision 55530-55540
Ligation 55550

Spermatocele
Excision 54840

Spermatocystectomy
See Spermatocele, Excision

Sphenoid Sinus
See Sinuses, Sphenoid

Sphenoidotomy
Excision
   with Nasal/Sinus Endoscopy ...31287-31288

Sphenopalatine Ganglion
Injection
   Anesthetic 64505

Sphincter
See Specific Sphincter
Anal
   See Anal Sphincter
Artificial Genitourinary
   See Prosthesis, Urethral Sphincter
Pyloric
   See Pyloric Sphincter

Sphincter of Oddi
Pressure Measurement
   Endoscopy 43263

Sphincteroplasty
Anal 46750-46751, 46760-46761
   with Implant 46762
Bile Duct 47460
Bladder Neck
   See Bladder, Repair, Neck

Sphincterotomy 52277
Anal 46080
Bile Duct 47460

Spica Cast
Hip 29305-29325
Repair 29720
Shoulder 29055

Spinal Accessory Nerve
Anastomosis
   to Facial Nerve 64866
Incision 63191
Injection
   Anesthetic 64412
Section 63191

Spinal Column
See Spine

Spinal Cord
See Cauda Equina; Nerve Root
Biopsy 63275-63290
Cyst
   Aspiration 62268
   Incision and Drainage 63172-63173
Decompression 63001-63003
   with Cervical Laminoplasty 63050-63051
Drain Fluid 62272
Exploration 63001-63044
Graft
   Dura 63710
Implantation
   Electrode 63650-63655
   Pulse Generator 63685
   Receiver 63685
Incision 63200
   Dentate Ligament 63180-63182
   Tract 63170, 63194-63199
Injection
   Anesthetic 62310-62319
   Blood 62273
   CT Scan 62284
   Neurolytic Agent 62280-62282
   Other 62310-62311
   X-Ray 62284
Insertion
   Electrode 63650-63655
   Pulse Generator 63685
   Receiver 63685
Lesion
   Destruction 62280-62282
   Excision 63265-63273, 63300-63308
Needle Biopsy 62269
Neoplasm
   Excision 63275-63290
Puncture (Tap)
   Diagnostic 62270
   Drain Fluid 62272
   Lumbar 62270
Release 63200
Reconstruction
   Dorsal Spine Elements 63292
Removal
   Catheter 62355
   Electrode 63660
   Pulse Generator 63688
   Pump 62365
   Receiver 63688
   Reservoir 62365
Repair
   Cerebrospinal Fluid Leak 63707-63709
   Meningocele 63700-63702
   Myelomeningocele 63704-63706
Section
   Dentate Ligament 63180-63182
   Tract 63194-63199
Shunt
   Create 63740-63741
   Irrigation 63744
   Removal 63746
   Replacement 63744
Stereotaxis
   Aspiration 63615
   Biopsy 63615

   Creation Lesion 63600
   Excision Lesion 63615
   Stimulation 63610
Syrinx
   Aspiration 62268
Tumor
   Excision 63275-63290

Spinal Cord Neoplasms
See Spinal Cord
Tumor
   See Spinal Cord, Tumor; Tumor
   Excision
      See Spinal Cord, Tumor; Tumor, Spinal
      Cord

Spinal Fluid
See Cerebrospinal Fluid

Spinal Fracture
See Fracture, Vertebra

Spinal Instrumentation
Anterior 22845-22847
   Removal 22855
Internal Fixation 22841
Pelvic Fixation 22848
Posterior Nonsegmental
   Harrington Rod Technique 22840
      Removal 22850
Posterior Segmental 22842-22844
   Removal 22852
Prosthetic Device 22851
Reinsertion of Spinal Fixation Device 22849

Spinal Manipulation
See Manipulation, Chiropractic

Spinal Nerve
Avulsion 64772
Transection 64772

Spinal Tap
See Cervical Puncture; Cisternal Puncture;
Subdural Tap; Ventricular Puncture
Drainage Fluid 62272
Lumbar 62270

Spine
See Spinal Cord; Vertebra; Vertebral Body;
Vertebral Process
Allograft
   Morselized 20930
   Structural 20931
Autograft
   Local 20936
   Morselized 20937
   Structural 20938
Biopsy 20250-20251
CT Scan
   Cervical 72125-72127
   Lumbar 72131-72133
   Thoracic 72128-72130
Fixation 22842
Fusion
   Anterior 22808-22812
   Anterior Approach 22548-22585, 22812
   Exploration 22830
   Lateral Extracavitary 22532-22534
   Posterior Approach 22590-22802

Excision
Trachea 31780-31781
Laryngoplasty 31582
Reconstruction
Auditory Canal, External 69310
Repair
Trachea 31780-31781
Tracheal
See Trachea Stenosis
Urethral
See Urethral Stenosis

Stensen Duct
See Parotid Duct

Stent
Indwelling
Insertion
Ureter 50605
Placement
Bronchoscopy 31631, 31636-31637
Colonoscopy .45387
via Stoma .44397
Endoscopy
Gastrointestinal, Upper 43256
Enteroscopy .44370
Proctosigmoidoscopy 45327
Sigmoidoscopy 45345
Transcatheter
Intravascular . .37205-37208, 37215, 37216
Extracranial 0075T-0076T
Ureteroneocystomy 50947-50948
Revision
Bronchoscopy 31638
Urethra 52282
Prostatic 0084T

Stent, Intravascular
See Transcatheter, Placement, Intravascular
Stents

Stents, Tracheal
See Tracheal Stent

Stereotactic Frame
Application/Removal 20660

Stereotaxis
Aspiration
Brain Lesion .61750
with CT Scan and/or MRI 61751
Spinal Cord .63615
Biopsy
Aspiration
Brain Lesion 61750
Brain 61750
with CT Scan and/or MRI 61751
Breast 76095
Spinal Cord .63615
Computer Assisted
Brain Surgery 61795
Orthopedic Surgery 0054T-0056T
Creation Lesion
Brain
Deep 61720-61735
Percutaneous 61790
Gasserian Ganglion 61790
Spinal Cord 63600
Trigeminal Tract 61791

CT Scan
Aspiration 61751
Biopsy 61751
Excision Lesion
Brain 61750
Spinal Cord 63615
Focus Beam
Radiosurgery 61793
Localization
Brain 61770
Radiation Therapy 0082T-0083T, 77432
Stimulation
Spinal Cord 63610

Sterile Coverings
See Dressings

Sternal Fracture
See Fracture, Sternum

Sternoclavicular Joint
Arthrotomy 23044
with Biopsy .23101
with Synovectomy 23106
Dislocation
Closed Treatment
with Manipulation 23525
without Manipulation 23520
Open Treatment 23530-23532
with Fascial Graft 23532

Sternocleidomastoid
Division 21720-21725

Sternotomy
Closure 21750

Sternum
Debridement 21627
Excision 21620, 21630-21632
Fracture
Closed Treatment 21820
Open Treatment 21825
Ostectomy 21620
Radical Resection 21630-21632
Reconstruction 21740-21742, 21750
with Thoracoscopy 21743
X-Ray .71120-71130

Steroid-Binding Protein, Sex
See Globulin, Sex Hormone Binding

Steroids
Anabolic
See Androstenedione
Injection
Urethral Stricture 52283
Ketogenic
Urine 83582

STH (Somatotropic Hormone)
See Growth Hormone

Stimulating Antibody, Thyroid
See Immunoglobulin, Thyroid Stimulating

Stimulation
Electric
See Electrical Stimulation
Lymphocyte
See Blastogenesis

Spinal Cord
Stereotaxis .63610
Transcutaneous Electric
See Application, Neurostimulation

Stimulator, Long-Acting Thyroid
See Thyrotropin Releasing Hormone (TRH)

Stimulators, Cardiac
See Heart, Pacemaker

Stimulus Evoked Response 51792

Stoffel Operation
See Rhizotomy

Stoma
Creation
Bladder 51980
Kidney 50551-50561
Stomach
Neonatal .43831
Temporary 43830-43831
Ureter 50860
Ureter
Endoscopy via 50951-50961

Stomach
Anastomosis
with Duodenum 43810, 43850-43855
with Jejunum . . .43820-43825, 43860-43865
Biopsy 43600-43605
Creation
Stoma
Temporary 43830-43831
Temporary Stoma
Laparoscopic 43653
Electrogastrography 91132-91133
Excision
Partial 43631-43639, 43845
Total 43620-43622
Exploration 43500
Gastric Bypass 43644-43645, 43846
Revision 43848
Incision 43830-43832
Exploration .43500
Pyloric Sphincter 43520
Removal
Foreign Body 43500
Intubation with Specimen Prep 91055
Nuclear Medicine
Blood Loss Study 78278
Emptying Study 78264
Imaging 78261
Protein Loss Study 78282
Reflux Study 78262
Vitamin B-12 Absorption 78270-78272
Reconstruction
for Obesity 43644-43645, 43842-43847
Roux-En-Y 43644, 43846
Removal
Foreign Body 43500
Repair 48547
Fistula 43880
Fundoplasty 43324-43325
Laparoscopic 43280
Laceration 43501-43502
Stoma 43870
Ulcer 43501
Saline Load Test 91060

DHA
See Dehydroepiandrosterone Sulfate
Urine 84392

Sulfation Factor
See Somatomedin

Sulphates
See Sulfate

Sumatran Mite Fever
See Scrub Typhus

Superficial Musculoaponeurotic System (SMAS) Flap
Rhytidectomy 15829

Supernumerary Digit
Reconstruction 26587
Repair 26587

Supply
Chemotherapeutic Agent 96545
  See Chemotherapy
Contact Lenses 92391, 92396
Educational Materials 99071
Low Vision Aids 92392
  See Spectacle Services
Materials 99070
Ocular Prosthesis 92393
Prosthesis
  Breast 19396
Spectacle Prosthesis 92395
Spectacles 92390

Suppositories, Vaginal
See Pessary

Suppression 80400-80408

Suppression/Testing
See Evocative/Suppression Test

Suppressor T Lymphocyte Marker
See CD8

Suppurative Hidradenitides
See Hidradenitis, Suppurative

Suprahyoid
Lymphadenectomy 38700

Supraorbital Nerve
Avulsion 64732
Incision 64732
Transection 64732

Supraorbital Rim and Forehead
Reconstruction 21179-21180

Suprapubic Prostatectomies
See Prostatectomy, Suprapubic

Suprarenal
Gland
  See Adrenal Gland
Vein
  See Vein, Adrenal

Suprascapular Nerve
Injection
  Anesthetic 64418

Suprasellar Cyst
See Craniopharyngioma

Surface CD4 Receptor
See CD4

Surface Radiotherapy
See Application, Radioelement, Surface

Surgeries
Breast-Conserving
  See Breast, Excision, Lesion
Conventional
  See Celiotomy
Laser
  See Laser Surgery
Mohs
  See Mohs Micrographic Surgery
Repeat
  See Reoperation

Surgical
Avulsion
  See Avulsion
Cataract Removal
  See Cataract, Excision
Collapse Therapy; Thoracoplasty
  See Thoracoplasty
Diathermy
  See Electrocautery
Galvanism
  See Electrolysis
Incision
  See Incision
Microscopes
  See Operating Microscope
Pathology
  See Pathology, Surgical
Planing
  Nose
    Skin 30120
Pneumoperitoneum
  See Pneumoperitoneum
Removal, Eye
  See Enucleation, Eye
Revision
  See Reoperation
Services
  Post-Op Visit 99024

Surveillance
See Monitoring

Suspension
Aorta 33800
Kidney
  See Nephropexy
Muscle
  Hyoid 21685
Vagina
  See Colpopexy

Suture
See Repair
Abdomen 49900
Aorta 33320-33322
Bile Duct
  Wound 47900

Bladder
  Fistulization 44660-44661,
       45800-45805, 51880-51925
    Vesicouterine 51920-51925
    Vesicovaginal 51900
    Wound 51860-51865
Cervix 57720
Colon
  Diverticula 44604-44605
  Fistula 44650-44661
  Plication 44680
  Stoma 44620-44625
  Ulcer 44604-44605
  Wound 44604-44605
Esophagus
  Wound 43410-43415
Eyelid 67880
  Closure of 67875
  with Transposition of Tarsal Plate 67882
  Wound
    Full Thickness 67935
    Partial Thickness 67930
Facial Nerve
  Intratemporal
    Lateral to Geniculate Ganglion 69740
    Medial to Geniculate Ganglion 69745
Foot
  Tendon 28200-28210
Gastroesophageal 0008T, 43405
Great Vessel 33320-33322
Hemorrhoids 46945-46946
Hepatic Duct
  See Hepatic Duct, Repair
Intestine
  Large
    Diverticula 44605
    Ulcer 44605
    Wound 44605
Intestines
  Large
    Diverticula 44604
    Ulcer 44604
    Wound 44604
  Small
    Diverticula 44602-44603
    Fistula 44640-44661
    Plication 44680
    Ulcer 44602-44603
    Wound 44602-44603
    Stoma 44620-44625
Iris
  with Ciliary Body 66682
Kidney
  Fistula 50520-50526
  Horseshoe 50540
  Wound 50500
Leg, Lower
  Tendon 27658-27665
Leg, Upper
  Muscle 27385-27386
Liver
  Wound 47350-47361
Mesentery 44850
Nerve 64831-64876
Pancreas 48545
Pharynx
  Wound 42900

Syrinx
Spinal Cord
    Aspiration 62268

System
Endocrine
    See Endocrine System
Hemic
    See Hemic System
Lymphatic
    See Lymphatic System
Musculoskeletal
    See Musculoskeletal System
Nervous
    See Nervous System

T

T Cell Leukemia Virus I Antibodies, Adult
See Antibody, HTLV-I

T Cell Leukemia Virus I, Human
See HTLV I

T Cell Leukemia Virus II Antibodies, Human
See Antibody, HTLV-II

T Cell Leukemia Virus II, Human
See HTLV II

T Lymphotropic Virus Type III Antibodies, Human
See Antibody, HIV

T-3
See Triiodothyronine

T-4 .84436-84439, 86360

T-7 Index
See Thyroxine, Total

T-8
See CD8; T-Cells, Ratio

T-Cell T8 Antigens
See CD8

T-Cells
CD4
    Absolute 86361
Count 86359
Ratio 86360

T-Phyl
See Theophylline

T3 Free
See Triiodothyronine, Free

T4 Molecule
See CD4

T4 Total
See Thyroxine, Total

Taarnhoj Procedure
See Decompression, Gasserian Ganglion, Sensory Root; Section

Tachycardia
Heart
    Recording 93609

Tacrolimus
Drug Assay 80197

Tag, Skin
See Skin, Tags

Tail Bone
Excision 27080
Fracture 27200-27202

Takeuchi Procedure 33505

Talectomy
See Astragalectomy

Talotarsal Joint
Dislocation 28570-28575, 28585
    Percutaneous Fixation 28576

Talus
Arthrodesis
    Pantalar 28705
    Subtalar 28725
    Triple 28715
Arthroscopy
    Surgical 29891-29892
Craterization 28120
Cyst
    Excision 28100-28103
Diaphysectomy .28120
Excision 28120, 28130
Fracture
    Open Treatment 28445
    Percutaneous Fixation 28436
    with Manipulation 28435-28436
    without Manipulation 28430
Repair
    Osteochondritis Dissecans 29892
    Osteotomy 28302
Saucerization .28120
Tumor
    Excision 27647, 28100-28103

Tap
Cisternal
    See Cisternal Puncture
Lumbar Diagnostic
    See Spinal Tap

Tarsal
Fracture
    Percutaneous Fixation 28456

Tarsal Bone
See Ankle Bone

Tarsal Joint
See Foot
Arthrodesis 28730-28735, 28740
    with Advancement 28737
    with Lengthening 28737
Craterization 28122
Cyst
    Excision 28104-28107

Diaphysectomy .28122
Dislocation 28540-28545, 28555
    Percutaneous Fixation 28545-28546
Excision 28116, 28122
Fracture
    Open Treatment 28465
    with Manipulation 28455-28456
    without Manipulation 28450
Fusion 28730-28735, 28740
    with Advancement 28737
    with Lengthening 28737
Repair 28320
    Osteotomy 28304-28305
Saucerization .28122
Tumor
    Excision 28104-28107, 28171

Tarsal Strip Procedure 67917-67924

Tarsal Tunnel Release 28035

Tarsal Wedge Procedure .67916, 67923

Tarsometatarsal Joint
Arthrodesis 28730-28735, 28740
Arthrotomy 28020, 28050
Dislocation 28600-28605, 28615
    Percutaneous Fixation 28606
Exploration 28020
Fusion 28730-28735, 28740
Removal
    Foreign Body 28020
    Loose Body 28020
Synovial
    Biopsy 28050
    Excision 28070

Tarsorrhaphy 67875
Median 67880
Severing 67710
    with Transposition of Tarsal Plate 67882

Tattoo
Cornea 65600
Skin 11920-11922

TB Test
Antigen Response 0010T
Skin Test 86580-86585

TBG
See Thyroxine Binding Globulin

TBS
See Bethesda System

TCT
See Thrombin Time

Td Shots
See Tetanus Immunization; Vaccines

Team Conference
Case Management Services 99361-99373

Tear Duct
See Lacrimal Duct

Tear Gland
See Lacrimal Gland

Hip, Adductor 27000-27003
Leg, Upper 27306-27307, 27390-27392
Toe 28010-28011, 28232-28234, 28240
Wrist 25290

TENS
See Application, Neurostimulation; Physical
Medicine/Therapy/Occupational Therapy

Tensilon Test 95857-95858

Tension, Ocular
See Glaucoma

Tentorium Cerebelli
Section 61440

Terman-Merrill Test 96100

Termination, Pregnancy
See Abortion

Test
Antiglobulin
    See Coombs Test
Aphasia
    See Aphasia Testing
Bender Visual-Motor Gestalt
    See Bender-Gestalt Test
Binet
    See Binet Test
Blood
    See Blood Tests
Blood Coagulation
    See Coagulation
Breath
    See Breath Test
Cervical Mucus Penetration
    See Cervical Mucus Penetration Test
Clinical Chemistry
    See Chemistry Tests, Clinical
Complement Fixation
    See Complement, Fixation Test
Exercise
    See Exercise Stress Tests
Fern
    See Smear and Stain, Wet Mount
Fetal, Nonstress
    See Fetal Non-Stress Test
Function, Vestibular
    See Vestibular Function Tests
Gel Diffusion
    See Immunodiffusion
Glucose Tolerance
    See Glucose, Tolerance Test
Hearing
    See Audiologic Function Tests
Hemagglutination Inhibition
    See Hemagglutination Inhibition Test
Ink Blot
    See Inkblot Test
Intelligence
    See Intelligence Test
Lung Function
    See Pulmonology, Diagnostic
Neutralization
    See Neutralization Test
Papanicolaou
    See Pap Smears
Pregnancy
    See Pregnancy Test

Quick
    See Prothrombin Time
Radioimmunosorbent
    See Gammaglobulin, Blood
Rorschach
    See Rorschach Test
Schilling
    See Schilling Test
Skin
    See Skin, Tests
Stanford-Binet
    See Psychiatric Diagnosis
Tuberculin
    See Skin, Tests, Tuberculosis

Test Tube Fertilization
See In Vitro Fertilization

Tester, Color Vision
See Color Vision Examination

Testes
Cryopreservation 89335
Nuclear Medicine
    Imaging 78760-78761
Undescended
    See Testis, Undescended

Testicular Vein
See Spermatic Veins

Testimony, Medical 99075

Testing, Histocompatibility
See Tissue Typing

Testing, Neurophysiologic
Intraoperative 95920

Testing, Neuropsychological . .96117

Testing, Range of Motion
See Range of Motion Test

Testis
Abscess
    Incision and Drainage 54700
Biopsy 54500-54505
Excision
    Laparoscopic 54690
    Partial 54522
    Radical 54530-54535
    Simple 54520
Hematoma
    Incision and Drainage 54700
Insertion
    Prosthesis 54660
Lesion
    Excision 54512
Needle Biopsy .54500
Repair
    Injury 54670
    Suspension 54620-54640
    Torsion 54600
Suture
    Injury 54670
    Suspension 54620-54640
Transplantation
    to Thigh 54680
Tumor
    Excision 54530-54535

Undescended
    Exploration 54550-54560
Unlisted Services and Procedures . .54699, 55899

Testosterone 84402
Response 80414
    Stimulation 80414-80415
Total 84403

Testosterone Estradiol Binding Globulin
See Globulin, Sex Hormone Binding

Tetanus 86280
Antibody 86774
Immunoglobulin 90389
Vaccine 90703

Tetrachloride, Carbon
See Carbon Tetrachloride

Tetralogy of Fallot . . .33692-33697, 33924

Thal-Nissen Procedure 43325

Thawing
See Frozen Blood Preparation
Cryopreserved
    Embryo 89352
    Oocytes 89356
    Reproductive Tissue 89354
    Sperm 89353
Previously Frozen Cells 38208-38209

Thawing and Expansion
of Frozen Cell .88241

THBR
See Thyroid Hormone Binding Ratio

Theleplasty
See Nipples, Reconstruction

Theophylline
Assay 80198

Therapeutic
Abortion
    See Abortion, Therapeutic
Apheresis
    See Apheresis, Therapeutic
Drug Assay
    See Drug Assay
Mobilization
    See Mobilization
Photopheresis
    See Photopheresis
Radiology
    See Radiology, Therapeutic

Therapies
Cold
    See Cryotherapy
Exercise
    See Exercise Therapy
Family
    See Psychotherapy, Family
Language
    See Language Therapy
Milieu
    See Environmental Intervention

Occupational
   See Occupational Therapy
Photodynamic
   See Photochemotherapy
Photoradiation
   See Actinotherapy
Physical
   See Physical Medicine/Therapy/Occupational
Therapy
Speech
   See Speech Therapy
Tocolytic
   See Tocolysis
Ultraviolet
   See Actinotherapy

Therapy
ACE Inhibitor Therapy
   See Performance Measures
Beta Blocker Therapy
   See Performance Measures
Desensitization
   See Allergen Immunotherapy
Hemodialysis
   See Hemodialysis
Hot Pack
   See Hot Pack Treatment
Pharmacologic; for Cessation of Tobacco Use
   See Performance Measures
Radiation
   See Irradiation
Speech
   See Speech Therapy
Statin Therapy, Prescribed
   See Performance Measures

Thermocauterization
Ectropion
   Repair 67922
Lesion
   Cornea 65450

Thermocoagulation
See Electrocautery

Thermogram
Cephalic 93760
Peripheral 93762

Thermographies
See Thermogram

Thermography, Cerebral
See Thermogram, Cephalic

Thermotherapy
Prostate 53850-53853
   Microwave 53850
   Radiofrequency 53852

Thiamine 84425

Thiersch Operation 15050
See Pinch Graft

Thiersch Procedure 46753

Thigh
Fasciotomy 27025
   See Femur; Leg, Upper

Thin Layer Chromatographies
See Chromatography, Thin-Layer

Thiocyanate 84430

Third Disease
See Rubella

Third Opinion
See Confirmatory Consultations

Thompson Procedure 27430

Thompson Test
See Smear and Stain, Routine

Thoracectomy
See Thoracoplasty

Thoracentesis 32000-32002

Thoracic
Anterior Ramus
   See Intercostal Nerve
Arteries
   See Artery, Thoracic
Cavity
   See Chest Cavity
Duct
   See Lymphatics
   Cannulation 38794
   Ligation 38380
      Abdominal Approach 38382
      Thoracic Approach 38381
   Suture
      Abdominal Approach 38382
      Cervical Approach 38380
      Thoracic Approach 38381
Empyema
   See Abscess, Thorax
Surgery
   Video-Assisted
      See Thoracoscopy
Vertebra
   See Vertebra, Thoracic
Wall
   See Chest Wall

Thoracocentesis
See Thoracentesis

Thoracoplasty 32905
with Closure Bronchopleural Fistula 32906

Thoracoscopy
Diagnostic 32601-32606
   with Biopsy 32602, 32604, 32606
   without Biopsy 32601, 32603, 32605
Surgical 32650-32665
   with Control Traumatic Hemorrhage ...32654
   with Creation Pericardial Window 32659
   with Esophagomyotomy 32665
   with Excision Mediastinal Cyst, Tumor
   and/or Mass 32662
   with Excision Pericardial Cyst, Tumor
   and/or Mass 32661
   with Excision-Plication of Bullae 32655
   with Lobectomy 32663
   with Parietal Pleurectomy 32656
   with Partial Pulmonary Decortication ..32651
   with Pleurodesis 32650

with Removal Intrapleural Foreign
   Body 32653
with Removal of Clot/Foreign Body ..32658
with Sternum Reconstruction 21743
with Thoracic Sympathectomy 32664
with Total Pericardiectomy 32660
with Total Pulmonary Decortication ..32652
with Wedge Resection of Lung 32657

Thoracostomy
Empyema 32035-32036
Tube, with/without Water Seal 32020

Thoracotomy
Cardiac Massage 32160
for Pacing Cardioverter-Defibrillator
Pads 33245-33246
for Post-Op Complications 32120
Hemorrhage 32110
Removal
   Bullae 32141
   Cyst 32140
   Defibrillator 33243
   Electrodes 33238
   Foreign Body
      Intrapleural 32150
      Intrapulmonary 32151
   Pacemaker 33236-33237
   with Biopsy 32095-32100
   with Excision-Plication of Bullae 32141
   with Lung Repair 32110
   with Open Intrapleural Pneumolysis .32124
Transmyocardial Laser Revascularization ..33140-
                 33141

Thorax
See Chest; Chest Cavity; Mediastinum
Angiography 71275
Bioimpedance 93701
Biopsy 21550
CT Scan 71250-71275
Incision
   Empyema 32035-32036
   Pneumothorax 32020
Incision and Drainage
   Abscess 21501-21502
   Deep 21510
   Hematoma 21501-21502
Strapping 29200
Tumor
   Excision 21555-21556
   Excision/Resection 21557
Unlisted Services and Procedures, Surgery .21899

Three Glass Test
See Urinalysis, Glass Test

Three-Day Measles
See Rubella

Throat
See Pharynx
Abscess
   Incision and Drainage 42700-42725
Biopsy 42800-42806
Hemorrhage 42960-42962
Reconstruction 42950
Removal
   Foreign Body 42809

Repair
    Pharyngoesophageal 42953
    Wound 42900
Suture
    Wound 42900
Unlisted Services and Procedures 42999

Thrombectomy
See Thromboendarterectomy
Aortoiliac Artery 34151-34201
Arteriovenous Fistula
    Graft 36870
Axillary Artery .34101
Axillary Vein 34490
Brachial Artery .34101
Bypass Graft
    Other than Hemodialysis Graft or
    Fistula 35875-35876
Carotid Artery .34001
Celiac Artery 34151
Dialysis Graft
    without Revision 36831
Femoral 34201
Femoropopliteal Vein 34421-34451
Iliac 34151-34201
Iliac Vein 34401-34451
Innominate Artery 34001-34101
Mesentery Artery 34151
Percutaneous
    Coronary Artery 92973
Peroneal Artery 34203
Popliteal Artery 34203
Radial Artery 34111
Renal Artery 34151
Subclavian Artery 34001-34101
Subclavian Vein 34471-34490
Tibial Artery 34203
Ulnar Artery 34111
Vena Cava 34401-34451
Vena Caval 50230

Thrombin Inhibitor I
See Antithrombin III

Thrombin Time 85670-85675

Thrombocyte (Platelet)
See Blood, Platelet

Thrombocyte ab
See Antibody, Platelet

Thromboendarterectomy
See Thrombectomy
Aorta, Abdominal 35331
Aortoiliofemoral Artery 35363
Axillary Artery .35321
Brachial Artery .35321
Carotid Artery 35301, 35390
Celiac Artery 35341
Femoral Artery 35371-35381
Iliac Artery 35351, 35361-35363
Iliofemoral Artery 35355, 35363
Innominate Artery 35311
Mesenteric Artery 35341
Peroneal Artery 35381
Popliteal Artery 35381
Renal Artery 35341

Subclavian Artery 35301-35311
Tibial Artery 35381
Vertebral Artery 35301

Thrombokinase 85260

Thrombolysin
See Plasmin

Thrombolysis
Catheter Exchange
    Arterial 37209, 75900
Cerebral
    Intravenous Infusion 37195
Coronary Vessels 92975-92977
Cranial Vessels 37195

Thrombolysis Biopsy Intracranial
Arterial Perfusion 61624

Thrombolysis Intracranial 65205
See Ciliary Body; Cornea; Eye, Removal, Foreign
Body; Iris; Lens; Retina; Sclera; Vitreous

Thrombomodulin 85337

Thromboplastin
Inhibition 85705
Inhibition Test .85347
Partial Time 85730-85732

Thromboplastin Antecedent, Plasma
See Plasma Thromboplastin, Antecedent

Thromboplastinogen
See Clotting Factor

Thromboplastinogen B
See Christmas Factor

Thumb
See Phalanx
Amputation 26910-26952
Arthrodesis
    Carpometacarpal Joint 26841-26842
Dislocation
    with Fracture 26645-26650
        Open Treatment 26665
    with Manipulation 26641
Fracture
    with Dislocation 26645-26650
        Open Treatment 26665
Fusion
    in Opposition 26820
Reconstruction
    from Finger 26550
    Opponensplasty 26490-26496
Repair
    Muscle 26508
    Muscle Transfer 26494
    Tendon Transfer 26510
Replantation 20824-20827
Sesamoidectomy 26185
Unlisted Services and Procedures 26989

Thymectomy 60520-60521
Sternal Split/Transthoracic
Approach 60521-60522
Transcervical Approach 60520

Thymotaxin
See Beta-2-Microglobulin

Thymus Gland 60520
Excision 60520-60521

Thyramine
See Amphetamine

Thyrocalcitonin
See Calcitonin

Thyroglobulin 84432
Antibody 86800

Thyroglossal Duct
Cyst
    Excision 60280-60281

Thyroid Gland
Cyst
    Aspiration .60001
    Excision 60200
    Incision and Drainage 60000
    Injection 60001
Excision
    for Malignancy
        Limited Neck Dissection 60252
        Radical Neck Dissection 60254
    Partial 60210-60225
    Secondary 60260
    Total 60240, 60271
        Cervical Approach 60271
        Removal All Thyroid Tissue 60260
        Sternal Split/Transthoracic
        Approach 60270
        Transcervical Approach 60520
Metastatic Cancer
    Nuclear Imaging 78015-78018
Needle Biopsy .60100
Nuclear Medicine
    Imaging 78010
    Imaging for Metastases 78015-78018
    Imaging with Flow 78011
    Imaging with Uptake 78006-78007
    Metastases Uptake 78020
    Uptake 78000-78003
Tumor
    Excision 60200

Thyroid Hormone Binding Ratio 84479

Thyroid Hormone Uptake 84479

Thyroid Stimulating Hormone (TSH) 80418, 80438-80440, 84443

Thyroid Stimulating Hormone Receptor ab
See Thyrotropin Releasing Hormone (TRH)

Thyroid Stimulating Immune Globulins 84445

Thyroid Stimulator, Long Acting
See Thyrotropin Releasing Hormone (TRH)

Thyroid Suppression Test
See Nuclear Medicine, Thyroid, Uptake

Thyroidectomy
Partial 60210-60225
Secondary 60260
Total 60240, 60271
   Cervical Approach 60271
   for Malignancy
      Limited Neck Dissection 60252
      Radical Neck Dissection 60254
   Removal All Thyroid Tissue 60260
   Sternal Split/Transthoracic Approach . .60270

Thyrolingual Cyst
See Cyst, Thyroglossal Duct

Thyrotomy 31300

Thyrotropin Receptor ab
See Thyrotropin Releasing Hormone (TRH)

Thyrotropin Releasing Hormone (TRH) .80438-80439

Thyroxine
Free 84439
Neonatal 84437
Total 84436
True 84436

Thyroxine Binding Globulin 84442

Tibia
See Ankle
Arthroscopy Surgical 29891-29892
Craterization 27360, 27640
Cyst
   Excision 27635-27638
Diaphysectomy 27360, 27640
Excision 27360, 27640
   Epiphyseal Bar 20150
Fracture 27759
Fracture
   Arthroscopic Treatment 29855-29856
      Plafond 29892
   Closed Treatment 27824-27825
   Distal .27824-27828
   Intercondylar 27538-27540
   Malleolus 27760-27766, 27808-27814
   Open Treatment 27535-27536,
                 27758-27759, 27826-27828
   Plateau 29855-29856
      Closed Treatment 27530-27536
   Shaft .27752-27759
   with Manipulation 27825
   without Manipulation 27824
Incision 27607
Osteoplasty
   Lengthening .27715
Prophylactic Treatment 27745
Reconstruction .27418
   at Knee 27440-27443, 27446
Repair 27720-27725
   Epiphysis 27477-27485, 27730-27742
   Osteochondritis Dissecans
      Arthroscopy 29892
   Osteotomy 27455-27457, 27705,
                      27709-27712
   Pseudoarthrosis 27727
Saucerization 27360, 27640

Tumor
   Excision 27635-27638, 27645
   X-Ray 73590

Tibial
Arteries
   See Artery, Tibial
Nerve
   Repair/Suture
      Posterior .64840

Tibiofibular Joint
Arthrodesis 27871
Dislocation 27830-27832
Disruption
   Open Treatment 27829
Fusion 27871

TIG
See Immune Globulins, Tetanus

Time
Bleeding
   See Bleeding Time
Prothrombin
   See Prothrombin Time
Reptilase
   See Thrombin Time

Tinnitus
Assessment 92625

Tissue
Culture
   Chromosome Analysis 88230-88239
   Homogenization 87176
   Non-neoplastic Disorder 88230, 88237
   Skin Grafts 15100-15121, 15342-15343
   Solid Tumor .88239
   Toxin/Antitoxin 87230
   Virus 87252-87253
Enzyme Activity .82657
Examination for Ectoparasites 87220
Examination for Fungi 87220
Expander
   Breast Reconstruction with 19357
   Insertion
      Skin 11960
   Removal
      Skin 11971
   Replacement
      Skin 11970
Grafts
   Harvesting 20926
Granulation
   See Granulation Tissue
Homogenization .87176
Hybridization In Situ 88365-88368
Mucosal
   See Mucosa
Preparation
   Drug Analysis 80103
Soft
   Abscess 20000-20005
Transfer
   Adjacent
      Eyelids 67961
      Skin 14000-14350
      Facial Muscles 15845

Finger Flap 14350
Toe Flap 14350
Typing
   HLA Antibodies 86812-86817
   Lymphocyte Culture 86821-86822

Tissue Factor
See Thromboplastin

TLC
See Chromatography, Thin-Layer
Screen 84375

TMJ
See Temporomandibular Joint (TMJ)
Prostheses
   See Prosthesis, Temporomandibular Joint

Tobacco
See Performance Measures

Tobramycin
Assay 80200

Tocolysis 59412

Tocopherol 84446

Toe
See Interphalangeal Joint, Toe;
Metatarsophalangeal Joint; Phalanx
Amputation 28810-28825
Capsulotomy 28270-28272
Fasciotomy 28008
Fracture
   See Fracture, Phalanges, Toe
Lesion
   Excision 28092
Reconstruction
   Angle Deformity 28313
   Extra Toes .28344
   Hammertoe 28285-28286
   Macrodactyly 28340-28341
   Syndactyly .28345
   Webbed Toe 28345
Repair
   Bunion 28290-28299
   Muscle 28240
   Tendon 28232-28234, 28240
   Webbed 28280
   Webbed Toe 28345
Tenotomy 28010-28011, 28232-28234
Unlisted Services and Procedures 28899

Toe Flap
Tissue Transfer .14350

Toes
Arthrocentesis 20600
Dislocation
   See Specific Joint
Magnetic Resonance Imaging
(MRI) 73721-73723
Reconstruction
   Extra Digit .26587
Repair
   Extra Digit .26587
   Macrodactylia 26590
Reposition to Hand 26551-26556
Strapping 29550
X-Ray 73660

Tolbutamide Tolerance Test 82953

Tolerance Test
Glucagon 82946
Glucose 82951-82952
   with Tolbutamide 82953
Heparin-Protamine 85530
Insulin 80434-80435
Maltose 82951-82952
Tolbutamide 82953

Tomodensitometries
See CT Scan

Tomographic Scintigraphy, Computed
See Emission Computerized Tomography

Tomographic SPECT
Myocardial Imaging 78469

Tomographies, Computed X-Ray
See CT Scan

Tomography, Computerized Axial
Abdomen
   See Abdomen, CT Scan
Head
   See Head, CT Scan

Tomography, Emission Computed
See Positron Emission Tomography
Single Photon
   See SPECT

Tompkins Metroplasty 58540
See Uterus, Reconstruction

Tongue
Abscess
   Incision and Drainage ..41000-41006, 41015
Biopsy 41100-41105
Cyst
   Incision and Drainage 41000-41006,
               41015, 60000
Excision
   Complete 41140-41155
   Frenum 41115
   Partial 41120-41135
   with Mouth Resection 41150-41153
   with Radical Neck 41135, 41145,
               41153-41155
Fixation 41500
Hematoma
   Incision and Drainage ..41000-41006, 41015
Incision
   Frenum 41010
Lesion
   Excision 41110-41114
Reconstruction
   Frenum 41520
Reduction for Sleep Apnea 0088T
Repair
   See Repair, Tongue
   Laceration 41250-41252
   Suture 41510
Suture 41510
Unlisted Services and Procedures 41599

Tonography 92120
with Provocation 92130

Tonometry, Serial 92100

Tonsil, Pharyngeal
See Adenoids

Tonsillectomy 42820-42826

Tonsils
Abscess
   Incision and Drainage 42700
Excision 42825-42826
   Lingual 42870
   Radical 42842-42845
   Tag 42860
   with Adenoids 42820-42821
Lingual
   Destruction 42870
Unlisted Services and Procedures 42999

Topiramate
Assay 80201

Torek Procedure
See Orchiopexy

Torkildsen Procedure 62180

TORP (Total Ossicular Replacement Prosthesis) 69633, 69637

Torsion Swing Test 92546

Torula
See Cryptococcus

Torus Mandibularis
Tumor Excision 21031

Total
Abdominal Hysterectomy
   See Hysterectomy, Abdominal, Total
Bilirubin Level
   See Bilirubin, Total
Catecholamines
   See Catecholamines, Urine
Cystectomy
   See Bladder, Excision, Total
Dacryoadenectomy
   See Dacryoadenectomy, Total
Elbow Replacement
   See Replacement, Elbow, Total
Esophagectomy
   See Esophagectomy, Total
Gastrectomy
   See Excision, Stomach, Total
Hemolytic Complement
   See Complement, Hemolytic, Total
Hip Arthroplasty
   See Hip, Total Replacement
Knee Arthroplasty
   See Prosthesis, Knee
Mastectomies
   See Mastectomy
Ostectomy of Patella
   See Patellectomy
Splenectomy
   See Splenectomy, Total

Touroff Operation 37615
See Ligation, Artery, Neck

Toxicology Screen 80100-80103

Toxin Assay 87230

Toxin, Botulinum
See Chemodenervation

Toxoplasma
Antibody 86777-86778

Trabeculectomies
See Trabeculoplasty

Trabeculectomy ab Externo
in Absence of Previous Surgery 66170
with Scarring Previous Surgery 66172

Trabeculoplasty
by Laser Surgery 65855

Trabeculotomy ab Externo
Eye 65850

Trachea
Aspiration 31720
   Catheter 31720-31725
Catheterization 31700
Dilation 31630-31631, 31636-31638
Endoscopy
   via Tracheostomy 31615
Excision
   Stenosis 31780-31781
Fistula
   with Plastic Repair 31825
   without Plastic Repair 31820
Fracture
   Endoscopy 31630
Incision
   Emergency 31603-31605
   Planned 31600-31601
   with Flaps 31610
Instillation
   Contrast Material 31708
Introduction
   Needle Wire 31730
Puncture
   Aspiration and/or Injection 31612
Reconstruction
   Carina 31766
   Cervical 31750
   Fistula 31755
   Intrathoracic 31760
Repair
   Cervical 31750
   Fistula 31755
   Intrathoracic 31760
   Stoma 31613-31614
Revision
   Stoma
      Scars 31830
Scar
   Revision 31830
Stenosis
   Excision 31780-31781
   Repair 31780-31781
Stoma
   Repair
      with Plastic Repair 31825
      without Plastic Repair 31820

Revision
Scars 31830
Tumor
Excision
Cervical 31785
Thoracic 31786
Unlisted Services and Procedures
Bronchi 31899
Wound
Suture
Cervical 31800
Intrathoracic 31805

Tracheal
Stent
Placement 31631
Tubes
See Endotracheal Tube

Trachelectomy 57530
Radical 57531

Tracheloplasty
See Cervicoplasty

Trachelorrhaphy 57720

Tracheo-Esophageal Fistula
See Fistula, Tracheoesophageal

Tracheobronchoscopy
through Tracheostomy 31615

Tracheoplasty
Cervical 31750
Intrathoracic 31760
Tracheopharyngeal Fistulization 31755

Tracheostoma
Revision 31613-31614

Tracheostomy
Emergency 31603-31605
Planned 31600-31601
Revision
Scar 31830
Surgical Closure
with Plastic Repair 31825
without Plastic Repair 31820
Tracheobronchoscopy through 31615
with Flaps 31610

Tracheotomy
Tube Change 31502

Tracking Tests (Ocular) 92545
See Ear, Nose and Throat

Tract, Urinary
See Urinary Tract

Traction Therapy
See Physical Medicine/Therapy/Occupational Therapy
Manual 97140
Mechanical 97012

Tractotomy
Medulla 61470
Mesencephalon 61480

Training
Activities of Daily Living 97535, 99509
Biofeedback 90901-90911
Cognitive Skills 97532
Community/Work Reintegration 97537
Home Management 97535, 99509
Orthoptic/Pleoptic 92065
Orthotics 97504
Prosthetics 97520
Self Care 97535, 99509
Sensory Integration 97533
Walking (Physical Therapy) 97116
Wheelchair Management/Propulsion 97542

TRAM Flap
Breast Reconstruction 19367-19369

Trans-Scaphoperilunar
Fracture/Dislocation
Closed Treatment 25680
Open Treatment 25685

Transaminase
Glutamic Oxaloacetic 84450
Glutamic Pyruvic 84460

Transcatheter
Biopsy 37200
Closure
Percutaneous
Heart 93580-93581
Embolization
Percutaneous 37204
Cranial 61624-61626
Occlusion
Percutaneous 37204
Cranial 61624-61626
Placement
Intravascular Stents 0075T-0076T, 37205-37208, 37215-37216
Therapy
Embolization 75894
Infusion 37201-37202, 75896-75898
Perfusion
Cranial 61624-61626
Retrieval 75961

Transcatheter Foreign Body
Retrieval 37203

Transcortin 84449

Transcranial
Doppler Study (TCP) 93886-93893
Stimulation, Motor 95928-95929

Transcutaneous Electric Nerve Stimulation
See Application, Neurostimulation

Transdermal Electrostimulation
See Application, Neurostimulation

Transection
Artery
Carotid 61610, 61612
Blood Vessel
Kidney 50100
Brain
Subpial 61567
Carotid
with Skull Base Surgery 61609

Nerve 64732-64772
Vagus 43640-43641
Pulmonary Artery 33922

Transesophageal
Doppler Echocardiography 93312-93318

Transfer
Blastocyst
See Embryo Transfer
Gamete Intrafallopian
See GIFT
Jejunum
with Microvascular Anastomosis
Free 43496
Preparation
Embryo 89255
Cryopreserved 89352
Surgical
See Transposition
Tendon
See Tendon, Transfer
Toe to Hand 26551-26556

Transferase
Aspartate Amino 84450
Glutamic Oxaloacetic 84450

Transferrin 84466

Transformation
Lymphocyte 86353

Transfusion
Blood 36430
Exchange 36450-36455
Fetal 36460
Push
Infant 36440
Blood Parts
Exchange 36511-36516
Unlisted Services and Procedures 86999
White Blood Cells 86950

Transfusion of, Blood, Autologous
See Autotransfusion

Transluminal
Angioplasty
Arterial 75962-75968
Atherectomies
See Artery, Atherectomy
Coronary Balloon Dilatation
See Percutaneous Transluminal Angioplasty

Transmyocardial Laser Revascularization 33140-33141

Transosteal Bone Plate
Reconstruction
Mandible 21244

Transpeptidase, Gamma-Glutamyl
See Gamma Glutamyl Transferase

Transplant
See Graft
Bone
See Bone Graft
Hair
See Hair, Transplant

Transplantation
See Graft
Allogenic
   See Homograft
Autologous
   See Autograft
Bone Marrow 38240-38242
Cartilage
  Knee
    Allograft 27415, 29867
    Autograft 27412, 29866
Chondrocytes
  Knee 27412
Conjunctiva 65782
Cornea
  Autograft/Homograft
    Lamellar 65710
    Penetrating 65730-65755
    for Aphakia 65750
Eye
  Amniotic Membrane 65780
  Conjunctiva 65782
  Stem Cell 65781
Hair
  Punch Graft 15775-15776
  Strip 15220-15221
Heart 33945
  Allograft Preparation 33933, 33944
Heart-Lung 33935
Heterologous
  See Heterograft
Intestines
  Allograft Preparation 44715-44721
  Allotransplantation 44135-44136
  Donor Enterectomy 44132-44133
  Removal of Allograft 44137
Liver 47135
  Allograft Preparation 47143-47147
  Heterotopic 47136
Lung
  Allograft Preparation ...32855-32856, 33933
  Anesthesia 00580
  Donor Pneumonectomy 32850
  Double, with Cardiopulmonary
    Bypass 32854
  Double, without Cardiopulmonary
    Bypass 32853
  Single, with Cardiopulmonary
    Bypass 32852
  Single, without Cardiopulmonary
    Bypass 32851
Meniscus
  Knee 29868
Muscle
  See Muscle Flaps
Pancreas 48160, 48550, 48554-48556
  Allograft Preparation 48551-48552
Parathyroid 60512
Renal
  Allograft Preparation 50323-50329
  Allotransplantation 50360
    with Recipient Nephrectomy 50365
  Autotransplantation 50380
  Donor Nephrectomy 50300-50320, 50547
  Recipient Nephrectomy 50340
  Removal Transplanted Renal Allograft .50370

Skin
  See Dermatology
Stem Cells 38240-38242
  Cell Concentration 38215
  Cryopreservation 38207
  Harvesting 38205-38206
  Plasma Depletion 38214
  Platelet Depletion 38213
  Red Blood Cell Depletion 38212
  T-cell Depletion 38210
  Thawing 38208
  Tumor Cell Depletion 38211
  Washing 38209
Testis
  to Thigh 54680
Tissue, Harvesting
  See Graft, Tissue, Harvesting

Transpleural Thoracoscopy
See Thoracoscopy

Transposition
Arteries
  Carotid 0037T, 35691, 35694-35695
  Subclavian 0037T, 35693-35695
  Vertebral 35691-35693
Cranial Nerve 64716
Eye Muscles 67320
Great Arteries
  Repair 33770-33781
Nerve 64718-64721
Ovary 58825
Peripheral Nerve
  Major 64856
Vein Valve 34510

Transthoracic Echocardiography
See Echocardiography

Transthyretin
See Prealbumin

Transureteroureterostomy 50770

Transurethral Balloon Dilation
Prostatic Urethra 52510

Transurethral Fulguration
Postoperative Bleeding 52606

Transurethral Procedure
See Specific Procedure
Prostate
  Incision 52450
  Resection 52612-52614
  Thermotherapy 53850-53853
    Microwave 53850
    Radiofrequency 53852

Trapezium
Arthroplasty
  with Implant 25445

Travel, Unusual 99082

Treacher-Collins Syndrome
Midface Reconstruction 21150-21151

Treatment, Tocolytic
See Tocolysis

Trendelenburg Operation
See Varicose Vein, Removal, Secondary Varicosity

Trephine Procedure
Sinusotomy
  Frontal 31070

Treponema Pallidum
Antibody
  Confirmation Test 86781
Antigen Detection
  Direct Fluorescence 87285

TRH
See Thyrotropin Releasing Hormone (TRH)

Triacylglycerol
See Triglycerides

Triacylglycerol Hydrolase
See Lipase

Tributyrinase
See Lipase

Trichiasis
Repair 67825
  Epilation, by Forceps 67820
  Epilation, by Other than Forceps 67825
  Incision of Lid Margin 67830
    with Free Mucous Membrane Graft .67835

Trichina
See Trichinella

Trichinella
Antibody 86784
Trichogram 96902

Trichomonas vaginalis
Antigen Detection
  Nucleic Acid 87660

Trichrome Stain 88313

Tricuspid Valve
Excision 33460
Repair 33463-33465
Replacement 33465
Repositioning 33468

Tridymite
See Silica

Trigeminal Ganglia
See Gasserian Ganglion

Trigeminal Nerve
Destruction 64600-64610
Injection
  Anesthetic 64400
  Neurolytic 64600-64610

Trigeminal Tract
Stereotactic
  Create Lesion 61791

Trigger Finger Repair 26055

Trigger Point
Injection
  One or Two Muscles 20552
  Two or More Muscles 20553

Esophagus
   Ablation 43228
Excision
   Femur 27355-27358
Facial Bone 21029-21030, 21034
Fallopian Tube
   Resection 58950, 58952-58956
Femoral 27355-27358
Femur 27065-27067
   Excision 27365
Fibroid
   See Leiomyomata
Fibula.......................27635-27638
   Excision 27646
Finger
   Excision 26115-26117
Foot 28043-28046
Forearm
   Radical Resection 25077
Gastrostomy
   See Lesion
Gums
   Excision 41825-41827
Hand
   Excision 26115-26117
Heart
   Excision 33120-33130
Hip 27047-27049, 27065-27067
   Excision 27075-27076
Humerus
   Excision 23150, 23220-23222, 24110
     with Allograft 23156, 24116
     with Autograft 23155, 24115
Ileum 27065-27067
Immunoassay for Antigen 86294, 86316
   CA 125 86304
   CA 15-3 86300
   CA 19-9 86301
Innominate
   Excision 27077
Intestines, Small
   Destruction 44369
Ischial
   Excision 27078-27079
Kidney
   Excision 50562, 52355
Knee
   Excision 27327-27329, 27365
Lacrimal Gland
   Excision
     Frontal Approach 68540
     with Osteotomy 68550
Larynx
   Excision 31300
     Endoscopic 31540-31541, 31578
     Incision 31300
Leg, Lower 27615-27619
Leg, Upper
   Excision 27327-27329
Localization
   Nuclear Medicine 78800-78804
Mandible 21044-21047
Maxilla 21030, 21034, 21048-21049
Maxillary Torus Palatinus 21032
Mediastinal
   Excision 39220
Mediastinum 32662

Meningioma 61512
   Excision 61519
Metacarpal 26200-26205, 26250-26255
Metatarsal 28104-28107
   Excision 28173
Neck
   Excision 21555-21556
   Radical Resection 21557
Olecranon
   Excision 24120
Olecranon Process
   with Allograft
     Excision 24126
   with Autograft
     Excision 24125
Ovary
   Resection 58950-58956
Pancreatic Duct
   Destruction 43272
Parotid Gland
   Excision 42410-42426
Pelvis 27047-27049
Pericardial
   Endoscopic 32661
   Excision 33050
Peritoneum
   Resection 58950-58956
Phalanges
   Finger 26210-26215, 26260-26262
   Toe 28108
   Excision 28175
Pituitary Gland
   Excision 61546-61548, 62165
Positron Emission Tomography
(PET) 78811-78816
Pubis 27065-27067
Radiation Therapy 77295
Radius 25120-25126, 25170
   Excision 24120
   with Allograft
     Excision 24126
   with Autograft
     Excision 24125
Rectum
   Destruction 45190, 45320, 46937-46938
   Excision 45160-45170
Resection
   Face 21015
   Scalp 21015
   with Cystourethroscopy 52355
Retroperitoneal
   Destruction/Excision 49200-49201
Sacrum 49215
Scapula
   Excision 23140, 23210
     with Allograft 23146
     with Autograft 23145
Shoulder
   Excision 23075-23077
Skull
   Excision 61500
Soft Tissue
   Elbow
     Excision 24075
   Finger
     Excision 26115
   Forearm
     Radical Resection 25077

Hand
   Excision 26115
Wrist
   Excision 25075
   Radical Resection 25077
Spinal Cord
   Excision 63275-63290
Stomach
   Excision 43610-43611
Talus 28100-28103
   Excision 27647
Tarsal 28104-28107
   Excision 28171
Temporal Bone
   Removal 69970
Testis
   Excision 54530-54535
Thorax
   Excision 21555-21556
   Radical Resection 21557
Thyroid
   Excision 60200
Tibia 27365, 27635-27638
   Excision 27645
Torus Mandibularis 21031
Trachea
   Excision
     Cervical 31785
     Thoracic 31786
Ulna 25120-25126, 25170
   Excision 24120
   with Allograft
     Excision 24126
   with Autograft
     Excision 24125
Ureter
   Excision 52355
Urethra 52234-52240, 53220
   Excision 52355
Uterus
   Excision 58140-58146
Vagina
   Excision 57135
Vertebra
   Additional Segment
     Excision 22116
   Cervical
     Excision 22100
   Lumbar 22102
   Thoracic
     Excision 22101
Wrist 25075-25077, 25135-25136
   Radical Resection 25077

Tunica Vaginalis
Hydrocele
   Aspiration 55000
   Excision 55040-55041
   Repair 55060

Turbinate
Excision 30130-30140
Fracture
   Therapeutic 30930
Injection 30200
Submucous Resection
   Nose Excision 30140

Turbinate Mucosa
Cauterization 30801-30802

Turcica, Sella
See Sella Turcica

Turnbuckle Jacket 29020-29025
Removal 29715

TURP
See Prostatectomy, Transurethral

Tylectomy
See Breast, Excision, Lesion

Tylenol
Urine 82003

Tympanic Membrane
Create Stoma 69433-69436
Incision 69420-69421
Reconstruction 69620
Repair 69450, 69610

Tympanic Nerve
Excision 69676

Tympanolysis 69450

Tympanomastoidectomy
See Tympanoplasty

Tympanometry 92567
See Audiologic Function Tests

Tympanoplasty
See Myringoplasty
Radical or Complete 69645
   with Ossicular Chain Reconstruction . .69646
with Antrotomy or Mastoidotomy 69635
   with Ossicular Chain Reconstruction . .69636
      and Synthetic Prosthesis 69637
with Mastoidectomy 69641
   with Intact or Reconstructed Wall . .69643
      and Ossicular Chain Reconstruction . .69644
   with Ossicular Chain Reconstruction . .69642
without Mastoidectomy 69631
   with Ossicular Chain Reconstruction . .69632
      and Synthetic Prosthesis 69633

Tympanostomy 69433-69436

Tympanotomy
See Myringotomy

Typhoid Vaccine 90690-90693
AKD 90693
Oral 90690
Polysaccharide 90691

Typhus
Endemic
   See Murine Typhus
Mite-Borne
   See Scrub Typhus
Sao Paulo
   See Rocky Mountain Spotted Fever
Tropical
   See Scrub Typhus

Typing, Blood
See Blood Typing

Typing, HLA
See HLA Typing

Typing, Tissue
See Tissue Typing

Tyrosine 84510

Tzank Smear 87207

U

Uchida Procedure
See Tubal Ligation

UDP Galactose Pyrophosphorylase
See Galactose-1-Phosphate, Uridyl Transferase

UFR
See Uroflowmetry

Ulcer
Anal
   See Anus, Fissure
Decubitus
   See Debridement; Pressure Ulcer (Decubitus);
   Skin Graft and Flap
Pinch Graft 15050
Pressure 15920-15999
Stomach
   Excision 43610

Ulcerative, Cystitis
See Cystitis, Interstitial

Ulna
See Arm, Lower; Elbow; Humerus; Radius
Arthrodesis
   Radioulnar Joint
      with Resection 25830
Arthroplasty
   with Implant 25442
Centralization or Wrist 25335
Craterization 24147, 25150-25151
Cyst
   Excision 24125-24126, 25120-25126
Diaphysectomy 24147, 25150-25151
Excision 24147
   Abscess 24138
   Complete 25240
   Epiphyseal Bar 20150
   Partial 25145-25151, 25240
Fracture
   Closed Treatment 25530-25535
   Olecranon 24670-24675
      Open Treatment 24685
   Open Treatment 25545
   Shaft 25530-25545
      Open Treatment 25574
   Styloid
      Closed Treatment 25650
      Open Treatment 25652
      Percutaneous Fixation 25651

with Dislocation
   Closed Treatment 24620
   Open Treatment 24635
with Manipulation 25535
with Radius 25560-25565
   Open Treatment 25575
without Manipulation 25530
Incision and Drainage 25035
Osteoplasty 25390-25393
Prophylactic Treatment 25491-25492
Reconstruction
   Radioulnar 25337
Repair
   Epiphyseal Arrest 25450-25455
   Malunion or Nonunion 25400, 25415
   Osteotomy 25360, 25370-25375
      and Radius 25365
   with Graft 25405, 25420-25426
Saucerization 24147, 25150-25151
Sequestrectomy 24138, 25145
Tumor
   Cyst 24120
   Excision . .24125-24126, 25120-25126, 25170

Ulnar Arteries
See Artery, Ulnar

Ulnar Nerve
Decompression 64718
Neuroplasty 64718-64719
Reconstruction 64718-64719
Release .64718-64719
Repair/Suture
   Motor 64836
Transposition 64718-64719

Ultrasonic
See Ultrasound

Ultrasonic Cardiography
See Echocardiography

Ultrasonic Procedure 52325

Ultrasonography
See Echography

Ultrasound
See Echocardiography; Echography
Abdomen 76700-76705
Arm 76880
Artery
   Intracranial 93886-93893
   Middle Cerebral 76821
   Umbilical 76820
Bladder 51798
Bone Density Study 76977
Breast 76645
Bronchi
   Endoscopy 31620
Chest 76604
Colon
   Endoscopic 45391-45392
Colon-Sigmoid
   Endoscopic 45341-45342
Drainage
   Abscess 75989
Echoencephalography
   See Echoencephalography
Esophagus
   Endoscopy 43231-43232

Eye 76510-76513
   Arteries 93875
   Biometry 76516-76519
   Foreign Body 76529
   Pachymetry 76514
Fetus 76818-76828
Follow-up 76970
for Physical Therapy 97035
Gastrointestinal 76975
Gastrointestinal, Upper
   Endoscopic 43237-43238, 43242, 43259
Guidance
   Amniocentesis 59001, 76946
   Amnioinfusion 59070
   Arteriovenous Fistulae 76936
   Chorionic Villus Sampling 76945
   Cryosurgery 55873
   Drainage
      Fetal Fluid 59074
   Endometrial Ablation 58356
   Fetal Cordocentesis 76941
   Fetal Transfusion 76941
   Heart Biopsy 76932
   Needle Biopsy 43232, 43238, 43242,
      45342, 45392, 76942
   Occlusion
      Umbilical Cord 59072
   Ova Retrieval 76948
   Pericardiocentesis 76930
   Pseudoaneurysm 76936
   Radiation Therapy 76950
   Radioelement 76965
   Shunt Placement
      Fetal .59076
   Thoracentesis 76942
   Tissue Ablation 76940
   Vascular Access 76937
Head 76506, 76536
Heart
   Fetal 76825
Hips
   Infant 76885-76886
Hysteronsonography 76831
Intraoperative 76986
Intravascular
   Intraoperative 37250-37251
Kidney 76770, 76778
Leg 76880
Neck 76536
Non-Coronary
   Intravascular 75945-75946
Pelvis 76856-76857
Pregnant Uterus 76801-76817
Prostate 76873
Rectal 76872-76873
Retroperitoneal 76770-76775
Scrotum 76870
Sonohysterography 76831
Spine 76800
Stimulation to Aid Bone Healing 20979
Umbilical Artery 76820
Unlisted Services and Procedures 76999
Uterus
   Tumor Ablation 0071T-0072T
Vagina 76830

Ultraviolet Light Therapy
Dermatology
   Ultraviolet A 96912
   Ultraviolet B 96910
for Dermatology 96900
for Physical Medicine 97028

Umbilectomy 49250

Umbilical
Artery Ultrasound 76820
Hernia
   See Omphalocele
Vein Catheterization
   See Catheterization, Umbilical Vein

Umbilical Cord
Occlusion .59072

Umbilicus
Excision 49250
Repair
   Hernia 49580-49587
   Omphalocele 49600-49611

Undescended Testicle
See Testis, Undescended

Unfertilized Egg
See Ova

Unguis
See Nails

Unilateral Simple Mastectomy
See Mastectomy

Unlisted Services and
Procedures 99499, 99600
Abdomen 22999, 49329, 49999
Allergy/Immunology 95199
Anal 46999
Anesthesia 01999
Arm 25999
Arthroscopy 29999
Autopsy 88099
Bile Duct .47999
Brachytherapy 77799
Breast 19499
Bronchi 31899
Cardiac 33999
Cardiovascular Studies 93799
Casting 29799
Cervix 58999
Chemistry Procedure 84999
Chemotherapy 96549
Chest 32999
Coagulation 85999
Colon 44799
Conjunctiva Surgery 68399
Craniofacial 21299
CT Scan .76497
Cytogenetic Study 88299
Cytopathology 88199
Dermatology 96999
Dialysis 90999
Diaphragm 39599
Ear
   External 69399
   Inner 69949
   Middle .69799

Endocrine System 60699
Epididymis 55899
Esophagus 43289, 43499
Evaluation and Management Services 99499
Eye Muscle 67399
Eye Surgery
   Anterior Segment 66999
   Posterior Segment 67299
Eyelid 67999
Fluoroscopy 76496
Forearm 25999
Gallbladder 47999
Gastroenterology Test 91299
Gum 41899
Hand 26989
Hemic System 38999
Hepatic Duct 47999
Hip Joint .27299
Home Services 99600
Hysteroscopy 58579
Immunization 90749
Immunology 86849
Injection 90799
Injection of Medication 90799
Intestine 44238, 44799
Kidney 49659
Lacrimal System 68899
Laparoscopy 38129, 38589, 43289, 43659,
   44238-44239, 44979, 47379, 47579, 49329,
   49659, 50549, 50949, 54699, 55559, 58578,
   58679, 59898, 60659
Larynx 31599
Lip 40799
Liver 47379, 47399
Lungs 32999
Lymphatic System 38999
Magnetic Resonance 76498
Maxillofacial 21299
Maxillofacial Prosthetics 21089
Meckel's Diverticulum 44899
Mediastinum 39499
Mesentery Surgery 44899
Microbiology 87999
Mouth 40899, 41599
Musculoskeletal 25999, 26989
Musculoskeletal Surgery
   Abdominal Wall 22999
   Neck 21899
   Spine .22899
   Thorax .21899
Musculoskeletal System 20999
   Ankle .27899
   Arm, Upper 24999
   Elbow .24999
   Head 21499
   Knee 27599
   Leg, Lower 27899
   Leg, Upper 27599
Necropsy .88099
Nervous System Surgery 64999
Neurology/Neuromuscular Testing 95999
Nose 30999
Nuclear Medicine 78999
   Blood .78199
   Bone .78399
   Endocrine System 78099
   Genitourinary System 78799
   Heart .78499
   Hematopoietic System 78199

Urethrectomy
Total
Female 53210
Male 53215

Urethrocele
See Urethra, Prolapse

Urethrocystography 74450-74455
Contrast and/or Chain 51605
Retrograde 51610
Voiding 51600

Urethrocystopexy
See Vesicourethropexy

Urethromeatoplasty 53450-53460

Urethropexy 51840-51841

Urethroplasty 46744-46746
First Stage 53400
One Stage
Hypospadias 54322-54328
Reconstruction
Female Urethra 53430
Male Anterior Urethra 53410
Prostatic/Membranous Urethra
First Stage 53420
One Stage 53415
Second Stage 53425
Second Stage 53405
Hypospadias 54308-54316
Third Stage
Hypospadias 54318

Urethrorrhaphy 53502-53515

Urethroscopy
See Endoscopy, Urethra

Urethrostomy 53000-53010

Urethrotomy 53000-53010
Direct Vision
with Cystourethroscopy 52276
Internal 52601, 52647-52648
with Cystourethroscopy
Female 52270
Male 52275

Uric Acid
Blood 84550
Other Source 84560
Urine 84560

Uridyltransferase, Galactose-1-Phosphate
See Galactose-1-Phosphate, Uridyl Transferase

Uridylyltransferase, Galactosephosphate
See Galactose-1-Phosphate, Uridyl Transferase

Urinalysis 0041T, 81000-81099
Automated 81001, 81003
Glass Test 81020
Microalbumin 82043-82044
Microscopic 81015
Pregnancy Test 81025
Qualitative 81005
Routine 81002

Screen 81007
Semiquantitative 0041T, 81005
Unlisted Services and Procedures 81099
Volume Measurement 81050
without Microscopy 81002

Urinary Bladder
See Bladder

Urinary Catheter Irrigation
See Irrigation, Catheter

Urinary Concentration Test
See Water Load Test

Urinary Sphincter, Artificial
See Prosthesis, Urethral Sphincter

Urinary Tract
X-Ray with Contrast 74400-74425

Urine
Albumin
See Albumin, Urine
Blood
See Blood, Urine
Colony Count 87086
Pregnancy Test 81025
Tests 81001

Urobilinogen
Feces 84577
Urine 84578-84583

Urodynamic Tests
Bladder Capacity
Ultrasound 51798
Cystometrogram 51725-51726
Electromyography Studies
Needle 51785
Residual Urine
Ultrasound 51798
Stimulus Evoked Response 51792
Urethra Pressure Profile 51772
Uroflowmetry 51736-51741
Voiding Pressure Studies
Bladder 51795
Intra-Abdominal 51797

Uroflowmetry 51736-51741

Urography
Antegrade 74425
Infusion 74410-74415
Intravenous 74400-74415
Retrograde 74420

Uroporphyrin 84120

Urothromboplastin
See Thromboplastin

Uterine
Adhesion
See Adhesions, Intrauterine
Cervix
See Cervix
Endoscopies
See Endoscopy, Uterus
Haemorrhage
See Hemorrhage, Uterus

Uterus
Ablation
Endometrium 58353-58356
Tumor
Ultrasound, Focused 0071T-0072T
Biopsy
Endometrium 58100
Endoscopic 58558
Catheterization
X-Ray 58340
Chromotubation 58350
Curettage 58356
Postpartum 59160
Dilation and Curettage 58120
Postpartum 59160
Ectopic Pregnancy
Interstitial
Partial Resection Uterus 59136
Total Hysterectomy 59135
Endoscopy
Endometrial Ablation 58563
Exploration 58555
Surgery 58558-58565
Treatment 58558-58565
Excision
Laparoscopic 58550
Partial 58180
Radical 58210, 58285
Removal of Tubes and/or
Ovaries 58262-58263, 58291-58293,
58552, 58554
Total 58150-58152, 58200, 58953-58956
Vaginal 58260-58270, 58290-58294,
58550-58554
with Colpectomy 58275-58280
with Colpo-Urethrocystopexy 58267
with Repair of Enterocele ...58270, 58294
Hemorrhage
Postpartum 59160
Hydatidiform Mole
Excision 59100
Hydrotubation 58350
Hysterosalpingography 74740
Incision
Remove Lesion 59100
Insertion
Heyman Capsule
for Brachytherapy 58346
Intrauterine Device (IUD) 58300
Tandem
for Brachytherapy 57155
Laparoscopy 58578
Lesion
Excision 58545-58546, 59100
Reconstruction 58540
Removal
Intrauterine Device (IUD) 58301
Repair
Fistula 51920-51925
Rupture 58520, 59350
Suspension 58400
with Presacral Sympathectomy 58410
Sonohysterography 76831
Suture
Rupture 59350

Suture
    Cystocele 57240, 57260
    Enterocele 57265
    Fistula 51900, 57300-57330
    Rectocele 57250-57260
    Wound 57200-57210
Tumor
    Excision 57135
Ultrasound 76830
Unlisted Services and Procedures 58999
X-Ray with Contrast 74775

Vaginal Delivery 59400, 59610-59614
after Previous Cesarean Delivery . . .59610-59612
    Attempted 59618-59622
Antepartum Care 59400
Cesarean Delivery after Attempted 59618
    Delivery Only 59620
    Postpartum Care 59622
Delivery after Previous
    Vaginal Delivery Only
        Postpartum Care 59614
Delivery Only 59409
External Cephalic Version 59412
Placenta 59414
Postpartum Care 59410
Routine Care 59400

Vaginal Hysterectomy 58552-58554

Vaginal Smear
See Pap Smears

Vaginal Suppositories
Induced Abortion 59855
    with Dilation and Curettage 59856
    with Hysterectomy 59857

Vaginectomy
See Colpectomy

Vaginoplasty
Intersex State 57335

Vaginorrhaphy
See Colporrhaphy

Vaginoscopy
Biopsy 57454
Exploration .57452

Vaginotomy
See Colpotomy

Vagotomy
Abdominal .64760
Highly Selective 43641
Parietal Cell 43641, 64755
Selective 43640
Transthoracic 64752
Truncal 43640
with Gastroduodenostomy Revision,
Reconstruction 43855
with Gastrojejunostomy Revision,
Reconstruction 43865
with Partial Distal Gastrectomy 43635

Vagus Nerve
Avulsion
    Abdominal 64760
    Selective 64755
    Thoracic 64752

    Incision 43640-43641
    Abdominal 64760
    Selective 64755
    Thoracic 64752
Injection
    Anesthetic 64408
Transection 43640-43641
    Abdominal 64760
    Selective 43652, 64755
    Thoracic 64752
    Truncal .43651

Valentine's Test
See Urinalysis, Glass Test

Valproic Acid
See Dipropylacetic Acid

Valproic Acid Measurement
See Dipropylacetic Acid

Valsalva Sinus
See Sinus of Valsalva

Valva Atrioventricularis Sinistra (Valva Mitralis)
See Mitral Valve

Valve
Aortic
    See Heart, Aortic Valve
Bicuspid
    See Mitral Valve
Mitral
    See Mitral Valve
Pulmonary
    See Pulmonary Valve
Tricuspid
    See Tricuspid Valve

Valve Stenoses, Aortic
See Aortic Stenosis

Valvectomy
Tricuspid Valve 33460

Valvotomy
Mitral Valve 33420-33422
Pulmonary Valve 33470-33474
Reoperation 33530

Valvuloplasty
Aortic Valve 33400-33403
Femoral Vein 34501
Mitral Valve 33425-33427
Percutaneous Balloon
    Aortic Valve 92986
    Mitral Valve 92987
    Pulmonary Valve 92990
Prosthetic Valve 33496
Reoperation 33530
Tricuspid Valve 33463-33465

Van Deen Test
See Blood, Feces

Van Den Bergh Test
See Bilirubin, Blood

Vancomycin
Assay 80202

Vanillylmandelic Acid
Urine 84585

Vanilmandelic Acid
See Vanillylmandelic Acid

Varicella (Chicken Pox)
See Vaccines

Varicella-Zoster
Antibody 86787
Antigen Detection
    Direct Fluorescence 87290

Varices Esophageal
See Esophageal Varices

Varicocele
Spermatic Cord
    Excision 55530-55540

Varicose Vein
Ablation 36475-36479
Removal 37720-37730, 37765-37785
Secondary Varicosity 37785
with Tissue Excision 37735-37760

Vas Deferens
Anastomosis
    to Epididymis 54900-54901
Excision 55250
Incision 55200
    for X-Ray 55300
Ligation 55450
Repair
    Suture .55400
Unlisted Services and Procedures 55899
Vasography .74440
X-Ray with Contrast 74440

Vascular Flow Check, Graft 15860

Vascular Injection
Unlisted Services and Procedures 36299

Vascular Lesion
Cranial
    Excision 61600-61608, 61615-61616
Cutaneous
    Destruction 17106-17108

Vascular Malformation
Cerebral
    Repair .61710
Finger
    Excision 26115
Hand
    Excision 26115

Vascular Procedure
Brachytherapy
    Intracoronary Artery 92974
Intravascular Ultrasound
    Coronary Vessels 92978-92979
Stent
    Intracoronary 92980-92981

Vascular Procedures
Angioscopy
    Non-Coronary Vessels 35400
Endoscopy
    Surgical 37500

Harvest
    Lower Extremity Vein 35572
Intravascular Ultrasound
    Non-Coronary Vessels 75945-75946
Thrombolysis
    Coronary Vessels 92975-92977
    Cranial Vessels 37195

Vascular Rehabilitation
See Peripheral Artery Disease Rehabilitation
(PAD)

Vascular Studies
See Doppler Scan, Duplex, Plethysmography
Angioscopy
    Non-Coronary Vessels 35400
Aorta 93978-93979
Arterial Studies (Non-Invasive)
    Extracranial 93875-93882
    Extremities 93922-93924
    Intracranial 93886-93891
    Lower Extremity 93925-93926
    Middle Cerebral Artery, Fetal 76821
    Umbilical Artery, Fetal 76820
Artery Studies
    Upper Extremity 93930-93931
Blood Pressure Monitoring,
24 Hour 93784-93790
Cardiac Catheterization
    Imaging 93555-93556
Hemodialysis Access 93990
Kidney
    Multiple Study
      with Pharmacological Intervention ..78709
    Single Study
      with Pharmacological Intervention ..78708
Penile Vessels 93980-93981
Plethysmography
    Total Body 93720-93722
Temperature Gradient 93740
Thermogram
    Cephalic 93760
    Peripheral 93762
Unlisted Services and Procedures 93799
Venous Studies
    Extremity 93965-93971
    Venous Pressure 93770
Visceral Studies 93975-93979

Vascular Surgery
Arm, Upper
    Anesthesia 01770-01782
Elbow
    Anesthesia 01770-01782
Endoscopy 37500
Unlisted Services and Procedures 37799

Vasectomy 55250
Contact Laser Vaporization with/without
Transurethral Resection
    of Prostate 52648
Non-Contact Laser Coagulation of
Prostate 52647
Reversal
    See Vasovasorrhaphy
Transurethral
    Cystourethroscopic 52402
Transurethral Electrosurgical Resection of
Prostate 52601, 52648

Vasoactive Drugs
Injection
    Penis 54231

Vasoactive Intestinal
Peptide 84586

Vasogram
See Vasography

Vasography 74440

Vasointestinal Peptide
See Vasoactive Intestinal Peptide

Vasopneumatic Device
Therapy 97016
See Physical Medicine/Therapy/Occupational
Therapy

Vasopressin 84588

Vasotomy 55200, 55300
Transurethral
    Cystourethroscopic 52402

Vasovasorrhaphy 55400

Vasovasostomy 55400

VATS
See Thoracoscopy

VDRL 86592-86593

Vein
Ablation
    Endovenous 36475-36479
Adrenal
    Venography 75840-75842
Anastomosis
    Caval to Mesenteric 37160
    Intrahepatic Portosystemic ...37182-37183
    Portocaval 37140
    Reniportal 37145
    Saphenopopliteal 34530
    Splenorenal 37180-37181
    to Vein 37140-37160, 37182-37183
Angioplasty 75978
    Transluminal 35460
Arm
    Harvest of Vein for Bypass Graft 35500
    Venography 75820-75822
Axillary
    Thrombectomy 34490
Biopsy
    Transcatheter 75970
Cannulization
    to Artery 36810-36815
    to Vein 36800
Catheterization
    Central Insertion 36555-36558
    Organ Blood 36500
    Peripheral Insertion 36568-36569
    Removal 36589
    Repair 36575
    Replacement *.........36578-36581, 36584
    Umbilical 36510
Endoscopic Harvest
    for Bypass Graft 33508

External Cannula
    Declotting 36860-36861
Extremity
    Non-invasive Studies 93965-93971
Femoral
    Repair 34501
Femoropopliteal
    Thrombectomy 34421-34451
Guidance
    Fluoroscopic 75998
    Ultrasound 76937
Hepatic Portal
    Splenoportography 75810
    Venography 75885-75887
Iliac
    Thrombectomy 34401-34451
Injection
    Sclerosing Agent 36468-36471
Insertion
    IVC Filter 75940
Interrupt
    Femoral 37650
    Iliac 37660
    Vena Cava 37620
Jugular
    Venography 75860
Leg
    Harvest for Vascular Reconstruction ...35572
    Venography 75820-75822
Ligation
    Clusters 37785
    Esophagus 43205
    Jugular 37565
    Perforation 37760
    Saphenous 37700-37735, 37780
    Secondary 37785
Liver
    Venography 75889-75891
Neck
    Venography 75860
Nuclear Medicine
    Thrombosis Imaging 78455-78458
Orbit
    Venography 75880
Placement
    IVC Filter 75940
Portal
    Catheterization 36481
Pulmonary
    Repair 33730
Removal
    Clusters 37785
    Saphenous 37720-37735, 37780
    Varicose 37765-37766
Renal
    Venography 75831-75833
Repair
    Aneurysm 36834
    Angioplasty 75978
    Graft 34520
Sampling
    Venography 75893
Sinus
    Venography 75870
Skull
    Venography 75870-75872
Spermatic
    Excision 55530-55540
    Ligation 55550

Splenic
    Splenoportography 75810
Stripping
    Saphenous 37720-37735
Subclavian
    Thrombectomy 34471-34490
Thrombectomy
    Other than Hemodialysis Graft or
    Fistula 35875-35876
Unlisted Services and Procedures 37799
Valve Transposition 34510
Varicose
    See Varicose Vein
Vena Cava
    Thrombectomy 34401-34451
    Venography 75825-75827

Velpeau Cast 29058

Vena Cava
Catheterization 36010
Reconstruction 34502
Resection with Reconstruction 37799

Vena Caval
Thrombectomy 50230

Venereal Disease Research Laboratory
See VDRL

Venesection
See Phlebotomy

Venipuncture
See Cannulation; Catheterization
Breast
    Cytology 0045T
Child/Adult
    Cutdown 36425
    Percutaneous 36410
Infant
    Cutdown 36420
    Percutaneous 36400-36406
Routine 36415

Venography
Adrenal 75840-75842
Arm 75820-75822
Epidural 75872
Hepatic Portal 75885-75887
Injection 36005
Jugular 75860
Leg 75820-75822
Liver 75889-75891
Neck 75860
Nuclear Medicine 78445, 78457-78458
Orbit 75880
Renal 75831-75833
Sagittal Sinus 75870
Vena Cava 75825-75827
Venous Sampling 75893

Venorrhaphy
See Suture, Vein

Venotomy
See Phlebotomy

Venous Access Device
Fluoroscopic Guidance 75998
Insertion
    Central 36560-36566
    Peripheral 36570-36571
Obstruction Clearance 36595-36596
    Guidance 75901-75902
Removal 36590
Repair 36576
Replacement 36582-36583, 36585
    Catheter Only 36578

Venous Blood Pressure
See Blood Pressure, Venous

Venovenostomy
See Anastomosis, Vein

Ventilating Tube
Insertion 69433
Removal 69424

Ventilation Assist ..94656-94657, 99504
See Pulmonology, Therapeutic

Ventricular Puncture 61020-61026,
                          61105-61120

Ventriculocisternostomy 62180,
                          62200-62201

Ventriculography
Anesthesia
    Brain 00214
    Cardiac 01920
Nuclear Imaging 78635

Ventriculomyectomy 33416

Ventriculomyotomy 33416

Vermiform Appendix
See Appendix

Vermilionectomy 40500

Verruca Plana
See Warts, Flat

Verruca(e)
See Warts

Version, Cephalic
See Cephalic Version

Vertebra
See Spinal Cord; Spine; Vertebral Body; Vertebral Process
Additional Segment
    Excision 22103, 22116
Arthrodesis
    Anterior 22548-22585
    Exploration 22830
    Lateral Extracavitary 22532-22534
    Posterior 22590-22802
    Spinal Deformity
        Anterior Approach 22808-22812
        Posterior Approach 22800-22804
Cervical
    Excision
        for Tumor 22100, 22110
    Fracture 23675-23680

Fracture/Dislocation
    Additional Segment
        Open Treatment 22328
    Cervical
        Open Treatment 22326
    Lumbar
        Open Treatment 22325
    Thoracic
        Open Treatment 22327
    Kyphectomy 22818-22819
Lumbar
    Excision
        for Tumor 22102, 22114
Osteoplasty
    CT Scan 76013
    Fluoroscopy 76012
    Lumbar 22521-22522
    Thoracic 22520-22522
Osteotomy
    Additional Segment
        Anterior Approach 22226
        Posterior/Posterolateral Approach ..22216
    Cervical
        Anterior Approach 22220
        Posterior/Posterolateral Approach ..22210
    Lumbar
        Anterior Approach 22224
        Posterior/Posterolateral Approach ..22214
    Thoracic
        Anterior Approach 22222
        Posterior/Posterolateral Approach ..22212
Thoracic
    Excision
        for Tumor 22101, 22112

Vertebrae
See Vertebra
Arthrodesis
    Anterior 22548-22585
    Lateral Extracavitary 22532-22534
    Spinal Deformity 22818-22819

Vertebral
Arteries
    See Artery, Vertebral
Body
    Biopsy 20250-20251
    Excision
        Decompression 63081-63103
        Lesion 63300-63308
        with Skull Base Surgery 61597
    Fracture/Dislocation
        Closed Treatment 22305
        without Manipulation 22310
    Kyphectomy 22818-22819
Column
    See Spine
Corpectomy 63081-63103, 63300-63308
Fracture
    See Fracture, Vertebra
Process
    Fracture/Dislocation
        Closed Treatment
        with Manipulation, Casting and/or
        Bracing 22315

Very Low Density Lipoprotein
See Lipoprotein, Blood

Vesication
See Bulla

Vesicle, Seminal
See Seminal Vesicle

Vesico-Psoas Hitch 50785

Vesicostomy
Cutaneous 51980

Vesicourethropexy 51840-51841

Vesicovaginal Fistula
See Fistula, Vesicovaginal

Vesiculectomy 55650

Vesiculogram, Seminal
See Vesiculography

Vesiculography 55300, 74440

Vesiculotomy 55600-55605
Complicated .55605

Vessel, Blood
See Blood Vessels

Vessels Transposition, Great
See Transposition, Great Arteries

Vestibular Function Tests
See Ear, Nose and Throat
Additional Electrodes 92547
Caloric Test 92533
Caloric Vestibular Tests 92543
Nystagmus
    Optokinetic 92534, 92544
    Positional 92532, 92542
    Spontaneous 92531, 92541
Posturography 92548
Sinusoidal Rotational Testing 92546
Torsion Swing Test 92546
Tracking Test .92545

Vestibular Nerve
Section
    Transcranial Approach 69950
    Translabyrinthine Approach 69915

Vestibule of Mouth
See Mouth, Vestibule of

Vestibuloplasty 40840-40845

Vidal Procedure
See Varicocele, Spermatic Cord, Excision

Video
Esophagus 74230
Pharynx 70371, 74230
Speech Evaluation 70371
Swallowing Evaluation 74230

Video-Assisted Thoracoscopic Surgery
See Thoracoscopy

Videoradiography
Unlisted Services and
Procedures 76120-76125

VII, Coagulation Factor
See Proconvertin

VII, Cranial Nerve
See Facial Nerve

VIII, Coagulation Factor
See Clotting Factor

Villus, Chorionic
See Chorionic Villus

Villusectomy
See Synovectomy

VIP
See Vasoactive Intestinal Peptide

Viral Antibodies 86280

Viral Warts
See Warts

Virtual Colonoscopy
    Diagnostic .0067T
    Screening 0066T

Virus
AIDS
    See HIV-1
Burkitt Lymphoma
    See Epstein-Barr Virus
Human Immunodeficiency
    See HIV
Influenza
    See Influenza Virus
Respiratory Syncytial
    See Respiratory Syncytial Virus
Salivary Gland
    See Cytomegalovirus

Virus Identification
Immunofluorescence 87254

Virus Isolation 87250-87255

Visceral Larval Migrans 86280

Viscosities, Blood
See Blood, Viscosity

Visit, Home
See House Calls

Visual Acuity Screen 99172-99173

Visual Field Exam 92081-92083

Visual Function Screen . . .0065T, 99172

Visual Reinforcement Audiometry 92579
See Audiologic Function Tests

Visualization
Ileal Conduit .50690

Vital Capacity Measurement . . .94150

Vitamin .84591
A 84590
B Complex
    See B Complex Vitamins
B-1 84425
B-12 .82607-82608
    Absorption Study 78270-78272
B-2 84252

B-6 84207
B-6 Measurement
    See Pyridoxal Phosphate
BC
    See Folic Acid
C 82180
D 82307, 82652
D, 25-Hydroxy Measurement
    See Calcifediol
D-2
    See Calciferol
D-3 82306
E 84446
K 84597
K Dependent Bone Protein
    See Osteocalcin
K-Dependent Protein S
    See Protein S

Vitelline Duct
See Omphalomesenteric Duct

Vitrectomy
Anterior Approach
    Partial 67005
Pars Plana Approach 67036
Subtotal 67010
with Endolaser Panretinal
Photocoagulation 67040
with Epiretinal Membrane Stripping 67038
with Focal Endolaser Photocoagulation 67039
with Implantation or Replacement
    Drug Delivery System 67027

Vitreous
Aspiration 67015
Excision
    Pars Planta Approach 67036
    with Epiretinal Membrane Stripping . . .67038
    with Focal Endolaser
    Photocoagulation 67039
Implantation
    Drug Delivery System 67027
Incision
    Strands 67030-67031
Injection
    Fluid Substitute 67025
    Pharmacologic Agent 67028
Removal
    Anterior Approach 67005
    Subtotal 67010
Replacement
    Drug Delivery System 67027
Strands
    Discission .67030
    Severing 67031
Subtotal 67010

VLDL
See Lipoprotein, Blood

VMA
See Vanillylmandelic Acid

Vocal Cords
Injection
    Endoscopy .31513
        Therapeutic 31570-31571

Voice Box
See Larynx

W

Wire
See Pin
Insertion/Removal
   Skeletal Traction 20650
Interdental
   without Fracture 21497

Wiring
Prophylactic Treatment
   Humerus 24498

Wirsung Duct
See Pancreatic Duct

Witzel Operation 43500, 43520,
                               43830-43832
See Incision, Stomach, Creation, Stoma; Incision
and Drainage

Womb
See Uterus

Wood Alcohol
See Methanol

Work Hardening 97545-97546
See Physical Medicine/Therapy/Occupational
Therapy

Work Related Evaluation
Services 99455-99456

Worm
See Helminth

Wound
Debridement
   Non-Selective 97602
   Selective 97597-97598
Dehiscence
   Repair 12020-12021, 13160
Exploration
   Penetrating
      Abdomen/Flank/Back 20102
      Chest 20101
      Extremity 20103
      Neck 20100
   Penetrating Trauma 20100-20103
Infection
   Incision and Drainage
      Postoperative 10180
Negative Pressure Therapy 97605-97606
Repair
   Complex 13100-13160
   Intermediate 12031-12057
   Simple 12001-12021
   Urethra 53502-53515
Suture
   Bladder 51860-51865
   Kidney 50500
   Trachea
      Cervical 31800
      Intrathoracic 31805
   Urethra 53502-53515
Vagina
   Repair 57200-57210

Wrist
See Arm, Lower; Carpal Bone
Abscess 25028
Arthrocentesis 20605
Arthrodesis 25800
   with Graft 25810
   with Sliding Graft 25805
Arthrography 73115
Arthroplasty 25332, 25443, 25447
   Revision 25449
   Total Replacement 25446
   with Implant 25441-25442, 25444-25445
Arthroscopy
   Diagnostic 29840
   Surgical 29843-29848
Arthrotomy 25040, 25100-25105
   for Repair 25107
Biopsy 25065-25066, 25100-25101
Bursa
   Excision 25115-25116
   Incision and Drainage 25031
Capsule
   Incision 25085
Cast 29085
Cyst 25130-25136
Decompression 25020-25025
Disarticulation 25920
   Reamputation 25924
   Revision 25922
Dislocation
   Closed Treatment 25660
   Intercarpal 25660
      Open Treatment 25670
   Open Treatment 25670, 25676
   Percutaneous Fixation 25671
   Radiocarpal 25660
      Open Treatment 25670
   Radioulnar 25660
      Closed Treatment 25675
      Percutaneous Fixation 25671
   with Fracture
      Closed Treatment 25680
      Open Treatment 25685
   with Manipulation 25259, 25660, 25675
Excision
   Carpal 25210-25215
   Cartilage 25107
Exploration 25040, 25101
Fasciotomy 25020-25025
Fracture 25600-25645
   Closed Treatment 25622, 25630
   Open Treatment 25628
   with Dislocation 25680-25685
   with Manipulation 25259, 25624, 25635
Ganglion Cyst
   Excision 25111-25112
Hematoma 25028
Incision 25040, 25100-25105
   Tendon Sheath 25000-25001
Injection
   Carpal Tunnel
      Therapeutic 20526
   X-Ray 25246

Joint
   See Radiocarpal Joint
Lesion, Tendon Sheath
   Excision 25110
Magnetic Resonance Imaging (MRI) 73221
Reconstruction
   Capsulectomy 25320
   Capsulorrhaphy 25320
   Carpal Bone 25394, 25430
   Realign.......................25335
Removal
   Foreign Body 25040, 25101, 25248
   Implant 25449
   Loose Body 25101
   Prosthesis 25250-25251
Repair 25447
   Bone 25440
   Carpal Bone 25431
   Muscle 25260, 25270
      Secondary 25263-25265, 25272-25274
   Tendon 25260, 25270, 25280-25316
      Secondary 25263-25265, 25272-25274
   Tendon Sheath 25275
Strapping 29260
Synovium
   Excision 25105, 25115-25119
Tendon Sheath
   Excision 25115-25116
Tenodesis 25300-25301
Tenotomy 25290
Tumor 25130-25136
   Excision 25075-25077
Unlisted Services and Procedures 25999
X-Ray 73100-73110
   with Contrast 73115

X

X, Coagulation Factor
See Stuart-Prower Factor

X, Cranial Nerve
See Vagus Nerve

X-Linked Ichthyoses
See Syphilis Test

X-Ray
Abdomen 74000-74022
Abscess 76080
Acromioclavicular Joint 73050
Ankle 73600-73610
Arm, Lower 73090
Arm, Upper 73092
Artery
   Atherectomy 75992-75996
Auditory Meatus 70134
Bile Duct
   Guide Dilation 74360
Body Composition
   Dual Energy Absorptiometry 0028T

X-Ray Tomography, Computed

See CT Scan

Xa, Coagulation Factor

See Thrombokinase

Xenoantibodies

See Antibody, Heterophile

Xenograft

Xenografts, Skin
See Heterograft, Skin

Xenotransplantation
See Heterograft

Xerography
See Xeroradiography

Xeroradiography 76150

XI, Coagulation Factor
See Plasma Thromboplastin, Antecedent

XI, Cranial Nerve
See Accessory Nerve

XII, Coagulation Factor
See Hageman Factor

XII, Cranial Nerve
See Hypoglossal Nerve

XIII, Coagulation Factor
See Fibrin Stabilizing Factor

Xylose Absorption Test
Blood 84620
Urine 84620

Y

Yeast
Culture 87106
Yellow Fever Vaccine 90717
Yersinia
Antibody 86793

Z

Ziegler Procedure
Discission Secondary Membranous
Cataract 66820

Zinc 84630

Zinc Manganese Leucine Aminopeptidase
See Leucine Aminopeptidase

Zygoma
See Cheekbone

Zygomatic Arch
Fracture
    Open Treatment 21356-21366
    with Manipulation 21355

YOUR SOLUTION TO CORRECT CODING